FORENSIC PATHOLOGY

Dr. Greeshma Sharma

ALLIED
HEALTH
PRESS

Forensic Pathology

Author: **Dr. Greeshma Sharma**

Allied Health Press
4164 Lakeshore Road
Burlington ON L7L 1A4
Canada
www.alliedhealthpress.com
Email: orders@arclereducation.com

ISBN: 978-1-77956-838-0

ABOUT THE AUTHOR

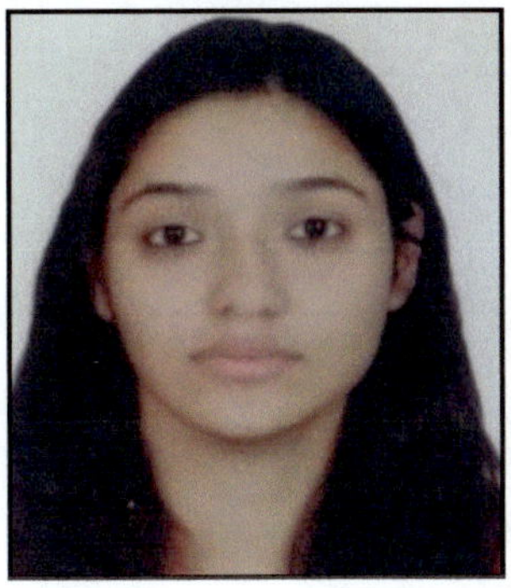

Dr. Greeshma Sharma, holds Ph.D. in Transfusion Medicine from PGIMER, Chandigarh, with a research focus on Neonatal Thrombocytopenia and Neonatal Alloimmune Thrombocytopenia (NAIT). She has completed her M.Sc. in Forensic Biotechnology from NFSU and a B.Sc. in Biological Sciences from Delhi University. She is currently working as a Project Research Scientist I under an ICMR-funded project on NAIT diagnosis and have previous experience as a Junior Research Fellow in DST-funded research. Some of her Publications include articles in Newborn Journal and Vox Sanguinis. She has qualified the UGC-NET (Forensic Science) and have received awards including the Harold Gunson Fellowship (ISBT 2020).

Brief Table of Contents

Getting Started with This Book

Chapter Openers

A list of Chapter Outline is presented providing a brief Introduction to what will be covered in the chapter.

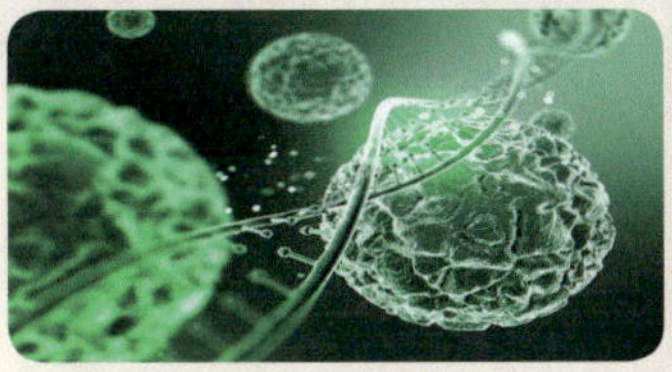

Introduction

Often referred to as the science of life, biology is a broad field of study aimed at comprehending the several kinds of life on Earth, from tiny creatures to sophisticated multicellular entities. Comprising several subfields, including molecular biology, ecology, and evolutionary biology, each of which advances our knowledge of living systems, this field clarifies the mechanisms controlling life events, including development, reproduction, and interaction with the surroundings, which is the central goal of biology. Moreover, biology fills in the void between the natural sciences and medicine by offering a necessary understanding of health, illness, and the interactions between organisms and their environments. Dealing with urgent global issues such as climate change, biodiversity loss, and new diseases depends on an awareness of these complex biological interactions, therefore highlighting the critical part biology plays in modern civilization. Fundamentally, biology explores and tests ideas about the living world using the scientific method. Through methodical observation and experimentation,

LEARNING OBJECTIVES

After studying this chapter, you will be able to:

1. Discuss the scientific method in biology;
2. Explain the cell theory;
3. Discuss the genetics and heredity;
4. Evolution and natural selection;
5. Focus on ecology and ecosystems;
6. Learn about human biology;
7. Evaluate the plant biology;
8. Explain the microbiology;
9. Focus on current trends in biology.

1.1. The Scientific Method in Biology

Learning Outcome

1. Describe the steps of the scientific method;
2. Focus on hypothesis formation;
3. Learn about experimental design.

Learning Outcomes

The beginning of each section of every chapter contains a set of Learning Outcomes that inform students of concepts they should understand. These outcomes help students understand what they should be able to do if they have mastered the material in that section.

Test Your Knowledge

Throughout each chapter, Test Your Knowledge cues you to note which topics have been covered and to self-test your understanding of the material presented.

Test Your Knowledge

1. Explain why correlation does not imply causation in scientific experiments.
2. How does the scientific method help reduce the influence of personal opinions in research?

Chapter Summary

The Summary Section appear at the end of each chapter and summarize main concepts covered throughout the chapter. These points provide key concepts in an engaging and meaningful way.

Summary

The investigation of biological principles highlights the importance of a comprehensive view of life by reflecting the intricate interactions that occur within living systems. The complexity of biology goes beyond individual species or systems, as this essay highlights; it also includes the interactions that mold ecosystems and affect biodiversity. Researchers can conduct in-depth analyses of metabolomic data using sophisticated technologies like MetaboAnalyst, which offer insights into the molecular mechanisms underlying these interactions. As demonstrated by the developments in MetaboAnalyst, for example, the integration of diverse omics data promotes a thorough understanding of metabolic pathways and helps identify important biological markers necessary for research on development and disease (Chong et al., 2018). Additionally, the phenomenon of ecological invasions is a key component of biological research and a vital field of study. The introduction of non-native species into unfamiliar habitats has significant ramifications and calls for multidisciplinary management strategies. Examining the origins and effects of these biological incursions, invasion science has become a crucial field that highlights the need to comprehend ecological dynamics and community interactions. As interest in biological invasions increases, new findings are emerging that put conventional ecological theories and practices to the test. The importance of incorporating various scientific viewpoints is shown by this developing discipline, which also highlights how invasive species shape ecosystems and advances our knowledge of ecological resilience (David et al., 2013). When taken as a whole, these discoveries from invasion science and metabolomics highlight the value of multidisciplinary biology research. Fostering cross-disciplinary collaboration and utilizing technological breakthroughs to improve our comprehension of intricate biological interactions are crucial as we look to the future of biological research. In addition to deepening our understanding of the complexities of life, this method lays the groundwork for tackling urgent environmental issues. Future studies can ensure the continued relevance of biology in a world that is constantly changing by acknowledging the interconnection of biological systems and opening the door to creative solutions that support sustainability and biodiversity conservation. We might imagine a thorough comprehension of life that serves both academia and society at large through ongoing investigation and integration of scientific knowledge.

Knowledge Assessment

The chapter includes material designed to review and reinforce each content. It includes Critical Thinking Questions to help test of your understanding of information presented in the chapter and Short answer Questions to review your understanding of the key concepts presented in the chapter.

Critical Thinking Questions

1. **Who is known as the "Father of Modern Biology"?**
   a. Aristotle
   b. Charles Darwin
   c. Gregor Mendel
   d. Louis Pasteur
2. **What is the basic unit of life?**
   a. Atom
   b. Molecule
   c. Cell
   d. Organism
3. **Which branch of biology studies the interaction of organisms with their environment?**
   a. Genetics
   b. Ecology
   c. Physiology
   d. Botany
4. **Which macromolecule is the main source of energy for living organisms?**
   a. Proteins
   b. Lipids
   c. Carbohydrates
   d. Nucleic acids
5. **DNA is primarily responsible for which function in living organisms?**
   a. Energy production
   b. Protein synthesis
   c. Storing genetic information
   d. Regulating body temperature

Short Answer Questions

1. What is biology, and why is it important to study biology?
2. What are the three main domains of life, and how are they different from one another?
3. Define homeostasis and give an example of how it works in living organisms.
4. What is the cell theory, and why is it fundamental to biology?
5. How do autotrophs and heterotrophs differ in the way they obtain energy?
6. What is the scientific method, and how is it applied in biological research?
7. Discuss how biology helps address global challenges such as climate change, disease, and food security.
8. Explain the levels of biological organization from the smallest unit to the largest. Provide examples at each level.
9. Describe the relationship between structure and function in biology, giving specific examples from cells or organs.
10. How has the discovery of genetics shaped our understanding of inheritance and variation among organisms?

Supplementary Materials

Key Terms: A list of key terms is given for quick reference

KEY TERMS FROM THIS CHAPTER

Annotation enrichment analysis	Biological structure	Cell
Cell theory	Cellular structure	Ecology
Ecosystems	Genetics	Human biology
Microbiology	Natural selection	Organism
Plant biology		

Further Resources: Recommendations for additional readings, websites, and multimedia resources.

References

1. Argelaguet, R., Velten, B., Arnol, D., Dietrich, S., Zenz, T., Marioni, J. C., Buettner, F., et al. (2018). Multi-omics factor analysis—A framework for unsupervised integration of multi-omics data sets. *Molecular Systems Biology, 14*. https://doi.org/10.15252/msb.20178124.
2. Bacher, S., Blackburn, T. M., Essl, F., & Genovesi, P. (2017). *Socio-Economic Impact Classification of Alien Taxa (SEICAT)*. https://core.ac.uk/download/286567949.pdf (accessed on 8th March 2025).
3. Barnett, R., Brace, S., Cucchi, T., & Dobney, K. (2013). *Divergent Evolutionary Processes Associated with Colonization of Offshore Islands.* https://core.ac.uk/download/20664364.pdf (accessed on 8th March 2025).

Detailed Table of Contents

CHAPTER 3

Postmortem Changes 61

CHAPTER 4

Autopsy Techniques 95

CHAPTER 5

Blunt Force Injuries 131

CHAPTER 6

Sharp Force Injuries 165

CHAPTER 7

Gunshot Wounds and Ballistics 195

CHAPTER 13

Identification of Human Remains 381

CHAPTER 14

Forensic Anthropology 405

CHAPTER 15

Emerging Technologies in Forensic Pathology 431

LIST OF FIGURES

PREFACE

Forensic Pathology combines legal inquiry and medical science in cases of death, trauma, and remains of humans. Pathologists determine cause, manner, and time of death from body, tissue, and scene data analysis. Routine postmortem alteration, pattern of injury, and toxicology assessment are employed for reconstructing events around death. *Forensic Pathology* brings together law enforcement, clinical medicine, and pathology to establish that medical findings support investigations of homicides, accidents, natural deaths, and unexplained or sudden deaths.

Advances in imaging technology, molecular diagnostics, and data analysis have augmented the toolkit available to forensic pathologists. From high-resolution postmortem CT scans to tissue injury biological markers, modern techniques enhance accuracy and speed. Medical professionals also need to learn to become experts at ancient autopsy techniques, recognize subtle trauma findings, and integrate multidisciplinary information. Whether in a medicolegal office, at the scene of a disaster, or in court, forensic pathologists uphold scientific integrity and ethical principles to ensure justice and public health.

Forensic Pathology is a comprehensive introduction to the principles, techniques, and practice of death investigation that blends foundational concepts with detailed coverage of specific kinds of injuries, special populations, and emerging technologies. Case examples and procedural checklists improve practice and learning, and legal issues chapters and interdisciplinary interaction chapters reinforce the broader context of forensic practice.

Chapter 1 outlines the scope and history of forensic pathology, including definitions of significant terms and the role of the forensic pathologist within the medicolegal process. It describes the causes of death and the guidelines governing medicolegal investigations.

Chapter 2 addresses medicolegal investigation of death, such as procedures at the scene, recovery of evidence, and liaison with police officials and forensic scientists. It addresses certification of death and legal reporting requirements. Chapter 3 describes postmortem changes—algor, rigor, and livor mortis—decomposition processes. Chapter 3 covers factors influencing these changes and estimating time since death.

Chapter 4 describes autopsy techniques, including external examination, incision of internal organs, tissue sampling, and documentation. Safety protocols, photography, and ancillary studies are covered. Chapter 5 discusses blunt force injury and distinguishes between abrasion, contusion, and laceration patterns. It explains how force amount, direction, and tool characteristics affect damage to tissues.

Chapter 6 addresses sharp force injuries—incised wounds, stab wounds, and defense wounds—and cites blade characteristics and wound morphology as the determinants to distinguish between types of sharp instruments. Chapter 7 addresses gunshot wounds and ballistics, including wound classification, range determination, and bullet trajectory analysis. It starts with an introduction to firearm mechanics and the preservation of gunshot evidence.

Chapter 8 addresses asphyxial deaths—strangulation, hanging, smothering, and drowning—and shows characteristic findings and differential diagnosis considerations. Chapter 9 addresses toxicology in forensic pathology, including specimen collection, common toxicants, analysis methods, and toxicological result interpretation in death investigations.

Chapter 10 addresses thermal injuries, including burns, scalds, and fatalities due to fire. It addresses assessment of burn depth, patterned trauma, and differentiation from other trauma. Chapter 11 discusses sudden natural deaths—cardiac, cerebrovascular, and metabolic disasters—with an emphasis on autopsy examination and the role of medical history.

Chapter 12 addresses pediatric forensic pathology, including child abuse, sudden infant death syndrome, and age-related factors in examination and reporting. Chapter 13 discusses methods of identification of human remains from dental records, fingerprints, DNA profiling, and anthropometric analysis.

Chapter 14 welcomes forensic anthropology with a discussion of skeletal analysis, bone trauma interpretation, and the reconstruction of biological profiles through different means. Chapter 15 presents the latest technology in forensic pathology, such as postmortem imaging, virtual autopsy, proteomic markers, and digital data management systems.

This book is addressed to forensic pathologists, pathology residents, medical examiners, and medicolegal office investigators. It will be of reference benefit to forensic scientists, legal counselors, and health care providers who deal with death investigations and court processes.

INTRODUCTION TO FORENSIC PATHOLOGY

1

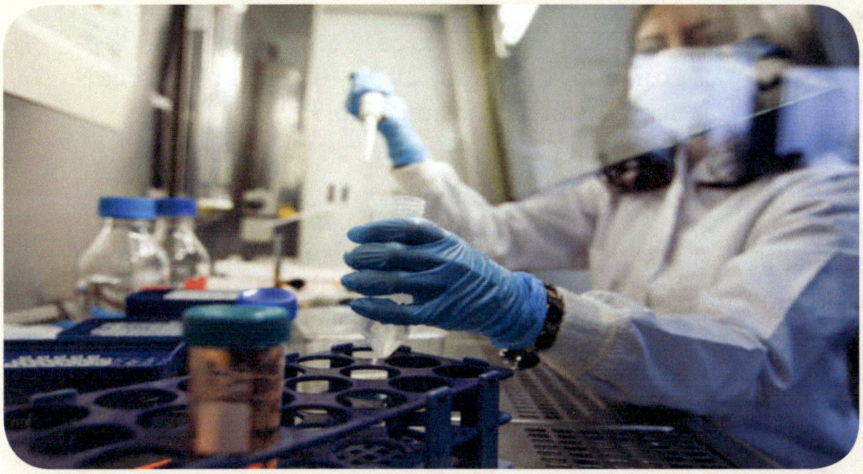

LEARNING OBJECTIVES

After studying this chapter, you will be able to:

1. Explain the history of forensic pathology;
2. Understand the role of forensic pathologists;
3. Know the techniques used in forensic pathology;
4. Describe the types of death investigated;
5. Know the legal and ethical considerations of forensic pathology;
6. Describe the challenges in forensic pathology.

Introduction

The field of forensic pathology contributes significantly to the medical and legal communities by illuminating the causes of death and injury using the application of medical knowledge. Its value has been more apparent in recent years due to the increased number of complex cases, like deaths from drugs and acts of violence. There are several ways in which forensic pathologists examine decomposed and intact bodies to ensure that investigations yield results with accuracy. The nature of such investigations is complex, as it adopts an interdisciplinary approach to harness the services of different specialists to enhance the reliability and accuracy of pathological evidence. As society increasingly recognizes the importance of forensic evidence to the justice system, the discipline needs to evolve further, growing its capacity to address contemporary challenges of crime and trauma analysis, and finally bring cases to closure for families and deliver justice in the justice system. In cases of drug-related deaths, forensic pathologists are also key to ascertaining the drugs implicated, as case studies have demonstrated in recent years. A specific instance involved a 30-year-old man whose demise resulted from the inhalation of toxic fumes, and as a result, there was a thorough forensic analysis of the chemicals in his system. In the example, toxicological processes such as gas chromatography and mass spectrometry were employed to detect the chemicals fentanyl and U-47700, which illustrate the extreme effects of unrestricted psychotropic compounds. This case shows the importance of not just determining the immediate cause of death but also understanding the broader context of the event, including the emergence of new drug trends and their implications for public health.

Conducting systematic toxicological analyses allows forensic specialists to provide essential information to both criminal justice and preventive health strategies, strengthening the role of forensic pathology in modern society. Pathological specimen study most commonly detects underlying health status and trauma that aid in legal investigation, making neuropathological changes knowledge vital to proper forensic investigation. The histological examination of brain tissue is capable, for instance, of providing significant information regarding seizure disorders and syndromes that accompany it, gaining insight into the victim's medical history. As noted in recent studies on epilepsy, standardized processes enable the gathering and examination of regions in the brain relevant to such conditions, thereby enhancing the efficacy and precision of results in forensic analysis. Categorization of these processes demonstrates the complexity involved in forensic pathology, with scientific accuracy being vital in delivering justice. Through diligent pathological analysis, forensic pathologists not only aid the criminal case adjudication process but also aid in advancing medical science, ultimately for the betterment of public safety and health outcomes (Figure 1.1).

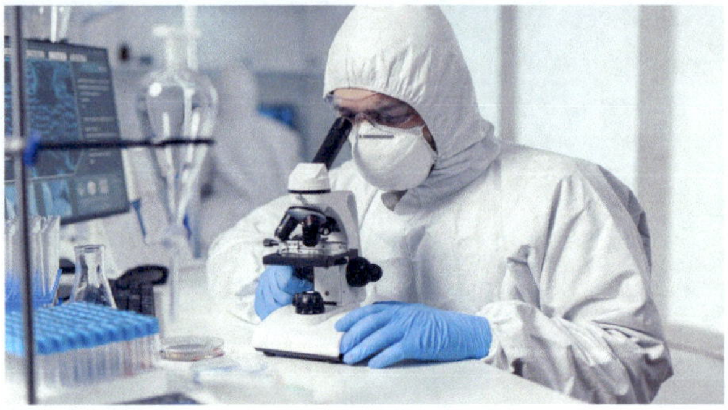

Figure 1.1. Forensic pathology.

Source: https://medlifemastery.com/wp-content/uploads/2023/09/Best-Medical-Schools-for-Forensic-Pathology.jpg.

Definition of Forensic Pathology

Forensic pathology plays a crucial role in both medicine and the law, marking the point where science and law intersect. Forensic pathology basically involves the use of medical science to analyze deaths that are unexpected or violent. Forensic pathology aims to establish the cause and the manner of death, something that can form critical evidence during criminal proceedings. Forensic pathologists conduct autopsies, scrutinizing the body and its systems for any evidence of trauma, disease, or toxicology. By applying rigorous scientific protocols, these experts aid in the determination of forensic truth, a theory encompassing objectivity of forensic examination and the broader legal implications of their conclusions (Klinkner et al., 2008). This kind of analysis can trigger criminal prosecution or eliminate wrongful suspicion of someone's death, underscoring the important function that forensic pathology has in justice systems within society. The delicacy of forensic pathology is more than mere determination of causes of death; it also encompasses the subtlety of interpreting such findings. Forensic pathologists must bring their medical expertise together with an understanding of legal requirements, typically presenting evidence to the court as expert witnesses. Having such a dual role demands not only an excellent understanding of biological and anatomical sciences, but also the ability to translate difficult scientific evidence into terms juries and judges can understand. The courtroom dynamics are also further complicated by the need to reconcile forensic realities with the larger paradigms of international law, especially in the event of cases of abuse of human rights or war crimes (Klinkner et al., 2008). It is important to ensure that forensic evidence allows for the presentation of a truthful narrative, makes the pathologist both a scientist and a storyteller of the legal narrative. The significance of definitions in forensic pathology must not be exaggerated, considering the fact that the topic is constantly evolving because of advancements in medicine and the law. An ordinarily accepted set of definitions of terms applied when dealing with injuries, deaths, and pathologic phenomena is essential in order to achieve uniformity in examinations and legal interpretations. Inconsistencies in definitions like operative deaths and anesthetic deaths can lead to misinterpretations in medico-legal situations at the cost of validity in forensic evaluation. Furthermore, forensic pathologists are often confronted with complex cases, such as distinguishing between natural and unnatural causes of death, whose implications can be tremendous in malpractice suits and wrongful death actions. So, as the discipline grows and advances, definition and understanding remain fundamental pillars supporting the critical discipline of forensic pathology so that it can rightly grow for future challenges, yet hold onto its central role in justice and health.

Significance in the Criminal Justice System

The integration of forensic pathology with the criminal justice system offers greatly enhanced tools to deliver justice by obtaining vital knowledge of the circumstances of death. Analysis of the body's evidence may help establish cause and manner of death, which are crucial elements that define law narratives. For instance, mass grave excavations, such as in the Cambodian context, are a testament to how forensic science is paramount in legal proceedings concerning historic atrocities. The Extraordinary Chambers in the Courts of Cambodia (ECCC) is an example of how new, sophisticated methods in forensic science can help uncover evidence of the atrocities that were perpetrated by the Khmer Rouge. With forensic pathologists examining remains, not only do they contribute towards the identification of victims, but also bring to the perpetrators of widespread human rights violations accountability, thereby enforcing the mandate of forensic pathology in the judiciary (Klinkner et al., 2008). Beyond the victim's cause of death identification, the impact of forensic pathology filters into jurors' perceptions and jurors' expectations in the justice system. The CSI effect has recently been a concern in research, whereby television dramatizations of forensic science generate unrealistic expectations of the presentability and availability of forensic evidence in real criminal cases. In an attempt to establish credibility, prosecutors then have to deal with the added burdens as a result of jurors' misapprehensions of what is realistically obtainable from forensic evidence. Consequently, media representation of forensic pathology can complicate jury deliberations in some instances, leading to unjust convictions or acquittals, as exemplified by the need for credible public education on forensic science (Alejo et al., 2016). This challenges forensic pathologists to be proactive in involving legal professionals and the media in describing their work and limitations. The importance of forensic pathology to the criminal justice system is further brought out by the role that it plays in providing closure to the victims' families and society in general. By determining the definitive cause of death, forensic pathologists are able to give definite answers that may ease the pain that grieving families endure. This function is most significant in the case of inexplicable disappearance or homicide, where the resolution of doubts allows healing. Secondly, the results of forensic examinations can also serve as significant deterrents to crime by illustrating tangible consequences of criminal behavior through legal accountability. As the criminal justice system evolves, the continued collaboration between legal agencies and forensic pathologists will be instrumental in instilling confidence, justice, and transparency in society (Klinkner et al., 2008) (Figure 1.2).

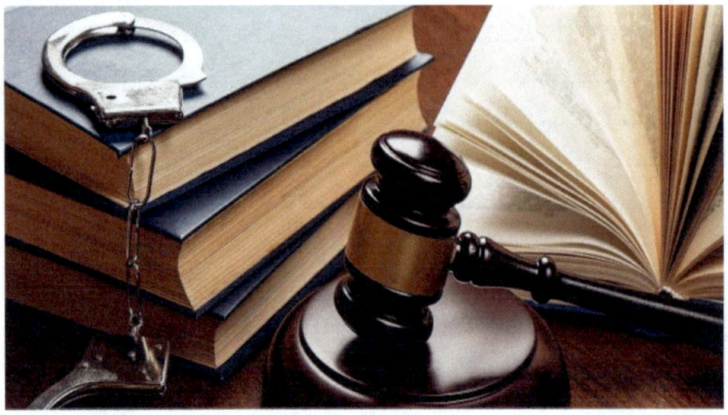

Figure 1.2. Forensics-enabled criminal justice system.

Source: https://images.news18.com/ibnlive/uploads/2023/12/criminal-justice-system-2023-12-9335d03e92c413ada366b67b157a43af-16x9.jpg.

1.1. History of Forensic Pathology

Learning Outcome

1. Describe the early practices in forensic medicine.
2. Understand the development of modern forensic pathology.
3. Learn about key historical figures and their contributions.

Forensic pathology is a well-storied discipline that is entwined with medical and legal advancements, paving the way to its use in contemporary processes of investigation. Its origins date back as early as ancient civilizations, when the bodies of the dead were subjected to examination by doctors to determine the cause of death, particularly in cases of suspicion. For instance, autopsy practice gained increasing importance in ancient Greece and Rome, and figures like Hippocrates advocated for the scientific investigation of the human body. It was not until the latter half of the 19th century, however, that forensic pathology became a real branch of medicine, influenced mostly by the efforts of the early giants such as Hans Gross, who pushed the improvement of crime investigations through science. This was a revolutionary shift, bringing together medicine, law, and scientific inquiry, thereby opening the way to modern forensic pathology's complexity. As forensic pathology developed, legal systems came to more fully appreciate the value of scientific evidence at trial. The 20th century witnessed substantial development in methodology and the technology available to the forensic pathologist, and their ability to provide accurate conclusions on cause and manner of death considerably improved. The implementation of forensic autopsy practices allowed pathologists to perform thorough analyses of various dimensions of death caused by lethal injuries and poisoning, and thereby led to more prudent judicial verdicts. Furthermore, advancements in imaging technology and toxicology opened new avenues for investigating deaths with hitherto unclear circumstances. As public interest in forensic science and crime became more prevalent, this era solidified the position of forensic pathology as a relevant field of the law, paving the way for the accreditation of organizations and well-established procedures that control the field now. In more recent years, the application of advanced technology and genetic analysis has further reshaped the field of forensic pathology. The creation of DNA profiling and multi-modal imaging techniques not only enabled forensic pathologists to determine causes of death but also to identify remains that would otherwise be unidentified. As noted by the ALRC Report 96, various activities encompassed in forensic examinations are considerably impacted by ethical, legal, and social concerns, which continue to evolve according to emerging scientific knowledge (Opeskin et al., 2025). Forensic pathologists currently face the ethical dilemma on one hand and the needs of justice on the other. The increasing range of forensic science, with ongoing debate surrounding topics such as consent and what implications will genetic information hold, remains imperative to the ethical application of forensic pathology in humans (Ahmed et al., 2017) (Figure 1.3).

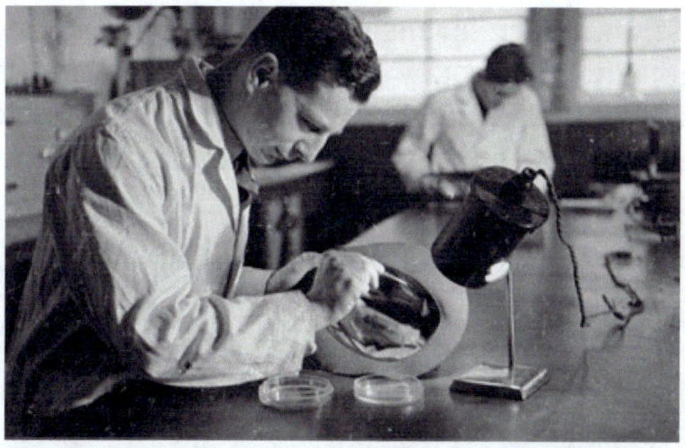

Figure 1.3. History of forensic pathology.

Source: https://08f043fb5b.clvaw-cdnwnd.com/65cf06e22b1051f5df11dfe70b7dd6da/200000203-48cca49c69/forensic-lab-technique-2.jpg.

1.1.1. Early Practices in Forensic Medicine

Forensic medicine's origins can be traced back to ancient civilizations, where early practitioners began to realize the importance of empirical evidence in solving crimes. Ancient Egyptians, for example, employed rudimentary forensic techniques in their mummification ceremonies, checking cadavers for signs of homicide. Likewise, the Chinese Tang Dynasty formulated protocols for performing autopsies, including evaluating wounds and the circumstances of death. These practices established the basis for scientific forensic techniques in medicine. While most of this earlier work was not nearly as scientifically rigorous as it is now, it was a significant step into understanding the medical side of criminal investigation, and a place was opened up for continued development in forensic pathology. Forensic medicine continued to gain much momentum during the Renaissance when medical professionals began to keep their observations in a systematic manner. In particular, the medicalization of the autopsy allowed physicians to delve into the cause of death more thoroughly, thereby enriching forensic science. In this period, an incident of an out-of-control physician who allegedly murdered his patients revealed the stringency in adequate death certification and forensic examination. Moreover, Legal Medicine, being an innovative discipline in Europe, began applying forensic information in judicial processes. The dialogue between expanding medical knowledge and law encouraged the development of more formalized practices that would ultimately be legally codified, an evolution toward the more scientific approaches that would characterize modern forensic pathology. Scientific procedure began to transform forensic medicine in the 19th century, spurred by a growing emphasis on evidence-based techniques. The development of toxicological testing became an invaluable resource, enabling forensic pathologists to detect poisons and drugs in specimens from autopsies. In one such landmark case, the detection of a toxic substance in a person who had passed away prompted a complete investigation, which stressed the importance of toxicological information in arriving at death causes involving criminal activity. Moreover, advances in anthropometric methods, such as Alphonse Bertillon's research, demonstrated the importance of body measurements in identifying a person. The integration of these methods not only enhanced forensic pathology skill sets but also emphasized more heavily the use of scientific studies in understanding human death and its implications for society, leading to enhancing legal processes against perpetrators.

1.1.2. The Development of Modern Forensic Pathology

The background of modern forensic pathology is complex, interlacing scientific advances with the requirements of the law. Forensic pathology, early on, was all about cause of death determination by comparatively rudimentary means, really in the domain of medical jurisprudence. It was not until the 19th century that a systematic and scientific one arrived, led by visionaries who instituted rigorous autopsy protocols. The establishment of pathology as an independent medical profession provided a foundation for modern forensic practice, enabling specialists to scrutinize deaths in a precise and detailed manner and provide reliable testimony in court. This initial transformation not only enhanced the quality of death investigation but also paved the way for the official introduction of medical science into the judicial system, making forensic pathology an integral subject in medical and legal education. The 20th century witnessed groundbreaking progress in forensic pathology, driven by technological advancements and increasing public interest in scientific evidence in the legal arena. DNA testing in the 1980s revolutionized forensic analysis, and for the first time, it became possible to attain record accuracy in the identification of victims and perpetrators. Moreover, the popularity of forensic science in popular media brought to the foreground an engaging portrayal of pathology work that focused its eyes on its importance in criminal justice. The global fascination led to the opening up of learning programs, as put forth in Stankiewicz et al. (2007), thus creating a robust pipeline of well-trained personnel who could handle the complexity of modern-day forensic cases. This extension in learning not only pushed the boundaries of forensic pathology but also focused on continued innovation and education in the discipline. As forensic pathology developed, so did the issues of ethics, becoming a focal point of concern. The profession continues to be focused on how evidence is collected, processed, and delivered during legal proceedings. Issues of consent, handling remains, and the risk of bias are also major concerns to be addressed. Professional standardization has also been accompanied by the formation of various organizations to direct and stimulate best practices in the field. The function of international conferences, as seen in the collaborative effort proposed by Stankiewicz et al. (2007), has also increased knowledge exchange and ethical discussion. Lastly, modern forensic pathology must balance scientific stringency with moral obligation, so that it plays a constructive role in the justice system while treating human beings with dignity (Figure 1.4).

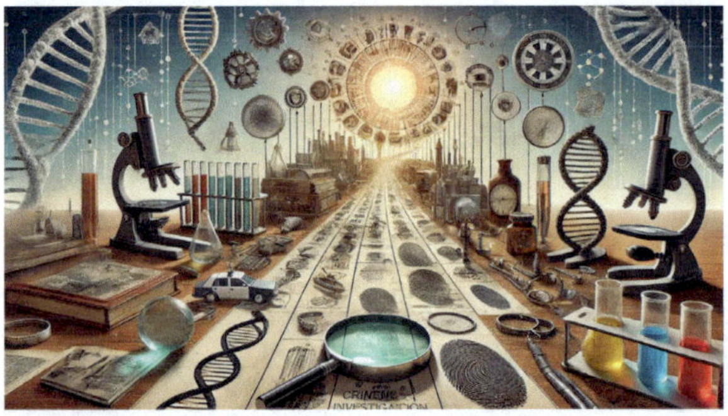

Figure 1.4. Forensic science timeline: a journey through the evolution of forensic investigation.

Source: https://cdn-ilbjbhl.nitrocdn.com/FyaMYitqUPNTCnovJEDCVNCvhqDiYUgo/assets/images/optimized/rev-0f7d9d8/sp-ao.shortpixel.ai/client/to_auto,q_glossy,ret_img,w_1536,h_878/https://simplyforensic.com/wp-content/uploads/2024/09/DALLE-2024-09-19-151109-A-detailed-and-engaging-wide-landscape-image-for-a-feature-post-titled-Forensic-Science-Timeline_-A-Journey-Through-the-Evolution-of-Forensic-Investi.webp.

1.1.3. Key Historical Figures and Their Contributions

Forensic pathology owes much to powerful historical figures whose writings have paved the way for modern practice. One such figure is Hans Gross, aptly referred to as the father of criminalistics. His magnum opus, Handbuch für Untersuchungsrichter, Polizeibeamte, Kriminalbeamte und Kriminaltechniker, published in 1893, emphasized the role of integrating various science disciplines in crime investigation. Gross was in favor of scientific methods of recovery and preservation of evidence, an idea that is the basis of modern forensic science. By advocating the application of scientific techniques to forensic analysis, Gross influenced forensic pathologists' approach to conducting investigations, stressing their necessity for interdisciplinarity and application of empirical research.

These ideas are still highly relevant to forensic pathology today (and indeed to medicine as a whole) (Varotto et al., 2024). Another figure of importance in the establishment of forensic pathology is Dr. Thomas Dwight, who may be regarded as the father of forensic anthropology. His efforts in the late 19th century were helpful in bridging the gap between forensic science and anthropology, particularly in analyzing human remains. Dwight's meticulous research and attention to the use of skeletal analysis for the purpose of age, sex, and ancestry estimation of unidentified remains provided valuable insights into human identification. His novel techniques have been of essential value in medico-legal proceedings where traditional methods of identification are lacking. Additionally, Dwight's research established anthropological benchmarks that continue to be utilized in the present day by forensic pathologists when they are analyzing remains in criminal and archaeological contexts, indicating the enduring relevance of his work in the broader forensic community (Varotto et al., 2024). In later times, the impact of the COVID-19 pandemic on forensic pathology has highlighted anew the enduring value of foundation workers and their output. Autopsies in this global health crisis have presented unique challenges, raising an interest in gaining knowledge of the pathological effects of the SARS-CoV-2 virus. Standard procedures established by pathologists, such as the requirement for meticulous examinations to ascertain causes of death, remain significant. As forensic pathologists grapple with the difficulties of diagnosing COVID-19 following death, the works of prior scholars emphasize the need to adapt forensic procedures to cope with new medical realities. The ongoing development of forensic practice indicates the need for responsiveness and adaptability in the area, ideas that were initially established by pathfinder figures like Gross and Dwight, and are required to advance the field in today's environments, like pandemics and epidemics of infectious disease.

Test Your Knowledge

1. Which ancient civilization is known for employing rudimentary forensic techniques during mummification?
2. What scientific method became a cornerstone of forensic medicine in the 19th century?

1.2. Role of Forensic Pathologists

Learning Outcome

1. Understand responsibilities during death investigations.
2. Collaborate with law enforcement and legal teams.
3. Understand the importance of an autopsy in determining the cause of death.

Forensic pathologists have a significant role at the intersection of law and medicine and generally work as medical examiners or deputy coroners. Their responsibilities involve determining the cause and manner of death in several different situations, particularly when the circumstances are uncertain or natural. Forensic pathologists, one of the most important parts of legal proceedings, perform autopsies, describe findings meticulously, and analyze tissue specimens to provide priceless evidence that can help validate or invalidate allegations of criminal activity. Their work does not remain limited to the autopsy table; they often appear in court, translating medical technical jargon into a language anyone can understand for judges and jurors. By playing this dual function, forensic pathologists both ensure the integrity of the scientific process and ensure that justice is being served by providing consistent expert evidence, which can influence legal outcomes. Toward that end, their services are irreplaceable to the development of an authoritative framework for the understanding of death in the context of law. The utilization of more advanced forensic techniques has further enhanced the capabilities of forensic pathologists to provide effective and comprehensive assessments. Developments in technology, such as imaging technology and genetic sequencing, currently complement established autopsy procedures to facilitate a much more intense analysis of remains. For instance, in recent disaster victim identification operations, the role of the forensic anthropologist—a related discipline—has been identified and reaped the benefits of multi-disciplinary collaboration. Previous DVI exercises have provided valuable lessons learned on the inter-relationship between forensic pathologists and specialists in all aspects of expertise, shaping their technique and approach to complex cases (Acharya et al., 2018). This collaborative effort not only provides depth to the study but also provides a clearer picture of the particular problems that arise in the process of forensic analysis, particularly in risky environments where accurate identification is required.

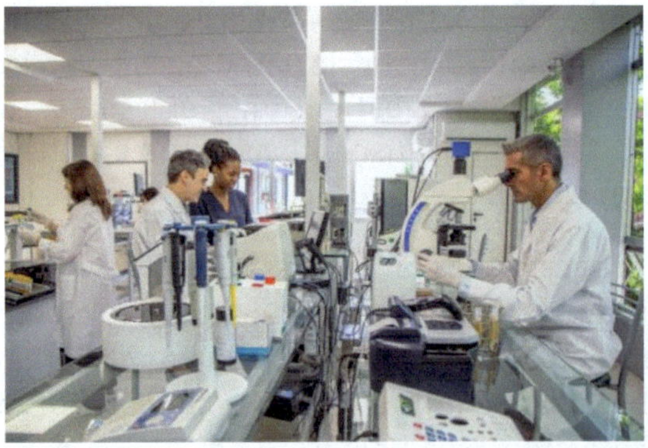

Figure 1.5. Role of forensic pathologists.

Source: https://www.umhs-sk.org/hs-fs/hubfs/forensic-pathology-lab.jpg?width=750&height=518&name=forensic-pathology-lab.jpg.

Additionally, forensic pathologists also act to ensure public health and safety by identifying disease and injury patterns that need to be investigated. For example, pathologists can detect groups of unexplained deaths that can foretell the greater health problems, such as an epidemic or bioterrorism. They also provide insight into the interpretation of toxicology results and can collaborate with public health officials to develop preventive strategies. In addition, while making conclusions in the field of law, as outlined within the context of international criminal law, for instance, the forensic analyses relating to the Srebrenica massacres, forensic pathologists create a forensic truth that is critical to justice (Klinkner et al., 2008). Their findings can be utilized to galvanize investigation and ensure transparency, and thereby make the work of forensic pathologists precious in the court and in society as well (Figure 1.5).

1.2.1. Responsibilities in Death Investigations

In forensic pathology, knowing one's role in death investigation is essential in the pursuit of justice and the integrity of the justice system. Forensic pathologists are tasked with determining the cause and manner of death, which entails meticulous examination of physical evidence and biological specimens. This role extends beyond identification; it involves meticulous examination of all of the observations that can be encountered in a case. The creation of a unifying account on which to construct a narrative through the gathering of evidence and the development of an explicable explanation is required in constructing that which can probably be termed a forensic truth. The formality of such inquiries can be seen in high-profile international cases, such as forensic exhumations in and following the events at Srebrenica, where the responsibility of the pathologists was not simply technical examination but also the presentation of evidence within a court setting (Klinkner et al., 2008). In addition, death investigation duties encompass ethical and precise reporting of the findings to the parties involved. Forensic pathologists can serve as expert witnesses, and thus need a level of accuracy in their testimony and reports. The Goudge Inquiry highlights the importance of such duties and addressing concerns regarding the quality and admissibility of forensic opinions, especially in high-risk matters like children (Donald et al., 2014). It is critical that the forensic expert has knowledge of the legal environment in which he or she practices, and that his or her opinion be based on proven, reproducible methods that can be validated. This two-pronged demand for scientific soundness and legal use underlines the pathologist's function as an indispensable translator between the worlds of medicine and law.

Beyond this, continuing professional education and application of quality control procedures are significant elements of the forensic pathologist's responsibility. Interfacing with the most current literature and emerging methodologies strengthens their practice as well as the validity of their results. The inclusion of ethics guidelines, as the Goudge Inquiry advised, establishes a culture of accountability that is essential to the integrity of forensic evidence in the courtroom (Donald et al., 2014). As forensic pathologists wade through the intricacies of death investigations, they must see to it that their practices are in accord with both science and law. In so doing, they strengthen the legal process and work toward the greater goal of justice—bringing clarity to cases that are riddled with uncertainty and giving families answers that are respectful of their loved ones (Figure 1.6).

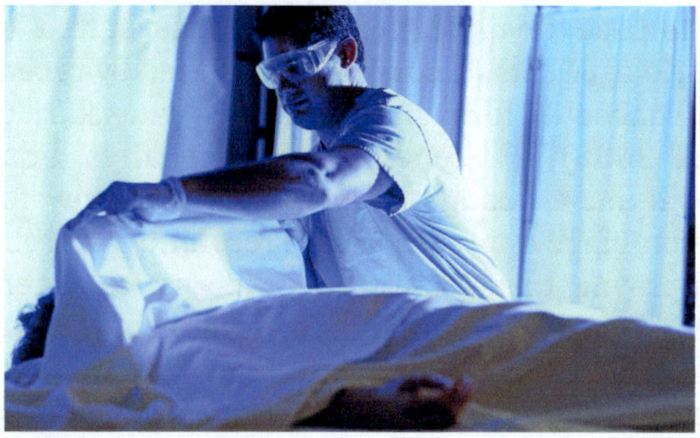

Figure 1.6. Death investigations: the role of medical examiners.

Source: https://www.policechiefmagazine.org/wp-content/uploads/GettyImages-1009504530-825x510.jpg.

1.2.2. Collaboration with Law Enforcement and Legal Teams

The sophisticated division of forensic pathology requires collaboration amongst forensic pathologists, police forces, and legal experts. Cooperative effort is required in managing investigations into violent, sudden, or suspicious death. Forensic pathologists provide critical information on the causation of death by using techniques like autopsy and toxicology to uncover evidence that police may not have the expertise to interpret. Therefore, law enforcement departments utilize this information in order to develop investigative plans that can potentially offer successful solutions to cases. Improved coordination enhances the integrity of evidence, which compels legal units to prepare trials in which well-documented studies could significantly shape judicial rulings. This exchange of information also transcends instant investigations, enhancing training and resource planning. Forensic pathologists are also involved in interagency workshops with police officers, enabling greater familiarity with the latest forensic methods and legal requirements of conclusions. For example, daily conversation about the application of dental information and DNA typing guides more informed investigative approaches suited to various circumstances, as exemplified by recent advances in forensic technology (Auerkari et al., 2008). These collaborations align both legal and investigative paradigms to allow for a combined approach in case resolution, thereby improving the effectiveness of the justice system as a whole. Coordination of legal components with forensic investigations is essential to ensure that collected evidence is meaningful and admissible in court. Legal professionals draw upon the skills of forensic pathologists to understand evidence that may be introduced in court, making sure it is put into context. Additionally, police have to ensure that their investigation procedures align with legal norms to avoid risking prosecutorial misconduct. Forensic pathologists will give evidence and provide expert assessment, filling any technical-humidity gap between forensic data and the legal discourse. Such inter-disciplinary cooperation not only increases the integrity of cases but also increases the credibility of forensic science as an appropriate tool of justice, reflecting on the indispensable role of cooperation between legal and forensic experts (Miwa et al., 2010).

1.2.3. Autopsy's Significance in Determining Cause of Death

Forensic pathology relies heavily on autopsies in the determination of the cause of death in cases that are suspicious. An autopsy allows forensic pathologists to conduct a thorough analysis of the body and organ structure and identify any physical evidence indicative of unnatural death. For example, visual inspection of injury, organ deformity, and extent of disease can provide vital information. Furthermore, when dealing with explosions or other traumatic deaths, complete documentation of patterns and types of injury plays a key role in interpreting the cause of death. This applies especially to unusual cases, such as explosion-sought suicide, where forensic pathologists must enable interagency cooperation and deal with issues of safety in the examination process (McLemore et al., 2016). Thus, the autopsy serves not only as a diagnostic process but as a method to reconstruct the history of an episode of death. In addition to the gross examination, biochemical analyses performed during autopsy can yield significant information not obtainable with routine morphological methods. Postmortem chemistry, which analyzes materials such as blood, urine, and cerebrospinal fluid, has also become increasingly integral to the determination of causes of death. Certain conditions, such as diabetic ketoacidosis or complex electrolyte abnormalities, may not be visible to the naked eye but can make a significant contribution to understanding a death. Such investigations may uncover underlying reasons for the lethal condition, which in turn could enhance understanding of the deceased's medical history and health conditions (Mangin et al., 2018). The integration of postmortem chemistry into forensic science not only enhances cause-of-death determinations but also aids the overall forensic investigation with invaluable scientific data. Moreover, autopsy findings hold significant public health and safety importance. When death is determined to result from homicide, suicide, or accidental overdose, information can direct health policy and prevention efforts. For instance, detecting trends in drug overdose or death due to certain diseases in certain populations may encourage public health authorities to allocate resources more wisely. This aspect points to the broader public impact of autopsies since they not only assist criminal investigations but also provide information that can save lives in the future. Basically, by careful analysis of physical evidence and biochemical changes, autopsies serve a twofold purpose: dispensing justice as well as informing improved programs of community health. Hence, the applicability of autopsy in forensic practice is much more profound than the specific case itself, culminating in a culturally educated ethos of mortality and public health (Figure 1.7).

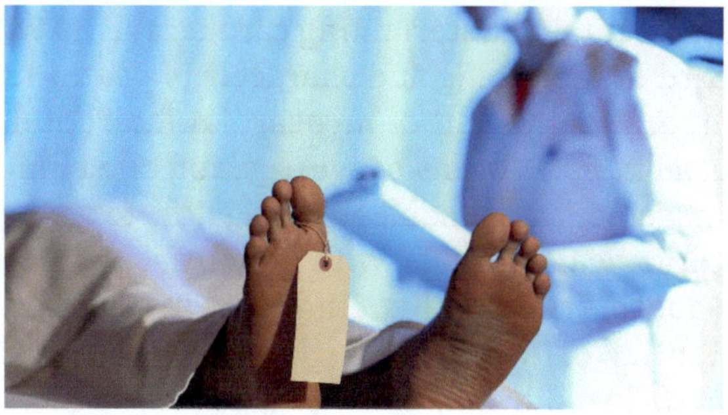

Figure 1.7. Autopsy in determining the cause of death.

Source: https://cdn.hswstatic.com/gif/body-autopsy.jpg.

Test Your Knowledge

1. What is the primary role of forensic pathologists in death investigations?
2. What is the importance of an autopsy in determining the cause of death?

1.3. Techniques Used in Forensic Pathology

Learning Outcome

1. Describe the autopsy procedures and methodologies.
2. Understand the use of toxicology in forensic investigations.
3. Know the application of advanced imaging technologies.

In forensic pathology, various techniques are employed in establishing the cause and manner of death, which are of immense significance in legal investigations and scientific information. Autopsy is one of the fundamental techniques, where pathologists carry out a thorough examination of the body to find external and internal injuries, illness, or irregularities that could be responsible for the death. The autopsy typically involves diligent inspection of organ systems, tissue biopsy for histological examination, and toxicologic examination to identify the possible substances that could have been responsible for the death. Furthermore, utilizing newer imaging technologies, such as X-rays or CT scans, forensic pathologists are now able to visualize internal structures without inducing invasive injury, thereby enhancing diagnostic sensitivity and having a better comprehension of the circumstances of death. Histopathology is also crucial in forensic examination, revealing cellular and tissue responses to injury or disease processes. By microscopic observation of tissue samples, forensic pathologists can find alterations that are characteristic of trauma, disease, or alcohol/drug use. For instance, identification of the infarction characteristics of myocardial ischemia, such as could be evidenced in a necrotic process, is instrumental in determining cardiac events with regard to the timing and character of death. This temporal definition of myocardial infarction is crucial in both forensic investigation and clinical management as it enables investigators to connect pathological findings with potential windows of death, thus enhancing the investigative potential of forensic specialists (Bello et al., 2015). In addition, emerging biomarkers and immunohistochemical staining techniques are revolutionizing forensic pathology's assessment of traumatic brain injuries. The identification of some proteins, such as the proteolytic fragment alpha-II Spectrin known as SNTF, illustrates the evolving character of diagnostic methods used to be applied to brain tissue following traumatic injuries. These markers are able to identify complexity in axonal injury that cannot be constructed with standard histological methods. For instance, studies have shown that SNTF is possible even in mild traumatic brain injury, thereby widening the definition of diffuse axonal injury, its clinical relevance, and potential effects (Cullen et al., 2015). Application of such advanced techniques not only enhances the validity of forensic examinations but also assures that the subtle mechanisms of trauma are addressed appropriately through judicial systems.

1.3.1. Autopsy Procedures and Methodologies

Techniques of autopsy form a significant component of forensic pathology and are utilized both legally and medically. Autopsy starts with a thorough external examination of the dead body, where the forensic pathologist inspects external trauma, the state of the body, and other such physical features relevant to the case. The initial step is crucial since it can instantly raise assumptions about the cause of death or homicide. Upon the external examination, a systematic internal examination is undertaken, which encompasses a structured dissection of major organ systems. These meticulous procedures are not only essential in establishing the cause of death but also very important in evidence collection, which can be vital in court hearings. The integration of newer technologies keeps refining such older techniques, advancing the field's potential for sound and valid determinations, consistent with the evolving environment of forensic pathology. The techniques utilized in autopsy procedures are increasingly evolving, especially with the availability of digital imaging technologies. Traditional methods have long focused on visual assessment of skeletal changes to estimate age at death, relying on established osteological markers such as cranial sutures and pelvic joints. However, the application of advanced imaging techniques, such as CT scanning and 3D reconstruction, has revolutionized how these assessments are conducted. For instance, they facilitate the development of virtual bone models that allow pathologists to study morphological changes without destroying physical samples. In addition, recent studies highlight quantitative analysis as a valuable tool in the process of uncovering changes in bone composition and density, with a more nuanced understanding of biological aging. The incorporation of advanced methods into normal practice not only enhances the scope of accuracy of autopsy findings but also the scope of forensic investigations, as is noted in research focusing on new data from imaging equipment (Acsádi et al., 2016). The need to adopt a diverse method while conducting autopsies cannot be overstated, especially in today's forensic environment. Expanding away from the domain of traditional post-mortem analyses, interdisciplinarity broadens input from various fields such as geoscience and materials science. Joint collaboration, for instance, partnerships with centers of excellence in high-level imaging and data analytics, bring added precision to forensic analysis by increasing contrast and resolution in imaging procedures. Such advancements represent a common direction toward more comprehensive analysis through new approaches that yield improved analysis of human remains. The convergence of different scientific disciplines has the potential to make educational extension services richer, as well as expand the universal pool of knowledge in the area of forensic pathology to keep professionals abreast of current trends and practices. Such a continuously evolving environment propels forensic pathology along, emphasizing the need for incessant research and collaboration among specialists (Ahmed et al., 2017) (Figure 1.8).

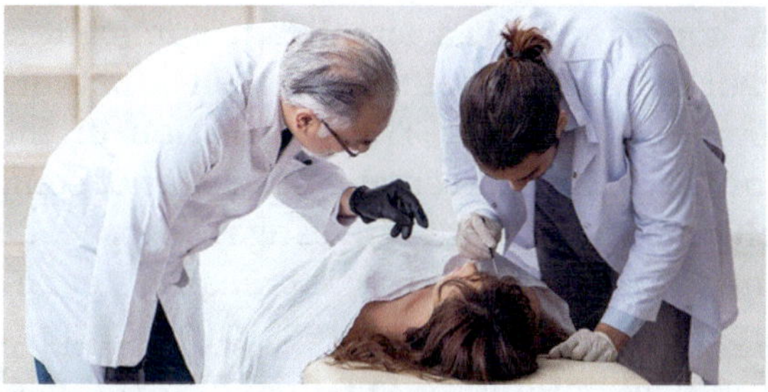

Figure 1.8. Forensic autopsy.

Source: https://www.diginerve.com/blogs/wp-content/uploads/2025/05/Forensic-Autopsy-Explained-Key-Types-Incisions-and-Procedures.webp.

1.3.2. Use of Toxicology in Forensic Investigations

The use of toxicology in forensic investigation is central to the process of unraveling the circumstances of unexplained deaths and criminal investigations. Practically, toxicology is essentially the scientific study of the effects of chemicals on biological organisms, which is widely used in cases of suspected poisoning or overdose. By testing body fluids such as blood, urine, and tissues, toxicologists can identify whether substances ranging from recreational drugs to toxic chemicals and metabolites are present. Not only does testing determine the cause of death, but it can also reveal potential foul play, especially in homicides. Toxicological results can also provide very useful information about a suspect's intent and behavior, such as in the case of serial criminals, where the information about chemicals found in the body of the victim can provide insight into the psychological profile of the perpetrator (Ho et al., 1994). Toxicology also has important applications in the legal process, influencing criminal investigations and judgments. Precision and credibility of toxicology testing are of prime concern; hence, rigorous regulations are established to avoid mishaps and ensure the evidence is court-admissible. Forensic toxicologists employ advanced methods such as gas chromatography and mass spectrometry to give precise quantitative results, differentiating between therapeutically acceptable levels of drugs and those likely to be harmful. This makes it possible to build a chronology of events leading up to death, essentially answering some of the most critical questions of intent and timing of drug administration. As forensic science becomes more popular across the globe, driven by partly popular interest as much as it is reflected in media portrayals, it guarantees that toxicology will be a part of comprehensive forensic pathology analysis (Stankiewicz et al., 2007). Within the broader forensic pathology framework, toxicology is not only utilized for determining the cause of death but also enables us to comprehend human behavior and any likely abnormalities in it. Toxicological analysis of victims or suspects may indicate drug abuse or drug abuse patterns, thereby guiding preventive strategies as well as therapeutic intervention for public health. Furthermore, there are some cases, such as serial killers, that unveil complex patterns of correlations between chemicals and mental states, illustrating how toxicology addresses mental health issues. The connection reveals the necessity of including toxicological information in forensic pathology because it provides a higher level of inference when interpreting evidence. Consequently, toxicology is imperative in revealing the various intricacies involving forensic examinations to enhance legal as well as academic practice in the field (Ho et al., 1994) (Figure 1.9).

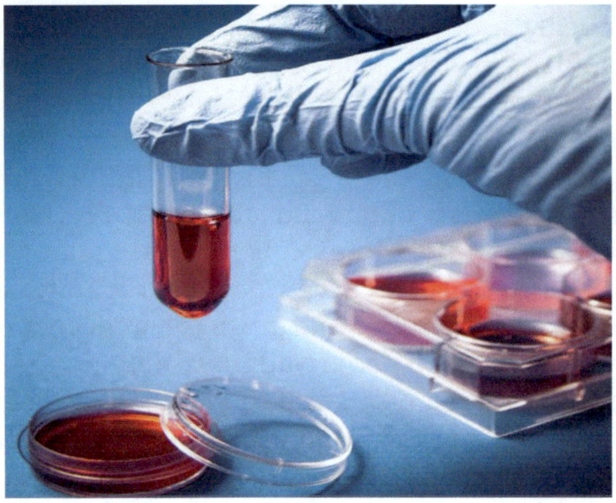

Figure 1.9. Forensic toxicology.

Source: https://www.fondelco.in/institute/assets/images/Toxicology2.jpg.

1.3.3. Application of Advanced Imaging Technologies

The field of forensic pathology has gained significantly from the application of new imaging technologies, which have enhanced the examination of complex cases with precision. Techniques such as confocal laser scanning microscopy (CLSM) represent a huge leap in technology, allowing for increased resolution and three-dimensional reconstruction of biological samples. This is very useful in the understanding of inflammatory reactions observed with many pathological conditions, such as myocardial infarction, as they allow semi-quantitative analysis and protein identification within the inflammatory cascade. The capacity for visualization and quantification of protein distribution and expression helps forensic pathologists analyze the dynamics of tissue damage and repair in furtherance of the common understanding of deaths resulting from unknown or violent causes (Cantatore et al., 2015). Micro-computed tomography (micro-CT) is also an area of major deviation in forensic imaging, specifically in cases involving skeletal remains or complicated trauma. The technology allows forensic experts to non-destructively analyze and realign severed bone structures recovered and scattered at crime scenes. Its application in cases of dismemberment reveals the intricate pattern of tool marks and processing of charred evidence, which are critical in piecing together the sequence of events of a victim's death. The high-resolution images created by micro-CT allow for strict scrutiny and are acceptable evidence in court, thus considering it a significant application of advanced imaging methods in forensic pathology (Baier et al., 2017). The integration of these innovative imaging technologies does not confine itself to improving the investigative procedure alone; it also includes increasing learning opportunities being offered to practitioners in forensic pathology. For instance, the use of three-dimensional modeling through printing technology allows for the physical portrayal of complex anatomical structures or injuries, thereby enabling both training and expert testimony cases. Through the translation of complex data into solid models, forensic pathologists are in a position to better describe their findings to juries and other involved parties in court. This mingling of learning and technology ultimately serves to emphasize the huge impact of advanced imaging in the advancement of forensic pathology, ensuring that professionals are equipped with the latest tools to enhance accuracy and understanding in their practices (Baier et al., 2017).

Test Your Knowledge

1. What is the primary purpose of an external examination during an autopsy?
2. Which technology has recently enhanced the methodologies of autopsy procedures?

1.4. Types of Death Investigated

Learning Outcome

1. Learn about homicides and their forensic implications.
2. Describe the accidental deaths and their analysis.
3. Understand the suicides and the role of forensic pathology.

Forensic pathology encompasses a variety of categories of deaths that must be examined to identify the cause and circumstances underlying them. Among them, natural deaths from progressive disease processes are routinely examined. Myocardial infarction (MI) is a stereotypical representative of this category of death, where the pathophysiology is complex cellular events triggered by ischemia resulting in cell death. The significance of awareness about MI is twofold: it offers knowledge to advance clinical treatment planning, and it is also critical evidence in forensic practice. The chronological dating of MI plays a significant role in the determination of timelines surrounding death, which can assist clinical and forensic pathologists in estimating the time of death and has extreme consequences on legal investigation and medical practice (Bello et al., 2015). Other than death due to natural causes, forensic pathologists also investigate accidental deaths resulting from accidents such as falls, drowning, or motor vehicle accidents. These cases typically require meticulous scrutiny of facts, such as the causes leading to death, to differentiate between negligence, mistake, or other reasons. Accidental deaths also rely not only on the physical evidence from the scene but also on autopsy reports that reveal the immediate cause of death. Forensic pathologists utilize a multi-disciplinary approach, integrating law enforcement officials, accident reconstructionists, and medical examiners to create an unambiguous image of the situation around the fatal incident.

Thorough investigation ensures that legal conclusions are appropriately made, addressing the medical and legal details of such deaths. In addition, homicidal and suicidal examinations comprise a significant component of forensic pathology. Such cases are typically complex and require advanced assessments of the physical evidence and the mental surroundings in which the death occurred. In homicides, pathologists not only provide the cause of death, but also give top-priority forensic information that can be employed for the identification and prosecution of criminals. Similarly, with suicide cases, having the ability to analyze the interplay between psychological conditions and the physiological mechanisms of death can be important in assessing the mentality of the victims during the time preceding the lethal process. The addition of post-mortem tissue analysis indicates active transcriptional regulation post-mortem, thus suggesting an active play of biological processes that forensic examiners must consider in their analysis (Aguet et al., 2018). Such detailed examinations underscore the intricacy of death investigation in forensic pathology (Figure 1.10).

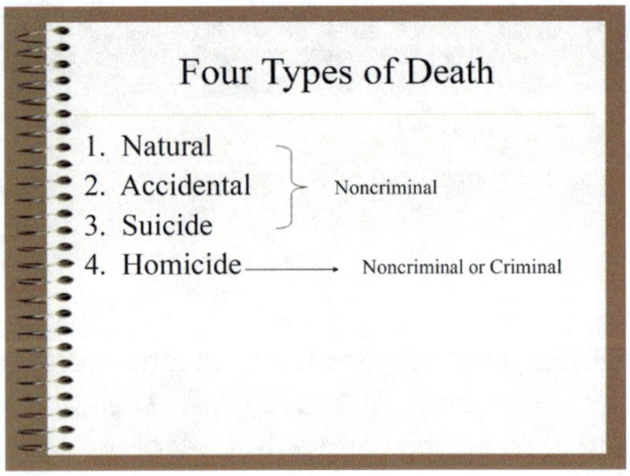

Figure 1.10. Types of death.

Source: https://slideplayer.com/slide/3903371/13/images/2/Four+Types+of+Death+Natural+Accidental+Noncriminal+Suicide.jpg.

1.4.1. Homicides and Their Forensic Implications

Homicidal investigation, in forensic pathology, involves unique situations that have a major impact on the methods applied in solving and detecting homicide. The reaction to the first homicide is most critical; forensic departments must record the crime scene properly, collect evidence, and maintain the integrity of the investigation. This first step is particularly important, as studies have shown that successful utilization of the first 48 hours makes a major difference in the clearance of homicide cases. Moreover, characteristics such as the location of the disposal site and the criminals' forensic knowledge contribute to investigators' awareness of the case.

Thus, early intervention by investigators and forensic pathologists can potentially affect the direction of the investigation and even attain quicker resolution of the case, highlighting the intricate dynamic between forensic practice and the efficacy of homicide case solution. Forensic consideration of homicides is not only a matter of detection, but also encompasses psychological and socio-environmental factors of criminal behavior. Forensic pathologists involved must consider numerous causes of homicide, including the mental health of victims and perpetrators. For instance, higher domestic violence rates in certain demographics, like military veterans, are of special concern. Based on research, conditions like situational PTSD and unworked-through trauma can put a strain on the relationship, culminating in violent outcomes. Specifically, the challenges of veterans adjusting back to life as civilians and the increasing rate of intimate partner violence underscore the necessity of readdressing these mental health challenges. This multidisciplinary response not only deconstructs the mystery surrounding the nature of human behavior in violent crime but also advocates for an interdisciplinary forensic pathology model that addresses mental health sensitivity as an essential element.

Further, forensic investigation of murders requires immense knowledge of various environmental conditions influencing the recovery and examination of evidence. It has been determined through research that the location where bodies are dumped has an influence on solving homicide cases effectively. Murders involving bodies disposed of in water can result in inconsistent levels of decomposition as well as challenging recovery, impacting the possibility of recovering useful forensic evidence. The distinction between indoor and outdoor homicides creates another level of complexity in cases because the two settings have varying factors in witness accounts and management of the crime scene. Correspondingly, a thorough examination of previously hardened homicide cases shows that a strategic approach to interpreting differences can optimize the efficiency of cold case examinations. The need for further research on individual trends around body disposal locations and the timing of evidence discovery is essential in a bid to improve investigative methods and improve future forensic practice in homicide cases, as evidenced by literature on serial killers and their victims (Raymer et al., 2019) (Figure 1.11).

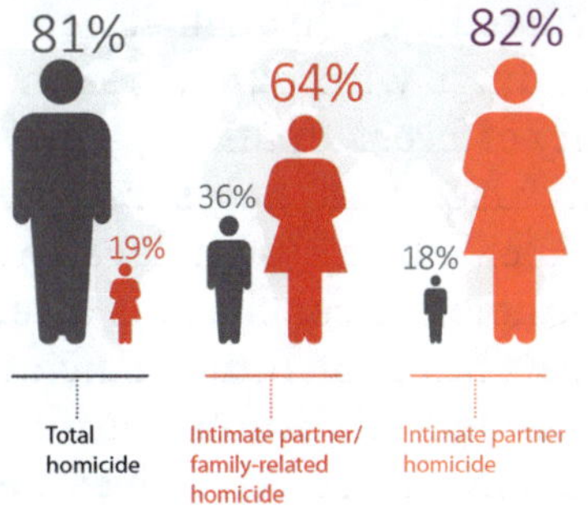

Figure 1.11. Global study on homicide.

Source: https://www.unodc.org/images/data-and-analysis/gsh/b1_total_homicide_share_final-01.png.

1.4.2. Accidental Deaths and Their Analysis

Unintentional deaths are an important area of investigation for forensic pathology, for the analysis of which includes an interdisciplinary approach that addresses a number of causative mechanisms along with situational variables. These deaths typically result from a cumulative effect of environmental hazards, human error, and occasionally underlying diseases that complicate the scenario. In forensic settings, pathologists carry out extensive investigations to classify the character of such occurrences, determining if they result from negligence, accidental occurrences, or other causes. For instance, data from Serious Case Reviews show that even though most accidental deaths result from severe physical violence or omission, the two categories need to be distinguished in order to institute effective preventive strategies and inform public health policies aimed at reducing such incidents (Belsky et al., 2011). Furthermore, there are some substances that bring about accidental deaths, particularly in the field of toxicology within forensic pathology. The case of Tetramethylenedisulfotetramine (TETS), a banned rodenticide, signifies the fatal outcome of accidental poisoning that continues even decades after its prohibition. Despite the fact that TETS was prepared in the 1930s, it is still linked with a number of accidental and intentional deaths on the basis of illegal distribution in some regions. Pharmacological properties of TETS carry high potential for inducing fatal convulsions through GABA antagonism, and this presents grave challenges to medical response and liability law for such casualties (Banks et al., 2014). It highlights the importance of toxicological profiles in the context of accidental death analysis to further enhance the capability of forensic pathologists to establish cause and effect. Moreover, the examination of accidental fatalities raises social and ethical questions of prevention and accountability. Each case has a unique set of circumstances in which law officials and medical examiners must frequently act in close collaboration. Forensic pathologists play a central part not only in the determination of the cause of death but also in confronting the broader social context of these tragedies.

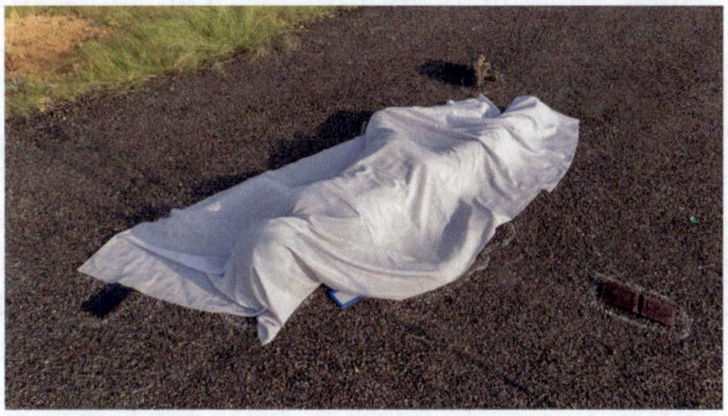

Figure 1.12. Road accident deaths.

Source: https://assets.telegraphindia.com/telegraph/2021/Feb/1613687161_shutterstock_1524998873.jpg.

Through the interpretation of patterns and causes, forensic analysis can assist in the prevention of unintended deaths by informing prevention strategies to reduce avoidable accidents. Public health interventions, public education campaigns, and policy changes can be the outcome of these analyses to prevent preventable accidents. In a sense, dealing with accidental deaths through forensic pathology is not only illuminating certain cases but can also significantly contribute to group safety practices and collective prevention policies (Belsky et al., 2011) (Figure 1.12).

1.4.3. Suicides and the Role of Forensic Pathology

Suicide is a grave public health concern, and forensic pathology plays a crucial role in understanding its complexities. Forensic pathology, as a medical science devoted to the investigation of death, prepares pathologists to determine the cause and mode of death, particularly in cases suspected to be suicide. Forensic pathologists make precise assessments post-mortem since accuracy is paramount in their consideration of a range of evidence, such as toxicology profiles and circumstantial details from the victim's life. Through a thorough analysis of such variables, pathologists can elucidate suicidal behavior within psychological and social frameworks, which is key to prevention planning. Moreover, findings from these studies can be employed to help shape mental health policy and resource allocation in a bid to reduce the frequency of suicide, an issue of reality in today's world. In addition to expanding our knowledge of the particular circumstances behind suicide, forensic pathology enlightens us about the broader issues involved with autopsy reports. Of special interest, forensic pathologists collaborate with law enforcement and mental health groups to gather data that may identify trends in the frequency of suicides and risk factors. As a case point, the Violence Policy Center states that an estimated 1200 Americans are murdered annually in murder-suicides, crimes in which a murderer kills one other person and then himself or herself (N/A, 2006). These statistics underscore the interdependent complexity of suicide and violence, highlighting the need for an integrated response to mental health that takes account of the role of firearms in these tragedies. Through its connection of forensic findings with public health initiatives, the specialty of forensic pathology both addresses individual cases and helps reduce the root causes of suicide on a system level. Additionally, forensic pathology's conclusions extend into the field of prevention of future suicides through intervention and education. Through pointing out the usually-stored narratives behind such events, forensic pathologists can contribute to important debates on mental health. Educating populations about the determinants leading to suicidal behavior—such as emotional distress, substance abuse, and access to dangerous means—is empowering people to identify crisis warning signs in themselves and others. .

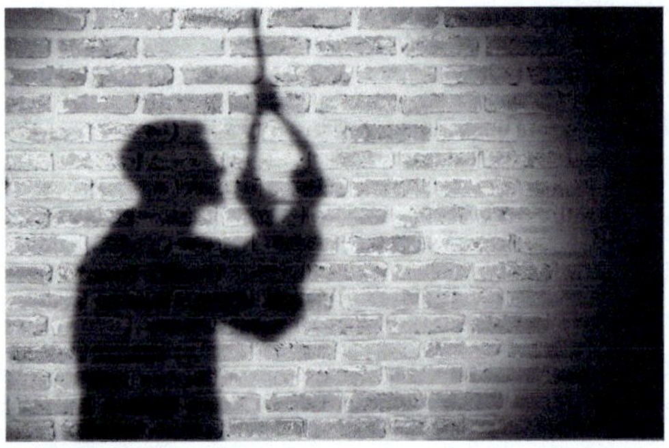

Figure 1.13. Suicide.

Source: https://imageio.forbes.com/specials-images/imageserve/5f53917b9eb85497be7087d8/Since-the-onslaught-of-the-pandemic--workplace-suicide-is-on-the-upswing-/960x0.jpg?format=jpg&width=960.

Furthermore, the rigorous analysis conducted by forensic pathologists can assist policymakers in effectively intervening against these determinants. As the legal and medical occupations increasingly collaborate, one hopes that heightened awareness and more focused interventions will not only enable improved forensic examination to be achieved but also be a forward-thinking measure for reducing the incidence of suicides and their devastating consequences (Nobus et al., 2004) (Figure 1.13)

Test Your Knowledge

1. What mental health condition is commonly associated with violent outcomes in domestic violence cases involving military veterans?
2. What primary factors contribute to accidental deaths?

1.5. Legal and Ethical Considerations

Learning Outcome

1. Describe the chain of custody and evidence handling.
2. Describe the ethical dilemmas faced by forensic pathologists.
3. Know the impact of forensic findings on legal outcomes.

In reflecting on the field of forensic pathology, legal and ethical considerations emerge as key factors influencing practice and policy. Forensic pathologists practice in a world governed not just by the standards of science but by statutes and ethical requirements to safeguard the rights of the deceased and their families. The need for ethics arises from the high-stakes implications of forensic findings in criminal cases, where the accuracy of autopsy results determines the outcome of justice. Ethical codes ensure that the dead individual's integrity is upheld, particularly when remains are analyzed for further research or exhumation. As cited in ALRC Report 96, affluent frameworks must take into account the ethical, legal, and social implications of forensic practices, with particular regard to assuring that modern-day practices are rooted in established moral principles (Opeskin et al., 2025). As forensic pathology further blurs the lines with advancements in genetic technology, more complexity arises in law. For instance, the use of DNA testing in criminal investigations is a double-edged sword; it enhances the potential to identify suspects and victims but creates concerns about privacy and consent. As genetic information is highly personal, ethical measures should be implemented to ensure its application so that it will not be abused or manipulated in legal proceedings. The structure put forth in juridical literature addresses such fears by insisting on the importance of informed consent, particularly when genetic information is kept or revealed. Ultimately, equilibrium must be found, pitting scientific progress against the requirement to maintain ethical standards and thus safeguarding that progress in forensic pathology serves the greater good of justice and societal values (Klinkner et al., 2008). The convergence of legal frameworks and forensic expertise introduces a further layer of complexity into the ethical nuances. How forensic evidence is interpreted and presented to judges and juries is capable of affecting not only trial decisions but also public confidence in the justice system. Legal tribunals, such as the International Criminal Tribunal for the former Yugoslavia, illustrate how high stakes become when forensic outcomes become legal judgments. The Srebrenica forensic exhumations are a strong example of how forensic truth is constructed and tested in court proceedings. Their presence in court serves to underscore the delicate balance forensic pathologists engage in, being both scientific experts and legal witnesses in a court of law and having the responsibility to convey complex results in plain terms. This dualism indicates the necessity for continued debate of legal and ethical boundaries in forensic pathology (Klinkner et al., 2008).

1.5.1. Chain of Custody and Evidence Management

Chain of custody is a critical principle in forensic pathology because it ensures the integrity and reliability of evidence during an investigation. This involves meticulous documentation of the acquisition and handling of physical evidence from the point that it is received at a crime scene to the point of presentation in court. Each individual who touches the evidence should be documented in such a way that there is an uninterrupted and reliable chain, preventing potential contamination or tampering. The advantage of a proper chain of custody is even more significant where the evidence is subject to challenge; a careless mistake will destroy the case. To enhance the process of chain of custody, one must incorporate standard procedures that not only provide accuracy but also foster interdisciplinary cooperation among forensic experts and law enforcement officials so that evidence can be secured appropriately and effectively for legal use. Proper procedures in evidence handling are crucial to ensure the quality and viability of forensic samples, especially in human pathology. Each choice from the point when evidence is collected will decide how well it will contribute to legal conclusions. Physical evidence may be influenced by how evidence is presented and where it is located. For instance, biological matter such as blood or tissue will have to be preserved under certain conditions so that they are not spoiled. Ignoring these standards will lead to deceptive results or total exclusion of valuable evidence, something that has far-reaching consequences for justice. Therefore, rigorous training and protocols in evidence handling must be put in place, particularly for first responders, who tend to be the first point of contact with the evidence, ensuring they are trained with the perspective to maintain the chain of custody correctly and effectively (Cecchi et al., 2023). Chain of custody and evidence handling constitute a unique challenge in forensic pathology. Successful collection and transport of evidence directly impact the validity of autopsy results and can potentially have a significant impact on forensic conclusions. In criminal investigations, with the concern for public health and potential for zoonotic exposure, proper management of a scene becomes absolutely critical. Forensic experts largely rely on the integrity of evidence that is gathered by on-scene workers, and thus a training system that has significant focus on maintaining the chain of custody is needed. Such interdependence necessitates adherence to a cycle of continuous improvement and systemic practices in recording, storing, and transmitting evidence. By establishing robust interdisciplinary alliances and utilizing standard documentation protocols, forensic pathology can make it possible for its findings to be grounded on scientifically justifiable practices, hence helping to deliver more precise judicial results (Anderson et al., 2013) (Figure 1.14).

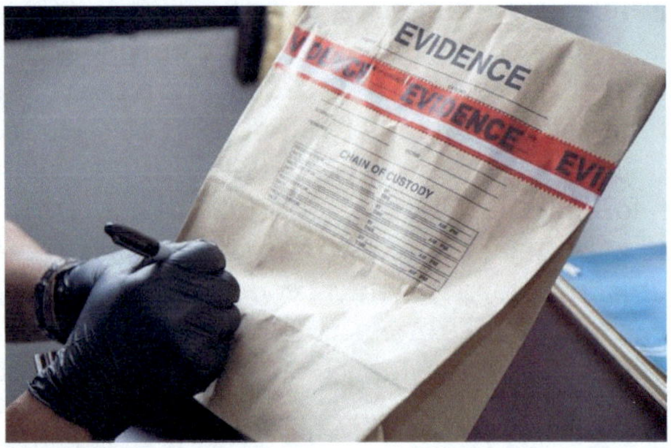

Figure 1.14. The responsibility and importance of maintaining the chain of custody.

Source: https://www.relialabtest.com/wp-content/uploads/2019/05/chain-of-custody.jpeg.

1.5.2. Ethical Dilemmas Faced by Forensic Pathologists

Forensic pathologists walk a tightrope of moral quandaries, where their work involves much more than simply establishing the cause of death. The presentation of human remains is one of the most important ethical dilemmas they encounter, as in the context of using three-dimensional (3D) printed models in court demonstrations. Although 3D prints can enhance understanding for juries and legal practitioners, they have the unforeseen consequence of perpetuating desensitization to death and trauma, becoming more prevalent. Recent studies indicate that while the public largely perceives such innovation as positive, there is a pressing need for ethical standards allowing the respectful use of technology so that dignity is preserved at every phase of the judicial process (Carew et al., 2021). This underscores the essential balance that forensic pathologists must maintain between technological advance and ethical practice. The second ethical issue is in the sphere of forensic pathologists' roles in immigration cases, notably age estimation in children. Since the age of majority in law varies so enormously from one legal jurisdiction to another, age determination in undocumented children can be of paramount legal and humanitarian importance. One particular study in Libya compared the validity of dental development indices as predictors of age, where both high sensitivity and specificity were observed in distinguishing between adolescence and adulthood (Cameriere et al., 2016). However, the ethical concern of misclassifying individuals can lead to disastrous consequences, including wrongful treatment or deportation. Forensic pathologists must be careful and adhere to strict ethical standards to prevent errors, ensuring that their conclusions do not put already vulnerable groups at risk of increased injustice. This is what makes the role emphasize the critical intersection between scientific knowledge, ethical standards, and the representation of marginalized communities. In addition to this, forensic pathology poses ethical questions regarding the application of consent and confidentiality. Forensic pathologists often work with cadavers without the affirmative consent of the deceased or their families for autopsy or utilization of body materials in research. This lack of consent invites ethical doubt, particularly where findings may affect criminal investigations or public health. The employment of openness in communication and consent processes is crucial to establishing rapport among forensic pathologists, communities, and families. Additionally, as newer technologies in forensic science emerge, such as genetic testing, safeguarding the privacy of personal information becomes more crucial. The ethical challenge of ensuring human rights while fulfilling professional requirements is a daunting paradox for forensic pathologists, making the need for updated ethical standards responding to these newer demands in practice more urgent (Figure 1.15).

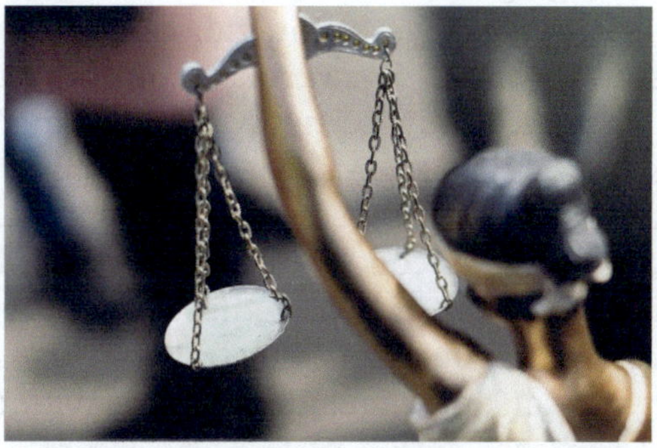

Figure 1.15. The ethical dilemmas in forensic science: Justice and privacy.

Source: https://img1.wsimg.com/isteam/ip/f300726b-ec8a-4a77-a7fc-542dfce792a6/blob.png.

1.5.3. Impact of Forensic Findings on Legal Outcomes

The role of forensic evidence in determining legal outcomes has been made even more significant, particularly with the innovations within forensic pathology and genetics that continue to unravel. Forensic evidence like DNA profiling and other genetic testing has greatly changed the criminal investigation landscape, allowing investigative agencies to link suspects to crimes in a more credible manner. The Australian Law Reform Commissions comprehensive report highlights the reality that genetic information is increasingly playing a key role in legal issues, as emphasized in its articulation of the ethical, legal, and social aspects of the New Genetics (Opeskin et al., 2025). This means that forensic reports are not just vital in verifying or dispelling evidence in the courts but also in providing knowledge for legal codes in regulating their application and, more directly, jury verdicts and court judgments. In addition to genetic evidence, structural neuroimaging techniques have assumed prominent roles in forensic evaluations, particularly in assessing the mental status of defendants. Offering the neurological underpinnings of behavior, neuroimaging aims to adduce a converging line of evidence regarding an individual's mens rea—the state of mind or awareness of criminality. Still, incorporation of neuroimaging in legal cases is not challenge-free, as indicated by the research implying that imaging interpretation could be influenced by biases (Ferracuti et al., 2018). As such, while these findings can powerfully support defense strategies or affect court verdicts, they must be handled with care. Proper interpretation of forensic information, especially neuroimaging-dependent evidence, is important for legal judgments. The impact of forensic findings on legal decisions is not only to provide evidence but to have an effect on public perceptions of justice and the efficiency of the legal system. With forensic science holding a greater stake in high-profile cases, public trust in legal institutions can come to rest upon the perceived reliability and accuracy of the forensic techniques. And, as forensic technology continues to advance, it exhibits a double-edged sword effect: enhancing the efficiency of justice systems while also creating ethical dilemmas over privacy and consent when collecting genetic data. Lastly, the jurisdiction of forensic evidence extends beyond the court context to legislative policy and social justice norms and accountability, thus reiterating the need for constant ethical scrutiny and surveillance in forensic application (Opeskin et al., 2025) (Figure 1.16).

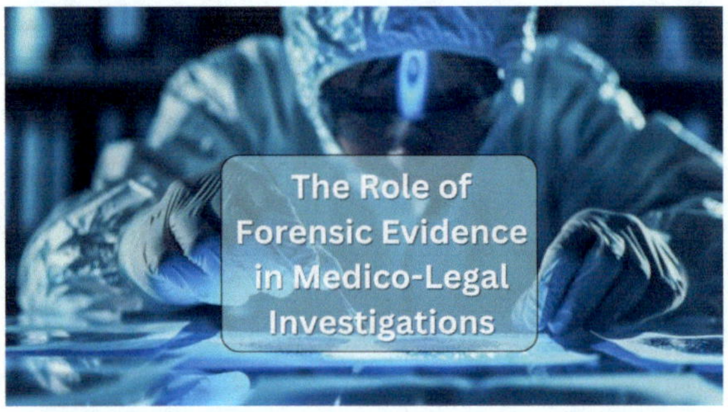

Figure 1.16. The role of forensic evidence in medico-legal investigations.

Source: https://legaleye.co.in/wp-content/uploads/2024/11/The-Role-of-Forensic-Evidence-in-Medico-Legal-Investigations.png.

Test Your Knowledge

1. What is the primary purpose of the chain of custody in forensic investigations?
2. What was a key finding of the Australian Law Reform Commission's report on genetic information?

1.6. Challenges in Forensic Pathology

Learning Outcome

1. Describe the limitations of current forensic techniques.
2. Know the issues related to misinterpretation of findings.
3. Know the impact of public perception and media on forensic work.

Forensic pathology is also critical to determine the cause and manner of death, but it is best suited to address significant challenges that complicate making an accurate diagnosis. Foremost among them is legal and medical interaction. For instance, in suspected child abuse, such as shaken baby syndrome, forensic pathologists have to navigate ethical and moral complexities while following the legal system. Diagnosis is often contingent on the development of specific physiological manifestations, such as subdural hemorrhage and diffuse axonal injury, but the absence of hard data can lead to divergent views among doctors and attorneys. This complexity underscores the need for forensic professionals to not only possess vast medical knowledge but also to possess an eagle-eyed vision regarding the legal context within which they operate, as misjudgments can be fatal to the subjects in such scenarios (Apostol et al., 2017). A second important challenge of forensic pathology is the rapid progress in medical science, which is often ahead of the established methods and procedures to evaluate new disorders in an effective manner. The changing nature of conditions such as amniotic fluid embolism (AFE) reflects this issue clearly. With a frequency of approximately 5.5 per 100,000 deliveries, AFE has an insidious clinical presentation characterized by the sudden onset of severe symptoms, including acute hypotension and hypoxia. Whereas scientists work diligently to delve into the pathophysiologic mechanisms underlying and the potential link to immune response, forensic pathologists must work to incorporate such scientific developments in their investigations and findings. The problem is that forensic practices need to be capable of keeping pace with evolving science to ensure experts provide informative and reliable outcomes to the legal system (Busardo' et al., 2015). Furthermore, the subjective aspect of forensic interpretation is also the source of most of the problems in this field. Human anatomy is intricate and varies from case to case, resulting in experts holding varying views regarding diagnosis and interpretation of findings. For example, in the case of diffuse axonal injury, the non-specificity of certain immunohistochemical markers has the potential to generate significant controversy over the causative mechanisms of injury seen. Experts are often required to reach conclusions on unqualified or conflicting evidence, which can generate controversy not only in the medical profession but also in legal practice. This subjectivity reinforces the imperative need for standardized protocols and training among forensic pathologists to enhance their ability to provide consistent, objective, and scientifically valid conclusions that are open to examination in medical as well as legal arenas. (Apostol et al., 2017).

1.6.1. Limitations of Current Forensic Techniques

The field of forensic pathology is continually evolving, but not without its drawbacks, particularly where investigative methods are concerned. At the forefront of the list of disadvantages is the overhyped nature of forensic science in the media, especially on television crime shows. The notorious CSI effect has the potential to generate unrealistic expectations from jurors regarding the presentation of forensic evidence in court. This effect thus increases the burden of proof for prosecutors and creates a leaning for the jury to acquit based on insufficient forensic evidence. The gap between what the public perceive forensic techniques can achieve and what they actually can do degrades their role within the justice system, highlighting the need for increased awareness of forensic science among jurors and legal professionals (Alejo et al., 2016). As forensic pathology grapples with these challenges, generating public awareness of the fallibility of forensic evidence is essential to allowing fair decisions in legal cases. Another problem with existing forensic practices is excessive reliance on structural neuroimaging in forensic evaluation. While neuroimaging advances have been hailed for their ability to provide objective information about defendants' mental states, in reality, the technologies fall short. Research has shown that the neuroimaging results, though promising, are subject to interpretive biases that can skew their applicability within legal realms. Cognitive biases hinder the unbiased evaluation of evidence, and without strict standards of procedure for applying and interpreting the data from neuroimaging, misrepresentation becomes more of a threat. This limitation can give rise to incorrect conclusions regarding the mens rea of a defendant, making the purity of judicial decisions increasingly complicated (Ferracuti et al., 2018). Therefore, it is crucial to introduce standardized protocols so that neuroimaging can be made a more dependable tool in forensic pathology. Moreover, forensic techniques are not without limitations in biochemical and physical analysis of evidence obtained at crime scenes. The traditional analytical methods of blood and fingerprints, even though they are the foundation of forensic science, are usually hindered by conditions such as contamination, environmental degradation, or improper sampling. The interpretation of such analyses also continues to be prone to fallibility and personal prejudice, which can eventually influence the validity of the results. Secondly, forensic practices have not yet become standardized, leading to various jurisdictions being inconsistent. Such a lack of consistency can undermine the validity of forensic evidence in a court, particularly when plaintiffs' rights and the freedom of defendants are involved. Thus, the incorporation of advanced scientific methods along with good standards and guidelines is essential to overcome the limitations available in current forensic practice so that forensic pathology can provide greater integrity as a means of assistance towards justice (Figure 1.17).

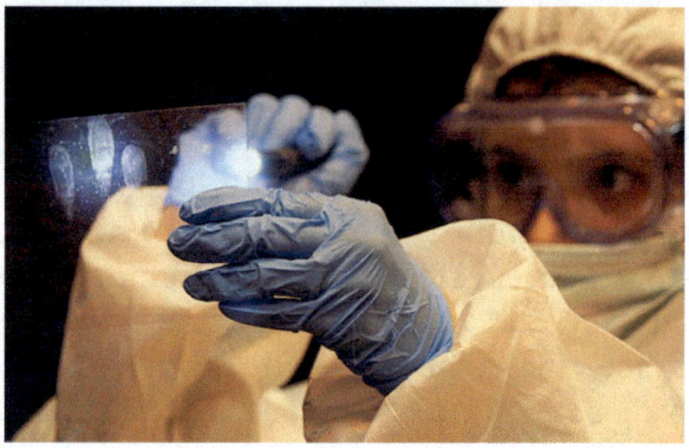

Figure 1.17. New forensic science techniques and technology.

Source: https://policeandsecuritynews.com/wp-content/uploads/2022/08/New-Forensic-Science-lead-image-675x437.png.

1.6.2. Issues Related to Misinterpretation of Findings

The discipline of forensic pathology is all too often plagued by misinterpretation of findings, particularly with the application of high-technology imaging. Neurostructural imaging, for instance, has gained favor for assessing defendants in criminal evaluations. While these methods are employed to provide objective evidence of a defendant's mental status, they inadvertently produce cognitive biases that distort conclusions about the findings. Misinterpretation can result from professionals overreliance on neuroimaging data and failing to consider correlating clinical data, thereby oversimplifying. The risks of these biases necessitate the development of accurate guidelines in order to ensure appropriate application and interpretation of neuroimaging data. The literature emphasizes the importance of integrated diagnostic methods based on anatomical context and cognitive sensitivities to act against the pitfalls in result misinterpretation in court cases (Ferracuti et al., 2018). Misinterpretations can also happen due to the investigation of physical evidence, for example, textile injury in cases involving sharp objects. A recent pilot study pointed to gaps in knowledge about the injury caused by trained users of such weapons and emphasized that not every knife attack leaves similar patterns of injury. If evaluators solely depend on available literature that sometimes tends to overemphasize stabbings, they might miss slight differences brought about by different weapon types. They might end up making wrong findings about the nature of an incident or the intention of the assailant.

Thus, there is a need to include empirical data from real observations of results within forensic practice to enhance accuracy of damage estimates. In the wake of forensic experts trying to properly interpret evidence, recognizing damage pattern variability is essential to avoid fallacies emanating from rigid structures (Carr et al., 2016). Misinterpretation of results could also have a significant effect on legal decision-making. When forensic data are misread or overinterpreted inappropriately, they lead to wrongful acquittals or convictions, revealing the high stakes placed on forensic pathology. The intricate dance of science and law demands that forensic practitioners adhere strictly to standards in evidence evaluation. Without adequate training to recognize the limits and situational nuances of forensic information, experts can contribute to judicial shortcomings. The need for continuous education on how best to utilize forensic practices is essential in the ability to address such issues. The emphasis on open methods, rigorous peer reviews, and correlative interpretation can help alleviate the risks posed by misinterpretation and thus enhance the power of forensic pathology in legal applications.

1.6.3. The Influence of Media and Public Opinion on Forensic Activities

The intersection of public imagination, media, and forensic practice plays a significant role in determining public understanding and expectations of forensic pathology in humans. Media, particularly through crime dramas and investigation programs, has sensationalized the activities of forensic experts, often depicting them as being infallible. This can lead to unjustified public hopes concerning the turnaround time and accuracy of forensic practice. People arrive to hold some notion of the omnipotent nature of forensic science, which overwhelms the richness and natural limitations of such a pursuit. Forensic pathologists in contemporary times grapple with balancing these hyperbolic portrayals of the rich reality of work at the crime scene and autopsy, as they must engage themselves in the molding of public perception in order to advocate realistic conceptions of their own. Public perception is also influenced by the way that forensic evidence is presented in the media as absolute truth. This can warp the image of forensic pathology, as the public will assume that the forensic evidence exists is essentially equivalent to absolute truth. The consequences of this assumption can be drastic, particularly in legal proceedings where juries may overestimate forensic evidence. Forensic pathologists are involved where evidence is in question or where evidence is subjectively interpreted, such as bruise features in assault cases. As found in literature, the multifactorial factors that influence bruising appearance and chronology demonstrate that no single photographic technique definitively establishes the amount of force used or bruise age (Baker et al., 2019). Thus, public and juror misconceptions have the potential to significantly influence trial outcomes and the dispensation of justice. Steps to halt the impact of public opinion on forensic science are vital to ensure the integrity of the field. Public education and outreach efforts can effectively de-mystify forensic pathology and clarify what can and cannot be accomplished by the field. Forensic professional organizations must also address misalignments between media representation and scientific reality. Such reports as the ALRC Report 96 have emphasized the importance of parameters for understanding the legal and ethical impact of forensic processes, which, in combination with public consultation, may reinforce professional authority (Opeskin et al., 2025). By enabling a well-educated public debate, forensic pathologists can ensure that what they do is subjected to the rigorous criticism it warrants, and in the end, make forensic science more effective and reliable in the legal system.

Test Your Knowledge

1. What are the consequences of misinterpreting forensic evidence in legal contexts?
2. According to the ALRC Report 96, what is crucial for improving the public understanding of forensic science?

SUMMARY

In summarizing an investigation of forensic pathology in humans, it is clear that the profession plays an essential role in the judicial system and public health. Through the diligent investigation of death, forensic pathologists not only offer clarity regarding the conditions of death, but also help to advance medical practice. This is particularly the case with anesthesia death, where there is a common accord regarding definitions of perioperative mortality that complicate legal interpretation. In literature, as noted, correct classification and identification of mechanisms for such deaths are paramount towards proper medical accountability and expanding patient safety protocols in anesthesiology. Hence, the use of forensic evidence in the health quality control will minimize instances of preventable deaths, proving that forensic pathology extends beyond inquiry and into teaching and prevention amongst the broader medical community (Argo et al., 2019). Moreover, the effect of forensic pathology resonates closely within the disciplines of criminology and criminal justice. Serial killer cases such as Jeffrey Dahmer's show the important role that autopsy reports and crime scene investigations play in unraveling why horrific crimes have been committed. The analysis of Dahmer's crime pattern identifies not only the multifaceted psychological dimensions of his behavior but also the forensic evidence to underpin a thesis based on unconscious emotions. The careful examination drawn up by forensic experts acts as a foundation where the twinned nature of such individuals can be understood, merging pathology with psychology to offer insights into violent conduct. Hence, the work of forensic pathology extends beyond the simple dispensation of justice in the short term, yielding important lessons in societal deficiencies and human psychological complexity (Ho et al., 1994). Finally, forensic pathology encompasses a wide range of complex and urgent issues that require continued participation from both the medical field and legal systems. As technologies and methods evolve, so too will the role of the forensic pathologist, requiring constant education and evolution. In addition, increasing concern with quality control in healthcare settings underscores the necessity for forensic expertise to guide policy and practice. By and large, therefore, as society wrestles with mortality, violence, and medical ethics concerns, the work of forensic pathology remains essential to bridge gaps between science, law, and public confidence. With meticulous scrutiny and compassionate understanding, forensic pathology can bring about a more secure, more informed society (Argo et al., 2019).

With the study of forensic pathology, there is a consideration required for the methodical analysis of various tissues of the body in a quest to identify the etiology of disease or death. A specific area of significant focus within this platform is the study of brain samples, particularly in the context of seizure disorder. The significance of these studies cannot be overestimated, as they illuminate the underlying pathology that could potentially have effects upon treatment modalities or provide closure for families. As underscored in the guidelines developed for ensuring that morphological studies are more accurate, optimization of brain dissection protocols results in diagnostic yield and precision. This is especially necessary where standard clinical work-up may be insufficient, hence guaranteeing that forensic pathologists can carry out careful assessments based on both neuropathological and clinical data (Jeans et al., 2015). Besides, forensic pathology advances go further into recognizing and identifying individuals based on unique physiological features. Among such notable fields of study is ear recognition, which has gained traction as a potential application in forensic practice. Unlike face recognition, which can be compromised by various factors, ear recognition offers a reliable backup that might be particularly effective where the face is obscured.

These biometric identification methods call for the inclusion of novel approaches in forensic science and thus enable a multi-dimensional approach to human identification. Though with certain challenges, such as occlusion of hair and variation in environmental factors, the recent research on this subject indicates fruitful directions for the improvement of forensic practice (Abaza et al., 2013). Finally, the intersection of histological studies with technological developments points to an interdisciplinary strategy for forensic pathology. Detection of pathological changes in tissue not only makes the diagnosis of disease possible but is also a key issue in forensic cases. The integration of traditional histopathological techniques with novel biometrics, such as ear identification, represents a paradigm shift in the methodology of forensic pathologists. As these fields continue to evolve, the collaboration between histopathology and advanced identification technologies will improve both the efficacy and precision of forensic analysis. Last but not least, this convergence may produce more conclusive evidence to inform legal judgments as well as public health interventions, serving as a source of pride for the dynamic development of forensic pathology in humans.

KEY TERMS FROM THIS CHAPTER

- Criminal justice system
- Drug-related deaths
- Forensic pathology
- Gas chromatography
- Mass spectrometry
- Public health
- Toxic fumes
- Death
- Forensic evidence
- Forensic science
- Injury
- Medical history
- Seizure disorders
- Toxicology

CRITICAL THINKING QUESTIONS

1. **What is the primary focus of forensic pathology?**
   a. Treating patients with chronic illnesses.
   b. Diagnosing genetic disorders in living individuals.
   c. Determining the cause and manner of death.
   d. Investigating infectious diseases in a population.
2. **Which of the following is a key responsibility of a forensic pathologist?**
   a. Performing autopsies to determine the cause of death.
   b. Collecting blood samples for transfusion purposes.
   c. Treating trauma patients in emergency departments.
   d. Conducting psychological evaluations of suspects.
3. **What does the term "manner of death" refer to in forensic pathology?**
   a. The anatomical location of injuries.
   b. The time it took for the person to die.
   c. The circumstances surrounding the death (e.g., natural, accidental).
   d. The medical history of the deceased.
4. **In cases of suspicious deaths, what is the role of forensic pathology?**
   a. To file legal charges against suspects.
   b. To collect and analyze evidence for legal investigations.
   c. To decide the criminal sentence in court cases.
   d. To treat injured victims of a crime.
5. **Which of the following is NOT typically examined during a forensic autopsy?**
   a. Toxicology reports.
   b. Examination of internal organs.
   c. Analysis of dental records.
   d. Genetic counseling for family members.

Short Answer Questions

1. Define forensic pathology.
2. Who is considered one of the pioneering figures in establishing forensic pathology as a recognized field?
3. What is the role of a forensic pathologist?
4. What techniques are used in forensic pathology?
5. What are the three categories of death?

Answer to Critical Thinking Questions

1. (c); 2. (a); 3. (c); 4. (b); 5. (d)

REFERENCES

1. Abaza, A., Harrison, M. A. F., Hebert, C., et al. (2013). A survey on ear biometrics. https://core.ac.uk/download/36778779.pdf (accessed on 12th July 2025).
2. Acharya, J., Adams, B. J., Anson, T., Bikker, J., Black, S., Black, S., Black, S. M., et al. (2018). The role of forensic anthropology in disaster victim identification (DVI): Recent developments and future prospects. https://core.ac.uk/download/195287881.pdf (accessed on 12th July 2025).
3. Acsádi, G., Knüsel, C. J., Leth, P. M., Lynnerup, N., Lynnerup, N., Rühli, F. J., Ubelaker, D. H., et al. (2016). Evaluating osteological ageing from digital data. https://core.ac.uk/download/76945934.pdf (accessed on 12th July 2025).
4. Aguet, F., Amador, R., Amadoz, A., et al. (2018). The effects of death and post-mortem cold ischemia on human tissue transcriptomes. https://core.ac.uk/download/157811337.pdf (accessed on 12th July 2025).
5. Ahmed, F., & Maisano, J. (2017). ToScA North America (6 – 8 June 2017, The University of Texas, Austin, TX) program. https://core.ac.uk/download/211334283.pdf (accessed on 12th July 2025).
6. Alejo, K. (2016). The CSI Effect: Fact or Fiction? https://core.ac.uk/download/70427279.pdf (accessed on 12th July 2025).
7. Anderson, J. S., & Williams, S. K. (2013). Norchem drug testing: A small company's lean journey: Working paper series–13-02. https://core.ac.uk/download/151422455.pdf (accessed on 12th July 2025).
8. Apostol, I., Belis, V., Calota, R. G., et al. (2017). Forensic and clinical diagnosis in shaken baby syndrome: Between child abuse and iatrogenic abuse. https://core.ac.uk/download/144553178.pdf (accessed on 12th July 2025).
9. Argo, A., Buscemi, R., Karch, S. B., Lanzarone, A., Roccuzzo, R., & Zerbo, S. (2019). Perioperative and anesthetic deaths: Toxicological and medico-legal aspects. https://core.ac.uk/download/224993621.pdf (accessed on 12th July 2025).
10. Asmundo, A., Baldari, B., Bertozzi, G., et al. (2020). Clinical-forensic autopsy findings to defeat COVID-19 disease: A literature review. https://core.ac.uk/download/327083240.pdf (accessed on 12th July 2025).
11. Auerkari, E. (2008). Recent trends in dental forensics. https://media.neliti.com/media/publications/282217-recent-trends-in-dental-forensics-522dfd43.pdf (accessed on 12th July 2025).
12. Baier, W., Burnett, B., Harrison, N. P., et al. (2017). Novel application of three-dimensional technologies in a case of dismemberment. https://core.ac.uk/download/74227383.pdf (accessed on 12th July 2025).
13. Baker, B., Carloway, C., Desmoulin, D., Dimitrova, F., et al. (2019). On the relationships between applied force, photography technique, and the quantification of bruise appearance. https://core.ac.uk/download/237453956.pdf (accessed on 12th July 2025).
14. Banks, C. N., Lein, P. J., Rogawski, M. A., et al. (2014). Tetramethylenedisulfotetramine. https://core.ac.uk/download/286729131.pdf (accessed on 12th July 2025).

15. Bello, S., Fineschi, V., Neri, M., et al. (2015). The meaning of different forms of structural myocardial injury, immune response, and timing of infarct necrosis and cardiac repair. https://core.ac.uk/download/54248087.pdf (accessed on 12th July 2025).

16. Belsky, B., Berkowitz, B., Blair, B., Bourget, B., et al. (2011). Fatal child maltreatment in England, 2005-9. https://core.ac.uk/download/44459.pdf (accessed on 12th July 2025).

17. Blanckaert, P., Coopman, V., Cordonnier, J., et al. (2016). A case of acute intoxication due to combined use of fentanyl and 3,4-dichloro-N-[2-(dimethylamino)cyclohexyl]-N-methylbenzamide (U-47700). https://core.ac.uk/download/84044061.pdf (accessed on 12th July 2025).

18. Busardo, F. P., Fineschi, V., Frati, P., et al. (2015). Amniotic fluid embolism pathophysiology suggests the new diagnostic armamentarium: β-tryptase and complement fractions C3-C4 are the indispensable working tools. https://core.ac.uk/download/54249007.pdf (accessed on 12th July 2025).

19. Cameriere, R., Dardouri, A. A. K., De Luca, S., et al. (2016). Third molar maturity index by measurements of open apices in a Libyan sample of living subjects. https://core.ac.uk/download/74211145.pdf (accessed on 12th July 2025).

20. Cantatore, S., De Carlo, D., Fineschi, V., et al. (2015). Confocal laser scanning microscope, Raman microscopy, and western blotting to evaluate inflammatory response after myocardial infarction. https://core.ac.uk/download/54248088.pdf (accessed on 12th July 2025).

21. Carew, R. M. (2021). An investigation into 3D printing of osteological remains: The metrology and ethics of virtual anthropology. https://core.ac.uk/download/480393497.pdf (accessed on 12th July 2025).

22. Carr, D. J., Cowper, E. J., Godhania, K., et al. (2016). A pilot study examining garment severance damage caused by a trained sharp-weapon user. https://core.ac.uk/download/42144462.pdf (accessed on 12th July 2025).

23. Cecchi, R., Gherardi, M., Marchetti, C., et al. (2023). On-site inspection form in veterinary cases: The Parma Veterinary Form. https://core.ac.uk/download/590395582.pdf (accessed on 12th July 2025).

24. Cullen, D. K., Johnson, V. E., Siman, R., et al. (2015). SNTF immunostaining reveals previously undetected axonal pathology in traumatic brain injury. https://core.ac.uk/download/46165322.pdf (accessed on 12th July 2025).

25. Donald, T., & Skellern, C. (2014). The relevance of the Goudge inquiry to the practice of child protection/forensic pediatrics. https://core.ac.uk/download/43353997.pdf (accessed on 12th July 2025).

26. Ferracuti, S., Miolla, A., Sartori, G., Scarpazza, C., et al. (2018). The charm of structural neuroimaging in insanity evaluations: Guidelines to avoid misinterpretation of the findings. https://core.ac.uk/download/188827245.pdf (accessed on 12th July 2025).

27. Gourley, S. J. (2016). Possible causes of increased domestic violence among military veterans: PTSD or mefloquine toxicity? https://core.ac.uk/download/58827124.pdf (accessed on 12th July 2025).

28. Ho, K. C., Jentzen, J., Johnson, L. T., et al. (1994). Destructive hostility: The Jeffrey Dahmer case: A psychiatric and forensic study of a serial killer. https://core.ac.uk/download/213059368.pdf (accessed on 12th July 2025).

29. Jeans, A., Katelaris, A., Klang, A., Pakozdy, A., Pakozdy, A., Pitkanen, A., Woznicka, A., et al. (2015). International Veterinary Epilepsy Task Force recommendations for systematic sampling and processing of brains from epileptic dogs and cats. https://core.ac.uk/download/36778779.pdf (accessed on 12th July 2025).

30. Klinkner, M. J. (2008). Forensic science for Cambodian justice. https://core.ac.uk/download/4897044.pdf (accessed on 12th July 2025).

31. Klinkner, M. J. (2008). Proving genocide? Forensic expertise and the ICTY. https://core.ac.uk/download/4897043.pdf (accessed on 12th July 2025).

32. Kojimoto, M., Matsubara, S., Nakatani, Y., & Takayanagi, I. (2010). New legislation for offenders with mental disorders in Japan. https://core.ac.uk/download/56644370.pdf (accessed on 12th July 2025).

33. Kotsyubinskaya, J., Kozan, N., & Zelenchuk, G. (2017). Express prediction of external distinctive features of a person using the program of dermatoglyphics for prediction. https://core.ac.uk/download/322516262.pdf (accessed on 12th July 2025).

34. Mangin, P., & Palmiere, C. (2018). Postmortem chemistry update part I. https://core.ac.uk/download/159155693.pdf (accessed on 12th July 2025).

35. McLemore, A. M., Prahlow, J. A., & Prahlow, S. P. (2016). Suicide by bomb, with decapitation. https://core.ac.uk/download/228066087.pdf (accessed on 12th July 2025).

36. N/A. (2006). American roulette: Murder-suicide in the United States. https://core.ac.uk/download/71339398.pdf (accessed on 12th July 2025).

37. Nobus, D., Evans, C., For, H., Hazelwood, R. R., Kronengold, E., Downing, L., et al. (2004). The iconography of asphyxiophilia: From fantasmatic fetish to forensic fact. https://core.ac.uk/download/337278.pdf (accessed on 12th July 2025).

38. Opeskin, B., Weisbrot, D., & Breen, K. (2025). Essentially yours: The protection of human genetic information in Australia. https://core.ac.uk/download/pdf/30672952.pdf (accessed on 12th July 2025).

39. Raymer, C. (2019). An investigation into summary data of solved North American serial killer cases to identify trends within murder and disposal locations and time between estimated death and recovery. https://core.ac.uk/download/222929066.pdf (accessed on 12th July 2025).

40. Schnabel, J. (2016). Realistic man, fantasy policeman: The longevity of Ruth Rendell's Reginald Wexford. https://core.ac.uk/download/305123640.pdf (accessed on 12th July 2025).

41. Stankiewicz, H. (2007). Investigating the worldwide popularity of forensics. https://core.ac.uk/download/56509355.pdf (accessed on 12th July 2025).

42. Varotto, E., Galassi, F. M., Aquila, I., Tarda, L., Ricci, P., Sacco, M. A., Gualtieri, S., et al. (2024). The fascinating world of forensic sciences: Multidisciplinary approaches in human remains and the role of forensic pathology in Calabrian experience. https://core.ac.uk/download/646504025.pdf (accessed on 12th July 2025).

MEDICOLEGAL DEATH INVESTIGATION

2

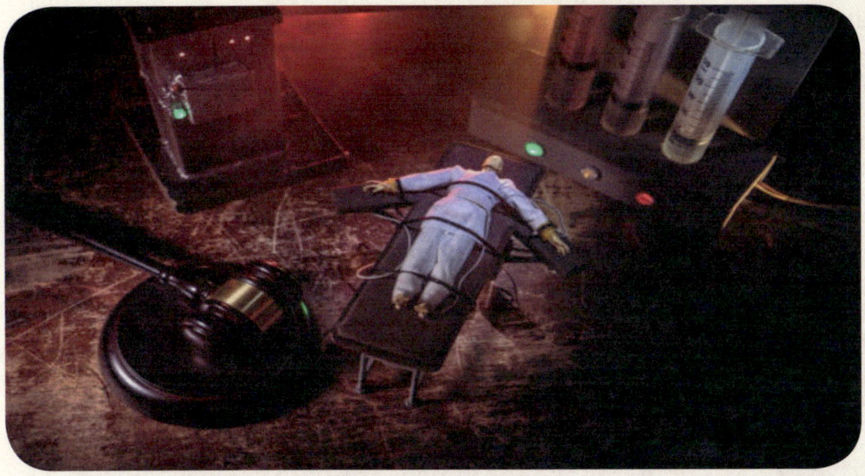

LEARNING OBJECTIVES

After studying this chapter, you will be able to:

1. Understand the roles and responsibilities of forensic professionals;
2. Describe the types of death investigations;
3. Know the autopsy process;
4. Understand the legal aspects of death investigations;
5. Describe the challenges in medicolegal death investigations.

Introduction

The medicolegal death investigation profession is essential to comprehending human mortality and its intricacies, and the ensuing legal implications. Since public health, criminal justice, and ethics have become issues for societies, the work of forensic practitioners becomes increasingly significant. This interdisciplinary discipline not only encompasses the methods for determining cause and manner of death but also addresses pivotal questions of systemic biases that affect investigations. It has been brought to light by recent studies that the discrepancies in identification rates among marginalized communities require a re-examination of medicolegal system practices. The urgency of speed in this case is evidenced by studies indicating that persons of color endure rates of identification delayed compared to whites, which points to potential weaknesses in the methodologies of forensic practitioners (Mace et al., 2022).

Moreover, the forensic anthropology specialty forms the core of the medicolegal system, with a specific focus on the differentiation between human and nonhuman remains. Misidentifications will likely result in significant delays in the investigatory process, both in recognition of the deceased and in the legal process. Research evidence indicates a high frequency of nonhuman skeletal remains occurring in casework, especially in areas dense with wildlife (Fourshee et al., 2022).

Forensic anthropologists have shown that a majority of nonhuman bones excavated are of similar size to human remains, thus being hard to identify (Fourshee et al., 2022). As such, it is important to enhance training for forensic anthropologists in the most common nonhuman taxa in order to make death investigations more accurate and efficient, thereby creating a more reliable medicolegal system.

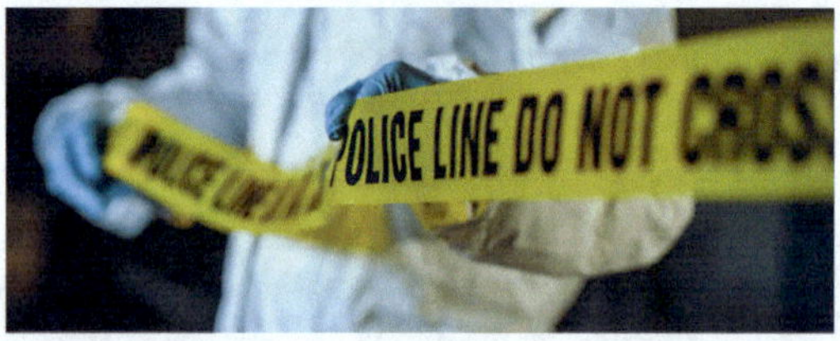

Figure 2.1. Medicolegal death investigations.

Source: https://dpjh8al9zd3a4.cloudfront.net/sites/default/files/styles/rti_masthead_with_image_large_image/public/2024-02/GettyImages-837664122_2500_updated.jpg.webp?itok=GgguHUiN.

In summary, enforcement of comprehensive training and awareness among forensic professionals is essential in addressing the prevailing imbalances in medicolegal death investigations. By recognizing systemic biases and enhancing identification procedures, the forensic community can work towards achieving a more equitable response in dealing with cases involving individuals of different backgrounds. With cumulative research and empirical data shaping these reforms, the medicolegal system can respond more effectively to the subtleties of human death and provide fair treatment to everyone, regardless of race or ethnicity, in investigations that profoundly impact their communities. Such efforts are essential to establish trust in forensic processes and provide justice to all individuals within the medicolegal system (Figure 2.1).

Definition of Medicolegal Death Investigation

Medicolegal death investigation is a term that refers to the multidisciplinary practice of determining the cause and the mode of death in cases that are sudden, unexpected, or suspicious in nature. In most instances, the investigation incorporates the involvement of forensic experts, law enforcement units, and medical professionals. The common objective is to determine the circumstances of a death to bring about clarification of the legal process, as well as for the comprehension of society. Medical examiners and coroners play pivotal roles in conducting autopsies, collecting data, and reporting, which are extremely valuable in providing guidance to legal judgments and public health viewpoints. Thus, medicolegal death investigation is characterized by more than clinical assessment, encompassing a broader socio-legal context aimed at securing justice and closure to bereaved families while improving the integrity of forensic practice. One of the characteristics of medicolegal death investigation is its emphasis on systematic collection and analysis of evidence for deaths. Such scientific investigation is typically into traumatic injuries and diseases that result in death, necessitating specialized expertise and technique. For instance, cases involving traumatic brain injury underscore the complexities of carrying out such investigations, where laboratory tests and biomarkers can complement diagnosis. The investigation of markers like βAPP and GFAP not only serves to identify cause of death mechanisms but also reveals underlying patterns capable of informing public health prevention (Frati et al., 2018). By this critical examination, medicolegal death investigation seeks to decrease uncertainty regarding cause and manner of death, enabling improved insight that can aid legal action as well as public health initiatives. Another crucial component of medicolegal death investigation is addressing systemic bias that could affect identification and analysis, particularly of marginalized populations. Disparities in unidentified individual processing, notably with People of Color, have been studied to reveal differences in rates of identification, with slower rates compared to their White peers. Adding to these disparities are societal inequalities, unconscious bias, and the terminology used by forensic practitioners in investigation processes (Mace et al., 2022). These issues require reexamination of current methods to increase fairness in the identification process so that outcomes are improved for all decedents. The medicolegal death investigation definition, therefore, not only encompasses the technical mechanism of analysis of death but also encompasses a critical critique of the social forces engaged in the forensic justice system, finally seeking fairness and justice in the medicolegal process.

Importance of Death Investigations in Legal Settings

The role played by death investigations in court cannot be overemphasized, as investigations determine the judicial process in cases of death. In cases of uncertain manner and cause of death, medicolegal investigators play a critical role in establishing facts that lead to criminal and civil trials. Sophistication of the investigations necessitates thorough knowledge of forensic science, law, and methods of investigation. Particularly, information gained by means of autopsy and examination procedures must be clearly documented and kept, as the information can directly influence legal rulings. The integrity of investigation techniques comes first; variations can lead to mistaken convictions or the release of guilty suspects. By doing so, the death investigation process not only seeks to uncover the facts of specific cases but also helps ensure the integrity of the system of laws itself. Above that, knowledge of challenges that confront medicolegal and coroner investigators is significant in order to improve the effectiveness of death investigations. Organizational nature stressors and burnout can significantly degrade an investigator's performance and decision-making capability. The lack of universal support systems for such professionals has been highlighted in recent studies, which present the need for redressal in the medicolegal system (Slack, 2020). It is necessary to treat these mental health problems, as a competent, fully operational workforce ensures more effective death investigations. Secondarily, understanding the lived realities of such investigators can reveal patterns that would improve their operational paradigm and provide them with the requisite resources to carry out their work. Increased organizational support, hence, not only serves investigators but eventually leads to more dependable determinations of cause and manner of death, thereby maintaining judicial integrity. The effect of dependable medicolegal death investigation transcends individual cases, and it affects the public health and safety environment as a whole. For instance, determining whether a death is a result of a crime or an accident directly affects the response of the community to potential threats to public safety. The distinction holds true even more so in instances of unidentified trauma, when postmortem examination yields critical details (Chapenoire et al., 2016). Under such challenging circumstances, the ability to correctly identify sources and times of trauma allows investigators to render more conclusive assessments regarding the cause of death, which can radically alter legal repercussions for involved parties. Through evidence-based standards for identification, death investigations are able to successfully overcome the confounding influences exerted by postmortem changes. Therefore, not only do such questions allow justice to be served in individual cases, but they also allow for an improved understanding of community safety and public health initiatives (Figure 2.2).

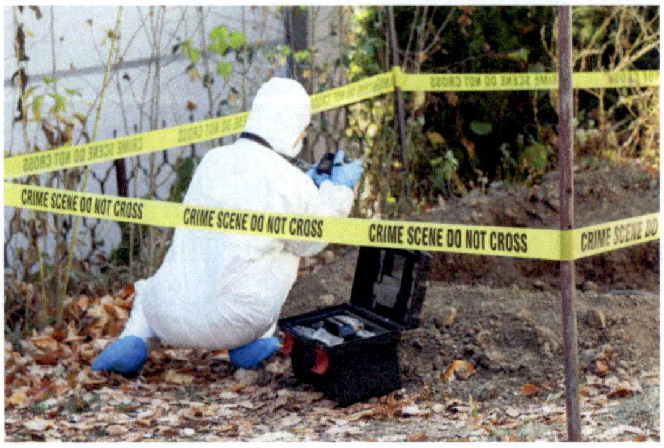

Figure 2.2. Importance of medicolegal death investigation.

Source: https://www.openaccessgovernment.org/wp-content/uploads/2021/09/dreamstime_xl_220627441-1068x712.jpg.

2.1. Roles and Responsibilities of Forensic Professionals

Learning Outcome

1. Understand the roles of medical examiners and coroners.
2. Describe the forensic pathologists and their functions.
3. Collaborate with law enforcement agencies.
4. law enforcement collaboration in death investigations.

The functions and roles of the forensic specialists are integral to the effective process of the medicolegal death investigation. Forensic specialists, including pathologists, forensic nurses, and investigators, not only carry out examinations but are also charged with safeguarding evidence. Forensic nurses, for instance, are likely to be at the intersection of healthcare and the justice system, offering medical care while collecting and preserving evidence in cases of violence or abuse. A study identified that many emergency nurses lack adequate forensic education needed to handle such cases adequately, which also indicates an acute need for specialist training and education in forensic procedures among healthcare professionals. This shortage poses a grave risk to the integrity of evidence collection, highlighting the urgent need for forensic special education to ensure that first-hand responders are efficient in managing forensic patients (Donaldson et al., 2020). In addition, forensic professionals also have to deal with a number of legal and ethical concerns when conducting death investigations. They need to maintain the integrity of the investigation while ensuring that they comply with the laws. In particular, forensic examiners must possess a thorough understanding of the evidence collection, preservation, and reporting laws. The work does not terminate at the first investigation because they often provide testimony in court to explain the results and procedures they employed while conducting an autopsy or investigating. Such a dual duty to scientific knowledge as well as the judicial system attests to the multifaceted character of their occupation. The increasing complexity of medicolegal cases demands a workforce with technical skills in death investigation alongside awareness of the legal context in which they operate (Thorpe et al., 2024). Secondly, the mental workload of working in forensic settings cannot be underestimated. Forensic workers routinely expose themselves to traumatic incidents and can experience burnout, compromising their work and decision-making abilities. The delicate management of death and trauma cases often leads to strong organizational stressors that affect job satisfaction and turnover among such professionals. Understanding the impact of such stressors enables organizations to design support systems that promote mental well-being and resilience among forensic professionals. Consequently, burnout and emotional exhaustion issues need to be addressed to ensure that there is an operational workforce in medicolegal death investigation, hence the forensic professionals are able to perform their duties and responsibilities with superior competence and emotional integrity (Thorpe et al., 2024) (Figure 2.3).

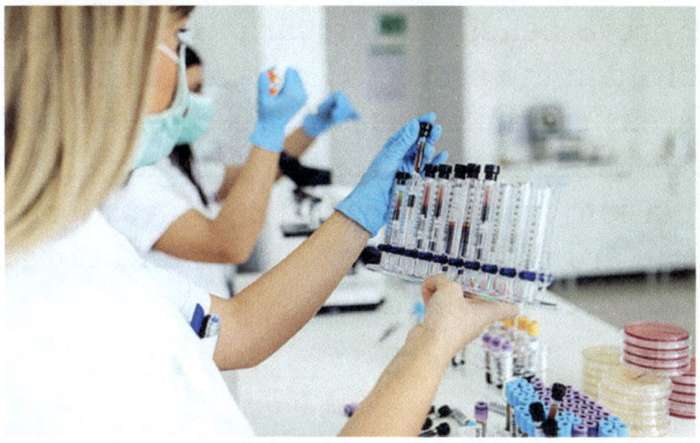

Figure 2.3. Roles and responsibilities of forensic professionals.

Source: https://nursingeducation.org/wp-content/uploads/2022/04/specialization-_0003_ForensicNurse.jpg.

2.1.1. Medical Examiners and Coroners

The roles of medical examiners and coroners are core to the medicolegal death investigation system, as they provide responses to questions of cause and manner of death in several scenarios. Medical examiners, typically forensic pathologists, conduct autopsies and use scientific techniques to offer an in-depth analysis of deaths, particularly suspicious or unexplained deaths. Their pathologic knowledge enables them to yield valuable information that may assist in criminal investigations or public health assessments. Coroners, however, need not always be medically trained and are usually elected officials. This may affect the quality and consistency of death investigations, emphasizing the need for adequate education and assistance to enhance their capacity, particularly in places where there are fewer skilled professionals. In recent years, the necessity for comprehensive training and support for county coroners has gained prominence, as can be seen from efforts in various regions. For instance, the Nebraska Department of Health and Human Services (DHHS) partnered with Support and Training for the Evaluation of Programs (STEPs) to assess and address county coroners' needs in the context of drug overdose death investigations. Surveys of the coroners in Nebraska offered valuable insight into their experience and the training gaps in this critical field. High-profile, at a response rate of around 27% on one survey, the data collected is a snapshot of how important it is to comprehend the distinctive issues for coroners, who operate with limitations of funds and specialization within the growing field of drug-related deaths (Cho et al., 2019).

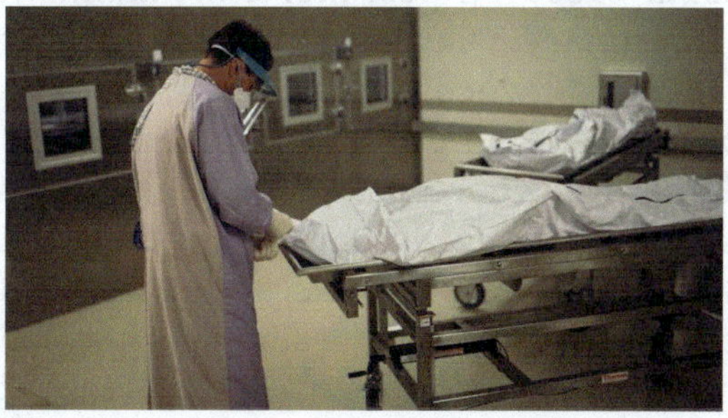

Figure 2.4. The medical examiner's office in New Mexico is considered the gold standard that all medical examiners should meet because it employs enough staff to investigate and perform autopsies on all sudden or violent deaths.

Source: https://media.npr.org/assets/img/2011/02/01/new-mexico-forensics2_wide-9408d8a1bcf85cbd99fdd892524be2939cf42396.jpg?s=900&c=85&f=webp.

Thus, the findings of these surveys reaffirm the necessity of implementing formal training programs and support mechanisms for coroners across the country. The surveys also indicated an emerging necessity for ongoing education pertaining to the complexities of drug overdose investigations, particularly since these types of cases typically intersect with public health issues as well as law enforcement strategies. By filling in training gaps highlighted in the surveys, state and local governments can significantly improve the accuracy and effectiveness of death investigations. This is important because not only do these improvements contribute to accurate certification of deaths, but also provide valuable information that can inform public health interventions and policies to reduce preventable substance use-related deaths (Ashley et al., 2020) (Figure 2.4).

2.1.2. Forensic Pathologists and Their Functions

Forensic pathologists play a pivotal role in medicolegal death investigations as medical experts who identify the cause and manner of death based on post-mortem examinations. Their primary role is conducting autopsies, an exacting process that involves detailed inspection of the body and associated physical evidence of the deceased person. In performing these autopsies, forensic pathologists not only establish injuries or diseases that would have caused death but also take samples and analyze them, possibly including toxicology tests that show the presence of drugs or poison. It is this proficiency that becomes an invaluable aid to guide legal investigation and testify in court, thus making a huge contribution to the judicial process. The general skills of forensic pathologists explain deaths otherwise buried in mystery, and thus become the unsung heroes of the interface between medicine and law in the determination of deaths. Practice and control of forensic pathology vary greatly in other parts of the world. For instance, the Police-led death investigation system prevalent in South Asian nations differs widely from the more formal United States Medical Examiners system. These differences impact the effectiveness and comprehensiveness of forensic examination and, consequently, public confidence in the justice system. The history and evolving practices of forensic medicine indicate massive variations in how investigations are conducted globally. South Asian forensic medicine has evolved since its start despite the issues that remain due to poor resources and professional control. According to recent studies, it is necessary to overcome such shortcomings for the betterment of the medical-legal system, which ultimately reflects in better outputs in death investigation that can prove beneficial for various stakeholders involved in the process (Iino et al., 2022). Even as forensic pathologists have a central position in the investigation process, the functionality and regulation of medicolegal death investigations overall are often lacking, with implications for the services provided.

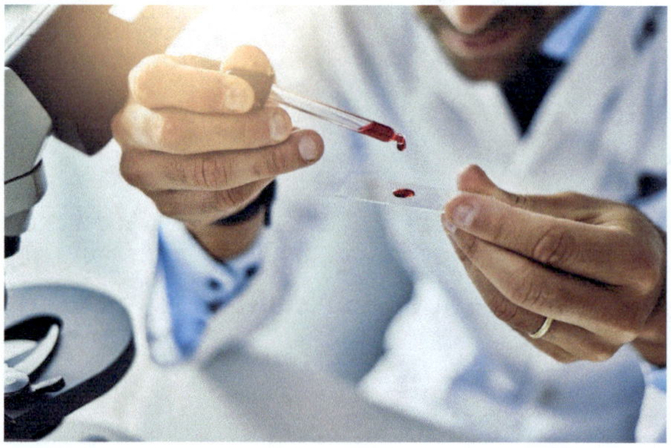

Figure 2.5. Forensic pathologists.

Source: https://s3-us-west-1.amazonaws.com/contentlab.studiod/getty/4efd8af7d87346918dff24a3870c6dab.jpg.

The absence of a standard training procedure and licensure for Medicolegal Death Investigators (MDIs) has created an ad hoc investigation policy, with heterogeneity of investigator experience. As is disclosed in the recent research, MDIs share varying perceptions regarding the importance of their work, but they are very dedicated to sustaining their safety and public safety. This contradiction stresses the need for uniform regulation and training protocols to enhance the quality of death investigations. These reforms would not only enhance the investigative process but also make the system more cohesive and reliable, addressing loopholes identified in current procedures (Vicks et al., 2019). These are vital changes for ensuring forensic pathology and the medicolegal death investigation system in general (Figure 2.5).

2.1.3. Law Enforcement Collaboration in Death Investigations

In a medicolegal death investigation, coordination between law enforcement agencies plays a critical role in ensuring that suspicious or unexplained deaths are brought under thorough and effective examination. By coordinated effort, the investigative process is made more robust by the harmonization of resources, experience, and expertise from various agencies, including police, coroner offices, and medical examiners. By facilitating interagency cooperation, law enforcement is able to effectively address the complexities associated with death investigations, such that all areas from scene processing through evidence collection and post-mortem analysis are addressed as needed. The harmony facilitated among such agencies not only leads to better investigation results but also fosters public trust in the whole system of justice, improving the image of accountability and transparency in dealing with death cases. The use of standard procedures for collaboration is needed to overcome challenges that commonly arise in death investigations. Differences in jurisdiction, training, and interpretation of legal mandates can hinder investigation and lead to inconsistency. Having clear guidelines and communication can allow law enforcement agencies to improve coordination and better manage cases. Technology adoption also serves to promote information sharing, as well as inter-agency collaboration. The use of databases and the internet allow for real-time sharing of investigation results and forensic data, further ensuring efficient effectiveness in inter-agency collaborations. As investigations become more complex, the adoption of new collaborative models is essential in order to promote justice for victims and their families. Burnout among medicolegal death investigators can have a significant impact on cooperative efforts and overall investigative outcomes. As per applicable studies, burnout has been linked to maladaptive habits and lower job satisfaction among medicolegal professionals (Thorpe et al., 2024).

Supportive network development and organizational stressor reduction by agencies are important for maintaining investigator well-being. With the stress being put on such professionals, it is now imperative that training programs and mental health services focus on the importance of resilience and self-care strategies. By establishing a more balanced working climate, agencies enhance not just the quality of life for investigators but also a more collaborative culture that consequently produces more complete and compassionate death investigations. Well-being-focused approaches can positively contribute to the dynamics of police cooperation within the multifaceted context of medicolegal death investigation (Vicks et al., 2019) (Figure 2.6).

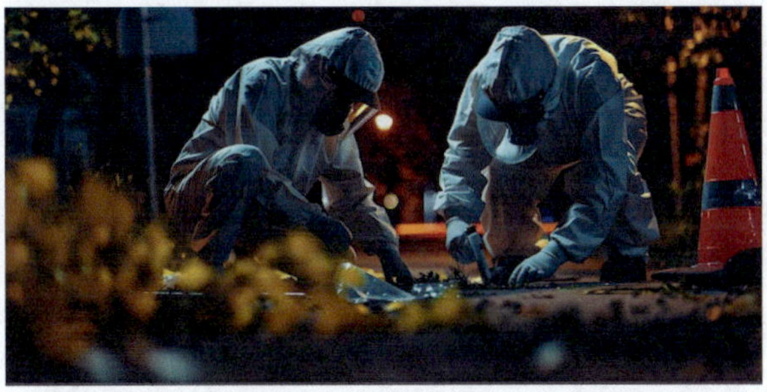

Figure 2.6. Collaborating at a crime scene, a police officer and a forensic scientist.

Source: https://img.freepik.com/premium-photo/collaborating-crime-scene-police-officer-forensic-scientist-working-together-concept-crime-scene-investigation-police-cooperation-forensic-science-evidence-analysis-law-enforcement_918839-42710.jpg

Test Your Knowledge

1. What is the role of the medical examiner?
2. What is the main function of a forensic pathologist?

2.2. Types of Death Investigations

Learning Outcome

1. Examine the natural deaths.
2. Know the investigative process for homicides.
3. Learn about accidental and suicidal deaths.

The discipline of death investigations comprises various methodologies, which are suitable for the specific context of death. One key type of investigation is the medicolegal autopsy, which is conducted when the cause of death is not known or is suspicious. Autopsies form the basis of ascertaining whether death results from natural causes, homicide, or accident. Nitty-gritty analysis is not just the physical evidence on the body but also toxicological analysis, which can reveal substances that may have led to the death of the deceased. Understanding the nuance in types of traumas—whether perimortem or postmortem—is crucial, as seen in the analysis of complex cases like the Yemenia plane crash. There, it was imperative to determine the source and timing of trauma so the cause of death could properly be evaluated and cognitive bias in the investigation could be avoided (Chapenoire et al., 2016). A second aspect of death investigation is the application of forensic anthropology, especially in cases involving skeletal remains. Forensic anthropologists are typically tasked with identifying human remains from nonhuman remains, and this ability is most critical in establishing an accurate context for a death scene. A routine analysis of a collection of bones from nonhumans, for instance, established the prevalence of mammalian remains such as deer and pigs, which are liable to be mistaken for human bones. This is a sign that there is a necessity for rigorous training in forensic anthropology to ensure accuracy in remains identification in medicolegal death investigations. Furthermore, more advanced educational courses centered on the distinction between human and nonhuman anatomy can significantly improve investigative outcomes, ensuring the integrity of the death investigation process (Fourshee et al., 2022).

Additionally, methods of death examination extend beyond the standard autopsy and anthropological methods, incorporating the discipline of forensic pathology to examine disease-related deaths. The specialty is dedicated to examining how diseases may have been factors in a person's death using clinical histories and existing medical records as references. In suspicious and unexplained deaths, the interface between disease conditions and physical evidence is explored in detail. For example, significant discoveries may be obtained through examination of the medical histories of victims who were undergoing unexplained complaints prior to dying. The identification of such correlations not only helps in establishing the cause of death but is also useful as an educational tool, affecting future medical interventions and public health policy. Thus, death investigations remain necessarily multidisciplinary in scope, calling on several disparate disciplines to arrive at more determinate conclusions (Figure 2.7).

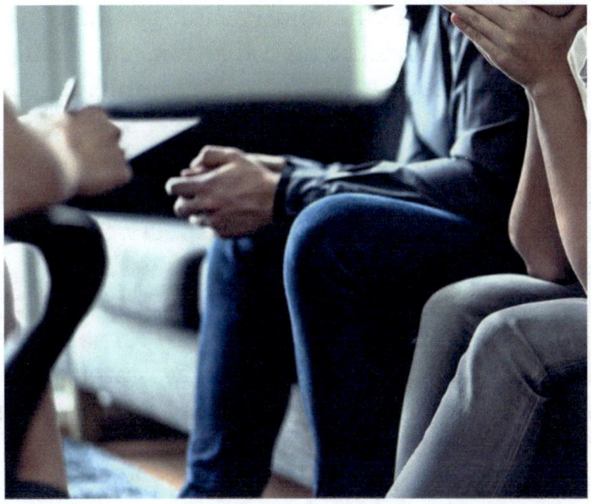

Figure 2.7. Types of death investigations.

Source: https://nita-wp.imgix.net/Private-Investigator-Professional-Development-Death-Investigation-Process-600x514.jpg?auto=format.

2.2.1. Natural Deaths and Their Examination

Natural deaths, generally due to pre-existing medical conditions, pose unique challenges to medicolegal examiners in determining the cause and mode of death. Natural deaths are not unrelated to foul play but require careful investigation to rule out all external causes of death. Sudden deaths may also result from heart disease, stroke, or infection, and demand complete autopsy procedures. An understanding of the pathophysiology of common diseases is also relevant to the forensic pathologist to distinguish anticipated natural causes from potential homicides masquerading as natural death. Additionally, thorough recording of clinical histories and death circumstances is a key aspect of successful medicolegal investigation, providing context that can guide additional examination and conclusion. Forensic anthropology can be included in the investigation of natural death in most jurisdictions when human skeletal remains are encountered. Forensic anthropologists are faced with cases where nonhuman bones, which are found near human remains, could potentially complicate cases. It is important to know if human or nonhuman skeletal material is available for analysis so that analysis can be credible, given that most mammalian skeletons can closely resemble adult human bones. As implied by research setting up a considerable percentage of the nonhuman remains in forensic settings, it would be crucial for forensic education courses to heighten training in the differentiation between these two forms of evidence. The information enhances more informed practice in medicolegal investigation and avoids relevant biological evidence from being improperly labeled, thus affecting case outcomes (Fourshee et al., 2022).

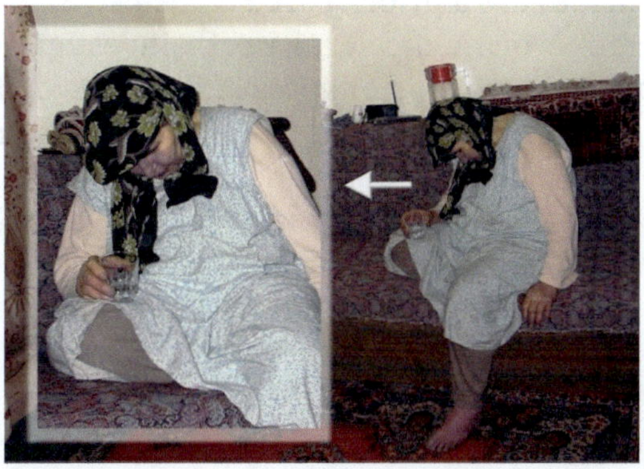

Figure 2.8. A seventy-six-year-old woman who had been living alone was found dead in her home in a sitting position and holding a glass in her hand. Note the livor mortis on the face, hands, and left foot due to the position of the deceased.

Source: https://cdnintech.com/media/chapter/19160/15123A45123/media/image32.jpeg.

Forensic DNA analysis is the focus of the investigation into natural deaths, particularly when extracting remains that are degraded or contaminated. Proper DNA sampling methods are crucial; high-quality or badly handled samples can result in inconclusive or misleading evidence. Forensic pathologists must navigate safely through medicolegal autopsy sampling intricacies, considering tissue degradation and potential extraneous biological contamination. This minute attention to sampling prevents, even in hostile environments, relevant evidence from being lost, but is preserved and subjected to analysis. Because the conditions under which natural death occurs differ from extended illness to extrinsic factors, accurate methodologies help facilitate proper forensic evaluation, thereby enhancing the quality of medicolegal inquiries (Kozma et al., 2018) (Figure 2.8).

2.2.2. Homicides and the Investigative Process

Homicides are a priority area of focus within the discipline of medicolegal death investigations since they are not only issues of loss of life, but also of the intricate process of untangling the circumstances surrounding each death. In the case of a homicide, law enforcement and forensic scientists must collaborate in retrieving and interpreting evidence in an orderly fashion. These details can be forensic medical reports, autopsy findings, and behavioral analysis, and collectively, aid in the construction of motives and suspects. The dynamic of homicide investigations is such that the process involves an interdisciplinary approach where forensic pathologists play a big role in ascertaining the cause and manner of death, alongside detectives who obtain eyewitness accounts and physical evidence. All this synergy contributes to the power of the investigative process and enhances the creation of the overall picture about the event, which is vital for legal proceedings and public safety. When investigating homicide cases, the personality traits and patterns of the perpetrators are typically under investigation. The FBI symposium on serial murder, for instance, dealt with serial killers' special features commonly exhibited by them and contributed further to what has been learned about this intricate crime. In exceptional cases, the Department of Forensic Medicine and Pathology illustrated how in-depth forensic investigations can divulge important information regarding both suspects and victims. The identified patterns guide the investigational techniques used by providing law enforcement with the means to link several cases and create profiles for suspects. Such data becomes vital in heightening the efficiency of homicide investigations and can ultimately lead to the apprehension of the perpetrators of serial murders, highlighting the importance of foresight and meticulous investigation within the medicolegal field (Holland et al., 2015). The medicolegal examination of homicides entails a substantial list of hardships, and the presence of serial crimes makes their occurrence even more intricate for law enforcement. The need for prompt and actual investigations is more pronounced due to the social responsibility to prevent further victimization and give justice to the victims.

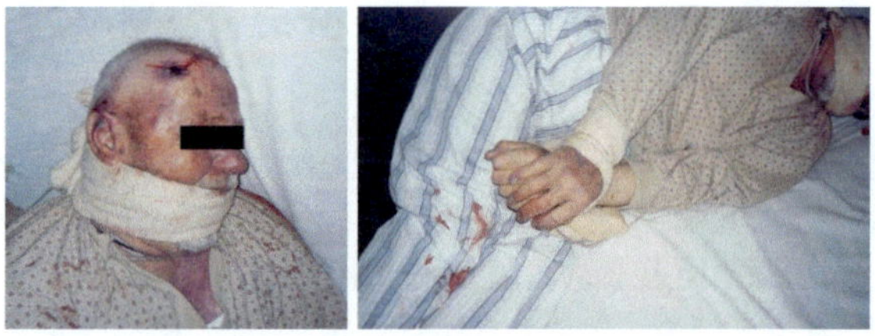

Figure 2.9. The murderer sometimes binds the victim's hands and mouth before killing the victim. A 65-year-old man was found dead in his bed; his hands and mouth were bound. The cause of death was strangulation and blunt head trauma.

Source: https://cdnintech.com/media/chapter/19160/1512345123/media/image4.jpeg.

The medicolegal death investigation system involves not only the scientific role of forensic pathology but also sociological and psychological forces of investigating the conduct and motives of people who kill. Through the analysis of complex murder patterns, particularly serial killer ones, forensic experts enhance their approaches in evidence analysis and criminal profiling. Continuous learning and refurbishment of forensic procedures are necessary as they can lead to pre-emptive identification of a series of murders as well as ease the application of advanced investigative measures, which are responsible for public safety and judicial outcomes (Justice et al., 2025) (Figure 2.9).

2.2.3. Accidental and Suicidal Deaths

The suicidal and accidental death process is quite challenging to medicolegal death investigations, where thorough examination is required to establish the circumstances and causes underlying such death. Accidental death typically arises from a variety of factors involving substance abuse, motor vehicle accidents, and work-related accidents. The role of toxicology in these investigations cannot be overstated, as it provides valuable information on the presence of alcohol or drugs that may have caused death. Past practice indicates that such drugs can be identified most accurately by full toxicological analysis, particularly when the postmortem blood samples are either not available or unreliable as a result of decomposition or trauma; therefore, secondary matrices such as bile may be an unexploited source under such conditions (Bottinelli et al., 2016). Suicidal deaths, however, demand a different type of investigation since they typically have complex psychological fundamentals. Awareness of the cause of suicide is as essential as awareness of how it was done. In the majority of instances, suicide perpetrators may be experiencing underlying psychiatric illnesses that are not apparent. This helps to underscore the necessity for a multidisciplinary medicolegal autopsy that combines forensic pathology with psychiatric evaluation. These comprehensive analyses not only aim to determine the cause and manner of death but also to identify preventable interventions for populations at risk. The decline in autopsy rates presents a crucial concern in this regard, as important information regarding the interconnectivity between suicidal behavior and mental health all too often goes unexamined (Frost et al., 2016). The intersection of accidental and suicidal deaths has important insights into public health patterns and the strength of prevention measures. As forensic professionals deal with such cases, the data compiled by detailed investigations is valuable to reveal underlying factors of great importance in society, from drug use patterns to mental health treatment deficits. This is particularly necessary because regions have varying rates of accidental and suicidal deaths, providing areas for targeted interventions and responses in public health. It is through the knowledge of the reasons behind such instances that policymakers can formulate efficient policies that aim at reducing mortality levels. With improved forensic science, it is equally vital to give high priority to postmortem examinations to comprehend the intricacies of such deaths and develop well-researched programs that can assist in the reduction of risks in society (Figure 2.10).

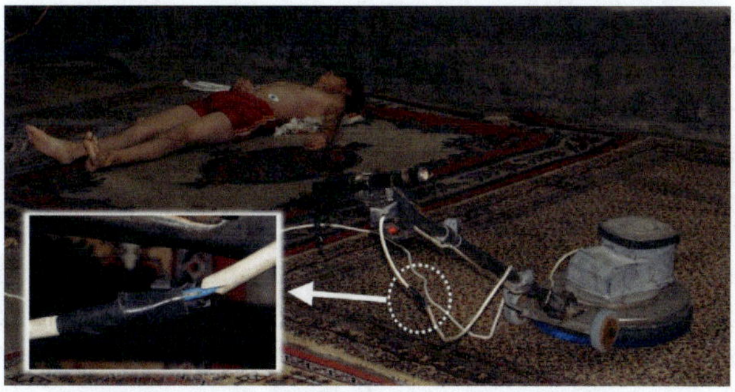

Figure 2.10. A 17-year-old worker died due to an electric shock in his workplace. The scene investigation revealed electrical leakage from the defect of the plastic sheath of the cable of the carpet washing machine.

Source: https://cdnintech.com/media/chapter/19160/1512345123/media/image23.jpeg.

Test Your Knowledge

1. What is an example of a natural cause of death?
2. Which alternative biological matrix can be used for toxicological analysis when blood samples are unreliable?

2.3. The Autopsy Process

Learning Outcome

1. Understand the purpose and significance of autopsies.
2. Describe the steps involved in conducting an autopsy.
3. Interpret the autopsy findings.

The autopsy process is an important aspect of the medicolegal analysis of death since it provides important information on the cause and mode of death. Forensic pathologists, during an autopsy, examine the body with great scrutiny, documenting any sign of trauma or disease. The examination is macroscopic and microscopic, with the former being injuries visible to the naked eye and the latter being tissue observation using a microscope. Good evidence collection is of utmost significance; tissue and body fluid samples are taken with care not to harm them. The sample integrity is key here since bad samples would get contaminated, and the findings of the investigations would be compromised ultimately. The thoroughness and integrity of the autopsy not only enhance the accuracy of determining the cause of death but also safeguard the process from the risk of legal disputes when findings could be challenged in court (Kozma et al., 2018). In addition to the traditional autopsy techniques, technological development such as postmortem computed tomography (PMCT) has provided a non-invasive alternative for examining internal structures. PMCT can reveal critical information, such as the identification of gas reservoirs in the body, which are signs of postmortem changes. The imaging modality allows forensic scientists to visualize injuries that may not be easily visualized under normal autopsy, thus improving the diagnostic process. Additionally, the likelihood of PMCT in aiding the recovery of volatile organic compounds (VOCs) from the gas reservoirs makes it even more promising. Information regarding the chemical composition of such VOCs can yield details of the activities that preceded the deceased's final hours and contribute to the overall death investigation story. Given the advancements, such non-invasive techniques could revolutionize the standard practices involved within the autopsy process (Focant et al., 2016). In addition, the multidimensionality of the autopsy process enhances its status in a legal context, especially in responding to questions raised during criminal investigations. While the autopsy is the physical evidence of death, it is also simultaneously a basis for forensic DNA analysis that allows the identification of persons and understanding of the conditions under which they died. This feature underscores the legal as well as social issues associated with the collection and storage of bio-samples during autopsy, compelling rigorous protocols to avert contamination. The integration of traditional methods with modern scientific innovation ensures that the procedure of autopsy is sound, delivering credible results. As the realms of law and medicine continue to cross paths, the importance of the autopsy process in medicolegal death investigations is likely to grow, emphasizing the need for ongoing research and development of new methods and technologies (Kozma et al., 2018).

2.3.1. Purpose and Importance of Autopsy

Autopsies in medicolegal death investigations have a multi-dimensional nature, beyond curiosity regarding the event of death. The primary role of autopsies is to establish a definite cause of death, particularly in scenarios where the manner of death is suspicious or ambiguous. The procedure is necessary for legal purposes as it provides a lucid picture that can establish criminal responsibility or insurance settlements. Besides that, autopsies also assist in public health through patterns of disease, which can further channel preventive efforts towards restricting subsequent deaths. Data obtained through post-mortem examination not only improves individual case understanding but also adds to epidemiology's knowledge base as a whole. Therefore, autopsies play a very important role in bridging the gap between medical expertise and legal procedure and thereby establishing their relevance in the whole context of death investigation. Beyond the determination of the cause of death, autopsies are significant in that they contribute to furthering medical education and scientific investigation. Autopsies are invaluable learning experiences for medical students and professionals alike, as direct exposure to pathological conditions helps reinforce theoretical knowledge. By presenting medical personnel and investigators with a broad spectrum of cases, autopsies encourage clinical expertise and trigger meticulous methodology in diagnosis. Furthermore, autopsy results may fuel current medical research, namely trends for causes of death, which could in turn fuel advances in treatment methods and prevention of health issues. Evidence indicates that high-quality standards and medicolegal death investigator training can result in a richer, informative autopsy report, thereby enhancing the profession's ability to manage high-profile cases and assist the legal system as well as the broader field of public health effectively (Vicks et al., 2019). Last but not least, knowledge of mental health issues for medicolegal death investigators further highlights the sensitive aspect of autopsies. This type of job can be a cause of a lot of burnout because the psychological toll can be so profound on investigators, who are supposed to confront mortality all the time. It is necessary to realize the role and significance of autopsies, not just for fact determination but also for providing a healthy atmosphere for those conducting these procedures. With growing appreciation for the need for resources that address stress reduction and resilience in investigators, it is vital to include protocols that guarantee their welfare.

This is particularly relevant because the literature emphasizes the need for regular training and psychological intervention to help investigators effectively work through what they experience and continue to provide high-level performance in their investigative work (Thorpe et al., 2024). Lastly, the worth of autopsies extends beyond the autopsy act itself; it encompasses the protection and improvement of both life and livelihood in death investigation (Figure 2.11).

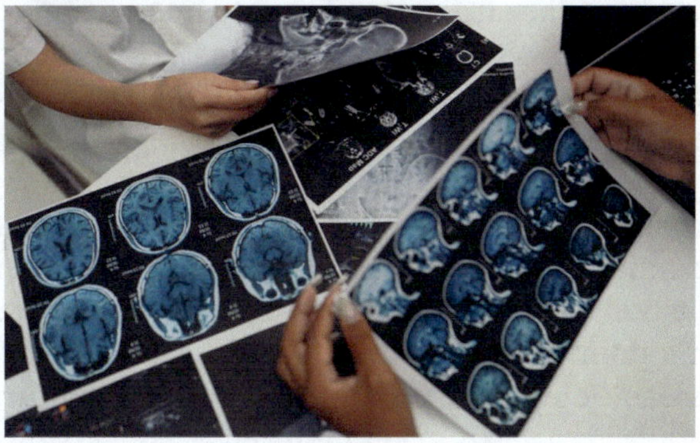

Figure 2.11. Purpose & procedures of a brain-only autopsy.

Source: https://www.1800autopsy.com/wp-content/uploads/2024/08/group-of-doctors-looking-at-x-ray-on-medical-confe-2023-11-27-05-06-06-utc-1080x675.jpg.

2.3.2. Steps Involved in Conducting an Autopsy

The process of performing an autopsy is sequential and systematic, beginning with a detailed analysis of the case history. The initial step is to gather information from the patient's background history, police reports, and other details pertinent to the death. A proper background picture is vital as it guides the forensic pathologists' approach. For instance, details about the deceased's past illnesses, medical history, and conditions under which death occurred can shed light on areas of interest during the examination. This first compilation of facts not only informs the forensic pathologists' questioning but also sets the stage for the autopsy, where the investigation can move in a focused and relevant way to the suspected cause of death. Following initial inspection, the second part of the autopsy process is external examination of the body. This is an essential part since it allows the forensic pathologist to observe evidence of trauma, initial impressions of putrefaction, and any other deviations without tainting the integrity of the body. During this inspection, accurate measurements and photographs are taken for documentation of the body's physical observations. This report serves as substantial proof in cases of homicide or suspicious death that require legal action. The external examination has a tendency to set the stage for the subsequent internal examination, where the pathologist will open the body's cavities. The pathologist's findings at this point begin to correlate with the histories already obtained, providing an overall picture required to verify accurate forensic conclusions. The final and most critical stage of the autopsy is internal examination and organ analysis. This involves careful dissection and examination of the body's major systems—cardiovascular, respiratory, gastrointestinal, and so forth, for any pathological alterations. Tissue may be harvested for histological study, and fluids may be sampled for toxicology, particularly if drug-related deaths are suspected. In Nebraska, the 2019 and 2020 surveys of county coroners by the Nebraska Department of Health and Human Services target additional training in handling death investigations of drug overdoses, with specialized knowledge on these autopsy parts (Ashley et al., 2020). The research shows training can be at the core of valid death investigations (Cho et al., 2019). Lastly, the findings from an autopsy not only aid in cause and manner of death determination but also contribute valuable information to public health data and policy.

2.3.3. Interpretation of Autopsy Findings

The analysis of autopsy results is a key component in medicolegal investigations into death, as it usually determines the cause and manner of death. Autopsy reports may result in the determination of trauma, disease, and other mortality-contributing factors. In particular, diligent observation of numerous body systems during an autopsy allows forensic pathologists to recreate incidents surrounding a death and, therefore, allow legal inquiries and public health interventions. Simple characterization of wounds as sharp, blunt, or thermal enhances the ability to solve indefinite cases and provides compelling evidence for use in a court of law. In addition, following progress in forensic techniques, for example, the combining of the application of the use of the thermal analysis method thermogravimetric analysis with chemometrics, the accuracy of estimating the postmortem interval can be increased, and autopsy results become even more informative and trustworthy in legal proceedings (Fabiano et al., 2017). Apart from routine findings, biochemical analyses can expand the information on autopsy results even further. There have been various biochemical markers detected, which are applicable in specific instances of death, for example, hypothermia. The glucose level, electrolytes, and other biomarkers in the biological tissue contribute to macroscopic and microscopic findings, enhancing sensitivity. These new techniques mirror the dynamic advancement of forensic pathology, in which classical autopsy methods are complemented by advanced biochemistry. Such synergy of fields serves to conquer postmortem diagnostic hurdles and enable a more complete examination of factors leading to death. Employing these new methods, the addition of these ultimately works to develop conclusions based on autopsy findings that are more accurate and establish more conclusive links between findings and the conditions under which death occurred (Mangin et al., 2018).

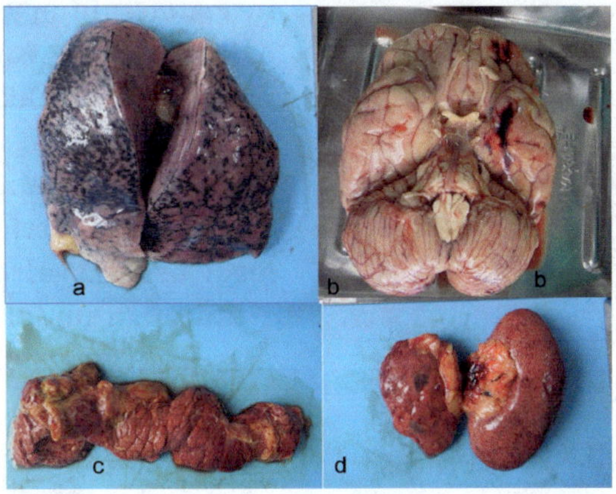

Figure 2.12. Gross findings of various organs during autopsy: (a) gross examination of lungs showing relatively unremarkable lungs with mild edema and consolidation; (b) gross examination of brain showing edema and subarachnoid hemorrhage; (c) gross examination of pancreas showing necrotic and hemorrhagic changes; (d) gross examination of kidneys showing contracted and flea-bitten kidneys.

Source: https://www.researchgate.net/profile/Brinda-Patel-12/publication/356565197/figure/fig2/AS:1094922870489091@1638061363403/Gross-findings-of-various-organs-during-autopsy-a-gross-examination-of-lungs-showing.png.

Multiple-factor explanation of the autopsy findings is important not only for causation, but also for public health evaluation and policy making. For example, an understanding of trends in drug-related fatalities and fatalities due to environmental conditions can guide preventive measures and budgetary planning. Detailed autopsy explanations are also pivotal for legal investigation that spurs accountability in events of wrongful fatalities or criminal activity. Therefore, the demand for trained and qualified forensic pathologists cannot be overemphasized since the integrity and accuracy of their interpretations can significantly influence judicial rulings. As research evolves, particularly in the field of novel forensic methods, the practitioners must stay abreast and integrate new information into their investigative processes so that the utility of autopsy findings in medicolegal death investigations continues to be enhanced (Fabiano et al., 2017) (Figure 2.12).

Test Your Knowledge

1. What is the purpose of autopsies?
2. What is the first step in conducting an autopsy?

2.4. Legal Aspects of Death Investigations

Learning Outcome

1. Describe the chain of custody and evidence handling.
2. Understand the role of death certificates in legal proceedings.
3. Describe the role of testimonies and expert witness contributions in medicolegal death investigation.

Legal aspects in death investigations play a core role in the medicolegal process, deciding the manner of dealing with cases and the rights of the parties involved. The general doctrine in this field is the responsibility to conduct thorough, impartial investigations of all sudden or suspicious deaths. This is necessary to ensure justice and to ensure the dead are accorded the dignity they deserve. Statutes and rules regulate the practice of medical examiners and forensic pathologists, prescribing their duties and procedures for gathering, examination, and reporting of evidence. Recent studies demonstrate that unequal identification rates of marginalized populations have direct implications in the area of ethics and fairness in the system. Forensic anthropologists must recognize the impact of their analyses on such differences, as in People of Color (POC), in which identification procedures took much longer than they did for White victims (Mace et al., 2022).

Another important aspect of the legal context for death investigation is the challenge of accurately estimating the postmortem interval (PMI). Legal cases often hinge on when death has occurred, in an attempt to influence charges in criminal cases or to resolve insurance claims. However, variations in decomposition can complicate these decisions, such that stringent methodologies based on current knowledge are very crucial. Acknowledging progress in understanding the biological and environmental influences on decomposition can render PMI estimates more accurate. Recent research has offered a conceptual model, which tries to incorporate such complexities and thus inform needed improvements to forensic models (Barton et al., 2024). The interdisciplinary approach encourages the collaborative working relationship between legal professionals, scientists, and investigators to come up with improved methodologies and reduce uncertainties concerning the timing of death investigation. Finally, tackling the legal aspects of death investigation requires a thorough understanding of social prejudices that could undermine the integrity of the investigation.

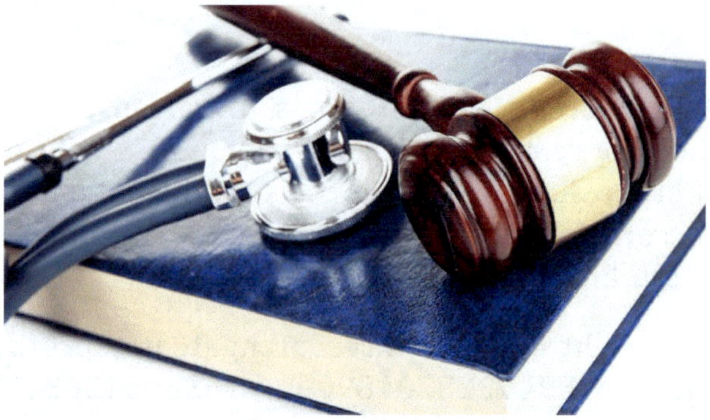

Figure 2.13. Investigates the medical and legal aspects of death.

Source: https://www.miamidade.gov/resources/images/news/medico-legal.png.

The legal system's historical response to minority communities has brought on systemic disparities, which affect the process of identification and investigation of deaths among such groups. The medicolegal staff working on such cases must address and counteract these biases so that investigations hold standards of justice for all, regardless of their ethnic or racial group. The interface between social attitudes and forensic science needs ongoing debate and transformation within the field. Through the promotion of awareness and the establishment of equitable practices, the medicolegal system may better represent the interests of all families and decedents, ultimately resulting in death investigations performed with integrity and respect (Mace et al., 2022) (Figure 2.13).

2.4.1. Chain of Custody and Evidence Handling

In a medicolegal death investigation, the chain of custody is important in preserving the integrity of evidence collected so that it may be retained as admissible in a court of law. Chain of custody refers to the meticulous documentation of storing and handling evidence from the moment that it is collected until it appears before a court. Each individual exposed to the evidence must document contact, hence preventing it from being contaminated or tampered with. This rigorous documentation is particularly critical in forensic cases of evidence, where even minor omissions can spoil the case's verdict. Without a well-documented chain of custody, establishing the authenticity and reliability of evidence will be challenging, which may lead to wrongful convictions or acquittals. The need for ensuring strict evidence handling protocols is emphasized in a number of studies on research that has revealed discrepancies in forensic protocol that could be due to inadequate training and supervision within legal and health systems. Evidence handling protocols in medicolegal death investigations also encompass the preliminary procedures performed by first responders, for example, police and medical personnel. These specialists should be trained to recognize, preserve, and collect vital evidence without degrading its quality. According to empirical research, the use of forensic nursing concepts, particularly in emergency care settings, has significant implications for managing evidence. These concepts not only enhance the quality of services provided to victims of violence but also improve the admissibility of evidence collected in the field (Brown et al., 2024). Forensic nurses play a significant role in documenting injuries, collecting biological evidence, and maintaining the chain of custody, all of which have immediate effects on the success of follow-up investigations and cases in the courts. Therefore, training these professionals regarding the nuances of handling evidence remains an important endeavor to support the safe and effective medicolegal process. Surveys of medicolegal death investigation practices identify a stark need for standardized training and procedures regarding evidence handling and chain of custody. Although most MDIs are confident in their professional position, the lack of formal regulation and accreditation highlights the weaknesses of the system (Vicks et al., 2019).

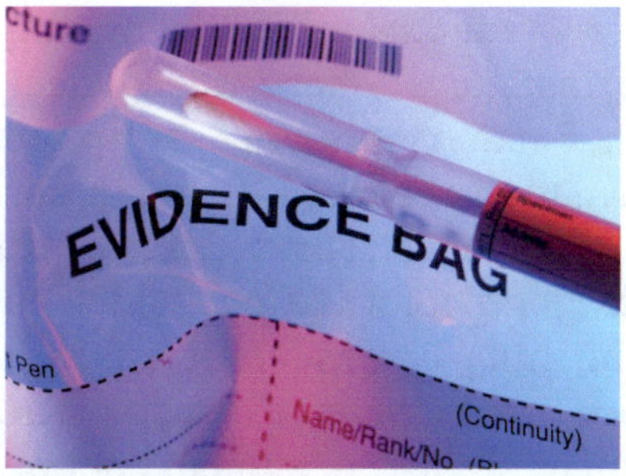

Figure 2.14. Chain of custody.

Source: https://www.thoughtco.com/thmb/8k6FFjuXsmNi-lui3oBS2ODlGKI=/1500x0/filters:no_upscale():max_bytes(150000):strip_icc()/bag-5c8909b5c9e77c0001f2ad4f.jpg.

Furthermore, inconsistencies in professionals' education make matters worse regarding a disjointed understanding of best practices in evidence handling that, in turn, could adversely affect the outcome of the investigations. Research highlights the necessity to develop standard training modules that merge detailed procedures for handling evidence and principles of the chain of custody. Through the closing of these gaps, the medicolegal field can improve death investigations, along with providing an incentive for increased responsibility in the retrieval and treatment of evidence, thereby preserving the integrity of the overall judicial process (Figure 2.14).

2.4.2. Role of Death Certificates in Legal Proceedings

The application of death certificates in legal proceedings is a significant field of medicolegal investigation of death. Death certificates are official declarations of cause of death for an individual, which are often required in numerous types of legal matters, including insurance claims, wills, and wrongful death litigation. Through the presentation of vital information regarding a death, death certificates have substantial legal weight. For instance, a clear determination of the cause of death assists in placing blame in those instances where negligence may be involved. Furthermore, the completeness of the information recorded on death certificates ensures that legal representatives can have access to good information, which is crucial for establishing claims or defenses in court. Therefore, the proper preparation and management of these documents not only affect families seeking closure but also affect ongoing investigations with legal implications. Other than their legal implications, death certificates are crucial in tracking public health and in research. They provide information that will be used to track mortality patterns, causes of death, and epidemiological research. For instance, comprehensive death certificates contribute to public health concerns, such as increased drug overdose deaths, helping policymakers make educated policy decisions about prevention and intervention. As demonstrated by Cho et al. (2019), analysis of data from death certificates has the potential to enhance the effectiveness of community health programs by identifying some areas or populations that need specific interventions. Integration of timely and precise data from death certificates is crucial in evaluating the efficacy of public health programs; thus, their relevance goes beyond particular legal issues. Such a dual-purpose role establishes the status of death certificates as more than legal documents but as instruments of the common good. This is tainted, though, by constraints in the standardization and precision of reporting by death certificates. Not regulating medicolegal death investigators leads to inconsistencies in the filling of death certificates, which can undermine their role in the court of law. In studies, it has been reported that the majority of death investigators operate without the necessary accreditation or license, which may be the source of inconsistency in the information contained in such critical documents (Vicks et al., 2019). The absence of standardized training guidelines can also add complexity to accurate cause-of-death reporting on death certificates. Stimulation of these deficits is essential as errors can cause conflict in court and affect the administration of justice. Therefore, the enforcement of full regulations and standardized death investigator training is essential to render death certificates more credible for use by the judicial system as well as public health programs (Figure 2.15).

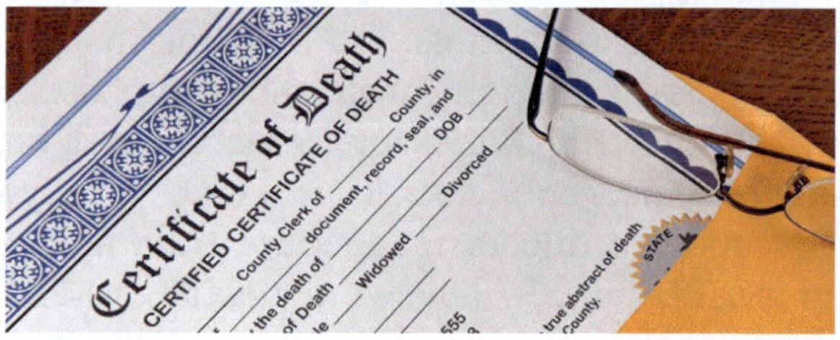

Figure 2.15. Death certificate.

Source: https://www.yourpathologist.org/wp-content/uploads/2023/09/0034593_Death_Certificate_1110x440.png.

2.4.3. Testimonies and Expert Witness Contributions

The role of expert testimonies and contributions of expert witnesses in medicolegal death investigation is multifaceted and holds great importance in the conclusion of legal proceedings.

In cases of suspicious deaths, witnesses may provide critical information regarding incidents of events leading up to the event, whereas expert witnesses, such as forensic pathologists, offer technical expertise to guide the interpretation of autopsy findings or injury patterns. These are critical viewpoints, acting as a bridge between the general comprehension and the complexity of judicial proceedings. They have the function of ensuring not just the completeness of investigations, but also the observance of pre-existing legal standards. The credibility of these accounts is decisive in determining the course of criminal and civil cases, and by extension, the courses of justice for victims and their families. Moreover, improvements in forensic science have also transformed the nature of expert witness testimonies in medicolegal cases greatly. With the increasing prevalence of technology, traditional testimonies increasingly struggle to be merged with physical evidence, such as DNA or internet traces. The launching of the Sexual Assault Evidence Kit (SAEK) is a clear example of this, showing how technoscientific evidence is now increasingly accepted as a valid witness in addition to human testimonies. The integration of such evidence attests to the evolution of medicolegal practice and the need for experts to change their testimonies to reflect such evolutionary changes in technology. Such a transformation raises concerns regarding the conflict between personal human testimony and scientific objective evidence, a conflict that is of utmost relevance to the attainment of fair legal verdicts in medicolegal cases, as analyzed in (Quinlan et al., 2013). Furthermore, the position of expert witnesses during medicolegal examinations is firmly anchored in cultural and societal bases that shape the definition of justice and evidence. A critical examination of forensic practices demonstrates how political ideology and social constructs such as gender narratives impact the understanding of credibility in testimony. It is crucial to comprehend this forensic culture, as it exposes the bias inherent in both witness statements and expert opinion. Media portrayal distorts these tendencies further, as sensationalized portrayals have the power to influence public thinking and, consequently, judicial trials. With the continued development of the argument around these practices, it is increasingly important to recognize how these influences bear on the integrity of evidentiary contributions and the pursuit of justice in the medicolegal environment, as indicated in (Bergers et al., 2023) (Figure 2.16).

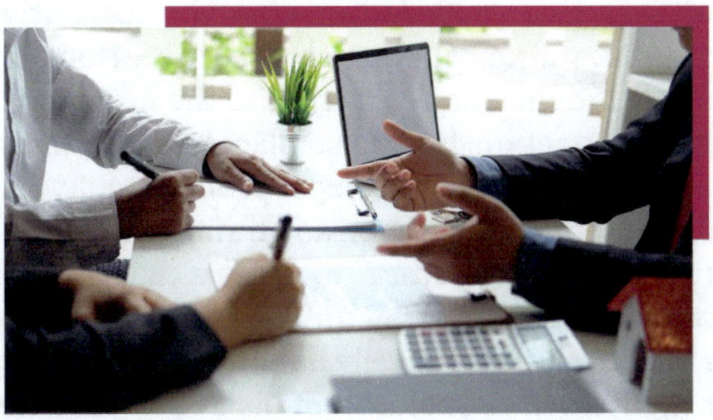

Figure 2.16. Expert witness testimony.

Source: https://omahaappraiser.com/wp-content/uploads/2023/12/Group-2-4.jpg.

Test Your Knowledge

1. What is the importance of a death certificate?
2. What is the primary role of witnesses in medicolegal death investigations?

2.5. Challenges in Medicolegal Death Investigations

Learning Outcome

1. Understand the issues of jurisdiction and authority.
2. Describe the ethical dilemmas faced by forensic professionals.
3. Know the advances in technology and their implications.

The medicolegal death investigation environment is plagued with an array of challenges that hinder efficient closure of cases. Most worrying is the absence of forensic training among first responders, particularly emergency nurses. A New Zealand study demonstrated that while nearly all emergency nurses (84%) valued the contribution of forensic knowledge to their work, few possessed the ability to carry out evidence preservation and the legislative guidelines underpinning clinical care. Not only does this deficiency compromise the integrity of the investigation, but it also places an inordinate burden on other medicolegal professionals. The need for greater education and training in forensic practice is most critical to ensure that all who are involved in investigating death are equipped to effectively and ethically handle the complexity of their work (Donaldson et al., 2020). Another critical issue in medicolegal investigation of death is professional burnout, which has far-reaching consequences for their practice and job satisfaction. The stressful characteristics of these investigations can lead to psychological distress, impairing the functioning of investigators and the coroner's office personnel. Organizational causes had a strong influence on job resiliency and compassion satisfaction in medicolegal and coroner investigators in the United States in a phenomenological study. The study emphasized establishing support systems and formulating a supportive work environment in order to combat burnout and enhance job satisfaction. Resolution of these mental health conditions not only improves personal well-being among investigators but also ensures the integrity of the medicolegal investigation process overall (Thorpe et al., 2024). Furthermore, increasing death investigation sophistication through technology and changing legal expectations is a continuing challenge to medicolegal professionals. The development of digital evidence and forensic technology requires that investigators absorb new procedures rapidly, placing pressure and responsibility on a demanding profession already. The question arises as to whether current training schemes are sufficient and doing enough to meet the evolving nature of forensic science. Absent curriculum revisions in schools to incorporate technological innovations and contemporary legal structures, researchers may find it hard to maintain accuracy and completeness in investigations. Thus, continuing education and resource allocation should be prioritized by institutions and organizations carrying out medicolegal death investigations to allow professionals to meet the evolving challenges they face (Donaldson et al., 2020).

2.5.1. Jurisdictional and Authority Problems

In a medicolegal death investigation, the complexity between jurisdiction and authority makes it extremely challenging to effectively administer justice. Jurisdiction is an issue that arises when deciding which legal system to apply based on the location of the death, the nature of the investigation, and the accountable legal authorities. Such an issue causes delays in the investigative process as well as complicates the process, particularly where multiple jurisdictions overlap. For instance, fatalities that take place in areas of conflict or regions with divergent legal systems pose unique challenges. Such divergences have the potential to hinder the delivery of justice to victims and their relatives, as various authorities will possess varying attitudes towards a sense of responsibility to investigate and prosecute, thus affecting the application of legal requirements and procedure in medicolegal death investigations. The jurisdictional issues are also informed by the power that has been invested in medicolegal death investigators (MDIs). While necessary to help determine the cause of death and collect vital evidence, MDIs are hampered by the lack of an overarching regulatory system. Power is awkward whenever MDIs operate without set guidelines determining their jurisdictional authority, and this can be at odds with law enforcers or other investigation agencies. Research stresses that MDIs are usually working in an unregulated profession, which determines the differences in training and working standards across jurisdictions (Vicks et al., 2019). These differences may cause variability in the quality of investigations into death, and thus affect subsequent legal proceedings as well as undermine public confidence in the justice system. In addition, decisions regarding jurisdictional and authority issues are also critical to further enhance the overall integrity of the medicolegal death investigation system. Loci vacant in the regulatory system and inconsistent enforcement of investigative practices can weaken the quality of death investigations. Hence, it is extremely significant to promote uniform procedures and establish clear jurisdictional boundaries that must be adhered to by MDIs and concerned authorities. These measures would go a great distance in improving not only the efficiency of death investigations but also the legal processes that are based on these outcomes. Evidence from various sources indicates the need for inter-institutional coordination among legal, medical, and law enforcement institutions so that an integrated medicolegal approach to death investigations is built (Angana et al., 2015). By producing a harmonized framework, the complexities of authority and jurisdiction can be more effectively managed, ultimately enhancing the pursuit of justice for those whose life was impacted by disputed or unsolved deaths (Figure 2.17).

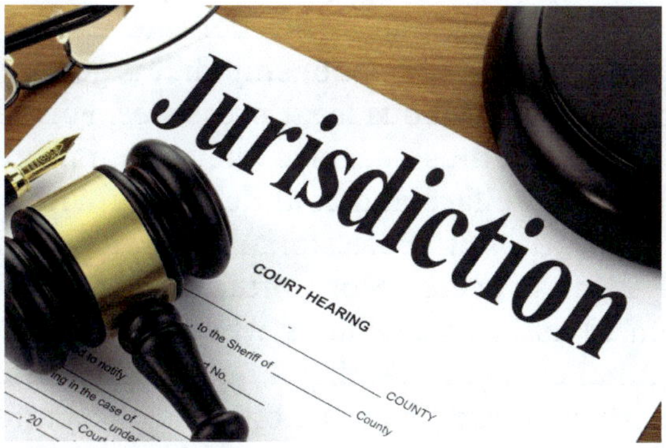

Figure 2.17. Issues of jurisdiction.

Source: https://img1.wsimg.com/isteam/ip/9092f379-0845-443a-8c5e-e2882ae1f6e0/jurisdiction.jpg.

2.5.2. Ethical Dilemmas Faced by Forensic Professionals

The multifaceted landscape of forensic medicine provides numerous ethical dilemmas that professionals have to contend with, particularly in relation to medicolegal inquiry into death. Forensic professionals must reconcile the responsibility to provide objective, accurate analysis with the potential for conflicts of interest that arise within the criminal justice system. This dilemma is greater when there is potential conflict between professional duty and personal belief. Experts must remain committed to the pursuit of truth, even where findings can have extensive social consequences, such as wrongful convictions or freeing potentially dangerous members of society. Without ethical commitment, public confidence in forensic science can be eroded, and thus, there is a need for continuous ethical training and sensitivity among experts within this sensitive profession. With forensic experts venturing into multidisciplinary activities, there is a potential risk of rising threats of ethical issues, and hence the need for a keen eye towards ethical standards in the face of evolving medicolegal investigation landscapes. Forensic psychiatry is particularly vulnerable to ethical issues due to the delicate nature of the patient-doctor relationship that is generally subject to extraneous legal pressures. Forensic psychiatrists must balance their commitment to patient welfare and confidentiality with the incorporation of professional observation into the legal process. Most often, this requires them to assess individuals who may be facing criminal charges, creating a dual loyalty where the psychiatrist's responsibility to the patient and the legal system may come into conflict.

These ethical codes informing the practice here emphasize beneficence and non-maleficence since practitioners are obligated to provide the best care in a way that does not involve themselves in practices that lead to human rights violations, such as capital punishment. These are some of the challenges that highlight the need to ground forensic practice on ethical foundations that are attuned to the fact of legal intervention and how it affects patient care (Niveau et al., 2018). Moreover, the integration of forensic nursing into death investigation units is emblematic of the complex ethical environment faced by professionals in the discipline. With continued growth in the field of forensic nursing, professionals are challenged to collaborate with other medical and legal agencies, posing communication barriers and moral conflicts. Torn between the responsibilities of reporting to law enforcement and safeguarding patient care, significant ethical tension can be generated. For example, forensic nurses may be confronted with the dilemma of whether to hold patient confidentiality or obey mandatory reporting legislation that compels disclosure of specific information. The need for increased interdisciplinary collaboration must be weighed against a keen awareness of such ethical dilemmas, particularly as the forensic nursing profession expands further. Through working on these subtleties through ongoing education and policy development, forensic practitioners can progress toward more ethical medicolegal death investigation practice (Rogers et al., 2023).

2.5.3. Advances in Technology and Their Implications

The use of advanced technology in medicolegal death investigation has revolutionized the practices in determining the cause of death. Digital forensics, imaging devices, and automized report platforms are some of the technologies that have improved the rate of efficiency and precision in investigations. For instance, 3D imaging allows investigators to generate precise replicas of crime scenes and bodies, which can be thoroughly searched for evidence that would have been overlooked in traditional methods. Moreover, computer forensic tools allow the thorough search of electronic evidence, which can reveal a great deal about a decedent's last moments. However, this shift towards technology is also matched by concerns over the accountability and dependability of these processes. As the field develops, the need for standard procedures and guidelines is greater than ever, to ensure that technological developments do not taint the integrity of the investigative process, illustrating the vital importance of regulation as highlighted in the existing body of literature (Vicks et al., 2019). Moreover, increasing reliance on technology in medicolegal death investigation has critical implications for the health of investigators, where burnout and job satisfaction are concerned. As tools and processes are increasingly automated, there is a risk that investigators will feel stressed by having to learn new technology and deal with the complexity of digital information. A study on burnout among medicolegal investigators provides crucial data regarding how organizational stressors affect job resilience and compassion satisfaction (Thorpe et al., 2024).

The problem of technological burnout highlights the importance of having proper support systems and training that equip investigators with the ability to successfully deal with such developments. Through understanding the relationship between technological dependence and the health of investigators, agencies can implement organizational programs that ensure an improved work environment, thus enhancing the quality of investigations undertaken. Lastly, while technological advancements promise improved outcomes in medicolegal death investigations, ethical concerns cannot be overlooked.

Employment of sophisticated surveillance and information-collection techniques requires complex issues of privacy and consent in investigations that involve sensitive personal information. When these technologies are utilized by investigators, the likelihood of interfering with the rights of the individual is a major point of concern.

The technology must balance advancement with ethical duty such that the rights of the victim and their family are not interfered with during the investigation process. As highlighted in debates within the research practice, having clear ethical principles within the use of technology in medicolegal settings is vital in ensuring responsibility and adherence to the investigative objective. The challenge of introducing technology ethically to the fold resonates with the call for ongoing debate and policy formulation within the pursuit of comprehensive medicolegal death investigation practice (Vicks et al., 2019) (Figure 2.18).

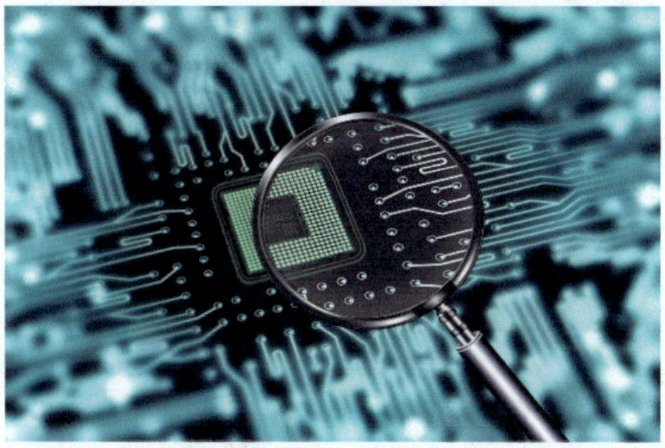

Figure 2.18. Digital forensic methods.

Source: https://www.openaccessgovernment.org/wp-content/uploads/2022/05/dreamstime_xxl_24807432-scaled.jpg.

Test Your Knowledge

1. What primary issue arises due to overlapping jurisdictions in medicolegal death investigations?
2. What is one of the critical roles of medicolegal death investigators (MDIs)?

SUMMARY

In summarizing a medicolegal death investigation tour, it is apparent that technological innovation is a key force driving the accuracy and efficiency of the field. Technologies such as iris recognition technology are significant improvements in postmortem identification and are more individualized than older methods like DNA analysis. A pilot trial had a very high match rate of approximately 80%, which suggested that this technology could potentially identify deceased individuals with reliability. Postmortem iris scanning also has the potential to lead to a universal identification database that would benefit forensic pathology and assist in cases involving missing persons or human trafficking. These advances not only highlight the imperative of continued research and development in forensic science but also the potential for the adoption of new methods into current practice to further medicolegal investigation (Sansola et al., 2015). Moreover, analysis of heat death illustrates the complex process of determining cause in medicolegal death investigations. Reliance on scene examination and exclusion of other explanations is necessary as the diagnosis of hyperthermia is not usually backed by conclusive macroscopic or microscopic features. The addition of postmortem biochemical analyses can also increase diagnostic potential, with valuable information being supplied by the physiological aftermath of overheating. By analyzing biochemical markers in combination with autopsy findings, investigators can construct a clearer image of the circumstances leading to death. The use of high-technology diagnostic techniques enhances the overall credibility of medicolegal investigations, so that heat-related deaths are properly diagnosed and placed in a larger investigative context (Mangin et al., 2018). The field of medicolegal death investigation is, in fact, becoming more refined with both technological advancement and thoughtful diagnostic practices. The efficacy of methods such as iris recognition for postmortem identification not only increases the process of establishing the identity but also the integrity of the investigations. Coupled with a commitment to using biochemical and immunohistochemical tests for challenging cases, the practice is able to handle challenges emerging from diverse death circumstances, particularly in diagnosing elusive causes of death. Lastly, a cross-disciplinary approach, whereby technology and investigative effort converge, holds the promise of the future of servant justice and forensic science in general, ensuring that each case will get the effort it deserves (Mangin et al., 2018; Sansola et al., 2015).

During medicolegal death investigations, identifying the difference between human and nonhuman remains is essential. Forensic anthropologists, often the professionals involved in these investigations, must thoroughly analyze skeletal remains to identify their species. The prevalence of nonhuman remains in cadaveric cases has been highlighted by the Office of the Chief Medical Examiner's Kenosha County study, which cataloged over 1940 nonhuman bones over a specified time period. This extensive store, comprised predominantly of mammalian remains, highlights the need for more widespread training in identifying nonhuman materials. By focusing on common nonhuman species like white-tailed deer, pigs, and domestic cows, forensic training programs can better educate practitioners to minimize misidentifications, and hence lead to more accurate and reliable death investigations (Fourshee et al., 2022). Another critical aspect of medicolegal death investigations is the establishment of death scene protocols. Upon reaching a scene, investigators ought to adhere to systematic guidelines that govern evidence collection and preservation. The application of the principles of forensic science assists these professionals in constructing a fact-based account of events leading up to a death. By employing methods such as careful photography, sketching, and note-taking, they record all details meticulously. The necessity of keeping the scene intact cannot be overstated, as it assists in maintaining the legitimacy of the evidence and withstands the scrutiny of a courtroom. Subsequently, such compliance with established procedures works to ensure that the process of investigation not only respects legal standards but also ensures the maximization of the thoroughness of the result (Brody et al., 2011). Furthermore, the impact of traumatic brain injury (TBI) plays a critical role in explaining certain deaths in medicolegal practice. Literature stipulates that there exists a relationship between acute TBIs and the prompt onset of neurodegenerative diseases, especially Alzheimer's disease. This correlation directs attention to the need for consideration of prior medical history and potential trauma when forensic pathologists determine the cause of death. The presence of amyloid-beta and tau protein pathologies within post-traumatic settings complicates cases further because these are factors that could influence the interpretation of predisposition conditions for death. Therefore, close scrutiny of clinical histories with respect to trauma can illuminate causative relationships, eventually leading to a more advanced strategy for medicolegal questions and the validity of follow-up assessments related to TBI and neurodegenerative disease (Brody et al., 2011).

KEY TERMS FROM THIS CHAPTER

- Accidental deaths
- Clinical assessment
- Forensic anthropology
- Implicit biases
- Investigation
- Medicolegal system
- Societal inequalities
- Biomarkers
- Evidence collection
- Heart disease
- Infections
- Laboratory tests
- Natural deaths
- Stroke

CRITICAL THINKING QUESTIONS

1. **What is the primary role of a medicolegal death investigator?**
   a. To collect evidence at crime scenes.
   b. To determine the time and cause of death.
   c. To establish the identity of the deceased.
   d. All of the above.
2. **Which type of death is most commonly investigated in a medicolegal context?**
   a. Deaths occurring in hospitals.
   b. Deaths under suspicious or unusual circumstances.
   c. Deaths due to natural causes in elderly individuals.
   d. All deaths, irrespective of circumstances.
3. **What is the first step in a medicolegal death investigation?**
   a. Conducting an autopsy.
   b. Documenting the death scene.
   c. Collecting toxicological samples.
   d. Determining the cause of death.
4. **What is the purpose of rigor mortis in medicolegal investigations?**
   a. To identify the deceased.
   b. To estimate the time of death.
   c. To confirm the manner of death.
   d. To determine the cause of death.
5. **Which professional is primarily responsible for conducting autopsies in medicolegal death investigations?**
   a. Medical examiner or forensic pathologist.
   b. Crime scene investigator.
   c. Coroner.
   d. Toxicologist.

Short Answer Questions

1. What is a medicolegal death investigation?
2. What is the importance of death investigations in legal contexts?
3. What is the primary role of forensic professionals in the medicolegal death investigation process?
4. List the different types of death investigations.
5. What is the primary purpose of the autopsy process in medicolegal investigations?

Answer to Critical Thinking Questions

1. (d); 2. (b); 3. (b); 4. (b); 5. (a)

REFERENCES

1. Ashley, P., Banman, A., Fraire, L., et al. (2020). DOP-Coroners' study 2020 final report: Assessing coroners' needs. https://core.ac.uk/download/346444209.pdf (accessed on 12th July 2025).
2. Barton, P. S., Carter, D. O., Dawson, B. M., et al. (2024). Bridging the gap between decomposition theory and forensic research on postmortem interval. https://core.ac.uk/download/622645352.pdf (accessed on 12th July 2025).
3. Bergers, L., Dirven, P., Ruberg, W., et al. (2023). Introduction. https://core.ac.uk/download/587381487.pdf (accessed on 12th July 2025).
4. Bottinelli, C., Bévalot, F., Cartiser, N., et al. (2016). State of the art in bile analysis in forensic toxicology. https://core.ac.uk/download/pdf/81153209.pdf (accessed on 12th July 2025).
5. Brody, D. L., Holtzman, D. M., LaFerla, F. M., et al. (2011). Controlled cortical impact traumatic brain injury in 3xTg-AD mice causes acute intra-axonal amyloid-β accumulation and independently accelerates the development of tau abnormalities. https://core.ac.uk/download/288812821.pdf (accessed on 12th July 2025).
6. Brown, M. (2024). The development, implementation, and evaluation of an online program for emergency nurses caring for victims of interpersonal violence: A mixed methods study. https://core.ac.uk/download/639243056.pdf (accessed on 12th July 2025).
7. Chapenoire, S., Claes, J., Crema, E. R., et al. (2016). Extensive unusual lesions on a large number of immersed human victims found to be from cookiecutter sharks (*Isistius* spp.): An examination of the Yemenia plane crash. https://core.ac.uk/download/77415271.pdf (accessed on 12th July 2025).
8. Chatterji, A. P., Fletcher, L. E., Kaur, M., & Altholz, R. (2015). Access to justice for women: India's response to sexual violence in conflict and social upheaval. https://core.ac.uk/download/75783197.pdf (accessed on 12th July 2025).
9. Cho, B. S., Harder, J., & Willmore, B. (2019). DOP-Coroners' study 2019 final report: Assessing coroners' needs. https://core.ac.uk/download/289232065.pdf (accessed on 12th July 2025).
10. Donaldson, A. (2020). New Zealand emergency nurses' knowledge about forensic science and its application to practice. https://core.ac.uk/download/322841929.pdf (accessed on 12th July 2025).
11. Fabiano, M. A., Fineschi, V., Frati, P., et al. (2017). New frontiers in thermal analysis: A TG/chemometrics approach for postmortem interval estimation in vitreous humor. https://core.ac.uk/download/98333908.pdf (accessed on 12th July 2025).
12. Focant, J. F., Grabherr, S., Perrault, K., et al. (2016). Postmortem internal gas reservoir monitoring using GC×GC-HRTOF-MS. https://core.ac.uk/download/77145287.pdf (accessed on 12th July 2025).
13. Fourshee, J. L. (2022). Differentiating human from nonhuman bone: Insights from a medical examiner's collection, Kenosha, Wisconsin. https://core.ac.uk/download/554010999.pdf (accessed on 12th July 2025).
14. Frati, A., Hyder, A. A., Palmer, A. M., Selassie, A. W., Buller, B., Roozenbeek, B., Murray, C. J., et al. (2018). Clinical-pathological study on β-APP, IL-1β, GFAP, NFL, Spectrin II, 8OHdG, TUNEL, miR-21, miR-16, miR-92 expressions to verify DAI-diagnosis, grade, and prognosis. https://core.ac.uk/download/154949003.pdf (accessed on 12th July 2025).

15. Frost, J. (2016). Forensic toxicology in Central Norway: Autopsy rates and findings with emphasis on codeine. https://core.ac.uk/download/646141145.pdf (accessed on 12th July 2025).
16. Holland, S. (2015). Unmasking serial murder: A comparison of a South African murder series with characteristics from the Federal Bureau of Investigation serial murder database. https://core.ac.uk/download/188770459.pdf (accessed on 12th July 2025).
17. Iino, M., Nakatome, M., Norbu, N., et al. (2022). Forensic medicine in South Asia: Comparison to the developed countries. https://core.ac.uk/download/544080091.pdf (accessed on 12th July 2025).
18. Justice, D. O. (2025). Needs assessment of forensic laboratories and medical examiner/coroner offices: A report to Congress. https://core.ac.uk/download/478917838.pdf (accessed on 12th July 2025).
19. Kozma, Z., Pádár, Z., & Zenke, P. (2018). Most common medico-legal autopsy-related human and nonhuman biological samples for DNA analysis. https://core.ac.uk/download/322434892.pdf (accessed on 12th July 2025).
20. Mace, G. (2022). Implications of ancestry estimation: An analysis of identification rates in unidentified persons cases. https://core.ac.uk/download/533928403.pdf (accessed on 12th July 2025).
21. Mangin, P., & Palmiere, C. (2018). Hyperthermia and postmortem biochemical investigations. https://core.ac.uk/download/159152225.pdf (accessed on 12th July 2025).
22. Mangin, P., & Palmiere, C. (2018). Postmortem biochemical investigations in hypothermia fatalities. https://core.ac.uk/download/159156050.pdf (accessed on 12th July 2025).
23. Niveau, G., & Welle, I. (2018). Forensic psychiatry, one subspecialty with two ethics? A systematic review. https://core.ac.uk/download/154916359.pdf (accessed on 12th July 2025).
24. Quinlan, A. G. R. (2013). Stabilizing the technoscientific witness: A history of controversy, medicolegal practice, and the Ontario sexual assault evidence kit. https://core.ac.uk/download/77106196.pdf (accessed on 12th July 2025).
25. Rogers, J. (2023). Bridging the gap between healthcare and law enforcement in the field of forensics. https://core.ac.uk/download/571293435.pdf (accessed on 12th July 2025).
26. Sansola, A. (2015). Postmortem iris recognition and its application in human identification. https://open.bu.edu/bitstream/2144/13975/8/Sansola_bu_0017N_11536_web.pdf (accessed on 12th July 2025).
27. Thorpe, A. J. (2024). Bearing the weight: A phenomenological exploration of burnout and stress among medicolegal investigators. https://core.ac.uk/download/639071767.pdf (accessed on 12th July 2025).
28. Vicks, A. (2019). Regulating medicolegal death investigations. https://core.ac.uk/download/232859026.pdf (accessed on 12th July 2025).

POSTMORTEM CHANGES

3

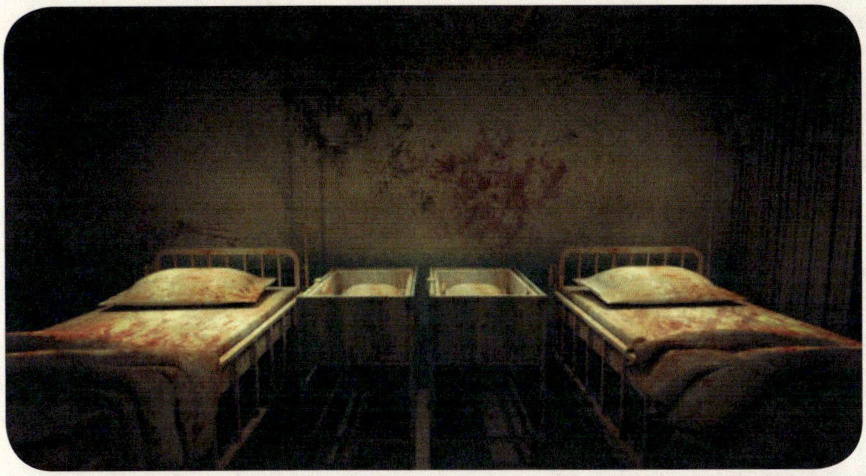

LEARNING OBJECTIVES

After studying this chapter, you will be able to:

1. Define the rigor mortis;
2. Define the livor mortis;
3. Explain the algor mortis;
4. Assess the decomposition stages;
5. Understand the impact of environmental factors on postmortem changes;
6. Describe the forensic implications of postmortem changes.

Introduction

The study of postmortem alterations in man involves a multifaceted set of biological, chemical, and physical reactions following death. The comprehension of these alterations is of vital importance to many fields, but most importantly to forensic science, where the establishment of the time of death can have far-reaching implications for investigations and legal cases. Decomposition is a significant indicator in postmortem studies, reflecting environmental conditions, the condition of the body at the time of death, and the underlying intrinsic biological processes at play. Qualitative assessment of rotting is generally quantified via various scales aimed at providing a standard process of categorizing the rotting stages. However, it should be known that there are limitations of such scales, particularly when utilized across different contexts, as mentioned in recent studies, stating that the sole application of such processes could result in statistically nonsignificant results, so that it becomes hard to have a proper understanding of postmortem intervals and their forensic significance (Santos et al., 2019).

Most importantly, postmortem change is influenced by an intricate set of external factors like temperature, humidity, and microorganism availability. They influence not only the rate of decomposition but also their visibility and whether these changes manifest as liquids, solids, or gases. Forensic anthropologists and medicolegal examiners employ qualitative and quantitative analysis to develop a more integrated understanding of decomposition processes. The confluence of advanced techniques, such as statistical examination of decomposition scales and cross-disciplinary studies, presents possibilities for enhancing the validity and accuracy of postmortem interval estimations. For example, systematic cadaver observations in different environments have the potential to yield salient points about decomposition, necessitating an integrated approach to forensic analysis. These advances are crucial in moving forward towards more accurate assessments within forensic environments and proving that medicolegal results stand the test of scrutiny (Santos et al., 2019). Future research will need to bridge gaps between forensic science and other branches of science to devise stronger methods for analyzing postmortem changes. This would entail tapping into advances in imaging methodologies and bioinformatics to gain insights into the biochemical transformations responsible for decomposition. One example would be making use of quantitative mapping methodologies, for instance, in studies involving neural myelination, to place focus on the biological processes occurring at cellular levels after death, thereby comprehending human degeneration more effectively. Emphasizing the multidisciplinary characteristic will not only enhance the current forensic techniques but also advance the quality of evidence generated in courts. By fostering interdisciplinary team collaboration, researchers are able to discover new frontiers in the examination of postmortem changes, ultimately enhancing current theory and further promoting the application of forensic science in legal frameworks (Figure 3.1).

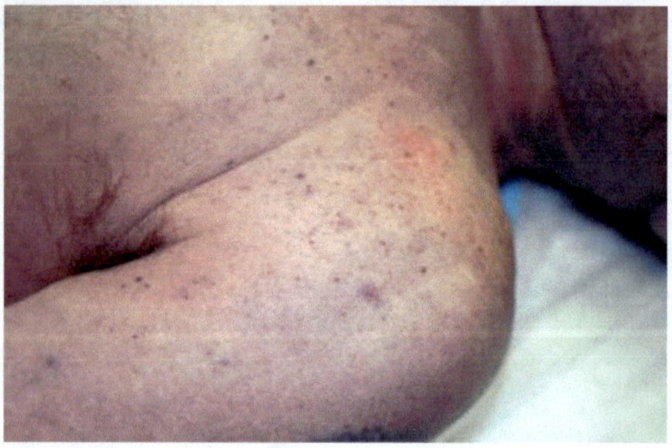

Figure 3.1. Postmortem changes.

Source: https://img.medscapestatic.com/pi/meds/ckb/49/9649tn.jpg.

Definition of Postmortem Changes

Postmortem changes are the biochemical and physiological changes that occur in the human body after death. The changes start almost immediately following the cessation of the heart function and can be of immense assistance to forensic examinations. Algor mortis, rigor mortis, livor mortis, and decomposition are the chief postmortem changes. Algor mortis, or the cooling of the body, typically results in a decrease of approximately 1.5°F an hour for the first 24 hours. Rigor mortis, which is the rigidity of muscles, usually sets in 2 to 6 hours post-mortem and persists up to 48 hours, which influences the determination of the time of death. Such changes are significant to forensic pathology because they enable useful deductions about the circumstances surrounding an individual's death. Furthermore, the physiological processes influencing postmortem alteration involve cellular and molecular changes, which contribute to the overall status of decomposition as well. Cellular respiration ceases, with energy exhaustion and tissue degradation that can be examined for further forensic details. The onset of decomposition shows a complex interaction of bacterial action, primarily by gut flora, which may also provide valuable information regarding time since death. This process is often marked by the onset of putrefaction, marked by typical odors and color changes. In addition, postmortem examination can reveal signatures of differentially co-expressed genes as observed in various studies, for example, on neurodegenerative diseases, describing biomolecular characteristics of postmortem biology and adding to the understanding of health prior to death (Casaccia et al., 2014). In the broad sense, the examination of postmortem changes also overflows into forensic genetics and investigative techniques. Knowledge of genetic differences can show underlying conditions that may have caused death. For example, genetic marker studies on epilepsy have provided insights into the interaction between genetics and postmortem phenomena and how certain gene expressions might influence the biochemical environment in the deceased's brain (Arumilli et al., 2017). This helps establish the importance of postmortem genetic investigations, as they can explain some of the diseases that were not evident during life. Last but not least, the definition and meaning of postmortem changes are not merely confined to appearances on the body; rather, they encompass a multidisciplinary system incorporating physiological, biochemical, and genetic investigation, leading to a general comprehension of human death (Figure 3.2).

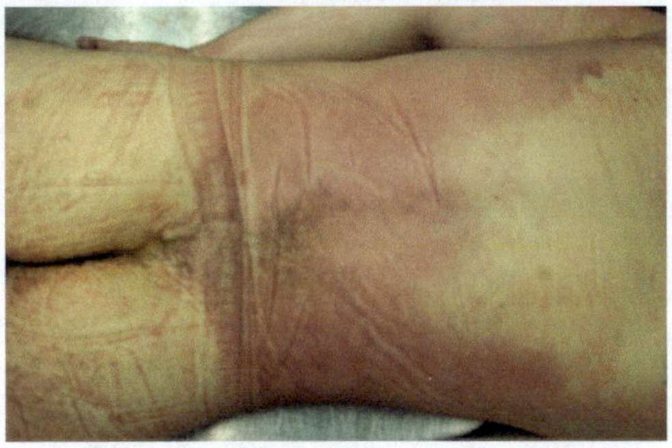

Figure 3.2. Livor mortis or lividity, on the posterior aspect of a body.

Source: https://ars.els-cdn.com/content/image/3-s2.0-B9780128000342000380-f0100038-10-9780128000342.jpg.

Importance of Studying Postmortem Changes

The study of human postmortem changes is crucial across various disciplines, particularly forensic science and medicine. The knowledge of the physiological changes that occur postmortem helps forensic scientists determine the cause and time of death, thus aiding criminal investigation. An integral component is the decomposition process, which occurs in phases that can provide useful information on the postmortem interval (PMI). By examining the sequence and type of changes—for example, the setting of rigor mortis or livor mortis—investigators can more accurately approximate the time elapsed since death. This kind of information is not only important in legal proceedings but also useful in epidemiology and public health statistics. Careful monitoring of these changes subsequently enhances our knowledge of human physiology and can potentially have a monumental impact in both legal and medical fields. Besides forensic uses, the study of postmortem changes also greatly aids medical research, such as the study of gene expression dynamics. It has been found that postmortem tissues are good sources for exploring patterns of gene expression, albeit these patterns tend to be greatly affected by processes initiated due to death and PMI. For instance, the effect of PMI may result in tissue-specific variations of gene expression, making biological analysis harder. However, scientists can control for these confounding effects through the correction of the appropriate covariates, making their results more valid. In addition, ante- and postmortem blood sample comparison has shown that there is a transcriptional cascade of events following the organism's death, indicating that postmortem changes are not random but indicative of ongoing biological processes, which may be of future biomedical interest (Aguet et al., 2018). Furthermore, postmortem change findings have wider significance outside of the immediate scope of forensic or medical science.

They play an important role in speeding up educational outreach and multi-modal imaging technology advancements. Institutes like the University of Texas High-Resolution X-ray CT Facility seek out these novel approaches to gain a better understanding of biological sciences at microscopic and macroscopic levels. With the application of advanced imaging techniques, researchers can visualize postmortem changes, providing responses that are central to outstanding questions in death examinations. Interdisciplinary investigations of these changes are facilitated by collaboration across the branches of science, providing a better appreciation for human biology in life and death. Lastly, the importance of studying postmortem changes opens new frontiers for research, studies, and teaching, and can give rise to groundbreaking advancements in forensic and biological sciences (Ahmed et al., 2017) (Figure 3.3).

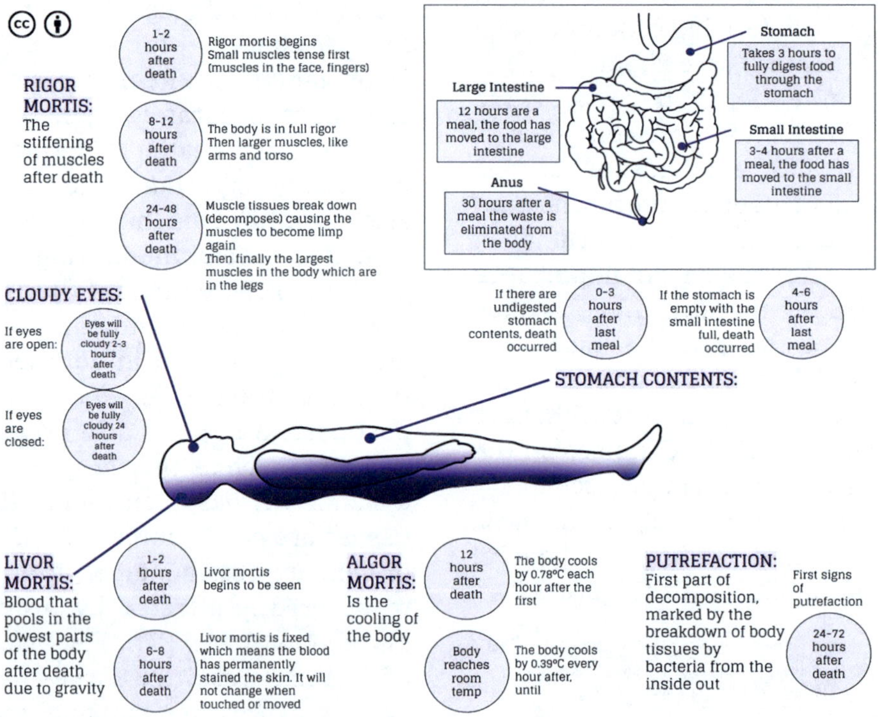

Figure 3.3. Post-mortem phenomena to estimate the time of death.

Source: https://upload.wikimedia.org/wikipedia/commons/1/16/Michele_Taylor_-_Forensics_Final_Project_%281%29.jpg.

3.1. Rigor Mortis

Learning Outcome

1. Understand the process of rigor mortis.
2. Describe the timeline of rigor mortis development.
3. Know the factors affecting rigor mortis.

The process of rigor mortis is an important feature of the postmortem changes that occur in humans following death. Rigor mortis involves the stiffening of the skeletal muscles, and this normally starts around two to six hours after death occurs. The molecular basis of rigor mortis lies in the abnormal aggregation of the contractile apparatus within muscle cells following the depletion of adenosine triphosphate (ATP), which is the energy molecule of cells. In the living tissue, the release of myosin from actin filaments during muscle contraction and relaxation is done by ATP. After death, ATP rapidly exhausts, and the state becomes one in which the actin and myosin filaments become locked together tightly. Stiffness manifests as rigidity and can be of high utility in providing information about the post-mortem time, and hence can be of use to forensic authorities. An understanding of the timing of rigor mortis can be highly valuable in postmortem interval estimation and the assistance of numerous legal cases. While rigor mortis has been associated with the cadaver's physical form, it should not be viewed in isolation from other comparable postmortem changes. As recent accounts have indicated, various biochemical modulations remain postmortem, affecting the overall process of decomposition. For instance, the upregulation of certain genes involved in inflammation and immunity is initiated within minutes of stopping biological function, potentially altering the timing of rigor mortis and subsequent changes such as livor mortis and algor mortis. Such expressions play a role in inflammatory responses, thus further making the traditional stages of decomposition more complex by affecting muscle rigidity and the speed at which rigor mortis occurs and resolves. Therefore, an integrated understanding of these tightly associated processes helps refine forensic practices and respect the complexity of postmortem biochemistry in deceased subjects (Claus et al., 2019). Rigor mortis will never last forever; it tends to peak most frequently between 12 and 24 hours post-mortem before fading away progressively over the next 24 to 48 hours. Factors such as ambient temperature, the condition of the individual at the time of death, and environmental conditions will all influence this timeline. For example, in warmer temperatures, rigor mortis can be reversed sooner, and with low temperatures, stiffness can persist longer.

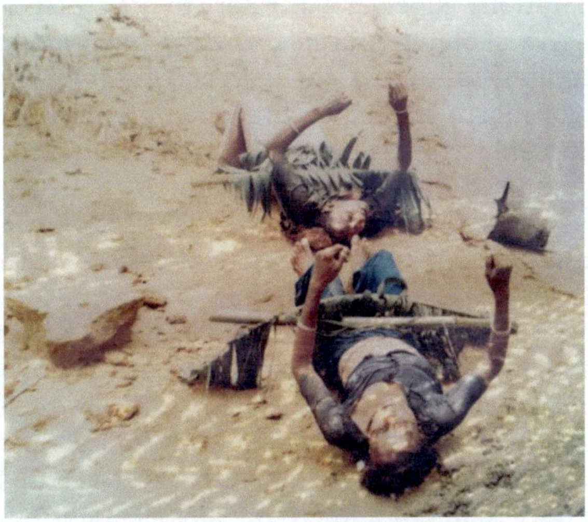

Figure 3.4. Corpses of victims of the 1991 Bangladesh cyclone in Sandwip displaying signs of rigor mortis.

Source: https://upload.wikimedia.org/wikipedia/commons/f/f3/People_Dead_1991_in_Sandwip.jpg.

For forensic purposes, these variations must be accounted for in the estimation of the time of death. Additionally, forensic taphonomy researchers support broad-based approaches to assessing rigor mortis in combination with other signs of decomposition. Understanding these variations enhances the reliability of the estimations of the postmortem interval, which is critical during criminal investigations. The greater the understanding of how environmental conditions are linked with patterns of decomposition, the better scientists can establish approaches to estimating the time of death within various environmental contexts (Hough et al., 2022) (Figure 3.4).

3.1.1. Definition and Process of Rigor Mortis

Rigor mortis is a well-documented process that occurs within the human body after death and is regarded as one of the significant postmortem alterations. Rigor mortis refers to the stiffening of the skeletal muscles due to biochemical changes following the arrest of the heart. Rigor mortis indeed occurs when the supply of adenosine triphosphate (ATP) is depleted, which is required to relax the muscles. Without ATP, myosin heads become irreversibly attached to actin filaments within muscle fibers and cause the stiffness characteristic of rigor mortis. This condition usually begins in the period of two to six hours postmortem, peaks between 12 and 24 hours postmortem, and gradually dissipates after approximately 48 hours, when breaking-down muscle tissues begin to run their course. Understanding rigor mortis is not only important to the biological sciences but also to forensic science since it aids in the estimation of postmortem interval and aiding in explaining the sequence of postmortem changes. Biochemical explanation of rigor mortis highlights the relationship between energy metabolism and muscle physiology. When metabolic activities of the body cease, there is a dramatic decline in ATP synthesis, mainly due to the lack of oxygen. This lack of energy induces the repeated attachment of myosin to actin without the normal cycle of contraction and relaxation that is seen in living muscle tissue. The stiffness begins in the smaller groups, such as those of the face and neck, before it progresses towards larger muscle groups such as those in limbs and trunk. By this course of stiffening, forensic scientists can determine clues about the postmortem interval. It has been extensively studied, and in recent evolution went beyond traditional techniques to more precise biochemical methods that track these physiological changes more specifically, revealing significant changes in forensic science (Johar et al., 2022).

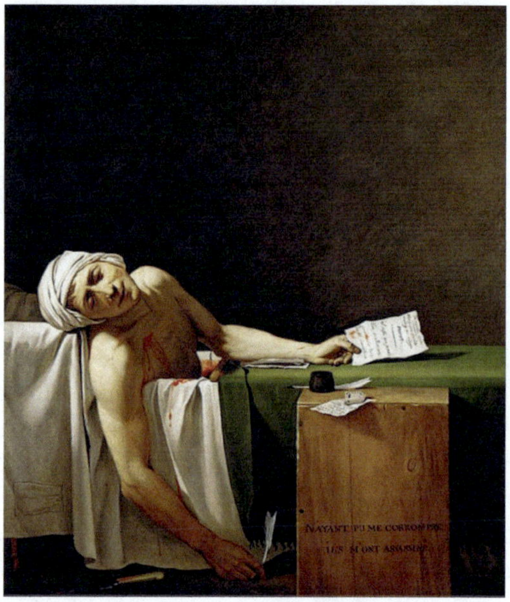

Figure 3.5. The death of Marat by French painter Jacques-Louis David in 1793. Rigor Mortis can be seen here by how the subject clutches the paper and quill.

Source: https://www.scienceabc.com/wp-content/uploads/2019/12/Jacques-Louis-David-La-Mort-de-Marat.jpg.

Aside from rigor mortis, other postmortem changes, including livor mortis and algor mortis, also play a critical role in providing context to the overall postmortem image. Livor mortis refers to the gravitationally affected settling of the blood, resulting in discolored dependent parts of the body. Livor mortis also assists in estimating the time of death since it will begin after a few hours of death and become fixed after about 12 hours. On the other hand, algor mortis is defined as the cooling of the body after death, where there is a uniform rate of heat loss that can further reduce estimates of time since death. Together, all three effects provide an encompassing framework for examining postmortem alterations, outlining the complexities of postmortem examinations needed in criminal justice and medico-legal purposes (Reisdorf et al., 2018) (Figure 3.5).

3.1.2. Timeline of Rigor Mortis Development

The timeline of rigor mortis development is one of the most critical considerations regarding postmortem changes in human beings. Rigor mortis typically begins between two to six hours after death, in which there is increased stiffness of the skeletal muscles. Upon the cessation of cellular respiration, there is ATP depletion, and this leads to irreversible binding of actin and myosin filaments in muscle tissue. The above illustrates how metabolic insufficiency relates to muscular rigidity. Significantly, factors such as environmental temperature and the individual's physical health upon death will also impact the onset and progression of rigor mortis. In warm temperatures, for instance, the development of rigor mortis can occur more rapidly. It is for this reason that knowledge of this timeline will be necessary for forensic science, where determining the time of death can prove to be crucial for legal reasons. With the advancement of rigor mortis, it typically reaches maximum stiffness between 12 and 24 hours post-mortem, leaving an important mark for forensic analysis. The rate of development of rigor mortis varies among different groups of muscles, with the small muscles becoming stiff before the larger muscles. The process reveals the complex interaction between fiber type within the muscles and biochemical processes in decomposition. In addition, the rigidity also starts to fade roughly 24 to 36 hours after death as the body enters the second phase of decomposition, also showing the temporary nature of rigor mortis. The phases highlight the importance of keen observation and recording in forensic investigations. By virtue of knowing this process, forensic professionals are better able to estimate the postmortem interval and sort out critical information embedded in the physical state of the corpse. Also, examination of the time scale of rigor mortis can provide the biochemical alterations leading to death. Rigor mortis development is not an isolated process but is part of a series of other postmortem processes, such as livor mortis and decomposition processes. Recent research employing metabolomic profiling has found striking diurnal variation in post-mortem tissue metabolites, which also correlated with the post-mortem interval, hence giving hints towards the timing of rigor mortis onset and ensuing processes of degradation (Kesharwani et al., 2025). This correlation highlights the necessity of considering rigor mortis on a multidimensional platform, incorporating environmental factors, biological variations, and state-of-the-art scientific processes. An integrated approach of this nature increases the precision of time-of-death estimates, which profoundly impacts forensic and legal procedures as well as scientific research into postmortem physiology.

3.1.3. Factors That Affect Rigor Mortis

The time of onset of rigor mortis, a postmortem process resulting from the stiffening of muscles, is influenced by a variety of intrinsic and extrinsic factors controlling its onset and duration. The intrinsic factors include the physiological state of the deceased at the time of death, such as age, sex, and disease. Young and fit subjects would develop rigor mortis more quickly due to more intense cellular processes, while older subjects or those with long-term illnesses would undergo alterations in this process due to depletion of energy reserves or muscle tissue breakdown. Basal metabolic rates can also differ according to these intrinsic factors, which influence ATP depletion, which forms the core process for relaxation of muscle. These nuances highlight the importance of being sensitive to distinctive circumstances of death within the background of rigor mortis while studying it within forensic science, thereby highlighting the importance of careful assessments during postmortem examination. Extrinsic factors also play a vital role in determining the duration and intensity of rigor mortis. Environmental temperature is one of the most important extrinsic factors, with increasing temperatures accelerating metabolic processes, thereby resulting in a quicker onset of rigor mortis. In contrast, colder temperatures delay its onset, and it becomes challenging to make exact times-of-death estimations. Climatic conditions also interfere with such determinations because the rate of tissue decay may be influenced by them, and the environment available for microbial activity within the body. For instance, in humid environments, the body decomposes at an accelerated rate of onset that, consequently, influences the time for rigor mortis. Such interactions of extrinsic factors demand vigilance during forensic examination to avoid misinterpretations about postmortem alterations in human beings, particularly in the legal arena where precise decisions are of paramount value. Advances in forensic science reveal that molecular alterations triggered after death are rich sources of information on rigor mortis and the prediction of the postmortem interval (PMI). As there is an ongoing investigation into degradation patterns of RNA, DNA, and protein in dead tissues, forensic scientists are gaining entry into biomarkers that likely will provide additional information in the traditional rigor mortis exam. Inference between intrinsic variables, like the individual's health at the time of death, and extrinsic variables, like environmental conditions, will be essential in interpreting molecular degradation accurately. This new approach complements the evolving paradigm for understanding postmortem change, as found in studies of the interrelations among biological markers, rigor mortis, and decomposition stages. Eventually, integrating all of these various factors—factors intrinsic, extrinsic, and molecular—may make PMI estimations more credible and lead to improved investigative outcomes in forensic science (Solanki et al., 2019; Proctor et al., 2007) (Figure 3.6).

Factors Affecting Rigor Mortis

Factors	Event	Effect	Circumstances
Temperature	Cold temperature	Inhibits rigor	Slower onset and slower progression of rigor
	Warm temperature	Accelerates rigor	Faster onset and faster progression of rigor
Activity before death	Aerobic exercise	Accelerates rigor	Lack of oxygen to muscles, the build up of lactic acid, and higher body temperature accelerates rigor
	Sleep	Slows rigor	Muscles fully oxygenated will exhibit rigor more slowly
Body weight	Obese	Slows rigor	Fat stores oxygen
	Thin	Accelerates rigor	Body loses oxygen quickly and body heats faster

Figure 3.6. Factors affecting rigor mortis.

Source: https://slideplayer.com/slide/3461303/12/images/4/Factors+Affecting+Rigor+Mortis.jpg.

Test Your Knowledge

1. What is the process of rigor mortis?
2. What are the factors affecting rigor mortis?

3.2. Livor Mortis

Learning Outcome

1. Understand the mechanism of livor mortis.
2. Describe the stages of livor mortis.
3. Understand the significance of forensic science.

Livor mortis, or postmortem hypostasis, is one of the first changes that occur in the human body after death. It is characterized by blood settling in dependent areas due to the force of gravity, and it begins shortly after circulation ceases and is potentially extremely telling about the time of death. When the blood pools, a pale purplish discoloration is formed on the surface of the skin. Livor mortis depends on several factors, including the body's position, ambient temperature, and the size and health of the subject at the time of death. The postmortem processes that are caused by livor mortis not only allow forensic experts to approximate the postmortem interval (PMI) but also allow them to ascertain the variation between categories of homicide, particularly concerning the position of the body in the criminal scene. Along with other postmortem manifestations, such as rigor mortis and decomposition, livor mortis plays a significant role in determining the PMI accurately. All these processes involve a certain time period, and their interactions offer forensic scientists a logical account of how long ago death occurred. While single variables could be subjected to variation based on external factors, adding livor mortis to factors like insect activity and body temperature gives a better approximation. As discussed in research analyzing different postmortem changes, the consistency of these signs is imperative in forensic practice and may be highly dependent on the environment surrounding the body, hence outlining the necessity of an extensive analysis of every aspect of factors contributing to postmortem changes in humans (Buras et al., 2006). Moreover, new research has identified the aroma of decay as a useful adjunct marker over traditional markers like livor mortis. When the body tissues decay, the release of stinky substances can be utilized to equate to the onset of postmortem changes, and a new approach to postmortem interval estimation is thereby provided. Decomposing odors have begun to be of interest for analysis in forensic science, referencing how temperature can influence the rate and structure of such compounds significantly (Love et al., 2001). While livor mortis remains a viable indicator in PMI determination, the addition of olfactory analysis to forensic practice can become even more precise in death investigations, enabling more sophisticated methods of time-of-death determination and providing valuable information on the conditions surrounding fatalities (Figure 3.7).

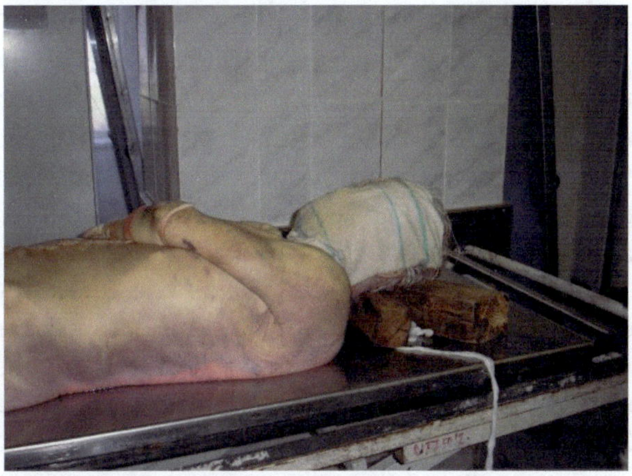

Figure 3.7. Livor mortis in a dead body.

Source: https://upload.wikimedia.org/wikipedia/commons/3/3e/%D0%9F%D1%8F%D1%82%D0%BD%D0%B0_%D1%82%D1%80%D1%83%D0%BF%D0%BD%D1%8B%D0%B5.jpg.

3.2.1. Definition and Mechanism of Livor Mortis

Livor mortis or postmortem hypostasis is a significant change observed in the body following death, in which there is venous congestion or pooling in the lower limbs under the influence of gravity. This takes place sometime following cardiac failure, preferably 20 minutes to two hours, and sets in within 12 hours of death. The process occurs when the withdrawal of circulation allows gravity to cause the blood to flow towards the most dependent areas of the body, producing a visible discoloration of the skin. The differential lividity patterns may provide critical information on the body's position during death, thereby informing forensic investigations. This condition is an instinctive sign employed by forensic pathologists to help determine the timing and cause of death, speaking to its importance in the general case of postmortem changes. The development of livor mortis is inherently related to the physical and biochemical changes in the body after death. Firstly, blood movement is obtained by the absence of heart contractions, creating a gravitational effect resulting in reddening of the skin in areas where blood pools. Red breakdown of blood also leads to the release of hemoglobin, which is also expected to cause purplish or reddish discoloration seen in decaying areas. It is mostly governed by ambient temperature, which has the tendency to enhance the rates of livor development and its subsequent fixation. Development of livor mortis usually occurs most frequently in a manner that follows a pattern in accordance with both the deceased individual's position at death as well as local environmental factors. Following knowledge of this mechanism is hence very important for both the biological and forensic aspects of death. The study of livor mortis not only serves as a time estimation aid but also as a marker for other postmortem changes that can occur, the complex interaction between body processes after death. Determination of fixed versus unfixed livor, for instance, can provide the forensic investigator with valuable information regarding the timing of death as well as the amount of postmortem movement of the body. Simultaneously, the process may be used for comparison with other processes such as rigor mortis and algor mortis that are also crucial in describing the circumstances of a person's death. Furthermore, the progress in forensic science in terms of the establishment of novel investigation methods emphasizes the importance of an extensive research of livor mortis and its application in forensic pathology (Piegari et al., 2018). Such interdisciplinarity ultimately enhances the validity of postmortem examinations, to the benefit of both human and veterinary forensic use (Wagensveld et al., 2020) (Figure 3.8).

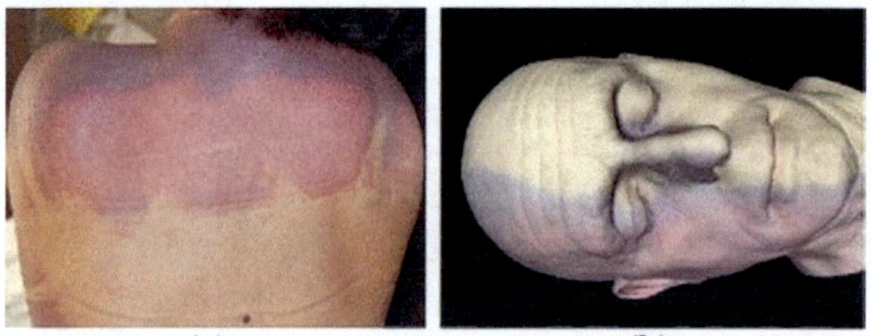

(a) (b)

Figure 3.8. (a) A photograph that highlights the pink and purple colorations of advanced livor mortis. Note that the coloration differences on the back are due to changes in the environmental temperature during livor mortis. (b) The colors of advanced livor mortis with high (bottom) and low (top) oxygen saturation.

Source: https://www.researchgate.net/publication/305040164/figure/fig9/AS:391312114241539@1470307486442/A-photograph-that-highlights-the-pink-and-purple-colourations-of-advanced-livor-mortis.png.

3.2.2. Stages of Livor Mortis

The understanding of the stages of livor mortis is significant to forensic science and the overall study of postmortem alterations in humans. Livor mortis or hypostasis is the accumulation of blood within the circulatory system when the heart no longer functions. It begins around 20 minutes to three hours post-mortem and causes a purplish-red discoloration of the skin of dependent portions of the body. In stage one, the pooling of blood remains temporary, and it is easy to re-arrange the dead body without altering the markings. With the gradual passage of time, distinct stages of livor mortis become more conspicuous and provide valuable information to forensic scientists regarding the post-mortem interval and the body position at the time of death. This critical aspect of postmortem alteration can thus be employed as a sign of the circumstances of the death of the subject. The subsequent development of livor mortis will typically occur within three to six hours post-mortem. During this time, discoloration becomes fixed, that is, the blood has coagulated and settled, and fixed the discoloration in the skin. From this point on, body movement fails to affect the established livor pattern. This residual livor is significant to forensic scientists because not only does it assist with the estimation of the postmortem interval (PMI), but it also aids in verifying the position of the body at the moment of death. Stabilization is based on a number of conditions, including ambient temperature and the physiological status of the person at death. Thus, when combined with the other postmortem changes, rigor mortis, and decomposition, livor mortis acquires considerable information regarding the cause and temporal sequence of death (Johar et al., 2022). During the later periods, which usually come after six hours, livor mortis still undergoes changes based on intrinsic and extrinsic causes. As the body further decomposes, the coloration can get darker, and the patterns will change depending on the surface that the body is resting upon. External temperature, humidity, and the health of the individual may decelerate or accelerate the process of livor mortis. Current studies have indicated that molecular changes in tissue can raise the accuracy of PMI estimation and validate the timetables according to livor mortis analysis. As scientists are investigating these biochemical methods, the integration of observation of livor mortis with contemporary techniques could lead to a better understanding of postmortem changes and factors influencing the rate of developing livor mortis (Solanki et al., 2019) (Figure 3.9).

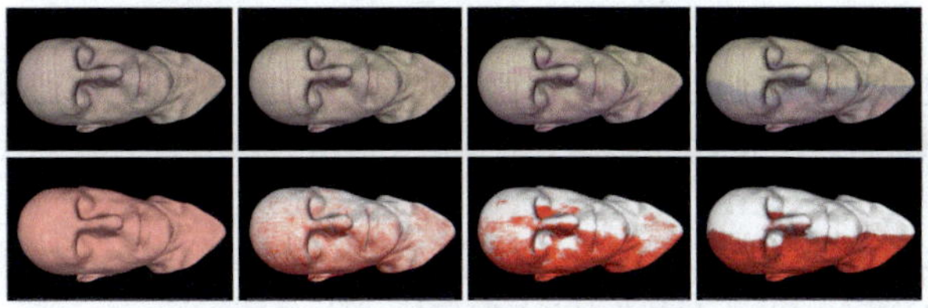

Figure 3.9. Stages of livor mortis.

Source: https://upload.wikimedia.org/wikipedia/commons/0/0d/Stages_of_livor_mortis.png.

3.2.3. Significance in Forensic Science

Forensic science is relevant because it has the ability to provide valuable information about postmortem changes in human remains. Knowledge of such changes is needed to calculate the postmortem interval, which could be a crucial characteristic in a legal case. Various environmental factors—temperature, humidity, and microbial activity—determine the rate of decay, and these must be accounted for, by forensic experts. For example, qualitative measurement of decomposition scales has been a specific area of interest in forensic research, as can be seen in the findings that assert that using just such scales could lead to statistically insignificant outcomes in some contexts. Such a divergence is an indicator for forensic professionals to combine various methodologies in order to obtain a strong measurement of postmortem intervals, one that truly mirrors the complexity of decomposition processes (Santos et al., 2019). The holistic way does not just reinforce the validity of forensic evidence but also preserves integrity in the process of investigation. Furthermore, the analysis of postmortem changes extends to earthy environments and to aquatic environments where decomposition occurs differently. It has been established that the fate of carcasses in marine environments can drastically differ from that in terrestrial environments. For example, coastal tetrapods as big as cetaceans have specific decompositional processes, and their knowledge is essential for forensic practitioners who work in adjacent fields. It seems that the corpses sink to the sea floor rather than blowing up from gas pressure, which was previously considered (Benecke et al., 2018).

The information is fundamental for both fossilization preservation records and the recovery of human remains in marine environments. With a comprehension of the taphonomy processes that govern decomposition, forensic scientists can provide significant inference into the cause and manner of death, finally aiding criminal investigations and informing paleontological knowledge. The use of forensic science to examine postmortem change thus represents a significant interstage transfer between legal inquiries and biological sciences. Through analysis of patterns of decay and evidence, forensic scientists can determine when and under what conditions human death takes place.

A multidisciplinary approach involving statistical models, environmental science, and biological understanding becomes vital in advancing our understanding of how varying conditions influence decay. These findings have repercussions in court, where reliable testimony of the postmortem interval can influence juries and judicial rulings. With advancing discipline, the continuous evolution of techniques and the exploration of new environments, terrestrial and aquatic, will yield progressively better forensic science applications (Santos et al., 2019; Benecke et al., 2018). This emphasizes the necessity for continuous investigation and interdisciplinarity in pursuing greater accuracy in forensic investigation (Figure 3.10).

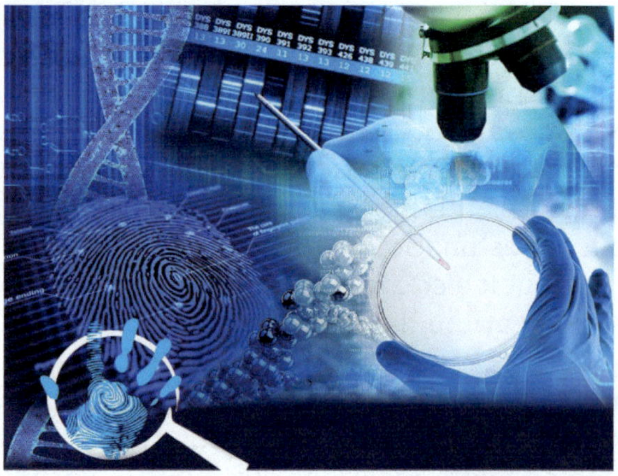

Figure 3.10. Significance of forensic science.

Source: https://www.legalserviceindia.com/legal/uploads/3rdyearlawstudentpresidencyuniversitybangalore_4764558229.jpg.

Test Your Knowledge

1. What is the mechanism of livor mortis?
2. What is the primary cause of livor mortis?

3.3. Algor Mortis

Learning Outcome

1. Define the algor mortis.
2. Describe the factors influencing body temperature postmortem.
3. Estimate time of death.

The algor mortis, or post-mortem cooling of the body, is a process that is of extreme significance in forensic science and the determination of time of death. After death, the body will begin cooling at around 1–1.5°F per hour until the ambient temperature of its surroundings is achieved. This anticipated drop in body temperature can be very informative as to the postmortem interval (PMI), particularly in the early stages after death. There are multiple factors, including environmental conditions, body composition, and clothing, that influence the rate of cooling and thus the accuracy of the estimates of PMI. Understanding of these factors is essential to forensic examiners who employ algor mortis as part of a battery of postmortem events to estimate time of death accurately. Furthermore, researchers working on the algor mortis phenomenon cross-talk with researchers working on the ecology of microbial community interaction in decomposition, or the necrobiome. In decomposition, there is a complex interaction of bacteria that begin to infect the human body within hours of death. These microbes, based on environmental factors and the initial state of the body, are accountable for most of the postmortem phenomena, such as temperature changes. According to available literature, there is appreciable and observable alteration in microbial communities throughout the decomposition process that could supplement temperature oscillation during algor mortis and be a double approach to estimating PMI. This connection emphasizes the importance of an advanced explanation of how algor mortis works in relation to other post-mortem biological mechanisms, as it can enhance the accuracy of forensic analysis (Dowell-Curby et al., 2017). Recent advancements in metabolomics profiling of post-mortem human tissues, such as the pineal gland, have revealed new avenues towards the knowledge of biochemical markers of algor mortis. These markers show big diurnal variations that agree with the post-mortem interval, and this suggests that metabolomics methods could complement traditional temperature-based estimations in estimating the time of death. Techniques like 1H-NMR spectroscopy facilitate the detection of post-mortem metabolic alterations, which provide forensic experts with some additional tools to make more accurate PMI estimates. This merger of metabolic and thermodynamic data shows an important development in forensic science because interdisciplinarity pushes the understanding of postmortem effects. With evolving investigation, such an approach promises to significantly increase the validity of determinations of the time of death since it highlights the interconnectedness between various postmortem changes, including algor mortis (Kesharwani et al., 2025) (Figure 3.11).

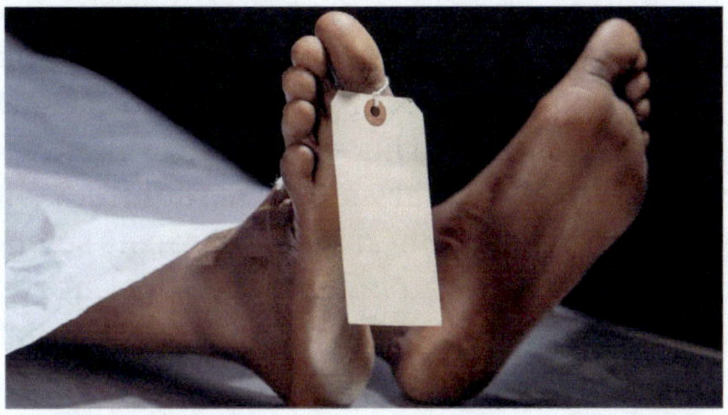

Figure 3.11. Algor mortis (postmortem cooling) and its significance in forensic investigations.

Source: https://cdn-ilbjbhl.nitrocdn.com/FyaMYitqUPNTCnovJEDCVNCvhqDiYUgo/assets/images/optimized/rev-0f7d9d8/sp-ao.shortpixel.ai/client/to_auto,q_glossy,ret_img,w_920,h_518/https://simplyforensic.com/wp-content/uploads/2021/08/Dead-rep-d_d-jpg.webp.

3.3.1. Definition and Explanation of Algor Mortis

Algor mortis refers to the postmortem cooling of the body, the process of which commences soon after death. Once the metabolic activity ceases, the body releases heat into the ambient environment, and the process is observed by the decrease in core temperature at a slow rate. Typically, algor mortis can become apparent at a rate of approximately 1 to 1.5° F per hour within the first 24 hours, but the rate is influenced by numerous variables, including ambient conditions surrounding the body and the body's makeup. The initial cooling is crucial for forensic investigation because the temperature of a dead body can say as much regarding the time when the individual died, which is also critical to establish the cause of death. Apart from external conditions, algor mortis may be influenced by physiological factors such as body size, clothing, and even the presence of objects near the body. For instance, a covered corpse may maintain warmth longer than an uncovered one due to insulation reasons. Moreover, conditions in the atmosphere, such as ambient temperature and wind, play significant roles in shaping the pace of heat dissipation. Awareness of such nuances makes a more accurate context for forensic experts, who are collecting evidence to estimate post-mortem time. This complexity illustrates why a multidisciplinary model is required, with input from biology, physics, and forensic science employed to accurately interpret postmortem change. Research has shown that algor mortis occurs in the body, often at the same time as other postmortem changes like rigor mortis and livor mortis. Collectively, these mechanisms create an ordinal series of changes in the body that can be utilized to assist in estimating the time of death. For example, while algor mortis focuses on temperature changes, rigors focuses on muscular stiffness, and livor focuses on blood settling. This dependency requires a complete postmortem examination. Forensic procedures, for example, non-invasive autopsy procedures, also facilitate investigations by providing accurate information regarding death, especially where normal autopsies are either unfeasible or not desirable (Wagensveld et al., 2020). Alongside these advances, decomposition research emphasizes temperature as a key factor and its role in the rates of decay, further reinforcing the significance of algor mortis in postmortem examination (Sharanowski et al., 2004) (Figure 3.12).

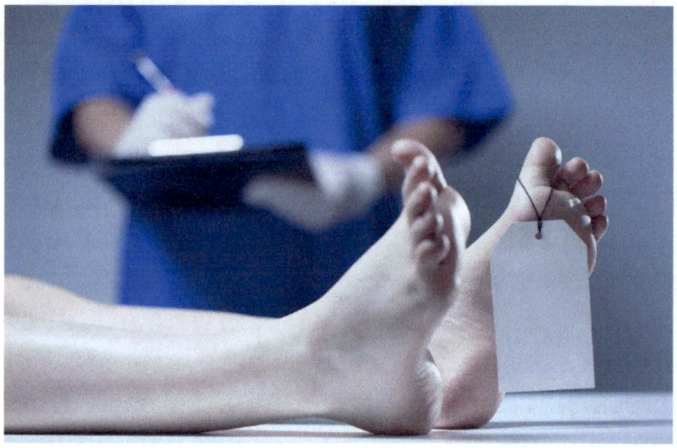

Figure 3.12. Algor mortis.

Source: https://mejorconsalud.as.com/wp-content/uploads/2018/09/algor-mortis-morgue.jpg?auto=webp&quality=7500&width=1920&crop=16:9,smart,safe&format=webp&optimize=medium&dpr=2&fit=cover&fm=webp&q=75&w=1920&h=1080.

3.3.2. Factors Influencing Body Temperature Postmortem

The mechanisms of postmortem body temperature are influenced by a myriad of factors that could make it difficult to ascertain the physiological status of the deceased. The most significant among these is the ambient temperature at the time of death and the exposure of the body to the environment afterward. Higher environmental temperatures will accelerate the rate of heat loss by mechanisms such as conduction and convection, while low temperatures could delay this process. In addition, ambient humidity can also control the thermal response of the body since it influences evaporative cooling. All these interactions validate the role of context in forensic examination as they are directly concerned with the estimated time of death. Particularly, physiological parameters such as direct sunlight or body position have a significant effect on cooling rates, further complicating forensic analysis in postmortem interval estimation. Additionally, individual physiological parameters at the time of death are the cause of affecting postmortem body temperatures. The metabolic state of the individual, conditioned by vitality at the time of death, has implications for thermal regulation even postmortem. For instance, a febrile or hyperthermic corpse at the time of death might retain more heat than a normothermic body, complicating time-related calculations since death. Body fat also contributes to retention or loss of heat; fat tissue is insulating and, as such, contributes to the cooling process experienced postmortem. Second, rigor mortis onset can interfere with metabolic processes and energy use soon after death, demonstrating that the physiological state at death can have a severe impact on the subsequent thermal dynamics. Finally, interactions among postmortem intervals and the above-listed factors create a complex web of influences that are to be assessed by forensic experts. External influences such as the clothing worn by the deceased change the cooling process; heavier clothing will lead to decreasing heat loss, while being lightly dressed leads to quicker cooling. Further, the time since death also must be considered along with ambient conditions and individual pre-mortem conditions in order to provide an overall picture concerning body temperature fluctuation. By integrating all these elements into their research, forensic scientists can make the time of death calculations more accurate, which is essential for criminal investigations. This accurate examination of postmortem body temperature variables underlines the intricacy of the postmortem process, one that each case must have a unique and delicate process to achieve rightful conclusions regarding the circumstances of death (Figure 3.13).

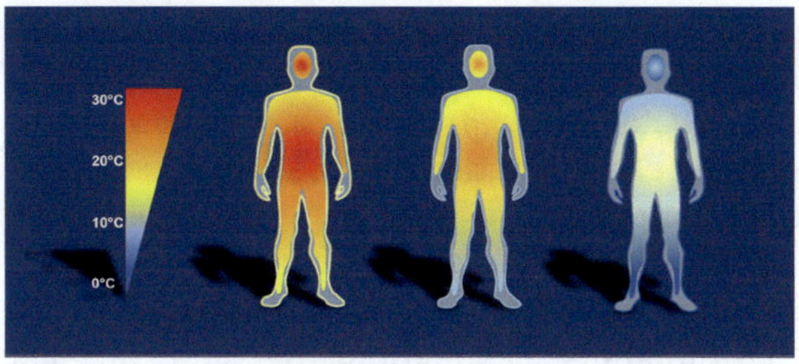

Figure 3.13. Postmortem temperature.

Source: https://dbe.unibas.ch/fileadmin/user_upload/dbe/04_Research/Forensic_Medicine___Imaging_Research/Bild_temperatures.png?1703067562.

3.3.3. Application in Estimating Time of Death

Determining the time of death is one of the most important procedures in forensic science, particularly in criminal investigations where timing can either make or break court cases. Some of the best ways forensic experts handle this is by analyzing postmortem changes like rigor mortis, livor mortis, and algor mortis. These are physiological responses within the body that provide forensic scientists with estimates of the postmortem interval (PMI). For instance, rigor mortis, or stiffening of the muscles after death, develops into a predictable timetable that is determined by temperature and body condition. By correctly viewing such physical indications of death, experts can establish a window in which death likely occurred, thereby helping to reconstruct what happened at the time of death. The biochemical and molecular analysis of postmortem tissues has been a crucial tool in the estimation of time of death, extending beyond traditional methods. The more recent studies showed the effect of the postmortem interval on the levels of expression of the genes, with certain genes varying in a tissue-specific fashion within hours of death. By analyzing such patterns, scientists are able to formulate a uniform model for forecasting the postmortem interval based on transcriptomic profile analysis from postmortem samples. As reported in studies that utilized cadaveric donor data, RNA expression changes are not the product of degradation processes alone; instead, they reflect active transcriptional regulation within the postmortem timeframe. These findings offer a sophisticated supplement to traditional physical methods to enable forensic specialists to more effectively construct time of death estimates, thereby improving the probative foundation of their inferences. In combination with gene expression profiling, biomarker identification also helps improve time of death estimates. These biomarkers, such as β-APP, GFAP, and IL-1β, were studied in postmortem traumatic brain injury and found to demonstrate significant alterations paralleling the injuries sustained before death. The expression levels of these proteins can be utilized as an indicator of the time of death when correlated with clinical data from the living patient. By integrating these biochemical markers with the traditional observational methods, forensic examiners enhance their ability to determine time periods of death more precisely. In addition, the recognition of active inflammatory response and cell apoptosis in postmortem tissues indicates the richness of biological processes after death, supporting the necessity for a multidimensional perspective in ascertaining the time of death and to improve the validity of forensic examination (Frati et al., 2018; Aguet et al., 2018).

Test Your Knowledge

1. What is algor mortis?
2. Which environmental factor most significantly affects postmortem body temperature changes?

3.4. Decomposition Stages

Learning Outcome

1. Understand the process of initial decay and autolysis marks.
2. Describe the putrefaction and its characteristics.
3. Describe the advanced decomposition and skeletal remains.

The process of decomposition is complex methodical, and takes place in several clear stages after an organism dies. Firstly, immediately after death, the body undergoes autolysis, where cell breakdown is initiated due to insufficient oxygen and its following enzymatic activity. In this phase, the tissues turn colorless, and gases produced by microbial flora accumulate, giving an inflated appearance. This early stage is significant, as it governs the course of the following processes. As decomposition goes on, the rate and extent of change may be influenced by environmental factors and proximity to organisms, with environmental variables like temperature and moisture playing key roles. The understanding of these early stages is significant in forensic science, as it can be applied in postmortem interval estimation and provides an insight into the overall process of decomposition. After autolysis, the body arrives at the active decay phase, where tissues are broken down rapidly by microbial action and infestation by insects. During this phase, the presence of putrid smells is observed as proteins and fats break down, calling scavengers and insects to the site. During forensic investigation, the active phase is crucial because forensic entomology depends on the pattern of insect infestation to offer decomposition timelines. The research on decomposition processes, particularly in various environments, has shown that the process might be significantly influenced by indoor conditions since decomposition of piglets in various environments has been studied in many researches.

These developments reiterate the need for integrative forensic procedures with regard to extrinsic variables of putrefaction because the application of qualitative scoring alone may generate statistically insignificant findings in the case of estimating postmortem time, rendering such methods inappropriate for courtroom use. Termination of the process of decomposition includes dry decay, where remains experience slow desiccation and skeletonization. At this stage, the majority of the soft tissue has decomposed, and what remains is primarily bones and hair. Scavenger activity and environmental factors also affect how quickly this stage is reached. Photographic documentation and recording are emphasized in current studies as a useful method for ascertaining the decomposition stages through time, particularly across various habitats. Advanced techniques, even those for assessing decomposition using 2D digital photography, have provided promising results in accurately capturing real-time changes. Such findings underscore the importance of adopting robust, open, and evidence-based approaches in forensic taphonomy. As forensic sciences evolve, the integration of multiple methods will enhance the accuracy of postmortem interval estimation and provide valuable information in legal and educational fields (Santos et al., 2019; Carter et al., 2018) (Figure 3.14).

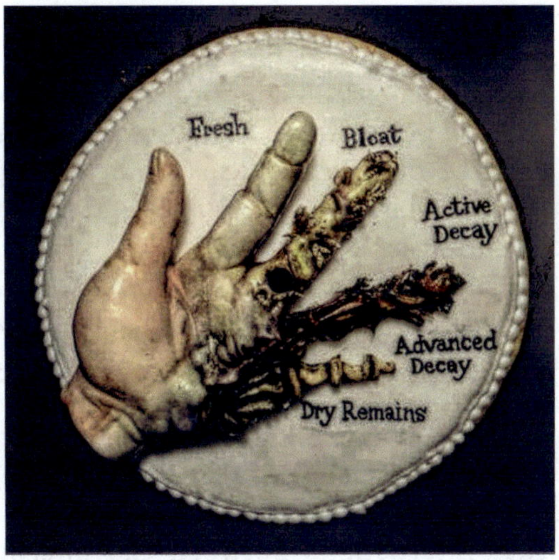

Figure 3.14. Decomposition stages.

Source: https://f4.bcbits.com/img/a3505343676_16.jpg.

3.4.1. Initial Decay and Autolysis

Early decay and autolysis form the onset of postmortem alterations in human corpses, beginning shortly after death. As biological activities cease, cells within the body begin to develop oxygen deficiency, which leads to a cascade of biochemical reactions. Among them is the activity of lysosomes disintegrating and releasing enzymes that start to break down cell materials, hence resulting in autolysis or self-digestion. This is a critical process because it is the transition from dead to living tissue and contributes significantly to breaking down the body as a whole. With the disruption of cell membranes, intracellular material leakage can produce an environment conducive to microbial growth and hence becomes interwoven with subsequent decay phases. Explanation of such processes provides some insight into the decomposition time course, which is extremely important in forensic science and estimating the postmortem interval (PMI), a field that has witnessed increased attention in recent studies (Solanki et al., 2019). Within a discussion of primary decay and autolysis, scientists have increasingly focused on the function of microbial communities in decomposition. There are numerous microorganisms present within the body, which get released and become active in the absence of physiological protection upon death. Microbial breakdown of the tissues can potentially alter the decomposing process by a significant margin, with variations based on inherent factors such as the person's age and health condition, and extrinsic factors such as temperature and humidity. They control the rate of both microbial growth and autolysis, which in turn influence the observable changes to the body. Recent studies have examined the intricate interactions between the microbial populations and the autolytic processes and offered possible ways of estimating PMI. By integrating an understanding of the autolytic changes and microbial activity, forensic science continues to refine its ability to estimate time since death (Spencer et al., 2013).

Also, the environmental conditions under which the decay process occurs should not be overstated when determining primary decay and autolysis. Various areas of the world have varied patterns of decomposition due to characteristic climatic patterns, which influence the pace and nature of such occurrences. For instance, a western Montana study discovered that lower temperatures can be very inhibitory to decomposition, leading to incomplete decay, such as mummification, towards the end of winter. The findings highlight the significance of regional models to consider postmortem alteration because what is practiced in current systems may not be applicable everywhere. By studying localized environmental conditions, researchers are able to learn how primary decay and autolysis proceed differently in various situations. Such details are refined to aid in accurately determining PMI and assist forensic anthropologists in solving human remains cases (Spencer et al., 2013).

3.4.2. Putrefaction and Its Characteristics

One of the most striking postmortem alterations, putrefaction, is the breakdown of body tissues by biochemical activity initiated by microbial processes. Occurring relatively soon after death, it is a testament to the body's susceptibility to the environment, particularly temperature and humidity. Putrefaction typically begins within 24 to 48 hours of death, since cellular autolysis and bacterial enzymes cause breakdown of tissues. The process is characterized by a sequence of visible events, including skin discoloration, which progresses from an early greenish hue to a more advanced state of breakdown. In forensic applications, such changes are invaluable for estimating the post-mortem interval when combined with other decomposition signs. Understanding the nuances of putrefaction helps forensic examiners establish more accurate timelines during postmortem examinations, which ultimately aid legal investigations in determining the circumstances of death. Putrefaction dynamics correlate directly with environmental factors, and these have a major impact on the rate and progression of decomposition. For instance, in high-humidity environments, microbial activity becomes more intense, leading to aggressive putrefaction, as can be illustrated by experiments on carcass exposure under varying environmental conditions. Such studies reveal that cadavers that decompose in water develop faster acceleration of putrefaction than those in dry conditions. Forensic use of this information is crucial since the postmortem interval may differ a lot based on the prevailing conditions. The decomposition phase can thus be employed as a decent indicator of the postmortem interval (PMI). Because forensic experts deal with environmental conditions during their analyses, the use of decomposition scales is beneficial, although there are certain restrictions present within such measurements, particularly indoors, where conditions that incline to exhibit less pronounced putrefactive changes are common (Santos et al., 2019). Additionally, the sophistication of the putrefaction emphasizes the requirements for multi-disciplinary approaches in forensic science with the integration of biological, chemical, and climatological data for holistic analysis. Research developments, like investigating alterations in intraocular pressure after death, further enhance understanding of how putrefaction and other physiological indicators interact with each other over time (Genero et al., 2019). Interdisciplinary convergence facilitates improved PMI estimations and overall discounting of forensic evidence. Through such interdisciplinary approaches, it is depicted that employing different methodologies in determining the credibility of postmortem analysis is essential. As the field evolves, the integration of detailed empirical data into forensic methodology remains paramount, enabling a clearer portrayal of the temporal aspects associated with human decomposition and facilitating the pursuit of justice in legal contexts (Figure 3.15).

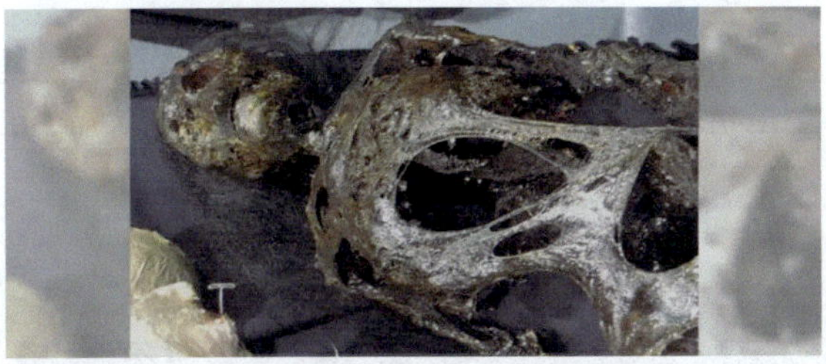

Figure 3.15. Putrefaction.

Source: https://media.geeksforgeeks.org/wp-content/uploads/20240122151809/Putrefaction.webp.

3.4.3. Advanced Decomposition and Skeletal Remains

Advanced decomposition is a series of chemical and biological mechanisms that significantly alter the skeletal remains. When human bodies decompose, they are exposed to various factors like environmental conditions, scavengers, and some trauma inflicted on the body. The interaction between these factors can accelerate or decelerate decomposition rates and later alter the visibility and integrity of skeletal trauma. For instance, research employing Sus scrofa domesticus as a model of human decomposition has established that different types of traumas, such as gunshot wounds, significantly influence the process of decomposition. Weather patterns in hot climates also render it hard to view and study such remains, thereby pointing towards the need for an integrated understanding of how trauma interacts with decomposition in the forensic context (Tieken et al., 2025). One of the important elements in examining skeletal remains is the role played by metabolomics, which provides insight into the biochemical reactions that occur after death. Application of this analytical chemistry technique has been important in the understanding of postmortem metabolic alterations and how they impact decomposition. Research at outdoor taphonomy sites has strongly indicated that the metabolic traces of decaying organic matter not only contribute significantly to the general understanding of the decomposition process but also aid forensic analysis. Importantly, human skeletal remains under investigation by metabolomics have shed significant insight into the release of metabolites into their surrounding soils and their applications for postmortem interval identifications and postmortem changes. This biochemical knowledge offers a comprehensive model for the elucidation of advanced decomposition and how it influences human bodies, thereby contributing value to forensic science (Hoeland et al., 2021). Furthermore, the elucidation of skeletal bodies in the context of advanced decomposition spills over into other disciplines of forensic science, particularly in the explanation of processes influencing decay. The analysis of intrinsic factors, that is, pathology prior to death, is pivotal in the creation of the postmortem environment and, therefore, the process of decomposition. The knowledge of how intrinsic and extrinsic factors, for example, the presence of diseases or drugs, interact with each other can supply critical information on the post-mortem interval and ensuing alterations to bone structures. Therefore, a compounded strategy that combines trauma analysis, biochemistry studies, and responsiveness to circumambient conditions is required for the accurate documentation of postmortem changes in dead bodies. The holistic approach finally enables forensic analysts to construct a more robust narrative of the conditions of putrefaction and the preservation of skeletal evidence (Tieken et al., 2025; Hoeland et al., 2021) (Figure 3.16).

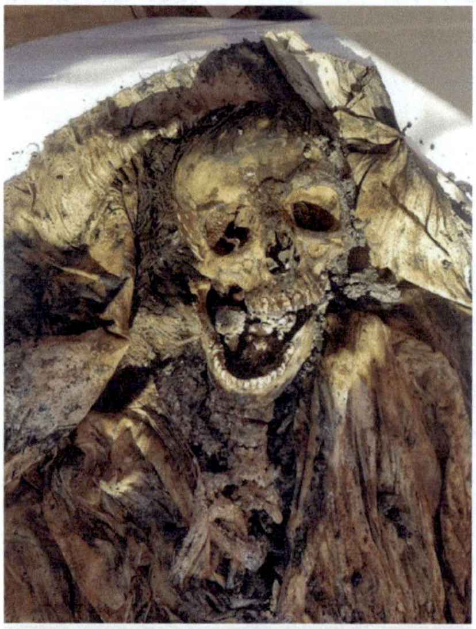

Figure 3.16. Skull and neck of the exhumed body showing an advanced stage of decomposition.

Source: https://www.researchgate.net/profile/Maman-Khurshid/publication/354859938/figure/fig1/AS:1072600587440128@1632739316271/Skull-and-neck-of-the-exhumed-body-showing-an-advanced-stage-of-decomposition.png.

Test Your Knowledge

1. Which cellular organelle is primarily responsible for releasing enzymes during autolysis?
2. What characterizes the process of advanced decomposition?

3.5. Environmental Factors

Learning Outcome

1. Describe the impact of temperature on postmortem changes.
2. Understand the role of humidity and moisture of postmortem changes.
3. Describe the influence of burial conditions.

The influence of environmental factors on postmortem decomposition in humans has an overall consideration of all the environmental factors that influence decomposition. Temperature and humidity are two of the key environmental factors that have a tremendous impact on the rate of decomposition. Increased temperatures will generally accelerate biological processes, leading to increased decay of tissues, while elevated humidity might promote bacterial and fungal growth involved in decomposition. Moreover, the presence of certain environmental microbiomes has the ability to speed up or slow down such changes by creating varying populations of decomposing organisms. Therefore, climate and regional ecosystem variation are of utmost significance in the determination of the exact timeline and nature of postmortem changes, providing a valuable context for forensic examination. Besides temperature and humidity, human activities are also responsible for shaping the environmental terrain upon which decomposition occurs. Human habitats have unusual issues, such as pollution and excessive artificial light exposure, that alter the typical decomposition process. Interference with natural circadian cycles by artificial light, for instance, impacts nocturnal scavengers' behavior that helps facilitate decomposition and, therefore, the process as a whole. Further, the study of human-altered land use patterns, like deforestation or urban growth, can give insight into how such environmental changes could affect the rates of organic breakdown and postmortem ecosystems. Those are facts that forensic experts must be aware of as they take the bigger ecological perspective in their practice. Finally, biogeochemical cycling's role in breakdown cannot be ignored. Nutrient supply, by the constitution of the soil and the microbiological flora, regulates the breakdown of dead organic matter. Some environmental toxins, enabled by human existence, further influence rates of breakdown and even the chemical signatures that persist in the deceased. Latest studies emphasize the interface between epigenetic modification and exposures to the environment and suggest a potential role for these processes in regulating the molecular integrity of deceased biological tissues. This increasing body of literature makes clear that knowledge of environmental effects is not just an addendum to the study of postmortem alterations but an integral component in the formulation of forensic techniques that aptly describe the circumstances of death, thus improving investigative results (Brown et al., 2020; Iannitelli et al., 2015) (Figure 3.17).

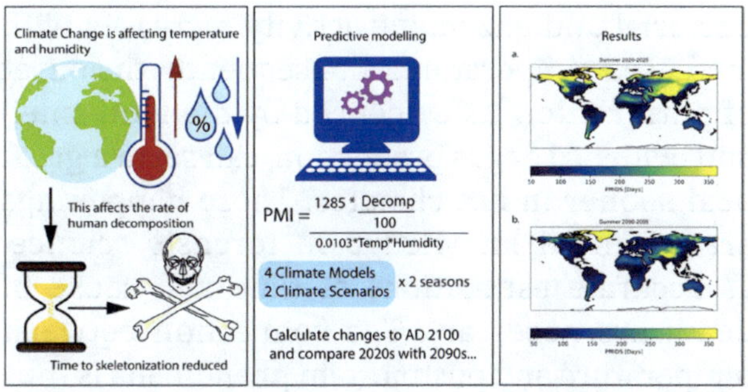

Figure 3.17. Predicted changes to the rate of human decomposition due to climate change during the 21st century.

Source: https://ars.els-cdn.com/content/image/1-s2.0-S2665910723000166-ga1_lrg.jpg.

3.5.1. Impact of Temperature on Postmortem Changes

The ambient temperature of a body in storage following death determines the pattern and rate of its breakdown. As the core body temperature falls after death, physiological processes decrease, leading to a sequence of postmortem changes that are markedly variable based on environmental temperature. For instance, the onset of rigor mortis, or rigidity of muscles, begins a few hours postmortem and is regulated by temperature. Under temperate conditions, rigor mortis can set in within hours, but under cold conditions, the process may take years. In the end, temperature fluctuation affects not only the timing of postmortem change but also influences the nature of decay itself. This association demonstrates the important position temperature holds as a fundamental component of forensic science, where ascertaining time of death relies on the knowledge of such physiological responses. Temperature is also an active force in other postmortem changes, such as livor mortis and decomposition, in addition to rigor mortis. Livor mortis, or the pooling of blood by gravity, is accelerated by heat, with more discoloration occurring within the skin. Under subject to higher temperatures, the body's tissues break down at a faster rate because bacterial and enzymatic activity increases with increased temperatures. Consequently, the onset of putrefaction, as evidenced by the fetid smell and evidence of gas production, can seem a great deal sooner in hot climates. These happenings are essential knowledge in forensic science, as accurate estimations of time and cause of death are necessary. The connection between temperature and postmortem phenomena is thus deserving of note for medical and legal purposes. Also, preservation or rapid decomposition of the remains may have significant impacts on criminal investigations and trials. Under cold storage conditions, postmortem alterations are reduced to a minimum, effectively halting decomposition and allowing extensive examination well beyond the time of death. Preservation may add important findings during the autopsy procedure, allowing more effective determination of cause and manner of death. Conversely, in weather exposure cases, their counterparts to temperature exposures are susceptible to rapid decomposition, with probabilities of cover-up of the evidence. The evidence highlights a strong relationship between temperature and postmortem alteration processes, highlighting the need for practitioners to be keen on thermal conditions during their analysis. As emphasized, appreciating temperature effects is essential to scientists in disciplines such as forensic pathology and anthropology because event reconstruction around death is the key to justice and accountability.

3.5.2. Role of Humidity and Moisture

The role of humidity and moisture in the situation of postmortem human decomposition is fundamental to the mechanism of how decomposition works. The body goes through a series of physical changes that are significantly dependent on environmental factors after death, such as humidity. High humidity can facilitate the process of decomposition by creating an improved environment for microbial activity and insect activity. It is high humidity that facilitates tissue decomposition because bacteria grow well in wet conditions and generate rapid putrefaction along with the formation of gases that lead to the characteristic smell of rot. Forensic practitioners need to therefore consider environmental humidity in estimating time of death, as it directly influences the rate and mode of decomposition. Apart from water, temperature fluctuation also plays an important role, to the extent that a complex interaction is observed impacting decomposition. The freeze-thaw cycle, for instance, has been found to induce bone decomposition in studies, and it suggests that extreme temperature variations also support the action of humidity. In hot, temperature-variable, humid conditions, as in western Montana, double effects in both the increase in expected rates of decomposition are seen, as characterized by research following both climatic variables and the associated effect on decomposition of organic material. These findings emphasize the need for a context analysis of postmortem alteration, noting that humidity not only affects soft tissue decomposition but also skeletal alteration by regulating various environmental conditions (Huey et al., 2013). Furthermore, humidity effects are not only applicable in initial decomposition but also in extended processes like mummification. In some cases, when a body is exposed to extremely dry environments, moisture loss can lead to mummification, which keeps the corpse intact for a long time. In most humid cases, however, the tendency for increased tissue moisture can result in quicker decay. The outcome reveals that, regardless of burial or surface environments, mummification is a striking outcome in arid and high-humidity climates, demonstrating a clear deviation from the typical process of decomposition. The discoveries are most significant for forensic applications, as they contribute to a baseline understanding of how environmental conditions variably affect postmortem changes in different geographic locations (Cato et al., 2019).

3.5.3. Influence of Burial Conditions

The postmortem processes in the human cadaver are also defined to a significant degree by burial conditions, which include a myriad of environmental factors. Some of these factors include soil texture, water saturation, temperature fluctuations, and microbial activity that regulate the intensity and rate of decomposition. For instance, anaerobic conditions established in the presence of waterlogged soils can dramatically slow down decomposition, instead providing a secondary process for tissue preservation. The intricate interaction among these environmental agents can produce variable outcomes in the preservation of soft tissues and skeletal remains. As previously documented, the chemical and biological conditions of the burial ground often determine the transparency and integrity of the remains with time, establishing that postmortem changes are not only biological reactions but also well entrenched in their physical surroundings. In addition to the immediate biochemical processes under burial conditions, postmortem alterations may also be affected by the geological history of the site. Variations in sedimentation rates and the earlier geological history of the area can create distinctive preservation environments. Bone fragments covered under sediments, for example, might have unique morphologies and chemical composition depending on the depositional history. Boreal or mountainous regions, with their specific climatic conditions, can also affect microbial processes and mineralization processes differently than they do in temperate regions. Understanding how these environmental and geological conditions interact before and after burial is important, as they can help to give insight into the state of preservation and potential for recovery of biological material in archaeological contexts, as evidenced from the information achieved through skeletal material reflecting both conditions of burial and pre-burial change (Alcalá Martínez et al., 2002). Besides, the biodeterioration processes initiated by microbial populations after burial are strong determinants of the final state of human remains. While microbial communities accelerate decomposition in environments that are rich in nutrients, they have a potential role in unique preservation conditions in environments that are poor in nutrients.

The examination of remains under alternating microbial influences also sheds light on the resistance of some tissue types, including glycosylated molecules that serve as indicators of preservation potential. Research into ancient mummification processes has revealed that millennia-old remains can retain glycan structures, providing us with information on preservation conditions that may otherwise be unavailable to archaeological investigation. These observations point to the stability of biological materials over centuries and show that conditions at burial are a governing factor in both decomposition and the preservation of complex biochemical profiles, further validating our understanding of postmortem changes in man (An et al., 2014) (Figure 3.18).

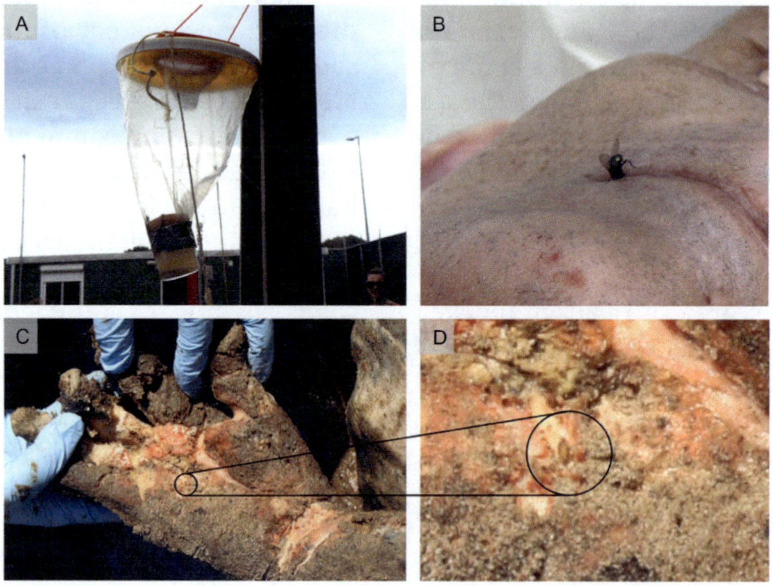

Figure 3.18. Entomological findings (A) Day 0 (day of burial), baited flytrap. (B) Day 0, female blow fly Lucilia sericata at the mouth corner of donor B. (C-D) Day 105 (second exhumation), a pupa of the scuttle fly Megaselia scalaris inside the right hand of donor B.

Source: https://www.researchgate.net/publication/346941411/figure/fig4/AS:11431281273993927@1724798268146/Entomological-findings-A-Day-0-day-of-burial-baited-flytrap-B-Day-0-female-blow.tif.

Test Your Knowledge

1. What is the impact of temperature on postmortem changes?
2. What is the role of humidity and moisture in postmortem changes?

3.6. Forensic Implications

Learning Outcome

1. Know the use of postmortem changes in criminal investigations.
2. Understand the importance of determining the cause of death.
3. Describe the ethical considerations in forensic studies.

In forensic pathology, the understanding of postmortem changes in human beings is crucial to determine the cause and mode of death. Traumatic brain injury (TBI) has been one of the central areas of inquiry, as it remains a significant cause of mortality and morbidity. In examining victims of death resulting from TBI, forensic pathologists look for certain biomarkers that can indicate the timing and nature of the injury. Research has shown that the availability of βAPP, GFAP, and other markers like IL-1β becomes appreciably elevated in cases of TBI, which can provide useful insight into the postmortem state of the brain. Further, identification of cell death by apoptosis, as measured by techniques like TUNEL, can enable forensic experts to distinguish between conditions prior to death and changes that occurred after death, hence rendering the sequence of events leading to death more determinable. Furthermore, the pathological changes following myocardial infarction (MI) also have serious implications in forensic investigation. MI is characterized by a sequence of events progressing from reversible ischemia to irreversible cell necrosis and resulting fibrosis, which can be crucial in autopsy findings. Pathologists are generally mandated to define the sequence of myocardial injury since it directly affects the investigation into the cause of death. Forensic analyses that can date the onset of MI can help ascertain whether the cardiac arrest occurred prior to death or due to other trauma, thus the need to differentiate between such circumstances for both legal and medical purposes. Additionally, understanding inflammatory processes involved in MI can aid in investigations of potential asphyxia or other causative factors in mortality. This integration into forensic practice enhances the ability to reconstruct events prior to death in a valid sense. By utilizing advanced neurobiological and cardiac markers, forensic professionals can make more precise determinations regarding the time of death and mechanisms involved. This is not only useful in criminal investigations, but has broader applicability to public health and safety in general, particularly in those communities where identification of the underlying causes of death is able to direct preventative interventions. Additionally, ongoing research into such pathobiological mechanisms will continue to refine forensic techniques so that practitioners can make use of emerging information in evaluating difficult cases. Thus, the forensic application of postmortem changes is significant, connecting medicine, law, and public health to foster a greater appreciation for human death.

3.6.1. Use of Postmortem Changes in Criminal Investigations

The use of postmortem changes in the course of criminal investigations plays a central role in determining the events surrounding a death. Forensic scientists study in depth various physiological and chemical changes that occur after death, all known as decomposition. The transformation not only indicates the amount of time passed since death but also determines whether foul play occurred. For instance, factors such as environment, temperature, and cause of death significantly influence the decomposition rate and need careful examination by investigators. Reliance on pre-existing scales of decomposition, as useful as they are, might be problematic when evaluating cadaver changes in diversified contexts. Hence, the addition of a multidisciplinary system that involves the combining of qualitative estimation and environmental elements is crucial in enhancing the postmortem interval (PMI) estimations' validity, rendering findings established during investigations scientifically sound and acceptable in courts of justice. Consistency of decomposition scoring systems is the main issue during forensic investigations, particularly in its impact on legal verdicts. One study highlighted that employing decomposition scales in isolation would yield statistically meaningless outcomes when estimating a body's condition, especially within controlled settings like indoors. For example, the research showed cadavers found indoors exhibiting early stages of decomposition, which creates a challenge for time-of-death estimates to be reliable. Such contrast heightens calls for interdisciplinarity in forensic taphonomy, where other scientific tests supplement traditional scoring techniques. As described in Santos et al. (2019), the variations in the rate of decomposition in various environments suggest that reliance on standardized scales may not be adequate to gain a comprehensive understanding of a case, hence advising investigators to utilize other methods to complement their conclusions and legal assumptions. Moreover, photographic evidence in forensic analysis has also gained prominence, particularly in assessing postmortem changes. As emphasized in more recent work, the use of 2D color digital photographs as an investigative tool has been promising in determining decomposition processes. Photographs' reliability to capture actual changes in cadaver status can support the evidentiary value of forensic analysis. The study reveals that methods employed in photographic evidence analysis can yield different outcomes, and therefore, there is a need to employ applicable scoring systems in determining accurate assessments. For instance, while a particular scoring system may not be optimal for photographical evaluation, another is likely to reflect better consistency with what can be seen through decomposition variations. This speaks to the dynamic and ongoing evolution of forensic science, where new guidelines require the introduction of photography as yet another resource within postmortem investigations and ultimately increase the capacity of forensic taphonomy (Carter et al., 2018).

3.6.2. Importance in Determining Cause of Death

Identification of the cause of death is very important in forensic pathology, particularly for legal and scientific purposes. Proper identification of the cause aids in identifying the circumstances of a death, which is important both in criminal investigations and in public health investigations. It assists authorities in providing closure to the deceased's family, as well as ensuring that any potential criminal activity is followed up on. Furthermore, it can be useful in epidemiological studies, determining mortality rate patterns that help form health policies. The complexity that arises from postmortem examination is facilitated by an in-depth analysis of multiple causes of death, with the significance underscored by expert training in forensic pathology to evaluate intricate cases effectively. In the determination of postmortem changes, the analysis of biological markers can help determine the cause of death successfully. For instance, estimation of postmortem interval using physiological changes such as rigor mortis and algor mortis helps determine the time of death, which would assist legal processes. Intraocular pressure measurement post-death has been recently found to be a valid parameter for the estimation of time since death, thereby allowing forensic scientists to determine the time of death with greater accuracy (Genero et al., 2019). These developments mirror the ongoing evolution of forensic techniques and indicate the importance of comprehensive postmortem analyses to arrive at accurate death determinations. Further, understanding the pathophysiologic mechanisms behind various causes of death is necessary in order to maximize clinical and forensic investigation. For example, myocardial infarction (MI) is a significant cause of death worldwide, and its pathological sequence provides insight into the time course of death (Bello et al., 2015). Recognition of the transition from reversible ischemic injury to irreversible myocardial cell death can elucidate the temporal correlation of death, which is key in distinguishing between natural and unnatural deaths. Greater understanding of these mechanisms not only enhances the validity of death investigations but also informs medical practice in formulating effective therapies and therapeutic interventions for cardiovascular disease. Thus, a thorough knowledge of postmortem changes is an integral component of the establishment of the cause of death and carries wide-ranging implications in both the forensic and the clinical field (Figure 3.19).

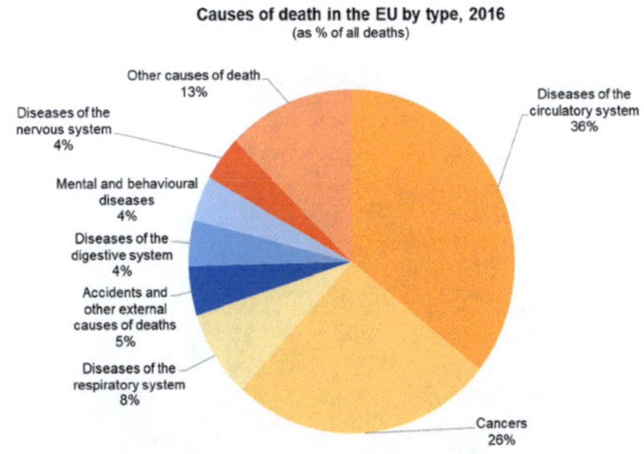

Figure 3.19. Causes and occurrence of deaths in the EU.

Source: https://ec.europa.eu/eurostat/documents/4187653/9834837/COD_2016_1/2ae221a6-87a0-4309-8693-9c3940c99c19?t=1562918638879.

3.6.3. Ethical Considerations in Forensic Studies

Ethical considerations are extremely significant in forensic studies, particularly when dealing with postmortem activities in human subjects. Scientists must achieve a balance between obtaining knowledge and the respect and dignity that is accorded to dead bodies, whether these are human cadavers or analog organisms such as pigs. Pig cadavers are globally accepted in forensic entomology and taphonomy due to the fact that they provide realistic models for carrying out decomposition studies. This practice has implications for ethics related to the well-being of non-human subjects, humane euthanasia, and how universally their findings can be applied to human biology. With the development of forensic science, it has become necessary to create and adhere to ethical principles that regard human and animal life while ensuring that findings derived are pertinent and useful in forensic investigations (Hall et al., 2019).

The ethical connotations of using human cadavers in forensic analysis make the issue more complex. Informed consent, especially when cadavers involve subjects whose bodies could have been donated to be utilized for scientific purposes, is essential. Researchers need to consider how to ensure the subjects themselves had agency over their decisions during their lifetimes and that there was not exploitation or abuse of their bodies. Additionally, religious and cultural beliefs surrounding death and the treatment of the deceased ought to be respected. Emotional impact on donor families and the public perception of forensic research add another layer to the ethical climate, necessitating cautious consideration and rigid ethical standards in research planning and conduct (Tieken et al., 2025). Furthermore, the combination of scientific investigation and ethics in forensic investigation includes the ethical requirement of scientists to report findings truthfully and openly. The potential consequences of their investigation, particularly in judicial proceedings, necessitate maintaining integrity and ethical accountability. Misrepresentation of findings on decomposition—affecting postmortem by trauma, environmental factors, or model cadaver choice—potentially endangers court trials extensively, thus preventing justice. Thus, it is the responsibility of researchers to uphold a high ethical standard whereby their contribution to forensic science does not inadvertently lead to harm, hence establishing a culture of ethical resilience that respects the deceased and upholds the trust of the public in forensic research (Tieken et al., 2025).

Test Your Knowledge

1. Which factor significantly affects the rate of decomposition?
2. What is intraocular pressure (IOP) used for in forensic investigations?

SUMMARY

In summary, research on postmortem changes provides profound insight into the biological and environmental processes involved in human decomposition. Awareness of those processes is not only relevant to forensic science but also to furthering human biological understanding. The study indicates that environments influence the rate and characteristics of decomposition and highlights the value of interdisciplinary research for forensic investigation. For instance, according to the findings of Santos et al. (2019), only decomposition scales used in cadaver condition analysis may yield inaccurate findings on postmortem intervals, hence implying that more scientific methods are needed for definite conclusions. Therefore, an integrated understanding of these factors enhances the ability to draw accurate conclusions regarding the time since death and the surrounding circumstances. Moreover, the interaction between postmortem changes and other mental conditions, such as major depressive disorder (MDD), adds a fascinating dimension to this subject. Importantly, cholinergic neurotransmission in the postmortem amygdala of MDD patients indicates that there are intricate interplays between mind and body deterioration upon death. The data that has been gathered through research, for example, findings in Argibay et al. (2015), shows that gender differences in the expression of neurochemistry can be used to further complicate understanding postmortem alterations. That data suggests that multidisciplinary methods of both forensic investigation and psychological testing are needed because they can aid in the interpretation of the effect of pre-mortem states on post-mortem states. Thus, postmortem studies need to consider a holistic understanding that includes psychological and biological assessments. Ultimately, ongoing postmortem research into changes of the human body will continue to advance and enhance our understanding of decomposition processes and their implications in forensic science. The integration of progress in genetic, biochemical, and environmental fields can encourage the methods used for postmortem interval estimation and comprehension of decomposition patterns. The perspectives outlined above, for instance, those in Santos et al. (2019) and Argibay et al. (2015), should lead to further studies on how various factors affect decomposition. Such analyses can, in fact, influence practices employed by forensic analysts and explain the complexities of the post-mortem human body. As the investigation continues, we can anticipate an increasingly sophisticated understanding of how both external environments and internal physiological states play a part in the complexities of postmortem alterations and thus improve the validity of forensic methods used in juridical procedures.

The postmortem changes in humans are a complex interplay of physiological processes that develop after death. Initially, rigor mortis is seen through muscle stiffening by the depletion of adenosine triphosphate (ATP), which leads to temporary firmness and stiffness of the body. This is followed by livor mortis, where blood settles in a pooling pattern, leading to small purplish discolorations on the skin. These body signs prove to be vital indicators to forensic examiners, assisting both in the estimation of postmortem interval as well as the detection of potential foul play. However, as highlighted by recent studies, total dependence on the conventional decomposition scales might be problematic. For instance, statistical insignificance obtained in investigations of various indoor environments emphasizes the importance of having integrated methodologies of forensic analysis with strength in determining the time since death and placing the evidence utilized during investigations (Santos et al., 2019). Furthermore, the environmental parameters controlling postmortem changes are considerably affected by environmental conditions. Temperature, humidity, and the existence of biological life may accelerate or decelerate the decomposition process, complicating the interpretation of forensic evidence. Environments vary to produce different decomposition rates, as seen in experiments that pit wet and dry environments against each other. In particular, bodies picked up indoors tend to have early decomposition, something that can obfuscate the time of death if misinterpreted. Thus, forensic experts are required to apply other scientific methods besides conventional decomposition analysis to deliver more precise outcomes. Recognizing such diversity allows forensic professionals to advance their methodologies, thereby achieving more credible outcomes in postmortem analysis and contributing to the global body of forensic science (Courchesne et al., 2019). Finally, the significance of learning postmortem changes goes beyond forensic examination; it contributes heavily to the understanding of human biology and health. What is learned through the study of decomposition can be used by medical science to better understand diseases and conditions that affect the processes of the body. By studying the phases of decomposition, scientists can make inferences about physiological changes at the time of death and any pre-existing health conditions. In addition, the interfacing of decomposition studies with cutting-edge science facilitates a comprehensive approach to human life cycles. This holistic approach, in addition to enhancing forensic methods, also sheds more light on post-mortem biological and environmental interactions. Fundamentally, studying postmortem changes provides insightful data to both the medical and forensic professions, an indication of the multidirectional essence of our engagements with death and life (Santos et al., 2019).

KEY TERMS FROM THIS CHAPTER

- Accuracy
- Algor mortis
- Forensic implications
- Genetic markers
- Livor mortis
- Postmortem changes
- Reliability
- Adenosine triphosphate
- Biological changes
- Forensic investigations
- Humidity
- Microorganisms
- Postmortem intervals
- Rigor mortis

CRITICAL THINKING QUESTIONS

1. **Which of the following is the correct sequence of postmortem changes?**
   a. Rigor mortis → Algor mortis → Livor mortis → Decomposition
   b. Livor mortis → Algor mortis → Rigor mortis → Decomposition
   c. Algor mortis → Livor mortis → Rigor mortis → Decomposition
   d. Decomposition → Rigor mortis → Livor mortis → Algor mortis
2. **What does the term "algor mortis" refer to?**
   a. The stiffening of muscles after death.
   b. The cooling of the body after death.
   c. The discoloration due to blood pooling.
   d. The decomposition of internal organs.
3. **Livor mortis typically begins to appear how long after death?**
   a. Immediately after death.
   b. 1–2 hours after death.
   c. 6–8 hours after death.
   d. 24 hours after death.
4. **What is the term for the settling of blood in the dependent areas of the body after death?**
   a. Algor mortis
   b. Livor mortis
   c. Rigor mortis
   d. Putrefaction
5. **What is marbling in the context of postmortem changes?**
   a. Stiffening of muscles due to rigor mortis.
   b. Discoloration caused by the decomposition of blood vessels.
   c. Cooling of the body resulting in pale skin.
   d. Swelling of tissues during putrefaction.

Short Answer Questions

1. What is a postmortem change?
2. What is rigor mortis?
3. What is livor mortis commonly referred to as?
4. What is the primary phenomenon described by algor mortis?
5. What advanced method has been found promising for assessing decomposition?

Answer to Critical Thinking Questions

1. (c); 2. (b); 3. (b); 4. (b); 5. (b)

REFERENCES

1. Abad Santos, J. (2019). Decomposition of pig carcasses at varying room temperature. https://core.ac.uk/download/228080080.pdf (accessed on 12th July 2025).
2. Aguet, F., Amador, R., Amadoz, A., et al. (2018). The effects of death and post-mortem cold ischemia on human tissue transcriptomes. https://core.ac.uk/download/157811337.pdf (accessed on 12th July 2025).
3. Ahmed, F., & Maisano, J. (2017). ToScA North America (6–8 June 2017, The University of Texas, Austin, TX) Program. https://core.ac.uk/download/211334283.pdf (accessed on 12th July 2025).
4. Alcalá Martínez, L., Andrews, P., Fernández Jalvo, Y., et al. (2002). Morphological taphonomic transformations of fossil bones in continental environments, and repercussions of their chemical composition. https://core.ac.uk/download/19725679.pdf (accessed on 12th July 2025).
5. Aleman, M., Byrne, B. A., Estell, K. E., et al. (2015). Pneumonia caused by Klebsiella spp. in 46 horses. https://core.ac.uk/download/323068316.pdf (accessed on 12th July 2025).
6. Allman, A., Annese, A., Lutti, A., Bailey, B., et al. (2012). Mapping the human cortical surface by combining quantitative T(1) with retinotopy. https://core.ac.uk/download/16220378.pdf (accessed on 12th July 2025).
7. Amendt, J., Bugelli, V., Campobasso, C. P., et al. (2020). A field study to evaluate PMI estimation methods for advanced decomposition stages. https://core.ac.uk/download/572838683.pdf (accessed on 12th July 2025).
8. An, H. J., Bereuter, T. L., Dimapasoc, L., et al. (2014). Glycosylated proteins preserved over millennia: N-glycan analysis of Tyrolean Iceman, Scythian Princess and Warrior. https://core.ac.uk/download/323070031.pdf (accessed on 12th July 2025).
9. Argibay, P., Bassi, S. C., Seney, M. L., et al. (2015). Elevated hippocampal cholinergic neurostimulation peptide precursor protein (HCNP-pp) mRNA in the amygdala in major depression. https://core.ac.uk/download/159285012.pdf (accessed on 12th July 2025).
10. Arumilli, M., Bathen-Noethen, A., Bhatti, S., et al. (2017). Generalized myoclonic epilepsy with photosensitivity in juvenile dogs caused by a defective DIRAS family GTPase 1. https://core.ac.uk/download/158346929.pdf (accessed on 12th July 2025).
11. Belhouari, A., El Abbadi, N., El Khasmi, M., et al. (2019). Relationship between 25-hydroxyvitamin D content and quality characteristics and lipid oxidation in raw and cooked camel meat during cold storage. http://agritrop.cirad.fr/595096/1/595096.pdf (accessed on 12th July 2025).
12. Bello, S., Fineschi, V., Neri, M., et al. (2015). The meaning of different forms of structural myocardial injury, immune response and timing of infarct necrosis and cardiac repair. https://core.ac.uk/download/54248087.pdf (accessed on 12th July 2025).
13. Benecke, M., Bux, R., Fornaro, P., et al. (2018). Float, explode or sink: Postmortem fate of lung-breathing marine vertebrates. https://core.ac.uk/download/159156116.pdf (accessed on 12th July 2025).
14. Brown, A. P., Ji, H., & Zhu, T. (2020). The emerging role of ten-eleven translocation 1 in epigenetic responses to environmental exposures. https://core.ac.uk/download/323070431.pdf (accessed on 12th July 2025).

15. Buras, K. L. (2006). Are enzymes accurate indicators of postmortem interval? A biochemical analysis. https://core.ac.uk/download/217400065.pdf (accessed on 12th July 2025).

16. Carter, D. O., Morgan, R. M., Rando, C., et al. (2018). The suitability of visual taphonomic methods for digital photographs: An experimental approach with pig carcasses in a tropical climate. https://core.ac.uk/download/144582757.pdf (accessed on 12th July 2025).

17. Casaccia, P., Emilsson, V., Fan, G., et al. (2014). Common dysregulation network in the human prefrontal cortex underlies two neurodegenerative diseases. https://core.ac.uk/download/323076793.pdf (accessed on 12th July 2025).

18. Cato, A. M. (2019). Macromorphological and microscopic effects of temperature in a controlled environment on the process of decomposition in bone. https://core.ac.uk/download/225563063.pdf (accessed on 12th July 2025).

19. Claus, S. P., Mora-Ortiz, M., Oregioni, A., et al. (2019). Thanatometabolomics: Introducing NMR-based metabolomics to identify metabolic biomarkers of the time of death. https://core.ac.uk/download/200749877.pdf (accessed on 12th July 2025).

20. Courchesne, E., Gazestani, V. H., Lewis, N. E., et al. (2019). The ASD living biology: From cell proliferation to clinical phenotype. https://core.ac.uk/download/323064765.pdf (accessed on 12th July 2025).

21. Dowell-Curby, J. (2017). A review of the microbiome associated with human decomposition. https://core.ac.uk/download/141488869.pdf (accessed on 12th July 2025).

22. Frati, A., Hyder, A. A., Palmer, A. M., Selassie, A. W., Buller, B., Roozenbeek, B., Murray, C. J., et al. (2018). Clinical-pathological study on β-APP, IL-1β, GFAP, NFL, Spectrin II, 8OHdG, TUNEL, miR-21, miR-16, miR-92 expressions to verify DAI-diagnosis, grade, and prognosis. https://core.ac.uk/download/154949003.pdf (accessed on 12th July 2025).

23. Genero, S., Gerometta, R. M. d. R., Larroza, G. O., et al. (2019). Variation of the intraocular pressure in relation to time of death: Contribution to the determination of the true postmortem interval (PMI). https://core.ac.uk/download/323211019.pdf (accessed on 12th July 2025).

24. Hall, M. J. R., Matuszewski, S., Moreau, G., et al. (2019). Pigs' vs people: The use of pigs as analogues for humans in forensic entomology and taphonomy research. https://core.ac.uk/download/334608154.pdf (accessed on 12th July 2025).

25. Hoeland, K. M. (2021). Investigating the potential of postmortem metabolomics in mammalian decomposition studies in outdoor settings. https://core.ac.uk/download/524887815.pdf (accessed on 12th July 2025).

26. Hough, M. (2022). Effect of coastal environments on the post mortem interval of a pig carrion: Implications for human decomposition. https://core.ac.uk/download/539106878.pdf (accessed on 12th July 2025).

27. Huey, T. N. (2013). Defining postmortem changes in Western Montana: A longitudinal study of the rate and sequence of surface and burial decomposition. https://core.ac.uk/download/267574429.pdf (accessed on 12th July 2025).

28. Iannitelli, A., Quartini, A., & Tirassa, P. (2015). Nerve growth factor, brain-derived neurotrophic factor, and the chronobiology of mood: A new insight into the "neurotrophic hypothesis." https://core.ac.uk/download/54533223.pdf (accessed on 12th July 2025).

29. Johar, D. K., Kumar, D., & Mungra, K. (2022). A systematic review on estimation of time since death from eyes. https://core.ac.uk/download/620835521.pdf (accessed on 12th July 2025).

30. Kesharwani, R. (2025). Post-mortem interval estimation through metabolomics of pineal gland. https://core.ac.uk/download/657073484.pdf (accessed on 12th July 2025).

31. Love, J. C. (2001). Evaluation of decay odor as a time since death indicator. https://core.ac.uk/download/588288266.pdf (accessed on 12th July 2025).

32. Nixon, G. (2017). Beyond the circle of life. https://core.ac.uk/download/131182523.pdf (accessed on 12th July 2025).

33. Piegari, G. (2018). New insights in veterinary forensic medicine and pathology. https://core.ac.uk/download/328815001.pdf (accessed on 12th July 2025).

34. Proctor, K. W. (2007). Estimating the early postmortem interval in domestic canines. https://core.ac.uk/download/268804644.pdf (accessed on 12th July 2025).

35. Reisdorf, A., & Wuttke, M. (2018). Re-evaluating Moodie's opisthotonic-posture hypothesis in fossil vertebrates Part I: Reptiles—the taphonomy of the bipedal dinosaurs Compsognathus longipes and Juravenator starki from the Solnhofen Archipelago (Jurassic, Germany). https://core.ac.uk/download/159149524.pdf (accessed on 12th July 2025).

36. Sharanowski, B. (2004). Initial studies in forensic entomology in Saskatchewan: Decomposition and insect succession on pig carrion in the prairie ecozone. https://core.ac.uk/download/226145888.pdf (accessed on 12th July 2025).

37. Solanki, M. (2019). Microbiome biomarkers–Post mortem interval. https://core.ac.uk/download/222929135.pdf (accessed on 12th July 2025).

38. Spencer, J. R. (2013). Defining postmortem changes in Western Montana: The effects of climate and environment on the rate and sequence of decomposition using pig (Sus scrofa) cadavers. https://core.ac.uk/download/267578045.pdf (accessed on 12th July 2025).

39. Tieken, A. C. (2025). Comparative analysis of gunshot trauma and decomposition in Southeast Nebraska. https://core.ac.uk/download/655998248.pdf (accessed on 12th July 2025).

40. Wagensveld, I. M. (2020). Hospital implementation and acceptance of minimally invasive autopsy. https://core.ac.uk/download/287757145.pdf (accessed on 12th July 2025).

AUTOPSY TECHNIQUES

4

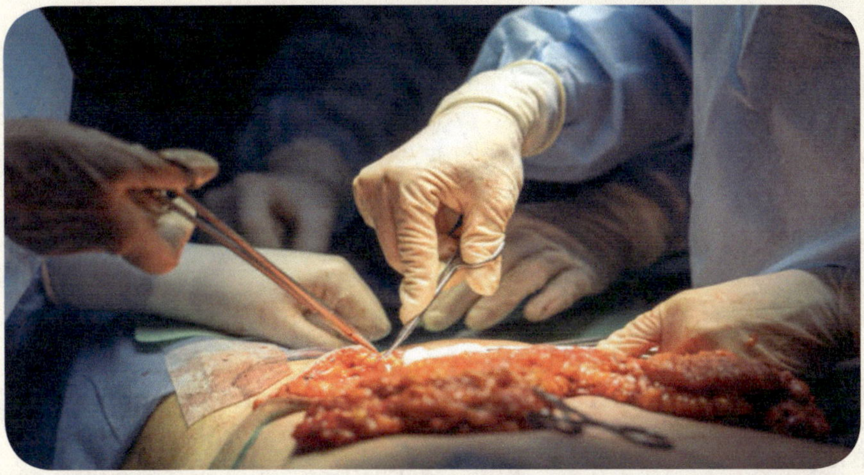

LEARNING OBJECTIVES

After studying this chapter, you will be able to:

1. Explain the historical background of autopsy;
2. Describe the types of autopsies;
3. Know the autopsy procedure;
4. Describe the tools and equipment used in autopsies;
5. Understand the role of the pathologist;
6. Know the legal and ethical considerations surrounding autopsy techniques.

Introduction

Autopsy techniques are a significant branch of forensic medicine and science responsible mainly for establishing the cause of death and disease pattern studies. Autopsy is more than just an intellectual exercise; it reveals information about the population's health, legal cases, and medical research advancements. By the methodical examination of post-mortem organs and tissues, forensic pathologists conduct an extended investigation that not only identifies pathological changes but also diagnoses underlying causes of death that were not identified or went unremarked during life. The discipline thus not only serves individual cases but also informs epidemiological studies on a larger scale, ultimately influencing policy and preventive healthcare measures. This call for greater transparency and methodological rigor in investigations is not limited to living subjects but is extended to autopsy techniques, which need rigorous reporting and replicability for their scientific validity (Percie et al., 2020). Autopsy technique continuously improves from conventional techniques to modern developments, and these have a significant impact on the approaches investigators employ when interpreting death. Traditionally, autopsies had been under suspicion, bedeviled by ethical issues and cultural taboos. However, current thought accepts that autopsies are an essential tool for shedding light on deaths with causes that are unclear, especially when there are injuries of a suspect nature or a threat to public health.

The addition of high-technology aids, including imaging and histopathology, has continued to extend the diagnostic roles of forensic pathologists. These technologies enhance the accuracy of evidence and are presently unavoidable in cases requiring a meticulous examination of body tissue. In addition, as forensic science continues to develop, the application of innovative methods presents a stimulating debate regarding optimal methods and ethical regulations for postmortem examination and disease identification, further emphasizing the need for high standards (Jürgen Rehm et al., 2017). In conclusion, the significance of autopsy techniques in humans comes out through their multifaceted use in medicine and law. The techniques facilitate a better understanding of the multifarious causes of death, hence equipping clinicians and legal experts with crucial information for sound intervention and policy making. In light of advances in the area, continuous reflection on methodological strategies, coupled with an affinity for adherence to established reporting standards, is of major importance. This combination ensures autopsy findings not only meet the rigorous standards of scientific research but also are worthy contributions to forensic pathology and public health advancements. As the autopsy procedure discussion continues, the embracing of transparency, ethical standards, and emerging technologies will be essential in furthering this life-saving practice's appreciation and significance (Figure 4.1).

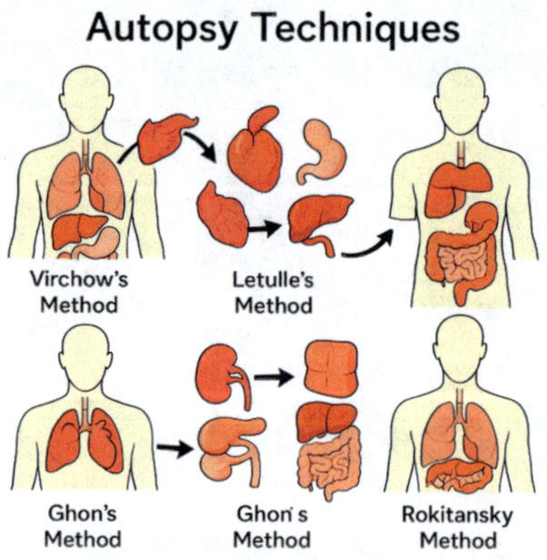

Figure 4.1. Autopsy techniques.

Source: https://www.diginerve.com/blogs/wp-content/uploads/2025/05/ChatGPT-Image-May-28-2025-04_38_22-PM.png.

Definition of Autopsy

Autopsy, the essence of forensic science and medicine, is the complete examination of the deceased body for the purpose of determining the cause and manner of death. The practice is normally undertaken by a pathologist who closely inspects the body, noticing its inner and outer features. Through the dissection of anatomical structures, examination of tissue samples, and sometimes the use of fancy imaging machines, autopsies give valuable information regarding pathologies that are not visible in a superficial examination. Data gathered not only assists legal investigations but also contributes to public health knowledge by identifying disease trends and possible health risks. Thus, the word autopsy is not a mere inspection; it is a multidisciplinary approach to understanding human death and disease processes, and hence carries importance in clinical as well as legal contexts. The technique of autopsies is again categorized into various types, viz., forensic and clinical autopsies. Forensic autopsies are conducted primarily in legal contexts, typically following suspicious or unexplained deaths. Here, the pathologist makes detailed documentation of evidence that may be vital in investigations using techniques that include toxicological screening for verification of poison or drug presence. Clinical autopsies, on the contrary, seek to uncover pathological findings that enhance clinical practice and medical knowledge. Autopsies have a standardized procedure of techniques and protocols such that the results will be valid and statistically reliable. This bifurcation of the forms of autopsy works to highlight the adaptability of the autopsy process, meeting both legal and medical investigation needs uniquely, providing a coherent model for the understanding of death. Additionally, a growing library of literature emphasizes the importance of emerging technologies in streamlining autopsy techniques. For instance, imaging methods such as magnetic resonance spectroscopy have been explored for their potential to reveal tissue metabolic changes, complementing the traditional autopsy's findings.

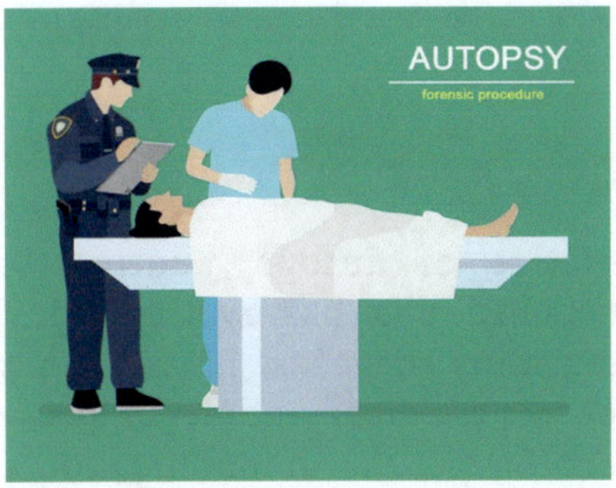

Figure 4.2. Autopsy.

Source: https://www.shutterstock.com/image-vector/flat-illustration-autopsy-murder-victim-600nw-517259449.jpg.

Later studies have shown how biochemical analysis, combined with non-invasive imaging, can provide a more advanced perspective of heterogeneous pathological disorders of organ systems (Agrawala et al., 2009). Also, the incorporation of new psychoactive substances in autopsy research raised questions regarding their impact on death, necessitating an expanded definition that encompasses newer chemicals and related dangers (Mannocchi et al., 2015). As medicine also evolves, so does autopsy definition, reflecting the procedures dynamic character in responding to contemporary health issues (Figure 4.2).

Importance of Autopsy in Forensic Science

The conduct of an autopsy is a fundamental cornerstone in forensic science, providing valuable information that can cast light on the circumstances surrounding the death of a person. Autopsies are not medical examinations; they are comprehensive evaluations that can identify underlying health issues, trauma, or even poisoning that may not be picked up by initial investigations. By using various techniques such as histopathological examination and immunohistochemistry, forensic pathologists can provide much information about the deceased. For instance, recent studies have indicated how autopsy findings can reveal the effect of diseases such as COVID-19 on the fertility of men by illustrating testicular abnormalities and immune reactions, thereby asserting the importance of autopsy findings in understanding both physiological and pathological processes (Li et al., 2020). Therefore, the ability to include clinical histories and autopsy reports enhances the potential for accurate death determination, thereby making the justice systems more effective. Furthermore, the value of autopsies goes beyond determining cause and mode of death; it enters into the domains of improving public health and safety. Forensic experts may trace patterns of death or injury through autopsy procedures that may suggest broader problems within society, such as patterns of violence, accidents, or emerging infectious diseases. Such systemic information can inform prevention and public health initiatives to mitigate mortality among particular populations or regions. Community health can be considerably improved as patterns established post-mortem are alleviated, contributing to evidence-based interventions in healthcare systems. Forensic anthropology, too, is enriched by autopsies through becoming interdisciplinary techniques that introduce nascent approaches, thus challenging and reconstituting the traditional discourses of death in society (Dennis et al., 2008). The multi-faceted importance of autopsies in forensic science, hence, stretches from case-by-case applicability to public health implications. Finally, the introduction of advanced autopsy techniques has initiated a paradigm shift in the usage and understanding of forensic science.

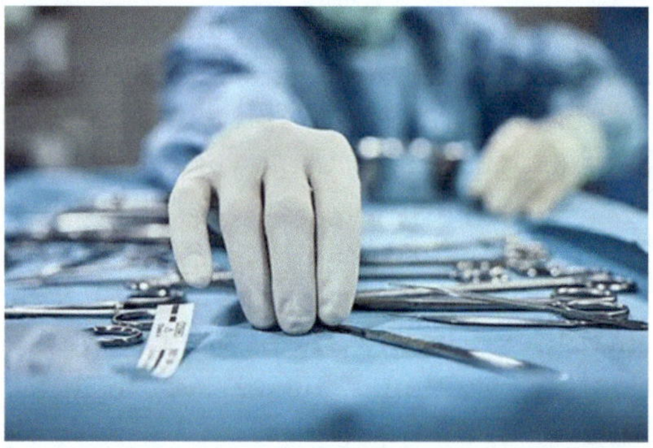

Figure 4.3. An autopsy (post-mortem exam or necropsy) is the examination of the body of a dead person and is performed primarily to determine the cause of death.

Source: https://images.medicinenet.com/images/article/main_image/surgery-prep.jpg?output-quality=75.

The advent of DNA analysis and quantitative methods has further entrenched the role of forensic pathologists beyond mere victim identification to reconstructive analytical investigation of death circumstances. Interdisciplinary collaboration among forensic anthropology, forensic taphonomy, and other paradigms of analysis continues to improve the investigative process by allowing a better grasp of the conditions of death. Such advances have broadened the scope of forensic science and increased its application in legal settings, so that the evidence submitted to courts is sound and scientifically valid. As forensic science develops and widens, the utility of autopsy techniques remains paramount in its capacity to stretch beyond the mechanical quantification of the body and into the tangled web of social, legal, and scientific understanding of life and death (Dennis et al., 2008). Thus, the role of autopsy in forensic science is paramount because it serves not only as an investigative tool but also a healing and justice instrument for society (Figure 4.3).

4.1. Historical Background of Autopsy

Learning Outcome

1. Learn about ancient practices and beliefs.
2. Understand the development of modern autopsy techniques.
3. Describe the key figures in the history of autopsy.

The practice of autopsy, dating back to ancient civilizations, has evolved significantly over thousands of years, having a profound influence on medical and legal procedures. In ancient Egypt, the mummification process showed some early understanding of anatomy and the human body, with priests cutting open corpses to prepare them for the next world. Autopsies were religious and practical, allowing for early understanding of the spread of disease. By. In the Greco-Roman period, doctors such as Hippocrates and Galen started conducting extensive research on the human body, which was a precursor to abandoning religious explanations of death for empirical observations. This was the start of practices employed in current autopsy, where scholars in academia started integrating dissection as a method of knowledge regarding human physiology and pathology, thus placing autopsies in a more prominent position in medicine and paving the way for forensic application in contemporary practice. The Middle Ages witnessed centuries of inertia in autopsy's scientific learning due to prevalent religious dogma discouraging dissection. However, the Renaissance heralded a fundamental revival in anatomy studies, spearheaded by those such as Andreas Vesalius. His work, De humani corporis fabrica, revolutionized the science of anatomy, incorporating personal observation and detailed descriptions of the human form. During this period, autopsies began acquiring popularity not only for their use in the realm of medicine but also in law. The necessity for proper investigations into death grew, and accordingly, medical knowledge entered the domain of law, and thus, autopsy became an important investigative tool in criminal cases and forensic science. This shift reflects the increasing recognition of the autopsy as essential in determining the cause of death and for legal culpability. Autopsy practices are now inherent to medical studies and forensic science, attesting to their time-honored relevance. The development of rigorous methodologies, such as cranial suture closure age studies, is evidence of the scientific advancement continually refining autopsy procedures (Buzdar et al., 2024). As forensic science has developed, so has its range of applications that encompass complex legal matters and encourage public health through comprehensive post-mortem examinations. This change serves the medical community and has profound implications for the judicial system, enabling responsible and precise death investigations. Legal and moral criteria that regulate autopsies are constantly shaped by experience, emphasizing society's dedication to knowledge of human mortality and responsibility in countless scenarios (Bence László Lukács et al., 2024) (Figure 4.4).

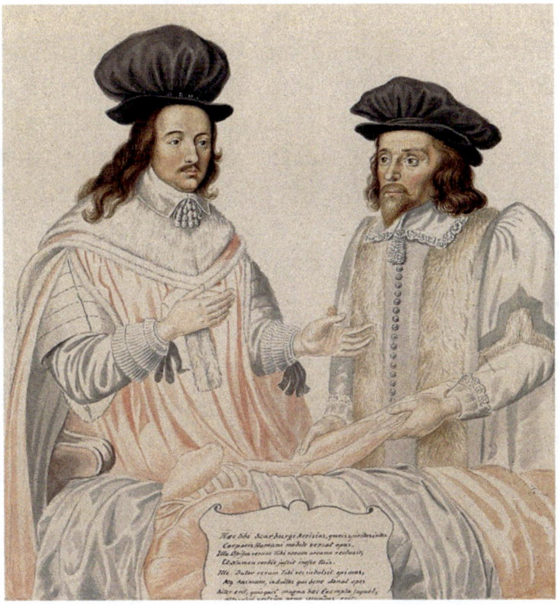

Figure 4.4. English physicians Charles Scarborough and Edward Arris performing an autopsy in 1651 (watercolor painted in 1818 by G.P. Harding from an original work in the Barber Surgeons' Hall, London).

Source: https://cdn.britannica.com/09/205609-050-7ABD6843/physicians-English-Charles-Scarborough-Edward-Arris-autopsy-1651.jpg.

4.1.1. Ancient Practices and Beliefs

Throughout history, various civilizations developed sophisticated practices with death and post-mortem examination of the deceased. Hepatoscopy is one such practice whereby ancient civilizations such as the Babylonians and the Etruscans employed the liver as a tool for divination to acquire knowledge about the future. The practice, hepatomancy, involved the inspection of the liver of sacrificed animals, predominantly sheep, after divination rituals. Ancient writing, like that of the Hebrew prophet Ezekiel, illustrates the significance afforded to the liver in religious and political contexts, which retained its perceived connection to supernatural power. This illustrates how deeply ingrained such beliefs , and are now categorized as being within anatomical study, and illustrates the ancient entanglement of science and superstition when attempting to ascertain mortality and health (Omar et al., 2021). As the body was studied for the sake of learning about death, ancient civilizations especially feared the act of dissection. Religious beliefs during those times tended to place the body in a position that it shouldn't be slain, and this contributed largely to shaping their idea of anatomy. This comingling of body and belief can be seen in the ancient Egyptian funeral rites, in which preservation of the body through mummification was at the heart of their approach to life after death. Egyptian priests, like their modern autopsy technicians' counterparts, were instrumental in preparing the dead for the hereafter and ensuring that no real changes were wrought in the body.

The cultural significance of maintaining the sanctity of the body was discovered to be crucial, linking traditional practices and our modern beliefs in terms of the necessity and morality of autopsy techniques (María Maixenchs et al., 2016). The progress in autopsy procedures also encountered hurdles from prevailing beliefs about the soul and the body's final fate. For instance, in Etruscan culture, the haruspex interpreted omens from animal guts, which was a shift from perceiving the body as a purely material entity to believing it as a vehicle carrying messages from gods. This shift occurred when there was an intricate coexistence between comprehending the material aspects of the body and the religious significance of death. With the continued evolution of autopsy practice during the Renaissance period, the ancient emphasis on interpretation of liver omens served as a precursor to more systematized anatomical investigation, revealing an early shift from mystical belief toward an emergent scientific interest that would ultimately inform today's autopsy practices (Omar et al., 2021).

4.1.2. Development of Modern Autopsy Techniques

The technology used to conduct autopsies has undergone a total transformation, particularly with the introduction of advanced technologies in the health sector. Autopsies were traditionally conducted primarily to ascertain the cause of death, and naked eye examination and rudimentary dissection procedures were used. The use of imaging devices such as computed tomography (CT) and magnetic resonance imaging (MRI) has revolutionized the practice. These modalities enable non-invasive visualization of structures in the body so that pathologists can diagnose conditions and diseases without dissecting cadavers. Not only does this preserve the body for families, but it also broadens the scope of information obtainable from an autopsy, thereby enhancing our understanding of pathological conditions. Growing reliance on these imaging modalities is a reflection of the trend towards a more systemic and advanced approach to examining human remains in the practice of modern medicine. In addition to the technological advancement in imaging, the incorporation of molecular biology as a component of autopsy techniques has been a major paradigm shift. Application of forensic genetics, as highlighted by emerging developments, has supplemented traditional autopsy methods by enabling more precise identification of genetic markers in deceased individuals. Polymerase chain reaction (PCR) and next-generation sequencing are among the methods employed by pathologists to extract and study DNA from biological traces in autopsy samples. This approach is not only for determining identity but also for determining cause and manner of death through further clarification of the genetic underpinnings of different diseases and conditions. Forensic genetics, therefore, has become a critical tool in autopsy examinations, making provision for more knowledge-based conclusions regarding deaths while contributing to the field of forensic science and criminal investigations at large (Kozma et al., 2018). Besides, the drive towards modernizing autopsies has also been fueled by the idea of interdisciplinary collaboration in which cutting-edge technology is merged with tried-and-tested medical expertise. Integration of artificial intelligence (AI) into pathology has begun, making it possible for better data analysis so that autopsy reports can be mapped against big medical history databases. This integration of AI with the autopsy technique can potentially yield insights that were unavailable through manual methods. Secondly, the emphasis on health equity explained in the United Nations' Sustainable Development Goals makes such innovative techniques necessary for attaining health equity and optimizing the quality of investigation across populations (Farooq et al., 2017). With such improvements, the practice of autopsy techniques will likely be transformed, leading to greater precision and efficiency in the determination of the cause of death as well as disease burden in populations.

4.1.3. Key Figures in the History of Autopsy

The history of autopsy techniques is in great part attributed to the innovators who played a key role in stabilizing the practice as a cornerstone of modern medicine. Andreas Vesalius is one such figure, a 16th-century anatomist whose detailed dissections and systematic observations formed the foundation of human anatomy learning. Vesalius challenged preconceived notions from ancient writings and advocated the merit of first-hand observation against speculation. His groundbreaking treatise, De humani corporis fabrica, not only explained anatomical structures but also advocated the use of autopsy as a procedure, providing a means to investigate the cause of death. This development towards empirical investigation set a precedent for later anatomists and pathologists, raising the scientific rigor accompanying autopsy procedures and ultimately having an influence on medical practice and education for centuries to follow. Another key proponent of autopsy development is the Italian physician Giovanni Morgagni, whose 18th-century contributions further etched the autopsy's role in medical diagnosis.

Morgagni's magnum opus, *De sedibus et causis morborum per anatomem indagatis*, emphasized the relationship between anatomical observations and processes of disease, providing a methodical process to consider pathology's relationship with clinical symptoms. His work highlighted not just the necessity of autopsies for verification of diagnosis but also their use in advancing medical knowledge through revealing underlying pathological conditions. The integration of autopsy findings with clinical practice changed the nature of the field, and Morgagni is a pioneering figure whose work continues to have relevance in current discussions regarding the role of autopsy in teaching and practice in the medical field. In the 19th century, Rudolf Virchow was a strong supporter of the autopsy, urging its application in medical research and public health. Referenced as the father of modern pathology, Virchow formulated the law of cellular pathology, where he said disease was a consequence of cell structure changes. His methodical process of postmortem examinations, coupled with his insistence on recording observations accurately, made the autopsy better. Virchow's impact was not only in describing the worth of autopsy to the mechanism of disease, but also in advocating for it as a tool for promoting public health. With his work, the autopsy had moved from procedural nicety to a necessary practice that produced valuable information not just for individual diagnoses, but also epidemiologic research, which guaranteed its worthiness in medical literature (Figure 4.5).

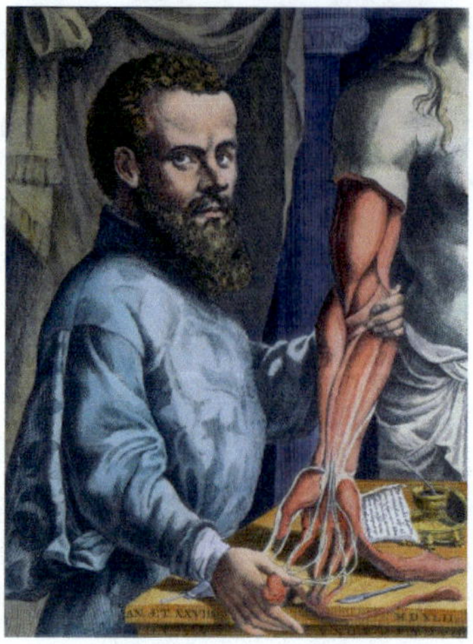

Figure 4.5. In the 16th century, Flemish physician Andreas Vesalius revolutionized the practice of medicine by providing accurate and detailed descriptions of the anatomy of the human body, which were based on his dissections of cadavers.

Source: https://cdn.britannica.com/83/92983-050-CDFD0992/Andreas-Vesalius-Flemish-practice-medicine-anatomy-human.jpg.

Test Your Knowledge

1. Which ancient cultures are known for practicing hepatoscopy?
2. Which ancient text mentions the significance of the liver in divination?

4.2. Types of Autopsies

Learning Outcome

1. Understand the clinical autopsy.
2. Define the forensic autopsy.
3. Describe the development of virtual autopsy techniques.

Understanding various types of autopsies is at the core of the broader scenario of forensic medicine and pathology. Clinically and generally, autopsies can be divided into clinical and forensic. Clinical autopsies serve mostly for educational and research purposes, providing information regarding disease processes, the effectiveness of treatment, and potential outcomes of patient management. These autopsies are most often performed in a hospital setting after death due to natural causes, so that doctors can correlate clinical information with findings after death. Forensic autopsies, in contrast, are conducted when a death occurs under suspicious conditions. Their primary purpose is the procurement of legal evidence and the determination of cause and manner of death, which may prove important in criminal investigations or court cases. Both types of autopsy are quite significant in assisting to boost medical information as well as maintain justice through thorough examination of deceased individuals. Autopsies can be further categorized based on their objectives, including diagnostic, educational, and research autopsies. Diagnostic autopsies are conducted to uncover concealed or hidden causes of death, thus assisting in affirming or supplementing previous medical diagnoses.

These autopsies are most likely to result in the development of better medical practice and a better understanding of various diseases. Autopsies for education, on the other hand, are primarily done for the education of doctors. By seeing the pathological changes following death, medical residents and students receive hands-on experience in correlating the clinical signs with pathological effects, which is required for their medical education. Investigative autopsies, however, are focused on gathering data for scientific investigation, and in most situations, they contribute substantially to the fields of epidemiology or research into specific diseases. Both subtypes point to the multiple functions performed by autopsy procedures in the enhancement of human health benefits. The practice of autopsy, moreover, has evolved in history and is also associated with medical technology progress and changes in attitudes of individuals toward death and postmortem procedures. Following the development of minimally invasive procedures, various new techniques have been created to carry out autopsies without disrupting the body. Imaging techniques, for instance, such as CT scans and MRI scans, have begun to supplement the conventional autopsy methods, allowing a non-invasive examination that is able to determine internal abnormalities without interfering with the corpse. This shift is particularly relevant in cases where there are religious or cultural complaints against conventional autopsies. Discussion concerning the ethical terrain of necropsy and consent illustrates how the balance between the advance of knowledge via science and being respectful of the dead and the family is tense. With the controversy on the types of autopsies abating, no letup, the demand for new techniques to meet medical and social requirements so that autopsies remain a realistic and informative procedure lingers (Figure 4.6).

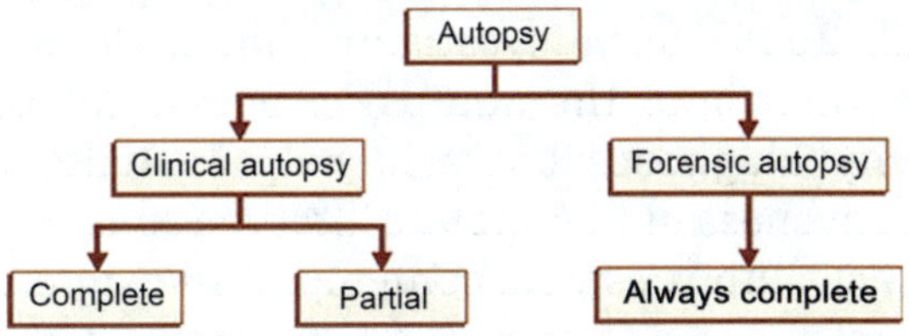

Figure 4.6. Types of autopsies.

Source: https://d45jl3w9libvn.cloudfront.net/jaypee/static/books/9789350254936/Chapters/images/119-1.jpg.

4.2.1. Clinical Autopsy

Clinical autopsy is a significant tool in the medical profession, employed to establish the causes of death and enhance medical practice. It is a process that is typically performed in hospitals with the purpose of gaining valuable information that may have proven hard to achieve through isolated clinical examination. By examining tissues and organs in close detail, pathologists can make diagnoses that may otherwise have been overlooked when a patient was alive, helping to advance clinical practices and guidelines. Clinical autopsies also yield demographic and epidemiological information, which can be applied to guide public health initiatives and assist with patient care. The findings of the study extend beyond case-by-case relevance, offering proof for subsequent medical interventions and expanding our understanding of disease progression. One of the most significant aspects of the clinical autopsy is its role as a link between pathological information and clinical observation. For instance, new technical advances in imaging techniques, such as amyloid imaging with positron emission tomography (PET), have revolutionized our view of neurodegenerative conditions like Alzheimer's disease. As well established in the literature, amyloid imaging can identify fibrillar beta-amyloid deposits related to cognitive impairment, thereby establishing an important link between biochemical markers and clinical symptomatology (Jagust et al., 2009). Such investigative methods, when integrated into the autopsy process, not only clarify diagnoses but also help evaluate the effectiveness of therapeutic interventions. Thus, clinical autopsies with contemporary diagnostic capacity provide increased understanding of disease processes and facilitate improved patient care. Beyond their utility for diagnosis, clinical autopsies have significant impacts on health care policy-making and research. By analyzing autopsy reports, researchers can define trends or patterns in the prevalence and progression of disease, thereby informing clinical practice guidelines and health policy. In HBV infections, studies have shown that HBV DNA can be sustained in other extrahepatic tissues, even when liver replication has ceased (Davidson et al., 1995). This shows the need to carry out comprehensive clinical autopsies to uncover such discoveries that would inform treatment and prevention protocols. Ultimately, clinical autopsies not only benefit individual patient knowledge but also enable aggregate medical knowledge, pointing towards a more intelligent and effective healthcare system.

4.2.2. Forensic Autopsy

Forensic autopsy is a critical scientific procedure in investigating unexplained death. Forensic autopsy, unlike normal hospital autopsies, specifically exists for legal investigation purposes, often under conditions of violence or suspicion. Forensic pathologists carefully examine corpses to ascertain cause and manner of death, taking tangible evidence that may aid criminal prosecutions. Such analyses not only encompass pathological reports but also toxicological analysis, which can pick up substance abuse or poisoning. Findings from a forensic autopsy can heavily influence the verdict in legal cases, and hence it is very important for professionals to maintain high standards during the process of analysis so that their findings will hold up in court (Jangid et al., 2024). In the last decade, the incorporation of newer imaging modalities, such as computed tomography (CT) and magnetic resonance imaging (MRI), has revolutionized forensic autopsy protocols.

Also referred to as virtual autopsy techniques, these tools facilitate a painless and thorough examination of the body without jeopardizing the physical evidence, providing crucial information about traumatic injury or underlying medical illnesses. Internal organs are observable to forensic examiners, and foreign matter can be identified, which could be the determining factor for the precise cause of death. However, although virtual autopsy techniques have numerous advantages, there are a few disadvantages too, such as the need for high-level equipment and training, which may not always be within the reach of every forensic center (Jangid et al., 2024). Age estimation based on cranial suture closure is also a critical part of forensic autopsy that highlights the interdisciplinary nature of the field. In accordance with studies, cranial suture closure varies greatly with age, and forensic pathologists can make educated estimates of the age at death of the individual. One of the studies employed a standardized scoring scale to measure the degree of suture closure in human cadavers and found that it generally occurs after the age of 60. This not only aids in identification in criminal investigations but also serves as an important variable in age-related legal prosecutions, pointing towards the central involvement of forensic autopsy in individual as well as communal contexts. Identifying the consequences of the above forensic procedures enhances the contribution of forensic autopsies to modern criminal justice systems (Figure 4.7).

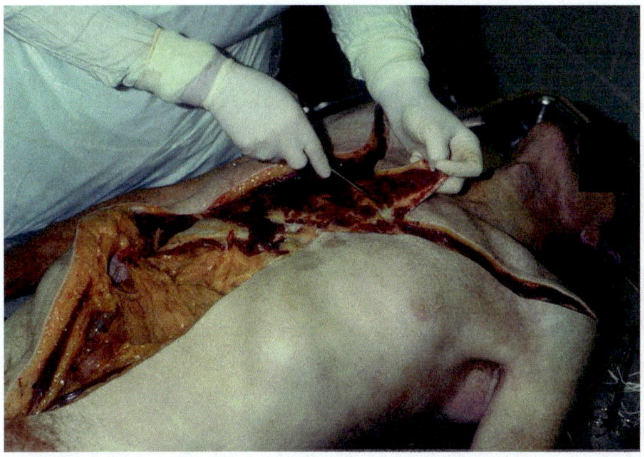

Figure 4.7. Forensic autopsy.

Source: https://media.springernature.com/lw685/springer-static/image/chp%3A10.1007%2F978-1-61779-058-4_7/MediaObjects/978-1-61779-058-4_7_Fig9_HTML.jpg.

4.2.3. Virtual Autopsy

The development of virtual autopsy techniques is a significant advance in forensic pathology that bridges the gap between traditional autopsies and modern imaging technology. Virtual autopsies employ non-invasive techniques such as computed tomography (CT) and magnetic resonance imaging (MRI) to create a three-dimensional reconstruction of the human body. With this, forensic pathologists can examine the internal structures and determine injury with extremely high precision without disrupting the integrity of the body. The fact that virtual autopsies are non-surgical not only respects the deceased but also provides useful information, which could prove useful in legal inquiries. Indeed, as forensic science progresses, virtual autopsy will prove an important instrument in demystifying complex cases where old-fashioned techniques may fall short, enabling us to have a better general idea of cause and manner of death. Besides, CT technology application has shown certain potential in wound ballistics, leading to enhanced complex trauma scenario analysis. By defining complex projectile trajectories and patterns of injury, virtual autopsy techniques improve the identification of gunshot wounds and other ballistic injuries, particularly in challenging cases with penetrating brain or abdominal wounds. With the current literature, this method's ability to image wound paths in unprecedented clarity surpasses traditional post-mortem analysis techniques, which lack the precision needed for such clarity. Furthermore, the inclusion of virtual autopsy into routine forensic practice can decrease the investigative process and aid in better trauma care. Hence, its incorporation into standard forensic procedure not only enables credible forensic conclusions but also signifies the medical imaging innovations that significantly enhance our understanding of human anatomy under various circumstances (Parvez et al., 2025). Apart from enhancing examination of adult corpses, virtual autopsy techniques are being weighed for their applicability in children's autopsies, particularly in exploring fetal heart anatomy.

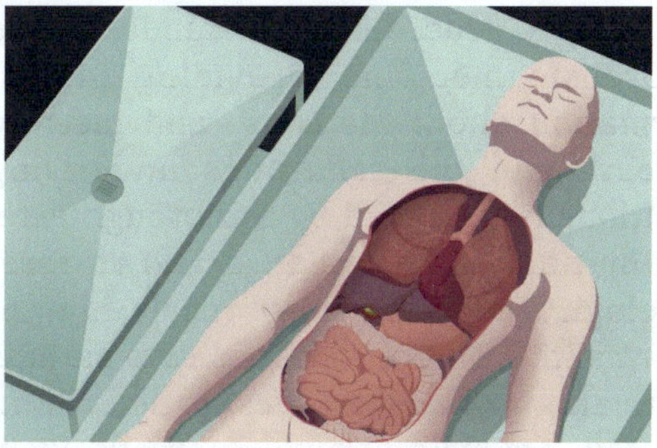

Figure 4.8. Virtual autopsy.

Source: https://media.australian.museum/media/dd/images/virtual_autopsy.5a7eb65.width-1200.27ff3a6.jpg.

A pilot study proved the feasibility of reconstruction of cardiac anatomy from histological sections of fetuses, pointing to the possibility of non-invasive means to validate suspected congenital heart disease. This new technique provides a valuable option when standard autopsy techniques are limited due to the minute size of anatomical structures. The precise visual depiction of important cardiac features via computer-aided 3D reconstruction ensures the promising role of virtual autopsy in pediatric pathology. As the resources for this technique keep improving, it can most likely redefine clinical practice for fetal examinations, ensuring proper preservation of crucial information about heart structures and their easy retrievability for future testing (Ruican et al., 2021) (Figure 4.8).

Test Your Knowledge

1. What is a clinical autopsy?
2. What is a forensic autopsy?

4.3. Autopsy Procedure

Learning Outcome

1. Prepare and consent for an autopsy.
2. Describe the external and internal examination during an autopsy.

The autopsy procedure is a standard practice in forensic medicine, providing important information about the cause and mechanism of death and the conditions underlying it. Traditionally preceded by a thorough external examination, the procedure allows forensic pathologists to inspect any visible injuries or abnormalities. This provides access to the internal examination, where the investigation continues in detail. Scalpels and saws are utilized for cutting to access internal organs systematically. Standard procedure is that vital organs such as the heart, lungs, and liver are thoroughly inspected, most commonly in combination with a histological work-up to determine disease that is not easily recognizable. The careful checks help to determine pathology fairly definitely and also generally have a significant influence on forensic conclusions as well as legal decisions. In addition to traditional methods, the inclusion of advanced technologies has also revolutionized the autopsy process. Modern practices have adopted techniques such as 3D imaging and virtual autopsy, which facilitate non-invasive examination. The use of imaging modalities enhances the visualization and assessment of internal structures without needing extensive physical dissection. This is particularly useful in situations where keeping the physical integrity of the body intact is paramount, for example, culturally or religiously. Also, applying artificial intelligence to the process of autopsy allows for the exploration of vast volumes of information, improving the precision of diagnosis and prognosis. By detecting trends and indicating abnormal results, AI enables a more neutral and efficient autopsy procedure that can potentially eradicate human prejudice (Kumar et al., 2024). Moreover, the anatomical discoveries disclosed during autopsies significantly influence subsequent medical and legal actions. For instance, some anatomical variations, including those of the tentorial notch, provide valuable information about neurosurgical implications. A human cadaver experiment confirms the importance of understanding these anatomical structures and their implications in performing medical interventions (Sharma et al., 2025). Not only can forensic pathologists employ such facts in determining the cause of death, but they can also instruct neurosurgeons on how to conduct interventions, hence making surgical procedures precise. As the science evolves, constant research and the advancement in autopsy techniques will always enhance both clinical and forensic outcomes, ultimately being the cornerstone of the practice of medicine and overall public health (Figure 4.9).

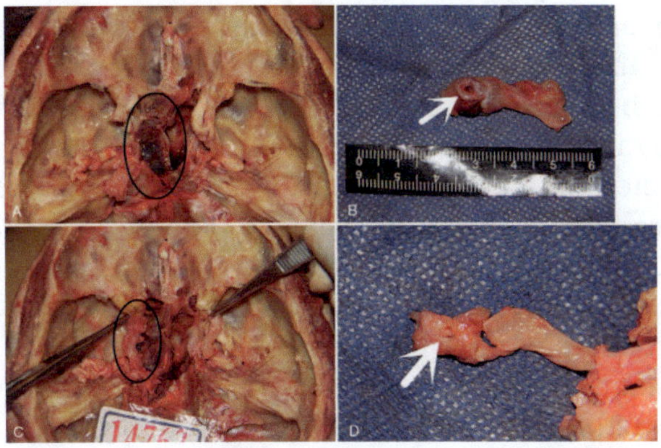

Figure 4.9. Autopsy findings and procedure. (A and B) A rupture pouch-like structure, pale and inflamed tissue at the breach, and blood accumulation and clot attachment on the front side of the left sphenoid sinus. (C and D) A pedicle-like structure extending into the left sphenoid sinus in the C3 segment (siphon curve) of the left internal carotid artery.

Source: https://www.researchgate.net/publication/357851682/figure/fig7/AS:1114361858916372@1642695979414/Autopsy-findings-and-procedure-A-and-B-A-rupture-pouch-like-structure-pale-and.ppm.

4.3.1. Preparation and Consent

The process of autopsy preparation includes several important aspects, of which consent and preparation are the most critical. Only after informed consent is provided by the deceased's family or legal guardian can any examination or autopsy be initiated. The fact that this step is required not only makes the process legally valid but also reiterates ethical considerations involving the autonomy of the deceased and the rights of the family. Having frank discussions with the grieving family about the purpose and significance of the autopsy can contribute significantly to the bereaved family. It is important that this be communicated by health personnel to the potential role of the autopsy in disease process knowledge, diagnosis confirmation, or public health information development. Informed consent is no longer an illegal technicality but instead a pillar of ethical practice whereby multidisciplinary autopsy management is respected and appreciated. On obtaining permission, careful preparation for the autopsy has to follow to ensure accuracy and integrity during the subsequent examination. This is typically the obtaining of relevant medical records, laboratory results, and imaging tests that provide contextual background information on the medical background of the decedent. This will aid the pathologist's inspection as well as help develop a template for disease process diagnosis or the cause of death. Making sure that the autopsy suite is properly equipped is also fundamental, with the diversity of instruments and technology available enhancing procedural efficiency as well as investigative capability. For instance, techniques like immunohistochemistry can reveal specific pathological markers relevant to the case at hand, such as SNTF as a potential biomarker of diffuse axonal injury, which once again underscores the importance of having the right equipment available during autopsy (Cullen et al., 2015). The affective environment in which autopsies are performed cannot be overstressed, as the stakes extend far beyond clinical and forensic considerations into affecting families and communities deeply. Psychosocial preparation of both the medical team and the family is needed in order to ensure that the procedure of autopsy is carried out with compassion and respect for the deceased individual. Pathologists and examiners must understand the significance of their role in providing closure and resolutions to grieving families; such an understanding enhances medical and legal system trust. Discussing their results in dialogue can prove to be a key element not only of healing but also in managing potential public health problems, as is shown by the growing acknowledgment of methods like DBS sampling in toxicological analysis in autopsy investigations (Kesel et al., 2012). Combined, the constituents of preparation and consent are the foundation of a professional and respectful autopsy process, bringing scientific investigation into conformity with ethical standards (Figure 4.10).

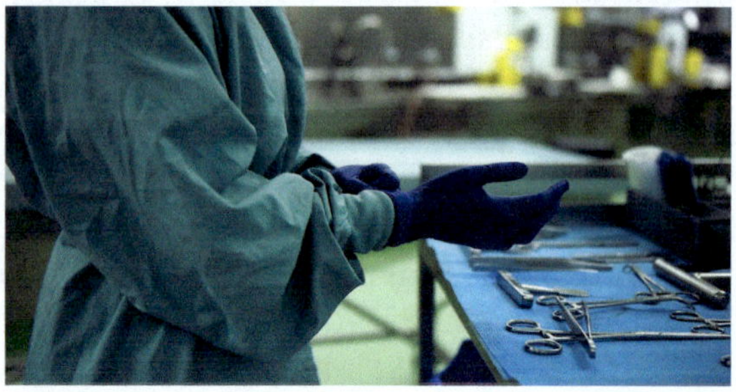

Figure 4.10. Preparation for an autopsy.

Source: https://media.post.rvohealth.io/wp-content/uploads/2024/09/close-up-doctor-pathologist-surgical-gloves-preparation-autopsy-1200x628-facebook.jpg.

4.3.2. External Examination

The external examination is a critical initial step within the autopsy process, providing a mass of information regarding the circumstances surrounding a person's death. This thorough investigation involves checking for evidence of trauma to the body in the form of bruising, abrasions, or ligature marks. These findings are crucial in differentiating between various causes of death and in guiding subsequent internal examination. In forensic investigation cases, especially cases of child homicide, external examination becomes more complex as a result of the increased need for sensitivity when handling vulnerable victims. A synergistic approach using traditional forensic methods and modern imaging and analytical technologies is critical to ensure that proper conclusions are drawn, perhaps deciding legal judgments in complex child death cases (Fragkou et al., 2025). Forensic pathologists use special protocols upon external examination to document and inspect the condition of the body in detail. This is all about the significant practice of photographing injuries and of being extremely thorough in taking notes that can be referred to later in court. The autopsy does not only include the visible external injuries; it also includes examination of the overall condition of the deceased, such as neglect or abuse. Particularly, healed rather than recent injuries may be used to signify the timeline of abuse or interactions' dynamics, probably causative of death. Furthermore, a competent external examination can determine key evidence in supporting the findings derived from follow-up internal examinations to enhance the interconnectivity of both stages of examination in the autopsy (Appuhamy, 2023).

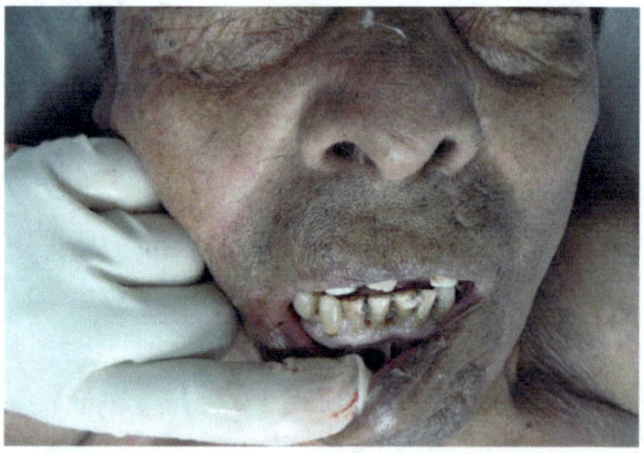

Figure 4.11. Denture with missing pieces and poor care conditions.

Source: https://cdnintech.com/media/chapter/81090/1512345123/media/F1.png.

Lastly, the external examination is the foundation upon which a complete autopsy is built. Careful consideration and documentation of external findings, including the assessment of normal variation and potential injury, allow forensic pathologists to construct a better image of the mechanisms that may have resulted in death. The multi-disciplinary practice of modern forensic analysis highlights the importance of collaborative interaction among pathologists, law enforcers, and legal practitioners in building complex cases. By using developments in conventional and newer technologies, such as imaging and molecular analysis, experts are able to significantly enhance the effectiveness and precision of third-party analyses. This integrated process not only aids in determining the cause of death but also becomes a key factor in facilitating justice and preventing incessant occurrences of violence or injury (Fragkou et al., 2025) (Figure 4.11).

4.3.3. Internal Examination

The inner examination during an autopsy is necessary to uncover the pathological findings that are not visible on the outside. This process of the autopsy is meticulously performed by forensic pathologists who inspect the structural condition of the internal organs and associated systems. Typically, the internal examination starts with a thorough anatomical inspection, and it includes inspection of the heart, lungs, liver, kidneys, and gastrointestinal tract to identify any signs of disease, trauma, or abnormalities. Not only does the examination reveal the direct cause of death, but it also has a tendency to show underlying conditions that might have precipitated the terminal event. The use of contemporary imaging technologies, such as computed tomography (CT) and magnetic resonance imaging (MRI), can improve the accuracy of the results during the internal examination, leading to a more comprehensive understanding of the deceased's health status. In some cases, internal examinations can identify critical information that would otherwise be missed through traditional methods. As an instance, in the case of biliary obstruction following organ transplantation, detailed assessment of the liver and biliary tree can show complications such as sludge or cast formation. They are particularly valuable because, if untreated, obstruction of the large bile ducts can lead to extensive necrosis and organ failure, as in studies where large casts blocked intrahepatic ducts (Hansbrough et al., 1977). The internal examination, thus, serves not only as a means for confirmation of provisional diagnoses but also as a means for identification of secondary complications, which may require further surgery and impact post-transplant management. Additionally, the careful inspection during the internal examination can extend beyond transient pathological changes and shape broader medical facts and practices. For example, studies on cardiovascular deaths among anabolic-androgenic steroid (AAS) abusing bodybuilders have shown lethal apoptotic changes in the cardiac tissue related to AAS abuse (Cecchi et al., 2017). The initial autopsy in such cases testifies to the importance of understanding the irreversible consequences of drug abuse on organ systems to enable sound future prevention and guide public health policy. Therefore, the internal inspection is important not only in the case of explaining death causes but also in the fact that it provides information for medical knowledge regarding disease processes, highlighting its importance within the larger context of the autopsy process in human beings (Figure 4.12).

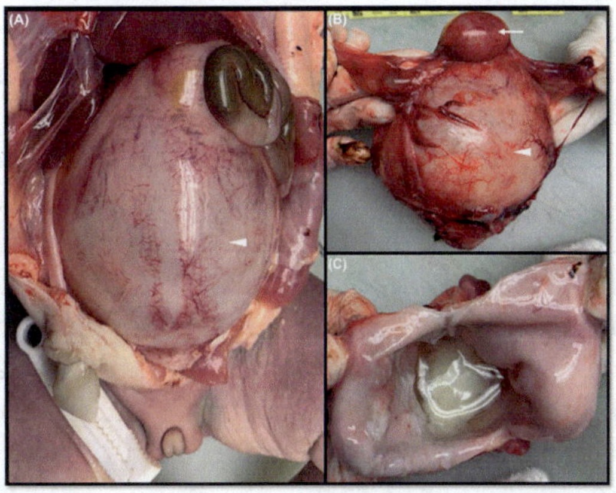

Figure 4.12. Internal autopsy examination of the fetus: (A) and (B) dilated uterus (arrow) and vagina (arrow head); (C) vaginal wall section with evidence of yellowish material inside.

Source: https://www.researchgate.net/publication/369107353/figure/fig4/AS:11431281136730635@1680574938063/Internal-autopsy-examination-of-the-fetus-Aand-Bdilated-uterus-arrow-and-vagina.jpg.

Test Your Knowledge

1. What documents are typically reviewed during autopsy preparation?
2. Which organ systems are typically inspected during an internal examination?

4.4. Tools and Equipment Used in Autopsies

Learning Outcome

1. Describe the basic instruments used in autopsies.
2. Describe the advanced technology used in autopsies.
3. Understand the importance of safety equipment and protocols in the context of autopsy techniques.

Success in carrying out an autopsy relies heavily on the equipment and apparatus utilized in the process. Some of the most critical instruments include scalpels, scissors, and forceps, which enable pathologists to dissect the body with thoroughness. Scalpels of various sizes with sharp blades enable one to make incisions with precision in order to dissect tissues carefully, while scissors are designed best for cutting through harder substances such as cartilage. Forceps are also employed in moving and gripping tissues for microscopic study. Other specialized equipment, such as bone saws, makes it possible to access bone structures when necessary, demonstrating the variety of tools necessary for comprehensive studies. The careful selection and maintenance of these tools are most important, as their effectiveness can have a profound influence on the quality of evidence during the autopsy process. Well-furnished autopsy rooms are no longer a luxury but a sine qua non to confirm accurate diagnoses as well as safe causes of death. In addition to the traditional equipment, newer imaging technologies have transformed autopsy practices with the availability of non-invasive modalities such as virtopsy. With this new method, MSCT and MRI are used to image internal organs without dissection. These scanners are particularly valuable in identifying fractures, gas production, and soft tissue pathology, frequently matching the effectiveness of conventional autopsy procedures. As studies of virtopsy progresses and expand, its value as a substitute or supplement to forensic investigation becomes increasingly obvious. The use of such technology in the autopsies may not only expedite the results in the mortuary but also decrease the emotional and physical burden on the grieving families involved. This innovation speaks of a fundamental shift in the way autopsies are conducted in modern forensic science, paving the way for sophisticated means. Additionally, there is a need for a complete autopsy protocol that includes the incorporation of various ancillary equipment that aids in the analytical procedure of the examination. Histological instruments and laboratory equipment are key aspects of the detailed analysis of tissue samples obtained during autopsy. For example, preservative liquids for tissues and microscopic slides are vital in examining the cellular structures under a microscope, thereby acquiring valuable information on root diseases or conditions. Toxicological analysis also has specialized equipment, such as mass spectrometers, to detect the presence of poison, drugs, or other substances in body fluids. The interaction between historical autopsy equipment and modern laboratory equipment is the evolution of forensic medicine, enhancing the overall efficiency and precision of the investigation process. With increasing innovations of procedures by forensic pathologists, the meticulous selection and use of the correct equipment and apparatus remain crucial in the attainment of correct and equitable results in human autopsy procedures (Figure 4.13).

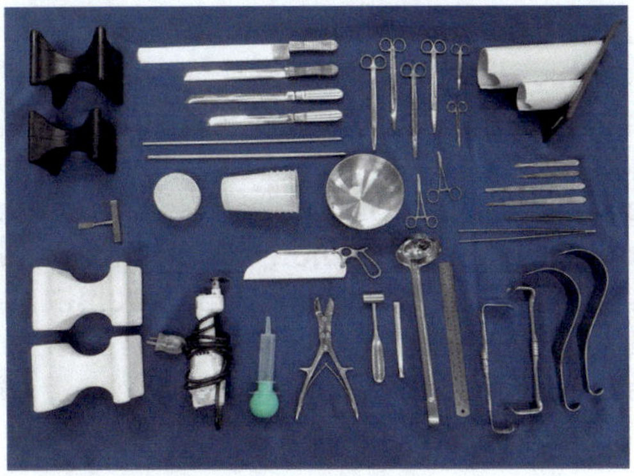

Figure 4.13. Autopsy tool kit.

Source: https://a1props.com/wp-content/uploads/2018/02/Autopsy-Tool-Kit-updated.jpg.

4.4.1. Basic Instruments (Scalpel, Scissors, etc.)

An autopsy involves the use of some fundamental tools, and each plays a critical role in cutting up and examining the human body. The scalpel, with its optimal use being for precision cutting, is obligatory upon initial penetration of the skin or organs. It has a sharp edge, which enables it to cut cleanly with little destruction of adjacent tissues, essential in performing adequate pathological examination. Likewise, surgical scissors have a crucial function during the process of dissection, allowing pathologists to navigate through tissues with precision and delicacy. Such tools are created to address various layers in the body, thus facilitating effective tissue separation and exploration. The realization of the specific handling and usage of such tools helps in ensuring that the autopsy is carried out effectively, thereby impacting the quality of findings that result from the investigation. Other than scalpels and scissors, forceps are the lesser-known heroes that enable organs and tissues to be removed and handled in an autopsy. Forceps exist in various forms, with some having serrated edges for better grip, while others have smooth edges for delicate work, such as the removal of small samples for histological analysis. Proper use of forceps allows forensic pathologists to handle soft tissues without causing additional trauma, which could compromise the integrity of samples tested.

This precision is particularly important when specimens are processed for microscopic study, where any external trauma can cover up microscopic information, thus impairing autopsy conclusions. Furthermore, inclusion of these basic tools in the autopsy process enhances the ability of the pathologists to perform comprehensive examinations that yield legal and medical information. As technology continues to evolve, the basic tools utilized in autopsy procedures are enhanced, embracing finer materials and ergonomic designs to become more effective. For instance, newer handles for scalpels can be designed with the ability to cut down on hand fatigue from long procedures, thus making the pathologists more efficient. Further, advances in instrument sterilization techniques offer guarantees that the instruments maintain their integrity and safety levels in forensic examinations. Even though traditional tools remain part of the autopsy process, ongoing innovation offers added advantages in terms of performance and ergonomics for the operators. This progressive enhancement in the quality and usability of basic tools highlights the necessity for consistent modifications in autopsy practices, ultimately leading to better results in the vital field of forensic science, as presented in literature on current high-tech developments in tissue handling and examination (Pazaitis et al., 2023) and surgical aspects (Filik et al., 2022).

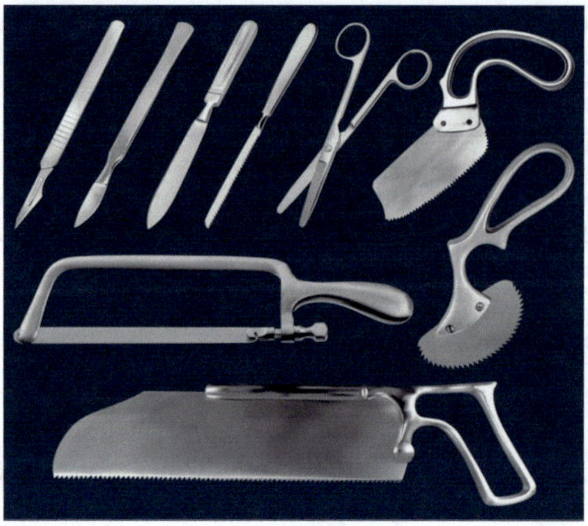

Figure 4.14. Basic instruments.

Source: https://www.shutterstock.com/image-vector/surgical-cutting-tools-set-600nw-1709318770.jpg.

4.4.2. Advanced Technology (CT Scans, MRI)

The advent of advanced imaging technologies such as Computed Tomography (CT) scans and Magnetic Resonance Imaging (MRI) has revolutionized human autopsy procedures. The modalities offer non-invasive techniques that enhance the visibility of internal structures, allowing forensic pathologists to access critical information without traditional dissection. By utilizing 3D reconstructions of the CT scans, physicians are able to analyze the anatomical structures of the body and diagnose fractures, foreign bodies, or other hidden abnormalities that are not apparent in a traditional autopsy. Not only does the utilization of such advanced imaging technology accelerate the diagnosis process, but it also ensures that the integrity of the cremation or burial remains intact, respecting the wishes of the families and the deceased. Apart from that, CT and MRI provide distinct advantages that supplement the accuracy and efficiency of post-mortem examination. For instance, the high-resolution images derived from these scans can expose trace pathological alterations in major organs, thus substantiating the determination of the cause of death. Where infectious diseases such as infective endocarditis are suspected, more advanced imaging can reveal internal conditions that older tests may miss, and more comprehensive analyses can be conducted. As assured by advancements inscribed in the newest medical guidelines, the integrative multidimensional approach based on these imaging technologies makes it possible for pathologists to adjust their research in relation to particular cases, which enhances clinical care quality along with the reliability of forensic evidence found in autopsies (Larry et al., 2015).

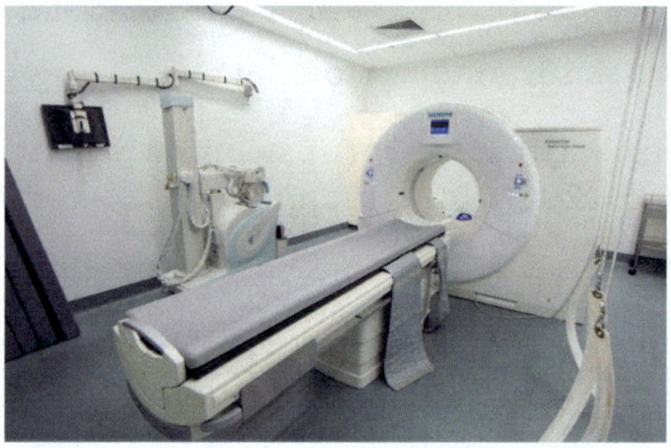

Figure 4.15. Forensic imaging technology helps virtual autopsies outnumber invasive post-mortem procedures.

Source: https://live-production.wcms.abc-cdn.net.au/e959cfe9ae830bb1df63fc614bf8ba91?impolicy=wcms_crop_resize&cropH=2592&cropW=3888&xPos=0&yPos=0&width=862&height=575.

In addition, the integration of advanced imaging technologies into autopsy procedures guarantees the solidity of the possibilities of interdisciplinary cooperation between medical professionals. Radiologists and forensic pathologists can together interpret sophisticated imaging data synergistically, enhancing the diagnostic process. The collaboration is especially valuable in cases that are multifactorial in nature, where the involved factors may be spread across multiple medical disciplines. Through the use of such advanced technologies, groups can collectively gain a more sophisticated perspective of the pathology involved and continue to develop autopsy methods to suit. Ultimately, the evolution of CT and MRI within autopsy practice not only sets a higher standard in forensic science but also assures sound, evidence-based findings when faced with the complexities of human demise (Humbert et al., 2022) (Figure 4.15).

4.4.3. Safety Equipment and Protocols

The importance of safety measures and equipment in the use of autopsy techniques cannot be overstated, since such preventive practices are critical in preventing both the medical team and the integrity of the autopsy from being compromised. Autopsies expose one to infectious material, and therefore, the use of personal protective equipment (PPE) such as gloves, masks, goggles, and gowns is necessary. With strict procedures established, like disinfection of equipment and surfaces on a regular basis, the risk of bloodborne pathogens and other contaminants is easily circumvented. Also, autopsy facilities must adhere to an entire disposal waste plan so that biological traces are handled in accordance with local law. This model not only protects medical professionals but also asserts the ethical responsibilities of conducting autopsies responsibly and safely, thus maintaining public trust (Shen et al., 2020). Apart from personal protective equipment, safety measures that are initiated during the conduct of autopsies are proper training and adherence to the regulations of regulatory authorities. Medical personnel, like pathologists and forensic scientists, need to be informed of best practices for handling the deceased as well as examination materials. These include guidelines published by groups interested in health and safety in medical environments, including proper sample collection and preservation techniques. This training is vital as it creates a safety culture within the forensic and medical centers, ultimately contributing to the overall quality and consistency of the autopsy findings. It also requires that workers be kept up to date with fresh safety protocols, particularly during public health crises, since changes may be necessary based on emerging information (Pelliccia et al., 2020). The integration of technological innovation into the autopsy process has also begun transforming safety measures. The introduction of robotic systems and advanced imaging technologies can potentially reduce direct handling of biological samples, thereby reducing the exposure risk for pathologists.

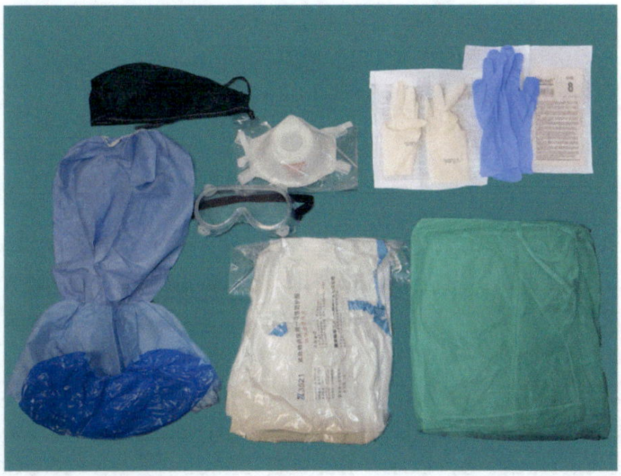

Figure 4.16. Personal protective equipment (PPE) used for a COVID-19 postmortem examination.

Source: https://www.researchgate.net/publication/342063050/figure/fig1/AS:902009280536578@1592067179564/Personal-protective-equipment-PPE-used-for-a-COVID-19-postmortem-examination-Head.ppm.

These technologies can diagnose and analyze samples remotely, providing additional layers of protection without sacrificing the integrity of the autopsy process. Besides, use of the systems, especially during periods of heightened health risk—such as the COVID-19 pandemic—persuades the high degree of adaptability for robotic use in overcoming conventional barriers faced in medical testing. Though security will remain a top concern, further research and development in such fields will likely yield new guidelines that guarantee safety and efficacy in autopsy procedures (Shen et al., 2020) (Figure 4.16).

Test Your Knowledge

1. What instruments are used in an autopsy?
2. What is the primary advantage of using CT and MRI in autopsy techniques?

4.5. Role of the Pathologist

Learning Outcome

1. Understand the responsibilities of the pathologist during an autopsy.
2. Interpret the findings in autopsy techniques.
3. Collaborate with law enforcement.

The pathologist stands in a central role in the use of autopsy techniques and functions as a critical bridge between postmortem examination and clinical practice. His or her proficiency in examining tissues and organs plays a crucial role in determining the cause of death, especially in difficult or complicated cases of infectious diseases, malignancies, or sudden unexplained death. For instance, autopsy findings can identify unsuspected conditions, and this gives essential additional information for public health. During the COVID-19 pandemic, the involvement of pathologists in postmortem examination underscores their worth, as they have modified to adhere to new biosafety protocols to analyze SARS-CoV-2's action in human tissues. The ability of the pathologist to assess macroscopic findings and microscopic changes offers an in-depth description of disease mechanisms, enabling a better understanding that can inform both clinical practice and epidemiological research (Calabrese et al., 2020). In addition, the duty of a pathologist includes investigation of some diseases and traumas that require proper investigation to understand the mechanisms behind them. In acute myocardial infarction (AMI), for example, pathologists analyze cardiac tissues in order to understand the mechanisms of ischemic reperfusion injury, a condition that is difficult to treat and to investigate in an admissible legal context. Such autopsies can provide vital information on the patient's condition at the time of death, substantiating a more solid comprehension of how conditions like AMI have a tendency to lead to sudden cardiac death. By means of injury pattern and cell change identification, pathologists provide for enhanced preventive strategies and therapy practices. Their findings can also inform medicolegal autopsies such that sudden deaths are thoroughly investigated to cast light on the order of events culminating in these deaths (Neri et al., 2017). Pathologists' collaboration with other healthcare professionals also optimizes the utility of autopsy findings. Via participation in multidisciplinary teams, pathologists provide knowledge that informs diagnosis and treatment modalities. Their input not only aids individual case analysis but also informs public health analysis overall. The sophisticated understanding of disease process set by autopsy studies informs epidemiological trends significant in the case of pandemics or public health crises. As evidenced in the COVID-19 pandemic, full autopsy procedures yield novel insights into the disease's impact on various body systems, hence shaping public health interventions. Hence, the pathologist's work is priceless in enhancing health outcomes and increasing medical knowledge through meticulous analysis and interpretation of postmortem information (Calabrese et al., 2020) (Figure 4.17).

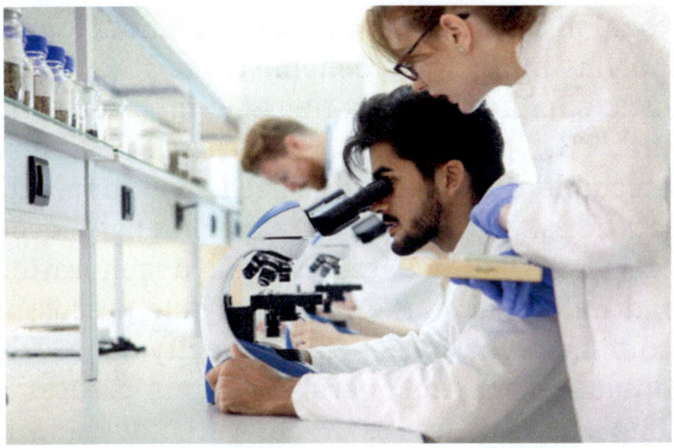

Figure 4.17. Role of the pathologist.

Source: https://www.aucmed.edu/sites/g/files/krcnkv361/files/styles/atge_3_2_crop_md/public/2022-03/Pathology.jpg?h=07294c09&itok=H5qjddhH.

4.5.1. Responsibilities During an Autopsy

Among these tasks are a range of essential activities required for the purpose of maintaining a legitimate diagnosis, completeness, and ethical integrity in death investigation. The primary role of the pathologist or medical examiner is to conduct a systematic examination of the body in strict compliance with protocols, enabling a reliable diagnosis. This involves an extremely meticulous review of physical and biological evidence, both external and internal examinations. The findings must be recorded by the pathologist in the form of minute notes and photographs, which become invaluable records for legal, medical, and educational purposes. With the further development of forensic science, the role to integrate modern technologies, such as neuroimaging, into the autopsy has also emerged, which can contribute towards a better understanding of the underlying causes of death. These responsibilities not only contribute to the determination of the cause of death but also to the credibility of forensic practice. In addition to the technical responsibilities of conducting the autopsy, there is also a moral aspect that practitioners must uphold in the sensitive process. Autopsies are emotionally upsetting for relatives of deceased patients, and pathologists must carry out their responsibilities with dignity and compassion. This calls for open communication with families regarding the basis for the autopsy and the potential implications of the findings. It is up to the medical examiner to clarify the autopsy's contribution to medical knowledge development without ever compromising the dignity of the deceased. The responsibility extends beyond providing valuable feedback to health practitioners regarding potential health hazards or risks that would affect public health, thus emphasizing the contribution of autopsies in the context of healthcare and prevention at large. Such a sense of ethical awareness ensures that the roles of the autopsy service are aligned with the desired expectations and values of society. Lastly, the evolving nature of autopsy techniques means that professionals need to keep up to date with technological developments as well as legal considerations impacting their responsibilities. Ongoing professional development is required, with developments in fields such as neuropsychology indicating the necessity of brain health and how it applies in cases involving degenerative diseases that may reveal intricate associations between pathology and behavior, impacting forensic conclusions. As suggested by the work of experts such as Dr. Ruben Gur, the profession that deals with autopsy tasks also increasingly interacts with legal investigation, particularly in the case of capital trials where thorough inquiry becomes paramount. Hence, the work involved in an autopsy not only demands technical competence and ethical duties but also commitment to ongoing professional development to enable adaptation to the sophisticated demands of contemporary forensic science. Comprehension of responsibility levels in autopsy is most important to maintaining the integrity and effectiveness of the overall forensic process (Figure 4.18).

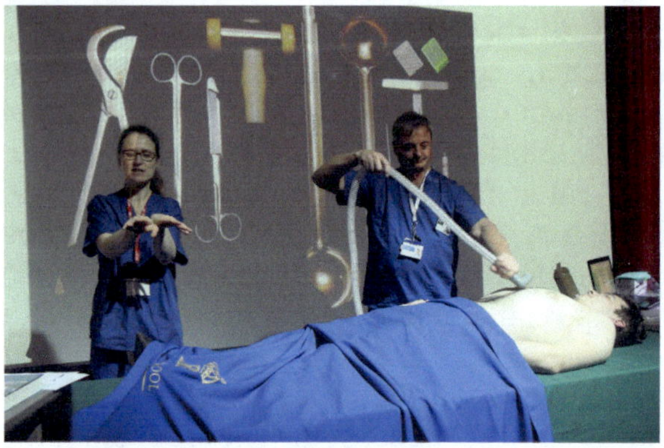

Figure 4.18. Responsibilities of pathologist during an autopsy.

Source: https://www.kingschester.co.uk/wp-content/uploads/2019/11/IMG_5007.jpg.

4.5.2. Interpretation of Findings

The interpretation of autopsy results is crucial to constructing medical knowledge and healthcare quality. The research on non-invasive and minimally invasive autopsy procedures, as stressed in recent literature, underscores the necessity to adapt post-mortem examinations to maximize family consent rates. In a review of new autopsy techniques conducted systematically, the study found that while conventional autopsies remain necessary, innovations based on radiological imaging and biopsies are becoming more popular. Surprisingly, a combination of CT and MR scans demonstrated acceptable correlation for the identification of the cause of death, yet the highest sensitivity was achieved using minimally invasive techniques. This means that such a transition can not only maintain diagnostic efficacy but also act as a mediator of ethical concerns surrounding autopsy consent, making post-mortem examination more palatable both for relatives and clinicians (Christe et al., 2016). The incorporation of biomarkers in traumatic brain injury (TBI) diagnosis at autopsy represents another example of the evolving context of post-mortem analysis. The research on SNTF as a potential biomarker for diffuse axonal injury stresses extensive methodologies. Applying immunohistochemistry to study brain tissue samples from patients with severe and mild TBI, proponents advocate for a less detectable diagnostic approach that supplants traditional markers. The experiment proved that SNTF could detect axonal degeneration that traditional markers, like amyloid precursor protein, might miss. This capacity to reveal populations of degenerating axons creates a comprehensive image of TBI pathology and is testimony to the value of integrating current evidence into conventional autopsy practice. Such revelations can significantly improve the comprehension of the consequences of brain injury post-mortem, paving the way for enhanced clinical intervention in surviving patients (Cullen et al., 2015). Interpretation of findings across various autopsy techniques thus entails the multidimensional quality that enables advances in medicine and remains attentive to ethics. The evolving discourse on minimally invasive autopsies and evolving biomarkers represents a paradigm shift in the perspective of pathologists and physicians with respect to post-mortem examinations. The availability of evidence affirming the efficiency of alternative tests and biomarkers provides testament to their ability to advance precision and dependability in the determination of the cause of death. To actually integrate these innovations into routine practice, continuous research and trials in bigger populations will be essential. With the progression of the discipline, it will no longer be enough to interpret results; to convert those results into workable knowledge that builds both forensic science and public health outcomes will also be needed. This integrative approach is critical for future human autopsy practice, where patient dignity and astute diagnosis can be balanced in harmony (Christe et al., 2016; Cullen et al., 2015).

4.5.3. Collaboration with the Police

The professional interaction between law enforcement agents and forensic scientists is indispensable in the context of death investigations, particularly where autopsy techniques are employed. Forensic pathologists are usually requested to provide not just medically significant information but also legally significant information. Professional interaction is particularly vital in suspicious or unexplained death, in which police attempt to reconstruct ~~in what manner~~ the event ~~took place~~. Cooperative communication between these agencies provides assurance that the autopsy reports direct investigation strategies and that any potential evidence is preserved and documented with utmost care. Additionally, the interdisciplinary communications foster improved understanding of the conditions at death, ultimately assisting in the pursuit of justice and case closure. With more advancements in forensic science, the incorporation of new methods has necessitated day-to-day coordination with the law enforcement community. New methods, such as microbial analysis for postmortem interval estimation, are becoming more mainstream in forensic analysis. With the ability to utilize microbial succession information, death investigation accuracy can be significantly enhanced, but its successful implementation also relies upon cooperation with law enforcement. Forensic experts must work very closely with investigators to ensure that samples are collected in a way that will benefit most in supporting scientific analysis. Moreover, law enforcement agencies' willingness to employ such new methods in their procedure can lead to quicker convictions in criminal cases. This collaboration of science and law enforcement is the best archetypal demonstration of the fundamental need for interdisciplinary collaboration in modern forensic practice, enriching our enhanced appreciation of death and supporting the judicial process. The role of working together to provide reliability to forensic evidence cannot be overemphasized, particularly in the field of autopsy practice and the broader investigation process. With more forensic agencies accepting digital forensic tools and techniques more often, as covered in the current study on computer forensics, there has become a greater need for cooperation. The necessity for expert examination of digital evidence, including which is derived from cybercrimes, demands close coordination with law enforcement to ensure investigators have the necessary data and tools to properly analyze evidence. Moreover, with the advancement of forensic technology, the police have to be receptive to these innovations and be in a constant state of changing to keep up with research and innovation. Thus, teamwork enhances the integrity and efficacy of the forensic test as a whole, strengthening the ultimate purpose of delivering justice with accurate and scientifically valid findings (Javed et al., 2022; Jessica, 2018) (Figure 4.19).

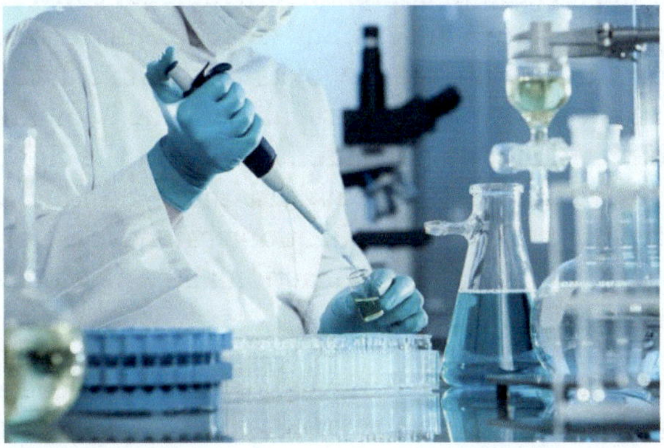

Figure 4.19. Forensic science for law enforcement.

Source: https://cdndailyexcelsior.b-cdn.net/wp-content/uploads/2024/06/Forensic-Science-Laboratory-FSL-Jammu.jpg.

Test Your Knowledge

1. Describe the responsibilities of the pathologist during an autopsy.
2. What role do forensic pathologists play in aiding law enforcement during death investigations?

4.6. Legal and Ethical Considerations

Learning Outcome

1. Learn about consent and family rights within the context of autopsy techniques.
2. Understand the confidentiality and privacy issues of autopsy techniques.
3. Describe the legal implications of autopsy findings.

The legal and moral concerns posed by autopsy techniques for humans are complicated and require careful examination. Autopsies serve a crucial role in determining causes of death, enhancing medical science, and promoting public health. However, these autopsies must be performed in compliance with legal controls that regulate consent and respect for human corpses. Legal frameworks are more likely to require explicit approval from next of kin, emphasizing the obligation to respect the rights and wishes of the dead and their families. A breach of such legal obligations can have severe repercussions, from civil action and litigation to ethical violations.

Thus, proper knowledge of the relevant laws is essential among professionals practicing autopsy to prevent infringement and ensure ethical practice in their routine activities. Ethically, autopsy practice raises various principles, including respect for autonomy, beneficence, and justice. The requirement of informed consent serves as an example of the ethical need to respect patients' and families' autonomy and their rights in medical decisions. Also, the implications of autopsies extend beyond the particular circumstances of death; they are a potential way of furthering medical knowledge, and thus to society as a whole. Ethical difficulties, however, arise when one considers the potential for exploitation or fancied disrespect of the dead and their families. As with the argument for artificial intelligence in medicine, a parallel exists with respect to the difficulties of confronting bias and consent while carrying out research with human subjects that involves a strong call for ethical thought in all scientific practice, including autopsies (Stacy et al., 2019).

In order to obtain the complex balance between ethical ideals and legal determinants, organizations performing autopsy procedures must possess robust ethical ideals and regulatory oversight. The Council for International Organizations of Medical Sciences (CIOMS) has established guidelines that emphasize the need for research to be scientific and of social importance, an element that can be applied to autopsy practice and its role in medical research (N/A, 2016). Autopsy procedures not only require prioritizing utmost importance to scientific inquiry but also involve a moral responsibility towards the deceased and their relatives. By giving similar treatment and informed consent, doctors are able to foster trust and transparency in the autopsy process, thus building a stronger legitimacy and social acceptance of these critical medical procedures. Implementing stringent training and accountability will further allow ethical conduct and compliance, safeguarding the dignity of participants.

4.6.1. Family Rights and Consent

The area of overlap between consent and family rights in autopsy procedures has profound ethical as well as legal consequences. Autopsies are useful tools for determining the cause of death, contributing to medical science, and enhancing public health. However, the procedural aspect of autopsies mandates that the family of the deceased or their representatives either give consent or be notified of the autopsy procedure. New social mores and legislation increasingly recognize informed consent not only as a bureaucratic mandate but also as a fundamental right of families. Thus, it puts greater weight on the importance of open discussion between healthcare providers and families regarding the purpose and intent behind an autopsy, thus establishing the family's right to be informed and exercise control over the post-mortem examination of their deceased relatives. Additionally, the impact of consent on families extends beyond direct emotional outcomes of loss. When a family provides consent for an autopsy, they unwittingly become participants in a complex procedure that includes medical practitioners, legal frameworks, and ethical standards. These procedures can control the way results are reported and how information is subsequently utilized. For instance, enhancing autopsy practices and adopting forensic science requires a clearer comprehension of how the family is considered in these processes. Autopsies that are compliant with consent procedures can result in trustworthiness and transparency, building rapport among healthcare providers and families. This is crucial for future consideration on how such post-mortem analysis might most effectively be used to the interests of broader public health, including review of the need for sensitivity and ethical responsibility in handling family rights and consent within autopsy procedure. Finally, the legal implications regarding consent and family rights in the context of autopsies demonstrate the requirement for reform and standardization within procedure. According to research on Sudden Unexpected Death in Epilepsy (SUDEP), there is a comparative lack of clarity in guidelines both for families and pathologists who conduct post-mortem examinations (Ackerman et al., 2017). Implementing more transparent legal frameworks would assist with the integration of family rights into autopsy practices, ensuring that families are properly informed regarding the purpose and aim of the autopsy. In addition, as technology advances with autopsy practice, the structures will also need to adjust accordingly, finding a balance between both the rights of families and the scientific demands of the medical community. This both/and strategy could lead to greater comprehension and application of consent, serving individual families as well as society as a whole (Figure 4.20).

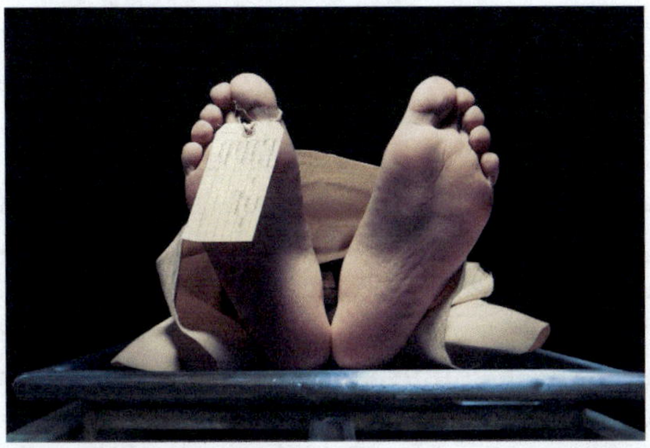

Figure 4.20. The family of the man dissected at the autopsy event says they didn't give consent.

Source: https://media.king5.com/assets/KING/images/b4bd2d44-c0fa-41cf-afab-e537f40cb2da/b4bd2d44-c0fa-41cf-afab-e537f40cb2da_1920x1080.jpg.

4.6.2. Confidentiality and Privacy Issues

In autopsy procedures, privacy and confidentiality concerns are of utmost significance, particularly in terms of the sensitive information involved in postmortem tests. Confidential treatment of personal records and medical histories is significant because autopsies can expose complicated dimensions of a person's life, health, and interfamily relationships. Autopsies provide high amounts of information, access to which becomes problematic. Poor strict data protection protocols can not only lead to breach of confidentiality but also lead to loss of confidence in medical practice. Everyone who takes part in postmortem examinations must take strict measures to safeguard individual privacy and thereby steer clear of any kind of distress due to unauthorized disclosures, which can have long-term emotional and social implications. Moreover, the recent discoveries in genetic testing following autopsy present a unique challenge to confidentiality. The identification of genetic markers for so many various diseases, including inherited cardiac disorders, indicates that there is a need for responsible and ethical management of genetic information. As highlighted in controversies surrounding postmortem genetic testing, the deceased as well as surviving relatives are required to give informed consent, which guarantees that they recognize the potential ramifications of genetic findings. Professional groups such as the European Society of Human Genetics call for the enactment of comprehensive guidelines that are privacy-respecting while inviting a teamwork-based system of genetic inquiry. It is critical that this balance is observed in promoting scientific knowledge and permitting adequate information exchange without compromising individuals' or families' privacy, which would happen inadvertently to enhance stigmatization and discrimination. Moreover, integrating AI in autopsy processes creates additional layers of complexity regarding confidentiality. AI applications can make diagnoses more accurate, but they can also inadvertently put biases or assumptions into patient data privacy. The ethical issues encompassed in AI technology implementation within autopsy settings cannot be disregarded, as they impose a fundamental scrutiny of data ownership, consent, and channels of abuse. Of supreme relevance is that AI solution deployment and implementation adhere to ethical guidelines, indicating compliance with patient confidentiality and informed consent. Engaging the public in debating matters related to these issues will have societal values represented in AI use in autopsy techniques, finally leading to trust and confidence in innovation, which can significantly influence healthcare outcomes for communities and people (Figure 4.21).

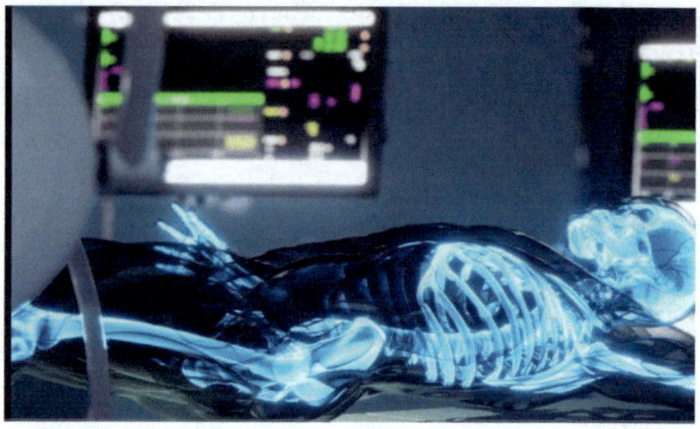

Figure 4.21. Privacy and confidentiality are vital in autopsy procedures due to sensitive postmortem data.

Source: https://imgengine.khaleejtimes.com/khaleejtimes/import/images/OF6AfzaYpNXHc9AxksUGPd8VIfE.png?width=1200&format=auto.

4.6.3. Legal Implications of Autopsy Findings

The juridical significance of autopsy results is multifaceted, influencing a broad spectrum of fields including criminal law, civil responsibility, and medical policy. Autopsy reports play a central role in submitting essential evidence in both criminal and civil cases, often deciding the proximate cause of death as defined by law. Consequently, for instance, a thorough examination can identify signs of foul play or negligence and lead to criminal prosecution or civil suit against responsible parties. Autopsy findings have the potential to affect the award of damages in wrongful death cases, and so it is really crucial that forensic pathologists ensure excellent standards during the examination process. Inconsistencies or perceived bias in the autopsy findings thus result in litigation threats, which jeopardize a case outcome and public trust in the justice system. In addition, autopsy findings can inform broader public health questions, as a critical instrument for epidemiologists and policymakers. Through determination of the cause and manner of death, autopsies can detect emerging health trends, such as rising rates of heart failure from substance abuse, including androgenic anabolic steroids (AAS).

Research suggests that chronic use of AAS may result in outstanding cardiac alterations, which are oftentimes confused with other illnesses, emphasizing the importance of employing appropriate autopsy procedures in identifying such patterns (Cecchi et al., 2017). The legal aspects extend to regulating agencies, whose deliberation process could involve such information while setting guidelines or policies for controlled substances. As such, conclusions made based on autopsy reports can not only impact individual cases but also inform legislative policies concerning public health and safety. Secondly, the fact that forensic science is now involved in legal processes also raises questions regarding the admissibility of autopsy reports in court proceedings. The increased reliance on neuroscience evidence in culpability and mitigation cases has placed more focus on expert testimony that connects forensic evidence to legal standards (Gur et al., 2016). Admissibility matters typically involve the autopsy expert's qualifications and the approach employed. Therefore, pathologists must not only possess technical knowledge but also legal skills to report their findings in the right manner and make them acceptable as credible reports prior to the court of law. With the dynamic interface between forensic science and law, there is a greater requirement for collaboration between forensic scientists and legal experts to navigate the intricacies of autopsy reports and their jurisprudence.

Test Your Knowledge

1. What is one potential outcome when a family consents to an autopsy?
2. What are the legal implications of autopsy findings?

SUMMARY

The culmination of autopsy technique learning, particularly with respect to human investigations, emphasizes the significance of such techniques in forensic science and medical research. Autopsies not only indicate the cause of death but also contribute to the advancement of medical knowledge in oncology and pathology. For instance, comparative examination of human and canine diseases illustrates the broad-based applicability of autopsy findings. Recent innovation has enabled the use of formalin-fixed tissues obtained from dog autopsies in order to extrapolate data pertinent to human cancer studies, affirming the utility of autopsy procedures as a tool for cross-species translation. Such innovation, as evidenced in research on osteosarcoma studies, shows that autopsies can be used to inform treatment regimes and improve outcomes in human patients (Jessica et al., 2025). Moreover, the importance of autopsy results extends beyond medicolegal research and evokes legal and ethical concerns. Autopsies, which are forensic in nature, are extremely important for criminal investigations because they serve to provide crucial evidence that is instrumental in the identification of unknown individuals and the resolution of death cases. Techniques like age estimation from closure of cranial sutures underscore once again how autopsy results can assist in forensic investigation, providing crucial information for legal intents. The ability to estimate age with comparative accuracy from cranial sutures not only aids in the identification of victims but also plays a crucial role in the formulation of timelines significant in the pursuit of justice (Buzdar et al., 2024). The importance of autopsy techniques in forensic analyses cannot be overestimated, as they are utilized for both investigation and education. Finally, the convergence of autopsy techniques in both medical and forensic science testifies to their varied significance. Continued research and methodical development will enhance the validity and reliability of autopsy findings and, ultimately, benefit society at large. Comparison with human cancer research on canine research gives us reason to believe that, in the future, when multidisciplinary research can pave the way for paradigm-breaking knowledge of disease pathology and treatment. Meanwhile, the utility of forensic autopsies in criminal investigations will persist in vindicating the application of such methods. Going forward, fostering collaboration between forensic scientists and medical researchers will be essential in maximizing the benefits derived from autopsy techniques, ensuring they continue to play pivotal roles in disease comprehension as well as justice realization.

Autopsy technique in humans is a critical intersection of medical science and forensic research, providing definitive data on causes of death and potential legal relevance. One basic observation in this regard is the necessity for proper and systematic processes in determining the validity of outcomes. These procedures not only optimize data assembly and analysis but also enhance the replicability of data in various studies. The ARRIVE guidelines represent a major framework for this purpose, placing focus on transparency and clear reporting of methodologies, which are both important to forensic pathologists and researchers. Although it has gained widespread support, the minimal effect of ARRIVE on publication behavior points to the need for continuous improvement in reporting quality, with the intricacies involved in autopsy investigations being clearly documented regularly (Percie et al., 2020). Another crucial matter is the integration of evolving technologies into traditional autopsy protocols, evolving to potentially revolutionize post-mortem examination. Virtual autopsies, through the use of imaging modalities such as CT and MRI scans, enable non-invasive inspection that has the potential to supplement or, in some cases, replace traditional invasive routines. These developments promise not merely to enhance diagnostic performance but also to alleviate some of the ethical concerns surrounding traditional autopsy methods. The creation of these technologies is reflective of a broader movement in medicine toward honoring patient and family desires and involving them in decision-making. Thus, the inclusion of modern imaging technologies as part of common autopsy practice is a significant step forward, supported by ethical reasons and combining scientific knowledge with qualifications in pursuing truth (Habib et al., 2015). Moreover, the educational nature of autopsy techniques cannot be overestimated since they play an important role in developing future generations of medical staff. Training programs that not only cover the technical skills of performing autopsies but also the critical thinking of making eulogized interpretations are required. These programs also need to emphasize the ethics of autopsy practice, including cultural presuppositions and family dynamics. By a complete understanding of autopsy techniques, medical training can go a long way in stirring public faith in forensic science and related medical sciences. This mode of learning, together with adherence to rules such as those the ARRIVE initiative has established, significantly enhances the quality and validity of outcomes that arise from autopsy procedures, ultimately leading to the development of excellence in culture within the medical profession (Percie et al., 2020).

KEY TERMS FROM THIS CHAPTER

- Artificial intelligence
- Biochemical analysis
- Community health
- Forensic autopsy
- Histopathological examinations
- Magnetic resonance imaging
- Polymerase chain reaction
- Autopsy
- Clinical autopsy
- Computed tomography
- Forensic taphonomy
- Immunohistochemistry
- Next-generation sequencing
- Trauma

CRITICAL THINKING QUESTIONS

1. **What is the primary objective of performing an autopsy?**
   a. To determine the time of death.
   b. To establish the identity of the deceased.
   c. To ascertain the cause, manner, and mechanism of death.
   d. To collect evidence for criminal cases only.
2. **What is the first step in conducting a medico-legal autopsy?**
   a. Opening the thoracic cavity.
   b. Examining the external features of the body.
   c. Performing toxicological analysis.
   d. Removing the brain for examination.
3. **What type of incision is typically used to open the thoracic and abdominal cavities during an autopsy?**
   a. Y-shaped incision.
   b. Linear midline incision.
   c. Horizontal incision.
   d. U-shaped incision.
4. **Which of the following is examined first in a standard autopsy procedure?**
   a. Internal organs of the abdomen.
   b. The brain and skull.
   c. External injuries, marks, and body condition.
   d. The heart and lungs.
5. **Which organ is usually dissected last during a cranial autopsy?**
   a. Brainstem.
   b. Cerebrum.
   c. Cerebellum.
   d. Spinal cord.

Short Answer Questions

1. What is an autopsy, in a short definition?
2. Which period marked the transition from spiritual to empirical observations in the study of the human body?
3. List the types of autopsies.
4. What equipment is used in an autopsy?
5. What is the role of the pathologist?

Answer to Critical Thinking Questions

1. (c); 2. (b); 3. (a); 4. (c); 5. (a)

REFERENCES

1. Ackerman, A., Agesen, A., Ahmad, A., Aiba, M., Annegers, J., Antoniuk, M., Atherton, J., et al. (2017). The past, present and future challenges in epilepsy-related and sudden deaths and biobanking. https://core.ac.uk/download/141438977.pdf (accessed on 12th July 2025).
2. Agrawala, A., Rehani, M., & Sharma, R. (2009). Detection of metabolites by proton *ex vivo* NMR, *in vivo* MR spectroscopy peaks, and tissue content analysis: Biochemical-magnetic resonance correlation: Preliminary results. https://core.ac.uk/download/pdf/288964.pdf (accessed on 12th July 2025).
3. Alley, T., Andrejevic, M., Apter, E., Citron, D. K., Clemens, J., Gandy, O. H., Humphries, P., et al. (2019). The profiling potential of computer vision and the challenge of computational empiricism. http://arxiv.org/abs/1904.10016 (accessed on 12th July 2025).
4. Appuhamy, P. (2023). A modified cosmetic technique for head and neck dissection in autopsy especially for bald-headed deceased. *Medico-Legal Journal of Sri Lanka.* https://www.semanticscholar.org/paper/8fd7c05d1d671f0cf0c8f3718716e98534856533 (accessed on 12th July 2025).
5. Baddour, L. M., Wilson, W. R., Bayer, A. S., Fowler, V. G., Tleyjeh, I. M., Rybak, M. J., Baršić, B., et al. (2015). Infective endocarditis in adults: Diagnosis, antimicrobial therapy, and management of complications. *Circulation, 132*, 1435–1486. https://doi.org/10.1161/cir.0000000000000296 (accessed on 12th July 2025).
6. Beck, J. A., Garg, A., Church, S. E., Mazcko, C., & LeBlanc, A. (2025). Spatial transcriptomics advances the use of canine patients in cancer research: Analysis of osteosarcoma-bearing pet dogs enrolled in a clinical trial. *Clinical Cancer Research: An Official Journal of the American Association for Cancer Research.* https://www.semanticscholar.org/paper/7b9e4b2412f66db68c5d9041ea9542ad3749e189 (accessed on 12th July 2025).
7. Buzdar, Z. A., Murad, T., Shabbir, S., Ahmed, A., Soomro, T. A., & Masood, R. (2024). Estimating age on the autopsy table: A postmortem study of forensic investigations. *Journal of Saidu Medical College, Swat.* https://www.semanticscholar.org/paper/fde681bc296472e9b38d3a4bc9801e2195d2b32b (accessed on 12th July 2025).
8. Calabrese, F., Pezzuto, F., Fortarezza, F., Hofman, P., Kern, I., Panizo, Á., von der Thüsen, J. H., et al. (2020). Pulmonary pathology and COVID-19: Lessons from autopsy. The experience of European pulmonary pathologists. *Virchows Archiv, 477*, 359–372. https://doi.org/10.1007/s00428-020-02886-6 (accessed on 12th July 2025).
9. Carter, S. M., Rogers, W., Win, K. T., Frazer, H., Richards, B., & Houssami, N. (2019). The ethical, legal and social implications of using artificial intelligence systems in breast cancer care. *The Breast, 49*, 25–32. https://doi.org/10.1016/j.breast.2019.10.001 (accessed on 12th July 2025).
10. Cecchi, R., Ciallella, C., LUCA, D. I., Natale, M., & Kimura, S. (2017). Ventricular androgenic-anabolic steroid-related remodeling: An immunohistochemical study. https://core.ac.uk/download/98348695.pdf (accessed on 12th July 2025).
11. Christe, A., Linden van der, A., Weustink, A. C., Weustink, A. C., Gatrad, A. R., Veress, B., Winters, B., et al. (2016). Non-invasive or minimally invasive autopsy compared to conventional autopsy of suspected natural deaths in adults: A systematic review. https://core.ac.uk/download/43291922.pdf (accessed on 12th July 2025).

12. Cullen, D. K., Johnson, V. E., Siman, R., Smith, D. H., et al. (2015). SNTF immunostaining reveals previously undetected axonal pathology in traumatic brain injury. https://core.ac.uk/download/46165322.pdf (accessed on 12th July 2025).

13. Davidson, D., Dejean, H., Hadchouel, H., Halpern, F., Hosoda, M., Jilbert, D., Korba, B., et al. (1995). Persistence of extrahepatic hepatitis B virus DNA in the absence of detectable hepatic replication in patients with baboon liver transplants. https://core.ac.uk/download/12205194.pdf (accessed on 12th July 2025).

14. Dirkmaat, D. C., Cabo, L. L., Ousley, S. D., & Symes, S. A. (2008). New perspectives in forensic anthropology. *American Journal of Physical Anthropology, 137*, 33–52. https://doi.org/10.1002/ajpa.20948 (accessed on 12th July 2025).

15. Farooq, S., Shahzad, I., Imran, M. A., Latif, S., Qadir, M., et al. (2017). How 5G wireless (and concomitant technologies) will revolutionize healthcare. https://core.ac.uk/download/143476480.pdf (accessed on 12th July 2025).

16. Fellmann, F., van El, C., Charron, P., Michaud, K., Howard, H., Boers, S. N., Clarke, A., et al. (2019). European recommendations integrating genetic testing into multidisciplinary management of sudden cardiac death. *European Journal of Human Genetics, 27*, 1763–1773. https://doi.org/10.1038/s41431-019-0445-y (accessed on 12th July 2025).

17. Filik, N., & FİLİK, F. (2022). Selected research and dramatic surgery fish cases of incisive complete in fish surgical. *Bulletin of Biotechnology, 4*, 30–35. https://doi.org/10.51539/biotech.1215628 (accessed on 12th July 2025).

18. Fragkou, K., Ketsekioulafis, I., Tousia, A., Piagkou, M., Bacopoulou, F., Ferentinos, P., Peyron, P., et al. (2025). From fragile lives to forensic truth: Multimodal forensic approaches to pediatric homicide and suspect death. *Diagnostics, 15*. https://www.semanticscholar.org/paper/63ebac527a63fda5f14ded21b3d1bd0f0e6cc6b9 (accessed on 12th July 2025).

19. Gur, A. G., Gur, A. E., Gur, O. M., Gur, et al. (2016). A perspective on the potential role of neuroscience in the court. https://core.ac.uk/download/144231732.pdf (accessed on 12th July 2025).

20. Habib, G., Lancellotti, P., Antunes, M. J., Bongiorni, M. G., Casalta, J.-P., Del Zotti, F., Dulgheru, R., et al. (2015). 2015 ESC Guidelines for the management of infective endocarditis. *European Heart Journal, 36*, 3075–3128. https://doi.org/10.1093/eurheartj/ehv319 (accessed on 12th July 2025).

21. Hansbrough, J. F., Porter, K. A., Putnam, C. W., Reid, et al. (1977). Biliary complications after liver transplantation: With special reference to the biliary cast syndrome and techniques of secondary duct repair. https://core.ac.uk/download/12203798.pdf (accessed on 12th July 2025).

22. Hou, D. (2024). Origin and development: History of storytelling. *Interdisciplinary Humanities and Communication Studies*. https://www.semanticscholar.org/paper/b206c4e73ebe3e15d41a88967f975dbc6298816c (accessed on 12th July 2025).

23. Humbert, M., Kovács, G., Hoeper, M. M., Badagliacca, R., Berger, R. M. F., Brida, M., Carlsen, J., et al. (2022). 2022 ESC/ERS Guidelines for the diagnosis and treatment of pulmonary hypertension. *European Respiratory Journal, 61*, 2200879–2200879. https://doi.org/10.1183/13993003.00879-2022 (accessed on 12th July 2025).

24. Ilg, G. (2013). The degeneration of the human mind: An analysis of Alzheimer's disease, a Kuhnian perspective. https://core.ac.uk/download/56325448.pdf (accessed on 12th July 2025).

25. Jagust, W. J., & Rabinovici, G. D. (2009). Amyloid imaging in aging and dementia: Testing the amyloid hypothesis *in vivo*. https://core.ac.uk/download/323081463.pdf (accessed on 12th July 2025).

26. Jangid, C., Dalal, J., Kumari, K., & Hamza, M. (2024). From traditional to virtual: The evolving landscape of autopsy techniques in forensic science. *Journal of Indian Academy of Forensic Medicine, 46*, 545–552. https://www.semanticscholar.org/paper/d00e7a7395688a53a02f2718e45257e1071ab12e (accessed on 12th July 2025).

27. Javed, A. R., Ahmed, W., Alazab, M., Jalil, Z., Kifayat, K., & Gadekallu, T. R. (2022). A comprehensive survey on computer forensics: State-of-the-art, tools, techniques, challenges, and future directions. *IEEE Access, 10*, 11065–11089. https://doi.org/10.1109/access.2022.3142508 (accessed on 12th July 2025).

28. Kesel, D., Ingels, A. S., Lambert, W., Stove, J., et al. (2012). Dried blood spots in toxicology: From the cradle to the grave? https://core.ac.uk/download/55802542.pdf (accessed on 12th July 2025).

29. Kirik, D., & Björklund, A. (2005). Histological analysis of fetal dopamine cell suspension grafts in two patients with Parkinson's disease gives promising results. *Brain: A Journal of Neurology, 128*(7), 1478–1479. https://www.semanticscholar.org/paper/4e32ebae1b6da85728997f1830c6701839951329 (accessed on 12th July 2025).

30. Kozma, Z., Pádár, Z., & Zenke, P. (2018). Forensic DNA technological advancements as an emerging perspective on medico-legal autopsy: A mini review. https://core.ac.uk/download/322434894.pdf (accessed on 12th July 2025).

31. Kraft, R., Fankhauser, G., Gerber, H., Hess, M., & Cottier, H. (1988). Age-related involution and terminal disorganization of the human thymus. *International Journal of Radiation Biology and Related Studies in Physics, Chemistry, and Medicine, 53*(1), 169–176. https://www.semanticscholar.org/paper/e0d8f065ceab9eb16256de2b5fef117457916023 (accessed on 12th July 2025).

32. Kumar, S., & Vats, S. V. M. (2024). A review article on the transformative impact of artificial intelligence-powered autopsy in forensic medicine. *International Journal for Multidisciplinary Research*. https://www.semanticscholar.org/paper/0fc74fb27376c6fde461d2d1c73ef7625cdabf73 (accessed on 12th July 2025).

33. Li, H., Xiao, X., Zhang, J., Zafar, M. I., Wu, C., Long, Y., Lu, W., et al. (2020). Impaired spermatogenesis in COVID-19 patients. *EClinicalMedicine, 28*, 100604–100604. https://doi.org/10.1016/j.eclinm.2020.100604 (accessed on 12th July 2025).

34. Lukács, B. L., & Veres, P. (2024). Innovative techniques for the storage and transportation of hazardous materials. *Advanced Logistic Systems–Theory and Practice*. https://www.semanticscholar.org/paper/8b87da42cfea7dbacf6eacb4ba82968ae07853cc (accessed on 12th July 2025).

35. Maixenchs, M., Anselmo, R., Zielinski-Gutiérrez, E., Odhiambo, F., Akello, C., Ondire, M., Zaidi, S., et al. (2016). Willingness to know the cause of death and hypothetical acceptability of the minimally invasive autopsy in six diverse African and Asian settings: A mixed methods

socio-behavioral study. *PLoS Medicine, 13*, e1002172–e1002172. https://doi.org/10.1371/journal.pmed.1002172 (accessed on 12th July 2025).

36. Mannocchi, G., Pantano, F., Romolo, F. S., et al. (2015). Recreational use, analysis, and toxicity of tryptamines. https://core.ac.uk/download/54534388.pdf (accessed on 12th July 2025).
37. Metcalf, J. L. (2018). Estimating the postmortem interval using microbes: Knowledge gaps and a path to technology adoption. *Forensic Science International Genetics, 38*, 211–218. https://doi.org/10.1016/j.fsigen.2018.11.004 (accessed on 12th July 2025).
38. Mousa, O. Y., & Kamath, P. S. (2021). A history of the assessment of liver performance. *Clinical Liver Disease, 18*, 28–48. https://doi.org/10.1002/cld.1100 (accessed on 12th July 2025).
39. Neri, M., Riezzo, I., Pascale, N., Pomara, C., & Turillazzi, E. (2017). Ischemia/reperfusion injury following acute myocardial infarction: A critical issue for clinicians and forensic pathologists. *Mediators of Inflammation, 2017*, 1–14. https://doi.org/10.1155/2017/7018393 (accessed on 12th July 2025).
40. Parvez, S., Chawla, H., & Yadav, H. (2025). Application of computed tomography in wound ballistics. *ARC Journal of Forensic Science.* https://www.semanticscholar.org/paper/841c31fc6da6329be60c52204c62cba60682ec1c (accessed on 12th July 2025).
41. Paxton, A., MacKay, A. P., AbouZahr, C., Chandra-Sekar, C., Hunger, C., Ronsmans, C., & Ronsmans, C. (2008). Measuring maternal mortality: An overview of opportunities and options for developing countries. https://core.ac.uk/download/177066.pdf (accessed on 12th July 2025).
42. Pazaitis, N., & Kaiser, A. (2023). TMA-Mate: An open-source modular toolkit for constructing tissue microarrays of arbitrary layouts. *HardwareX, 14*, e00419–e00419. https://doi.org/10.1016/j.ohx.2023.e00419 (accessed on 12th July 2025).
43. Pelliccia, A., Sharma, S., Gati, S., Bäck, M., Börjesson, M., Caselli, S., Collet, J. P., et al. (2020). 2020 ESC guidelines on sports cardiology and exercise in patients with cardiovascular disease. *European Heart Journal, 42*, 17–96. https://doi.org/10.1093/eurheartj/ehaa605 (accessed on 12th July 2025).
44. Percie du Sert, N., Ahluwalia, A., Alam, S., Avey, M. T., Baker, M., Browne, W. J., Clark, A., et al. (2020). Reporting animal research: Explanation and elaboration for the ARRIVE guidelines 2.0. *PLoS Biology, 18*, e3000411–e3000411. https://doi.org/10.1371/journal.pbio.3000411 (accessed on 12th July 2025).
45. Rehm, J., Gmel, G., Gmel, G., Hasan, O. S. M., Imtiaz, S., Popova, S., Probst, C., et al. (2017). The relationship between different dimensions of alcohol use and the burden of disease—an update. *Addiction, 112*, 968–1001. https://doi.org/10.1111/add.13757 (accessed on 12th July 2025).
46. Ruican, D., Petrescu, A., Ungureanu, A., Marinaş, M. C., Pirici, D., Istrate-Ofiţeru, A. I., Rosu, G., et al. (2021). Virtual autopsy and confirmation of normal fetal heart anatomy in the first trimester using three-dimensional (3D) reconstruction of histological sections. *Romanian Journal of Morphology and Embryology, 62*, 101–108. https://www.semanticscholar.org/paper/9848a8f884b7570c7441de12c4e3b81a3a1a23f3 (accessed on 12th July 2025).
47. Sharma, D., Kaul, R., & Agrawal, D. (2025). Morphometric analysis of tentorial orifice and its anatomical variations as relevant to transtentorial herniation: A preliminary cadaveric study. *Indian Journal of Neurotrauma.* https://www.semanticscholar.org/paper/c29ce247ff452bcbe26ee94df72894d635fc242d (accessed on 12th July 2025).

48. Shen, Y., Guo, D., Long, F., Mateos, L. A., Ding, H., Xiu, Z., Hellman, R. B., et al. (2020). Robots under COVID-19 pandemic: A comprehensive survey. *IEEE Access, 9*, 1590–1615. https://doi.org/10.1109/access.2020.3045792 (accessed on 12th July 2025).

49. Vretenarova, T., Atanassov, T., & Todorova, K. (2025). Surgery–from the barber-surgeon era to modern times. *Bulgarian Society of Medical Sciences Journal.* https://www.semanticscholar.org/paper/d9b54438da1a4d3f2dae7ee2ae131a922a169779 (accessed on 12th July 2025).

50. Zakaria, A. B., Zuki, M., Ibrahim, A., Okene, A., Mustapha, M., & Noordin, N. (2012). Applicability of virtopsy in veterinary practice: A short review. https://core.ac.uk/download/42992189.pdf (accessed on 12th July 2025).

BLUNT FORCE INJURIES

5

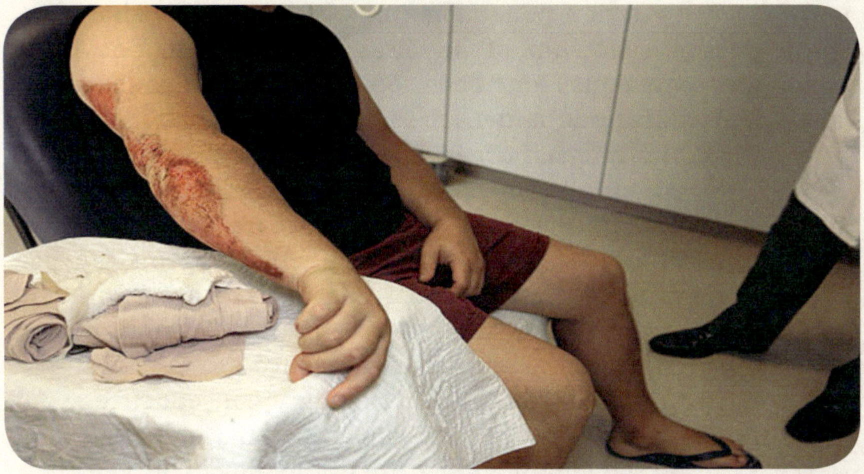

Introduction

Understanding blunt force injuries in humans is essential to the practice of medicine, psychology, and trauma science. Blunt force injuries are caused by impacts to the body that do not penetrate the skin or support tissues, in contrast with penetrating injuries that have the potential to directly damage structures and organs. These kinds of injuries can be the result of a large number of types of incidents, like falls, auto accidents, and assaults. They are capable of producing a variety of injuries, from minor bruising to severe internal injury, possibly resulting in long-term disability or fatalities. Increasingly, scientists are studying the biological and psychological effects of such injuries, mainly focusing on how they can affect an individual's recovery trajectory and general well-being. The influence of blunt trauma on the brain is particularly appalling, as it has the potential to cause the same outcomes that are induced by blasts or penetrating trauma. The latest studies have shown that traumatic brain injury (TBI) has been induced without any direct head impact owing to the exposure of the body to blast

LEARNING OBJECTIVES

After studying this chapter, you will be able to:

1. Describe the types of blunt force injuries;
2. Understand the mechanisms of injury associated with blunt force trauma;
3. Know the common causes of blunt force injuries;
4. Describe the symptoms and diagnosis of blunt force injuries;
5. Know the treatment options for blunt force injuries;
6. Understand the legal and forensic implications of blunt force injuries.

pressure waves, emphasizing the complexities involved in understanding brain injuries. For instance, the mechanisms of causing mild to moderate TBI included head acceleration and transmission of pressure waves through the thoracic cavity into the brain. The evidence supports the hypothesis that this blunt force trauma may result in widespread neurological injury, and it is important to bear this in mind while devising preventive strategies for vulnerable populations, such as troops and assault victims (Courtney et al., 2008). Besides, the effects of blunt trauma injuries extend beyond their direct physical impact as they can cause long-term psychological effects.

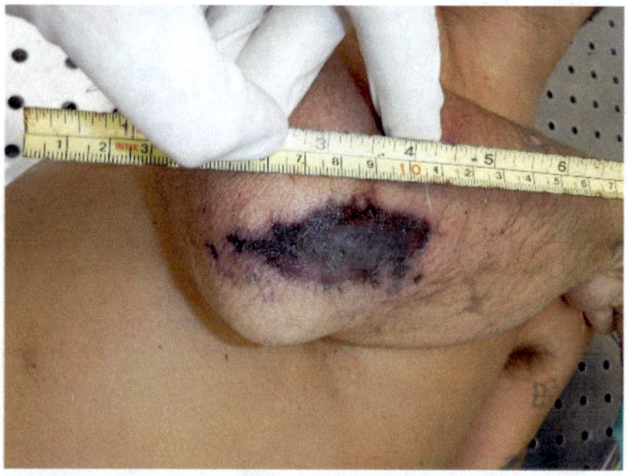

Figure 5.1. Skin injury consisting of the traumatic removal or detachment of the epidermis due to friction (shearing) or pressure (crushing) mechanisms.

Source: https://www.pathologyoutlines.com/imgau/forensicsbluntforceGitto01.jpg.

Their victims often develop symptoms of post-traumatic stress disorder (PTSD), anxiety, and depression, which further complicate their healing. Besides, correlation of remote blunt force trauma, as with projectile injury, and consequent cerebral damage, manifests a need for careful assessments following blunt force exposure. Studies have demonstrated correlations between serious blunt force injury and the occurrence of neurological disorders, including epilepsy, following a trauma (MP et al., 2008). Therefore, identifying the physical and the psychological effects of blunt force trauma is necessary for successful treatment regimens and continuing research investigations aimed at shedding light on their broader health consequences in human populations (Figure 5.1).

Definition of Blunt Force Injuries

Blunt trauma injuries, which are trauma inflicted by a non-penetrating object or surface, show a spectrum of physical injury to the body, which has long been separated into contusions, abrasions, and more severe forms like fractures and internal organ injury. Blunt injuries occur when a body part impacts against anon-penetrating force that produces a number of different tissue reactions depending on the velocity of the impact and surface area. The awareness of blunt force injuries extends to their insidious nature; they have the potential to inflict profound physiological consequences, including hemorrhage and inflammation, based on the length and nature of the blow. This calls for instant medical assessment, since blunt force assaults can advance exponentially if left untreated, resulting in further morbidity, even fatality. Physiologic pathways of blunt force trauma involve intricate inflammatory processes in the traumatized tissue. Following trauma, a cascade of biologic activity occurs, from the release of pro-inflammatory mediators to activation of immune cells reacting to tissue injury. Surprisingly, microglia, the central nervous system's resident immune cells, were responsible for playing pivotal roles such as mediating neuroinflammatory responses following blunt force trauma to the spinal cord and head. While the word "neuroinflammation" tends to be derogatory in clinical contexts, it is important to note that these inflammatory responses also contribute to recovery processes through healing and restoration of homeostasis. Therefore, duality in neuroinflammation emphasizes context, course, and duration as predictors in discerning the implications of blunt force injuries, particularly with regard to the central nervous system (Damon et al., 2016). Clinicians and researchers have to evaluate blunt force injuries comprehensively, both their immediate physical health effects and their longer-term physical health effects. Proportionality in terms of the severity of such injuries demands individualized therapy and rehabilitation. For instance, shallow contusions might require minimal treatment, while fractures or grievous internal harm demand advanced medical care, including surgery. Moreover, the psychological impact of blunt force trauma must not be overlooked, where the victim may endure long-term emotional or cognitive impairment following the trauma, particularly when there is a severe neuroinflammatory response (Damon et al., 2016). To this extent, an in-depth appreciation of the definition and consequences of blunt force trauma is crucial in developing meaningful prevention strategies and enhancing clinical outcomes among victims of this condition (Figure 5.2).

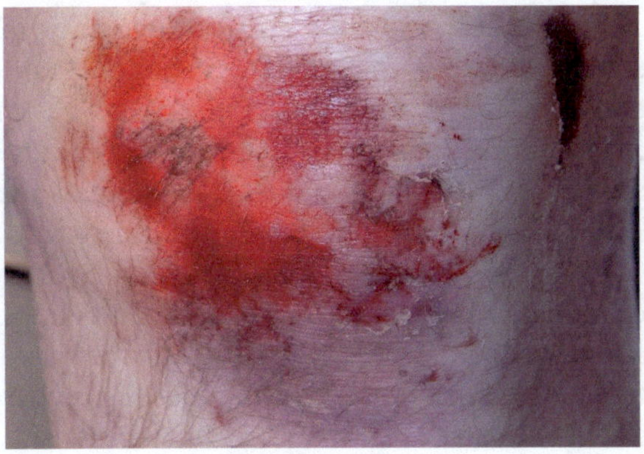

Figure 5.2. Abrasion on the knee.

Source: https://img.medscapestatic.com/pi/meds/ckb/34/9734.jpg.

Importance of Studying Blunt Force Injuries

The significance of learning about blunt force trauma must be realized not merely by medical professionals but also by the public safety and legal systems. Blunt force trauma refers to a wide spectrum of traumas from contusions, lacerations, and fractures through numerous kinds of incidents such as auto accidents, falls, and physical assaults. An examination of such injuries allows medical professionals to create better diagnostic tools and treatment guidelines to reduce morbidity from such trauma. Furthermore, accurate documentation and knowledge of the mechanisms behind blunt force injuries can make interventions more effective to prevent such accidents and further help in a broader public health policy on injury prevention and safety awareness. Additionally, the applicability of this discipline reaches into legal and forensic applications, in which an understanding of the medical ramifications of blunt trauma is crucial. In many cases, having the ability to fairly assess the cause and nature of the injuries can have monumental legal implications. Forensic experts rely on meticulous analyses of blunt trauma injuries to provide valid evidence during testimony in court, to ascertain whether death was accidental, self-inflicted, or homicide. Studies in this field promote a better appreciation of injury patterns, which is necessary for effective investigations and ultimately ensures that justice is maintained in society. The legal evidence, a number of times, depends on this clinical knowledge, emphasizing the significant role that the examination of blunt force injuries assumes in both criminal justice and public health systems. Finally, the study of the long-term effects of blunt force injury is critical in elucidating its broader health impact. Blunt force injuries can cause chronic pain, psychological trauma, and reduced quality of life. Examination of such results offers useful insights into the rehabilitation process and supports the creation of a full range of care strategies. Evidence indicates that results for patients who have incurred blunt force trauma can vary considerably depending on the nature and extent of the injury, and therefore, a specific approach to treatment is vital. Furthermore, public health intervention needs to incorporate research on the mental health impacts of such injuries, as they can lead to depression, anxiety, and post-traumatic stress disorder, similar to any other traumatic experience (Kennedy et al., 2015). In-depth investigation into the psychological impacts of blunt force injuries guarantees comprehensive treatment and care for victims, paving the way to recovery and resilience (Figure 5.3).

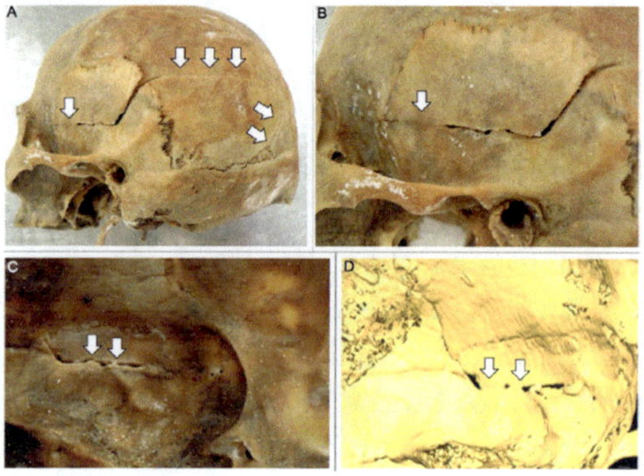

Figure 5.3. Fracture of the left parietal bone after a car accident 25 years ago. The bony bridges (arrows) on the ectocranial (A and B) and endocranial (C and D) surfaces. (D) illustrates the endocranial surface in a 3D reconstruction from CT scan data.

Source: https://www.dovepress.com/article/fulltext_file/70423/aW1n/fig1.jpg.

5.1. Types of Blunt Force Injuries

Learning Outcome

1. Describe the contusions.
2. Understand the abrasions.
3. Describe the fractures.

The classification of blunt trauma by force relies on a variety of conditions, including the kind of impact as well as the physiological damage that follows. Of the injury types that are most often encountered, the bruise or contusion is perhaps one of the most common. Contusions occur when blood vessels are damaged beneath the skin, and this causes the coloring of the skin and also swelling. Contusions most often result from direct blows or contact with soft tissues, and while they are often innocuous, the more significant presentation can inhibit usual function and require medical evaluation. Additionally, abrasions, which represent superficial damage from rubbing against a rough surface, typically accompany contusions in traumatic situations. Familiarity with the mechanisms of these injuries is important to ensure functional treatment regimens and prevention strategies in practice settings. Yet another important kind of blunt force injury is a laceration, which is a tearing of the skin and underlying tissue. In contrast to abrasions, lacerations are deeper in injury and tend to cause extensive bleeding and possible infection. They result from impact with sharp-edged objects, but can happen even when blunt force is used in a situation where the skin is stretched beyond its elasticity. For example, lacerations are frequently sustained in auto crashes where victims bounce back into the interior body parts of a vehicle. Besides their immediate physical impact, lacerations can also have long-term psychological scars in case of extensive damage. Health professionals need to be well-equipped with the implications of laceration injury so that they can properly provide adequate care and assistance to victims. Fractures, closed or open, are yet another severe category of blunt force trauma. Closed fractures are where bone is broken but not shattered to the point of breaking the skin, while an open fracture is where there exists an open wound through which the exposed bone is visible. They typically occur due to high impact, such as falls, crashes, or sports accidents, and need immediate medical care. The severity of fractures has a wide range; minor fractures might simply need to be immobilized, but compound fractures might need to be operated on in order to heal and avoid such complications as infection. It is important to understand the effects of these severe injuries because they can have a serious impact on an individual's recovery time and overall lifestyle. In addition, a significant volume of literature on allied health outcomes, including those related to accompanying mental illness, may result after severe trauma, highlighting the need for multifaceted care approaches that cater to physical and emotional demands (Kennedy et al., 2015; Azevedo et al., 2012).

5.1.1. Contusions

Contusions, or bruising, are the most common manifestation of blunt trauma in the form of bleeding around tissues without disruption of the skin's integrity. This is generated when small blood vessels rupture due to an impact force that compacts the deep tissues. Contusions are less evident than abrasions or lacerations because they do not breach the skin's integrity, although great damage may be incurred behind the skin. Physical presentation of contusions evolves over time, ranging from red to purple and eventually yellowish-green when the body begins to degrade the pooled blood in the tissue. Clinical understanding of the contusion mechanism is necessary, since contusions can be a sign of deeper injuries, particularly those in high-impact sports or road traffic accidents. Physiological response to contusions involves complex processes like inflammation and healing of the tissue. Following trauma, inflammatory mediators such as growth factors and cytokines are secreted into the injured tissue to heal, but also to induce pain and inflammation. It is a critical process of healing tissues, but it leads to complications if there is excessive inflammation. In severe cases, contusions predispose patients to secondary complications such as compartment syndrome, where increased pressure in muscle compartments compromises blood flow and nerve function. It is important that medical physicians understand the intricacies of contusions for the determination of the extent of injuries sustained, especially where early intervention can prevent secondary injuries with blunt force trauma. Blunt force injury has been explored in recent studies to examine the impact of contusions on more general physiological systems, including the central nervous system (CNS). Spinal cord contusions, for instance, have been found to lead to irreversible damage due to tissue contusion from external forces, which underscores the need for successful treatment protocols. Model studies of spinal cord injury have revealed the kinetics of secondary injury processes and provided the possibility of therapeutic intervention aimed at activating self-regeneration in damaged tissue. Looking at the biological response of tissue adjacent to contusions, like the location of neural stem cells during regeneration, shows the growing overlap between injury care and advanced medical science. With growing knowledge of contusions comes greater capacity for optimizing patient outcome and refining treatment procedures for blunt trauma injuries in the human body (Shibuya et al., 2009; Hurwitz, 1984) (Figure 5.4).

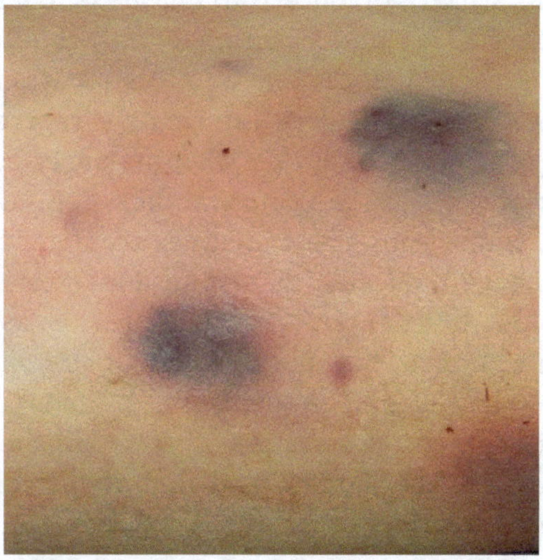

Figure 5.4. Two contusions on the skin of the chest.

Source: https://img.medscapestatic.com/pi/meds/ckb/35/9735.jpg.

5.1.2. Abrasions

Abrasions, which are generally considered to be superficial skin trauma, are caused by the rubbing action between the skin and outer surfaces in cases of blunt trauma. Abrasions in most situations occur in the event of a fall, collision, or sports contact, where the skin gets rubbed against coarse surfaces. Unlike more severe forms of trauma, abrasions affect only the epidermis and sometimes the superficial dermis, causing pain, color change, and swelling but frequently little bleeding. The mechanisms of abrasions are important for their treatment in the short term as well as their significance in forensic use. They can serve as indicators of the severity and type of force employed, and information on the dynamics of the event and the gravity of the other associated injuries (Knüsel et al., 2013).

Though apparently less grave than deeper wounds or punctures, abrasions can lead to complications if infected. The exposed body surface is a potential entry point for disease agents, which is of concern in clinical examination. Furthermore, under forensic anthropology, the presence, location, and distribution of abrasions can be very informative regarding the conditions of injury. For instance, some distributions can indicate whether an injury is accidental or not. These analyses are significant, as they provide depth to our understanding of blunt force interaction and provide useful information for traumatic event reconstruction. The skin reaction in such injuries must also be documented because it can reflect the impact,surface motion, and underlying forces involved (Knüsel et al., 2013). Additionally, the similarity in the interaction between abrasions and blunt force trauma is highlighted by the mechanical forces underpinning their creation. Impact is responded to by the body through intricate interactions of the applied force, the contacted area, and the characteristics of the skin. The interaction implies that abrasions should lie on a continuum and be affected by an array of variables, such as the area of contact and impact velocity. Understanding the types of these relationships allows clinicians and researchers to more accurately assess the severity of the trauma. Forensic investigation of patterns of abrasions can distinguish wounds caused by a self-inflicted injury from those caused by another, again emphasizing the need for careful assessment in clinical and forensic settings (Kroman et al., 2007). Thus, abrasions are a fascinating element of blunt trauma injuries, deserving extensive study within the greater field of trauma analysis (Figure 5.5).

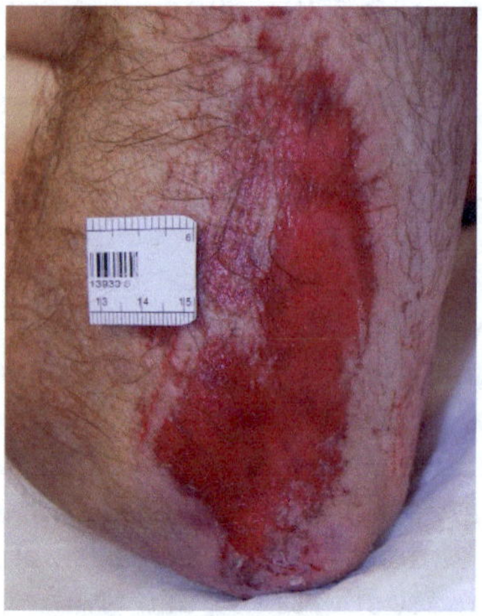

Figure 5.5. Abrasion on the elbow.

Source: https://img.medscapestatic.com/pi/meds/ckb/33/9733.jpg.

5.1.3. Fractures

Fractures, a natural consequence of blunt trauma injuries, significantly affect the quality of life, from transient annoyance to permanent disability. When trauma occurs, the extent and type of fracture are based on various factors, such as the intensity of the force applied, the location where the force was applied, and one's bone density. Specifically, fractures of the hand, which occur frequently from daily activities and sports trauma, need to be treated immediately and diagnosed properly to obtain optimal results. The standard way of diagnosing fractures involves imaging modalities, foremost X-rays, which are responsible for diagnosing the occurrence and nature of the fracture. But as Medaramatla et al. (2024) indicate, these imaging protocols occasionally fail to detect small fractures, highlighting the necessity for radiographic technology advancements to enhance early diagnosis and treatment. One interesting use of fracture analysis is in forensic medicine, particularly in suspicious cases of blunt force trauma. The pattern and nature of the fracture may provide vital clues regarding the causative forces involved in a particular injury, which can aid forensic experts in reconstructing the event and identifying suspects. For example, recognizing the variations between fracture patterns caused by blunt objects and those caused by accidents or falls is important in knowing the context of an injury. Studies such as those highlighted in Chen (2023) illustrate the intricate relationship between forensic analysis and fracture mechanics, in which quantitative research provides an enhanced understanding of fracture patterns and wound production to provide a successful outcome in criminal proceedings. Handling fracture care, the integration of sophisticated diagnostic methods is essential to enhance treatment outcomes. New approaches, such as hybrid models using deep learning algorithms in X-ray interpretation, are in the pipeline to improve diagnostic accuracy and speed. As explicated in Medaramatla et al. (2024), the new models have been developed to correctly diagnose fractures, preventing misdiagnosis and resultant complications. In addition, comprehensive educational interventions for medical professionals in the detection of various types of fractures can stimulate appropriate interventions, which ultimately minimize the severity of injury. Complemented by advancements in diagnostic techniques and forensic analysis, the significance of studying fractures in the broader context of blunt force injuries is thereby justified, hence the need for continued research and development in both medical and forensic sciences (Figure 5.6).

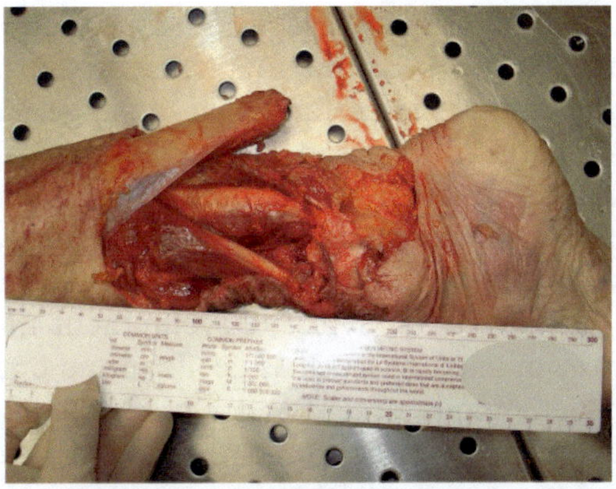

Figure 5.6. A bone lesion develops when the intensity of a trauma exceeds the bone's resistance. An open fracture of the left leg is shown.

Source: https://www.pathologyoutlines.com/imgau/forensicsbluntforceGitto04.jpg.

Test Your Knowledge

1. What is a contusion?
2. What imaging technique is most commonly used to identify fractures?

5.2. Mechanisms of Injury

Learning Outcome

1. Understand the impact forces.
2. Describe the acceleration-deceleration forces.
3. Understand the compression forces.

Understanding the mechanisms of injury associated with blunt force trauma is essential to advance clinical practice and forensic science. Blunt force injuries result from a range of impacts, such as falls, impacts, and attacks. These injuries most commonly lead to contusions, abrasions, and fractures. A review of the biomechanical principles associated with such injuries is useful in terms of learning about the thresholds for tissue damage. More specifically, transferred kinetic energy upon impact is the factor that determines the extent of injury. Improved knowledge of responses of the tissue to variations in force can be used to design protective devices. Development in the sciences of imaging, such as acoustic and optical imaging methods, urges further research into the mechanisms of injury. Data from such studies are priceless in the context of both preventative design and maximizing medical treatment for trauma patients across all levels of practice. For forensic analysis, scientific interpretation of blunt force trauma through the use of scientific methods is important. Specifically, analysis of the bruising pattern is crucial because these are cardinal signs of the dynamics of assault. Recent advancements in forensic techniques, including the use of alternate light sources (ALS), have shown potential to enhance the visibility of bruises, which is critical for documentation and forensic examination. Reviews indicate that while narrowband wavelengths can be used to enhance detection and visualization of bruises compared to white light, their efficacy is contingent upon the specific conditions of the examination. As an example, there are several factors, such as the history of the bruise and whether or not there are associated skin features, that can impact results. Continued development and validation of such methods is crucial to their utilization in routine forensic practice, demonstrating the importance to extending the knowledge about blunt force trauma.

The significance of properly understanding the dynamics of blunt force injury extends into the development of occupational and recreational safety protocols. Protective equipment, from helmets to pads, is designed based on current understanding of the impact dynamics upon human tissue. In this case, investigation, such as the development of human head phantoms that are able to accurately model and analyze cavitation effects in blunt impacts, becomes essential. Measurement with such phantoms has shed light on the need to investigate how energy dissipates in living tissues when it hits them, thereby acquiring valuable information about injury thresholds and safety measures. Use of acoustic imaging techniques to identify cavitation events further bridges the gap between theory and practice. These advances in biomedical research can be used to design more protective technology that might decrease the prevalence and severity of blunt force trauma across environments, from sports to the military (Eric et al., 2024; Tyr et al., 2024) (Figure 5.7).

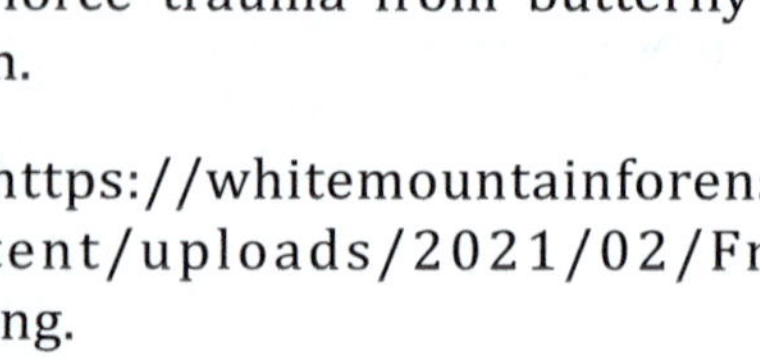

Figure 5.7. Interpreting injury mechanisms of blunt force trauma from butterfly fracture formation.

Source: https://whitemountainforensic.com/wp-content/uploads/2021/02/Fracture-pattern.png.

5.2.1. Impact Forces

It is worth learning about impact forces when handling blunt force injuries since impact forces are the fundamental mechanism of the physiological injury that the human body experiences during violent encounters. When a body is hit by an object, it will undergo an interaction force that can lead to deformation of tissues, fracture of bones, and injuries to internal organs. The direction and magnitude of impact forces directly influence the severity of the resulting damage. For instance, faster velocity collisions tend to cause more severe injuries, as a result of higher energy transfer, which overtaxes the body's capacity to absorb and distribute such stresses. Additionally, variables such as the size of impact, properties of object surfaces, and angle of impact all have significant roles in determining the outcomes of a collision, and the subject gestures towards the intricacy of analyzing blunt force trauma in forensic contexts. The mechanisms through which impact forces contribute to blunt force injury can be explained by looking into traumatic brain injury caused by blast pressure waves. Experiments have shown that mild to moderate TBI may occur along various pathways, including head acceleration or direct exposure to such wave events, which travel through the thorax to the cranial space. The findings underscore the importance of understanding how forces of impact from the outside world, like explosive blasts, can cause neurological damage through pressure waves that disrupt the structural integrity of the brain. While traditional views of blunt force trauma focus on the direct mechanical force, the addition of pressure wave dynamics, as seen in the study of research related to blasts, recognizes an additional element to the complexity of determining the effect of forces on human health, particularly brain injury (Courtney et al., 2008). Further impact force studies on blunt force injury also entail the utilization of experimental models to replicate human skeletal reaction to various types of trauma. New materials, such as polyurethane plates and spheres, have been used in recent forensic anthropology breakthroughs as a potential analogue for human bone in ballistic research.

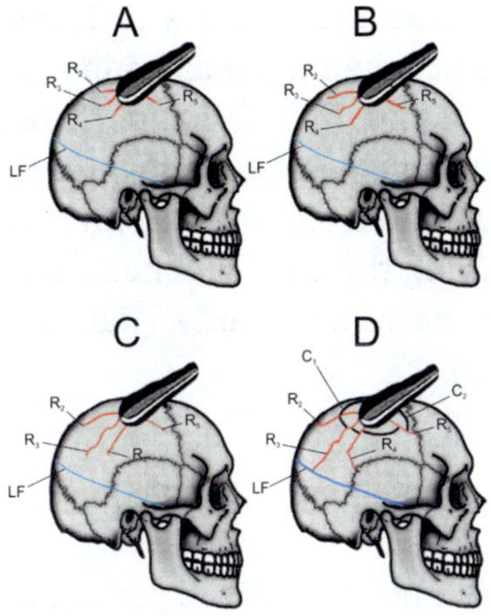

Figure 5.8. Mechanism of blunt force trauma on the vault A) Low velocity impact on the skull causing fracture formation at the impact point due to initial bending of the cranial vault with peripheral out-bending; inward displacement of the bony fragment due to plastic deformation; small fragments remaining in place suggest that the impact took place while soft tissue was present. B) Radiating fractures in the area of out bending which start at one or more points distant to the impact site, progressing both towards the impact point and in the opposite direction (away from it); C) The radiating fractures stop when they meet the sutures (e.g., R1). D) Formation of concentric fractures perpendicular to the radiating fractures. Image credit: Iakovos Ouranos.

Source: https://www.researchgate.net/publication/334209308/figure/fig5/AS:11431281272666740@1724189840880/Mechanism-of-blunt-force-trauma-on-the-vault-A-Low-velocity-impact-on-the-skull-causing.tif.

These tests attempt to reproduce impact conditions that are difficult to test in human cadavers due to ethical restrictions or lack of resources. Although these surrogate materials may demonstrate macroscopic results of impact force, caution is necessary; the response of the artificial material to stress may be different from that of actual human bone at the microstructural level. As research continues to bridge the gap between experimental results and actual human injury outcomes, the dynamic interaction of impact forces remains at the forefront as a focus area for strengthening forensic science and explaining the consequences of blunt force trauma in the human body (Ball et al., 2015) (Figure 5.8).

5.2.2. Acceleration-Deceleration Forces

In the analysis of blunt force injuries, acceleration-deceleration forces are also paramount in how impacts from the external environment affect the human body. Acceleration-deceleration forces happen with sudden velocity changes, either in a collision or from some other type of impact. If a person or object decelerates rapidly or changes direction, the inertial response of the body's internal structures may cause injury. Precisely, the amount of injury that such incidents typically will cause often will depend upon the magnitude of the forces involved, as greater accelerations more typically cause catastrophic damage. Force interaction is essential in forensic anthropology, where trauma to bone is viewed as a continuum rather than as classification, as presented in recent literature on bone fracture patterns and engineering input correlation (Kroman et al., 2007). The nature of acceleration-deceleration forces is the cause of various types of blunt force injuries, particularly in the event of a high-impact crash. For example, in automobile crashes, the occupants experience forces that can lead to injuries ranging from bruising to fracture, depending on the speed of the vehicle and the strength of the seatbelt and airbag. The complexity of such forces also involves variation in surface area between the body and the impact object, which could differentiate between blunt and sharp trauma. The subtle understanding of how acceleration and deceleration interact with the body's anatomy provides essential information to health professionals and forensic experts, information they can use to attribute the cause of the injuries due to accidents or attacks (Kroman et al., 2007). In addition, acceleration-deceleration forces have not only caused physical injuries; they can also cause traumatic brain injuries (TBI) in situations such as blasts or explosions. In modern combat, for instance, the stresses of a blast can cause severe brain damage even if there is no direct impact.

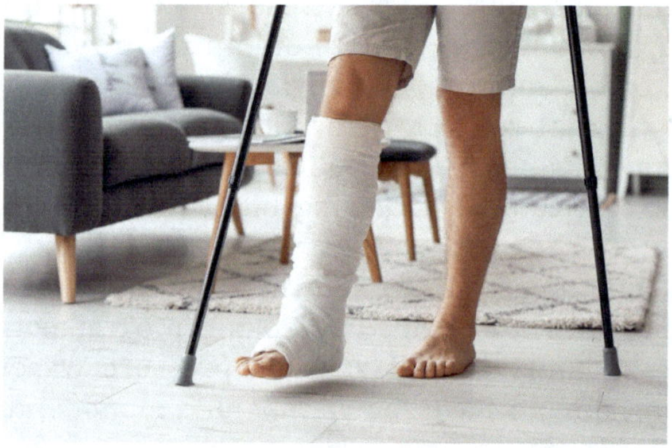

Figure 5.9. A figure showing the mechanisms of acceleration–deceleration and rotational head injury.

Source: https://www.researchgate.net/profile/Agnes-Tiwari/publication/251235271/figure/fig1/AS:298074464374784@1448077898523/A-figure-showing-the-mechanisms-of-acceleration-deceleration-and-rotational-head-injury.png

This is an area of research that has become key as researchers attempt to identify the long-term neurological consequences experienced by individuals who have been so harmed. Despite growing recognition of blast-induced TBI, scientific studies of its pathophysiology are few, with a need for more studies to investigate its effects on human health. Appreciation of acceleration and deceleration dynamics is crucial in meeting this challenge and promoting injury prevention measures across various settings (Figure 5.9).

5.2.3. Compression Forces

The mechanism of compression forces is a crucial component of the pathophysiology of blunt force trauma in humans. Compression forces are produced when two or more bodies crush against each other, producing rigid body deformation or tissue injury. In trauma, the forces are created through various mechanisms, such as motor vehicle collisions, falls, or collisions. Their impact can cause a range of injuries from bruising and hematoma to more severe effects such as fracture and organ damage. Familiarity with the nature and implications of compression forces is significant in forensic applications as they assist in reconstructing the event and assessing patterns of injury. As an example, non-invasive animal models of osteoarthritis have proven the way in which such forces induce adaptation processes in joint injury and provided valuable biomechanical insights into equivalent human injury (Pitsillides et al., 2015). The study of compression forces on human anatomy has urgent implications for the medical and legal professions. When compression occurs due to an acute blow, the body's tissues may respond in different ways depending on the location and degree of the force. Of concern is bone, which is very sensitive to such trauma and produces conditions such as post-traumatic osteoarthritis that develop over a long time due to compression. Animal model studies have also been employed to demonstrate that even non-invasive methods, such as cyclic tibial compression loading, can provide valuable insight into the manner in which the injuries occur (Pitsillides et al., 2015). Furthermore, the understanding of these forces not only informs clinical treatment regimens but also streamlines the accuracy of forensic evaluation, assessing how compression-induced injury correlates to specific instances of blunt force trauma. Furthermore, the challenges of replicating human response in laboratory settings illustrate the complexity of deconstructing blunt force trauma from compression. Traditional methods, traditionally relegated to the realm of animal models, are challenged regarding their applicability due to physiological differences. Alternative methods, such as polyurethane plates replicating human bone, have offered new avenues for inquiry by offering researchers a better-controlled context upon which to explore the force of blunt impact. These proxies are limited, however, in that they can only duplicate macro bone response; wide microscopic fluctuations caution against uncritical extrapolation to human trauma. Human anatomy needs to be replicated in sound standards and models for the development of scientific knowledge, as well as the establishment of sound forensic practice in the context of blunt force trauma.

Test Your Knowledge

1. What are the impact forces?
2. What are the compression forces?

5.3. Common Causes of Blunt Force Injuries

Learning Outcome

1. Learn about motor vehicle accidents.
2. Describe the Falls and physical assaults.

Blunt force trauma is a public health problem of immense size, more often than not the result of a broad spectrum of accidents and episodes. Motor vehicle accidents are the most common cause, significantly contributing to blunt trauma hospitalization and fatality. In such incidents, victims undergo impacts on various regions of the body, injuring them with entities such as contusions, fractures, and internal injuries to organs. The mechanisms of car crashes range from frontal collisions with other vehicles to secondary collisions, such as hitting the dashboard, windshield, or side windows. Additionally, the speed at which the collisions occur compounds the forces in action, and understanding the biomechanics is necessary in order to effectively treat the injuries. With the continually rising prevalence of incidents involving vehicles, additional research and preventive measures are essential in an attempt to lower the prevalence of blunt force trauma due to transport-related accidents. In addition to motor vehicle accidents, falls are also a common cause of blunt force trauma, particularly among the vulnerable population, such as the elderly. The falls are likely to occur in most environments, such as at home, in the workplace, and outdoors, and usually result in major complications such as hip fractures or head injuries. The conditions under which one has a fall can vary significantly, with differing factors such as height, ground, and the physical condition of the individual being significant predictors. For instance, older people are more susceptible to heightened vulnerability because of conditions like diminished balance and frailty, which can exacerbate the risk of severe injury upon falling. It is essential to identify the situations under which falls occur so that targeted interventions and educational programs for minimizing their occurrence may be established, particularly for vulnerable groups. Effective strategies can range from environmental modifications to balance training exercises, all with the intent of preventing disabling injury while preserving mobility. Athletic activities are also major venues of blunt trauma injuries, usually seen with contact sports such as football, rugby, and boxing. Such injuries can be produced by direct impact, tackles, or falls and are susceptible to not only acute trauma but also to long-term sequelae such as concussion. The following sports passion led to the frequent occurrence of injuries, calling for efficient management measures that include prevention, quick response procedures, and restoration. Prevention equipment like pads and helmets can reduce the severity of blunt trauma injuries; timely use, however, depends on compliance with the sport-specific manner of usage. With the increasing popularity of contact sports, an acute need for establishing guidelines for safe competition grows in significance so athletes can keep on competing without raising the level of injury risk (Figure 5.10).

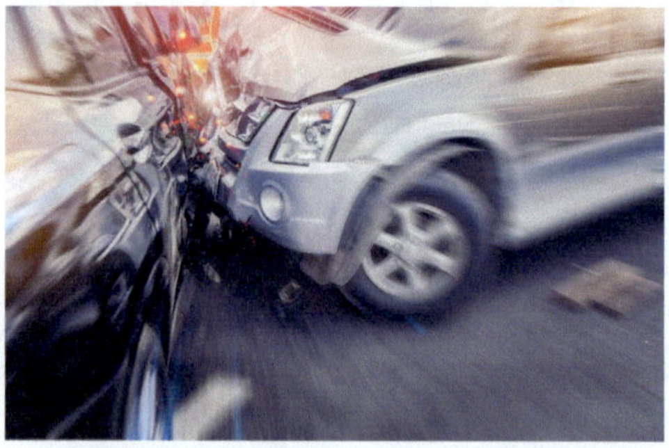

Figure 5.10. Car accidents can cause blunt force trauma to the chest.

Source: https://www.banksjones.com/wp-content/uploads/2024/06/Car-Accidents-Can-Cause-Blunt-Force-Trauma-to-the-Chest.jpeg.

5.3.1. Motor Vehicle Accidents

Motor vehicle accidents (MVAs) are a public health issue, often producing blunt force trauma injuries that may lead to serious body system trauma. Injuries typically result from deceleration forces imparted during an accident, which produce significant impacts to the occupants within the car. Typical presentations of these injuries include fractures, contusions, and concussions, which are predominantly related to the head, neck, and thoracic regions. The consequences of MVAs are not merely corporeal; they impose significant emotional and psychological burdens on victims and families. In the design of effective prevention measures and emergency response protocols, the mechanisms of blunt force injury in motor vehicle crashes must be considered. As continuous research evolves, it serves to further clarify the interaction between vehicle design, occupant protection systems, and the type of injuries sustained during crashes. The role of blunt trauma injury in motor vehicle accidents also encompasses internal injuries that are not easily visible but have important implications for patient outcomes. For instance, chest injury can result in serious conditions such as blunt cardiac injury, which could result from the severe deceleration forces in an accident. An example case illustrates the way a 28-year-old man suffered a rupture of the papillary muscle after receiving direct blunt-force trauma to his chest during an MVA. The resultant mitral valve dysfunction illustrates the difficulty of diagnosing cardiac injuries that may accompany external traumas. The intricacy of injuries sustained during MVAs complicates treatment even further, with medical practitioners having to treat both overt and latent indicators of trauma. Early and accurate diagnosis of such conditions is vital to provide for early intervention and better survival rates for victims. Forensic examination is also important in determining the actual cause of injuries sustained during motor vehicle crashes. In certain cases, for instance, investigating a 19-year-old male who died as a result of an accident, initial results may indicate death due to an accident. But forensic analysis revealed that the victim sustained extreme blunt force trauma, which was indicative of foul play rather than an accident. Failure of normal secondary injuries in being thrown out of the car led to suspicion of the scene being fabricated to resemble an MVA. These kinds of cases highlight the value of thorough forensic analysis not only to ascertain the cause of death but to establish the conditions of the event as well. Not only is this an act of justice, but it also further the understanding of how blunt force trauma occurs in various scenarios, illuminating the greater societal relevance of car safety and avoiding accidents (Figure 5.11).

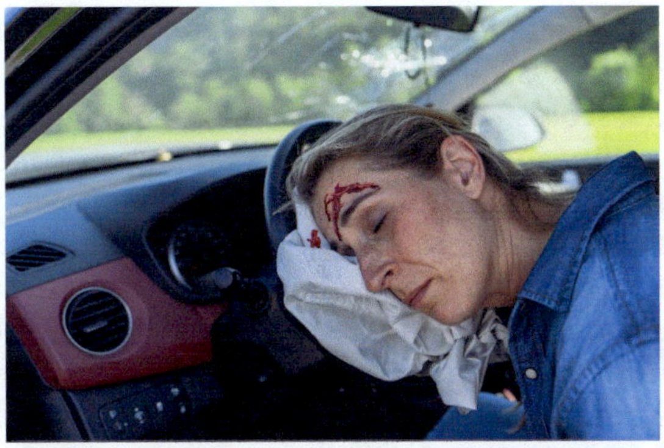

Figure 5.11. Motor vehicle accident.

Source: https://aica.com/wp-content/uploads/2024/09/Common-Injuries-from-Car-Accidents-What-to-Watch-Out-For.jpg.

5.3.2. Falls

Falls are a significant public health problem in elderly populations, where the incidence causes blunt trauma injuries. Falls can lead to injuries ranging from as mild as bruises to as severe as fractures and head injuries, which have a significant impact on quality of life. A fall biomechanics is an abrupt deceleration at impact, which may be responsible for massive tissue damage and disruption of physiological processes. Research has indicated that the contributing factors are diminished muscle strength, compromised balance, and environmental hazards like slippery floors and inadequate lighting, all of which increase the risk of falls for the elderly. They must be addressed not only to prevent injury but to enhance overall well-being in elderly people, as falls can undermine mobility and independence, ultimately exacerbating frailty and comorbidities in the elderly. Further, the psychological effect of falls should not be overlooked. The fear of falling would automatically limit people from participating in activities, leading to a sedentary lifestyle that decreases physical strength and balance ability even more. This vicious circle can cause subsequent falls to be more probable, and this is a vast cost for healthcare systems as the need for medical interventions becomes larger. Furthermore, the connection between a lack of physical activity and various conditions underscores the importance of remaining active as a means of reversing the impacts of falls. Muscle-strengthening and balance-improving exercise interventions not only reduce the rate of falls but also improve mental health, thereby guaranteeing an improved quality of life in the elderly. Multidisciplinary treatments integrating environmental adaptation and exercise may be effective in the prevention of falls and their subsequent effects on health. While treating the multifactorial nature of falls, due regard should be afforded to the role of adipose tissue and its contribution to physical health. Transformed adipose tissue is recognized to propel chronic ailments such as type 2 diabetes mellitus (T2DM) and cardiovascular disease (CVD), which are linked with the increased threat of falls and injury from falls. With declining metabolic function, patients become less active and more frail and have a greater risk for falls. It is essential to establish comprehensive fall prevention interventions that target these interrelationships. The prescription of exercise and structured physical activity, in addition to treating balance and muscle decline, can be a therapeutic approach towards metabolic optimization as well. Treatments addressing the underlying etiology of falls within a totalistic framework can be rewarding, reducing blunt trauma injury incidence and healthier aging populations (Figure 5.12).

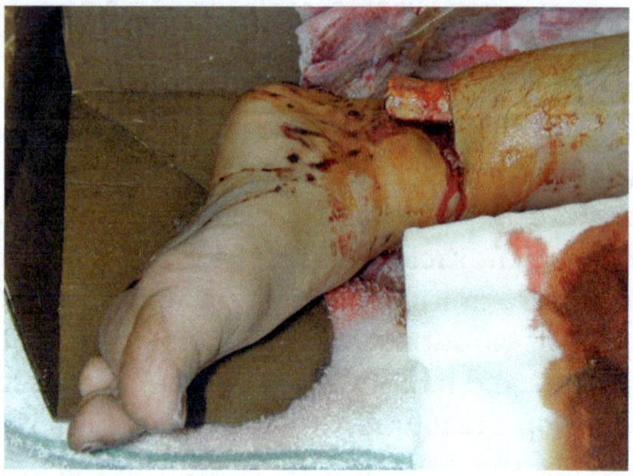

Figure 5.12. Compound fracture dislocation of the ankle following a fall from a height.

Source: https://08f043fb5b.clvaw-cdnwnd.com/65cf06e22b1051f5df11dfe70b7dd6da/200000078-a8a8ca9a33/Compound_fracture_dislocation_left_ankle.jpg.

5.3.3. Physical Assaults

Physical attacks are, however, of a general nature and encompass all types of violent acts that cause harm to individuals and, in most instances, have physical and psychological impacts. Physical attacks are of numerous kinds, including striking, kicking, or using weapons, and all such types are wide concerns for public health and security. Victims of physical assault usually present with blunt force trauma, which is characterized by injury due to pressure or collision, in contrast to laceration or puncture. Such injuries range in severity and character depending on a number of factors, including the weapon, force applied, and location of impact, typically resulting in bruises, fractures, or contusions, which require complete medical examination and treatment. Furthermore, the application of law enforcement to minimize physical assaults highlights the complexity involved in managing violent altercations.

Mechanisms such as pepper spray (OC) have been frequently used by police officers to neutralize hostile targets temporarily. While OC has been shown to reduce violent behaviors in most reported circumstances, its effectiveness is not absolute. For instance, scientific studies have established that the effective range is typically limited to below two meters, and a three-to-five-second delay before effects are visible is perilous in high-pressure encounters. In addition, collateral strikes against other officers have been experienced in 24% of the incidents, with the observation that while OC may be utilized for less threatening environments, it is not well-suited to counter the complexity of high threatening environments, including those with armed attackers (Bertilsson et al., 2017). In even more violent instances of brutality, explosive devices have been utilized as a tool of mass brutality and casualties, further complicating the act of physical assault. Blast trauma has analyzed what is most important of the details surrounding injuries inflicted by such an act, such as how shrapnel plays a magnifying role in injury over the blast itself. Experimental studies with controlled subjects, such as feral pigs, illustrate the devastating impact of explosives on the appendicular skeleton with rising traumatic amputation and fractures caused by other materials like shrapnel. These findings highlight the imperative of forensic science in understanding the dynamics of blunt force trauma and provide important context for medical professionals who treat injuries due to both interpersonal violence and collective conflict, particularly in an age defined by increasingly widespread use of explosives in human rights abuses (Lane et al., 2018) (Figure 5.13).

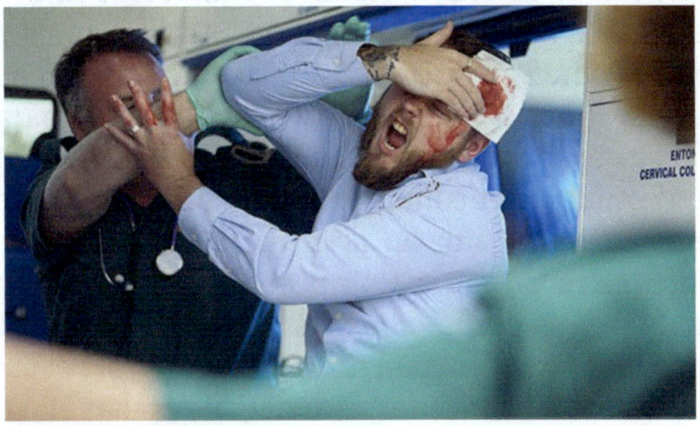

Figure 5.13. Physical assaults.

Source: https://dm1zcrsul8wju.cloudfront.net/sites/rcn_nspace/files/styles/full_width_banner/public/Aggression_tile_iStock_0.jpg?itok=VXQSaCa9.

Test Your Knowledge

1. Describe the Motor vehicle accidents.
2. What do you mean by physical assault?

5.4. Symptoms and Diagnosis

Learning Outcome

1. Understand the physical examination findings.
2. Describe the imaging techniques.
3. Understand the process of differential diagnosis.

Identification of symptoms of blunt force injury is important for early diagnosis and appropriate management of trauma. Characteristic signs include localized bruising, swelling, and pain at the site of injury, which are reflections of underlying tissue injury. In some cases, patients may present with an array of systemic signs, such as fever, indicating potential infection or, in extreme cases, shock secondary to blood loss. Physical examination is likely to reveal lacerations, contusions, or deformities that allow clinicians to assess the extent of the injury. More image resolution modalities, such as X-rays, CT scans, or MRIs, can be used to visualize internal injuries such as fractures or organ damage. An understanding of the intricacy of presentation of symptoms is significant since trivial signs can lead to undetected complications, highlighting the importance of appropriate examination and history taking while reaching a diagnosis. Blunt trauma injuries are primarily diagnosed based on an alliance of clinical assessment and diagnostic imaging. After a thorough patient history and physical examination, practitioners generally utilize radiologic imaging to assess trauma severity and character. For instance, while X-rays are most effective in the diagnosis of bone fractures, CT scans provide a broader image, which identifies damage to soft tissue, blood vessels, and organs that may not be immediately apparent. Furthermore, it is essential to check for vital signs so that the extent of the injury can be established. Anomalies of hypotension or tachycardia could indicate internal bleeding or shock and warrant immediate action. Re-revaluation and constant monitoring are important since patients often have delayed symptoms that only manifest as the clinical presentation evolves, in accordance with the dynamic nature of the diagnosis of blunt trauma injuries. Besides physical signs, the psychological impact of blunt trauma injuries may have significant effects on rehabilitation. Patients may also experience emotional distress, anxiety, or post-traumatic stress disorder (PTSD), further complicating the overall clinical picture.

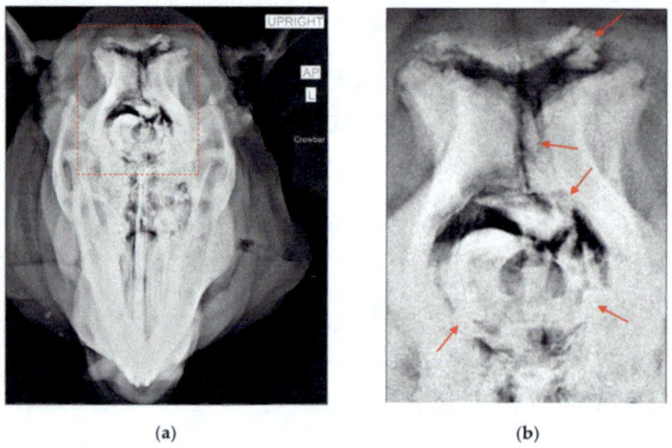

Figure 5.14. Radiographic image of sample CBH1. (a) Pre-burn radiograph of a specimen after manual trauma with a crowbar. Red dotted lines denote the area containing blunt force trauma. (b) Close-up image of the area within the red rectangle. Red arrows point to areas of incomplete fractures as a result of blunt force trauma, with associated fragments still attached.

Source: https://www.mdpi.com/biology/biology-11-00087/article_deploy/html/images/biology-11-00087-g001.png.

It is crucial that health practitioners remain vigilant for these psychological symptoms in conjunction with physical assessment and referral to the appropriate mental health care providers. In interdisciplinary care systems, collaboration among specialists—trauma surgeons to psychologists—can maximize patient outcomes and guarantee an integrative rehabilitative approach. Such combined therapy, in aiming at the body's immediate restoration, also aims at restoring the emotional and psychological health consequences of trauma, with acknowledgment that the best recovery is both of body and mind. Integrating these considerations generates holistic care, ultimately providing healthier long-term recovery from blunt force trauma (Figure 5.14).

5.4.1. Physical Examination Findings

A thorough physical examination is crucial in the identification and assessment of blunt force trauma injuries in humans due to its ability to detect subtle and apparent evidence of trauma. In the initial evaluation, clinicians should observe the patient's vital signs, neurological function, and outward signs of injury. This involves a systematic head-to-toe examination to assess for tenderness, edema, or deformity. For instance, evidence such as bruising, laceration, and abrasion may direct the mechanism of injury and guide further imaging. Systematically examining the cranial and cervical spine areas is important, particularly since blunt force trauma is often the cause of intracranial injury, which may be difficult to identify on initial examination. The outcome of the physical examination may also provide prognostic information regarding the severity of the trauma and the likely path for the patient. Coupled with the physical findings, determination of the Glasgow Coma Scale (GCS) is an important component of the evaluation of head injury severity. The GCS allows professionals to quantify changes in consciousness, which is imperative when considering interventions. Based on research with traumatic brain injury, variations in GCS scores tend to be related to intracranial lesions and other poor outcomes (Asikainen et al., 2014). Since patients have differing levels of consciousness, monitoring for change over time is important. Physical exam results combined with GCS assessments not only give information about the type of blunt force trauma but also guide treatment. Accurate early assessment can be beneficial in the triage of patients, especially in emergent presentations where timely intervention can have a profound effect on clinical outcomes. In addition, meticulous documentation of physical examination findings is crucial for future medical, legal, and research functions. Documentation of accurate information regarding the nature and pattern of injuries makes it easier to construct a logical sequence of events. For instance, different blunt trauma injuries will appear differently depending on the object and the force involved, and this can be literally crucial in determining fault or determining what did occur. Research has shown that certain techniques, including the spring-captive bolt gun in use in veterinary environments, provide useful comparisons for the nature and effect of blunt trauma and emphasize humane approaches to address injury (Boom et al., 2014). Lastly, a vigilant approach to physical examination results is accountable for a firm basis in blunt force injuries, offering the essence of effective clinical management and academic endeavor in this field (Figure 5.15).

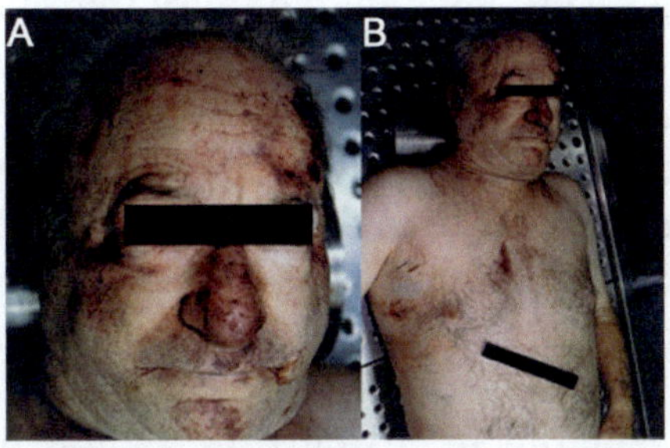

Figure 5.15. External examination photographs. (A) Multiple blunt force injuries of the head, probably sustained in the secondary attacks while the victim was on the ground. (B) Abrasion with surrounding hematoma on the right front side of the thorax (probably initial injury—running headbutt) with visible surgical incisions on the right thoracic wall.

Source: https://www.researchgate.net/profile/Nikica-Sprem/publication/268208575/figure/fig1/AS:290271507042305@1446217528224/External-examination-photographs-A-Multiple-blunt-force-injuries-of-the-head-probably.png.

5.4.2. Imaging Techniques

Diagnosis of blunt trauma injuries in man relies heavily on the application of sophisticated imaging techniques, which have also become central to the diagnosis and assessment of trauma levels. Techniques such as computed tomography (CT), magnetic resonance imaging (MRI), and ultrasonography offer non-surgical means to visualize internal injuries, allowing health professionals to assess injury to the brain and other vital structures. CT scans are at an advantage in emergencies to detect hemorrhage and fractures, providing real-time information to guide treatment. MRI, although not as available in acute cases, is better for the detection of subtle brain tissue abnormalities and diffuse axonal injury (DAI), a common finding in blunt trauma. Its ability to quantify certain tissue properties extends the information on injury path and potential recovery trajectory, providing a comprehensive view that is critical for effective clinical management and optimizing patient outcomes. One imaging modality that has been increasingly attracting attention over the past few years is diffusion tensor imaging (DTI), a focused MRI tracing the direction and integrity of white matter tracts in the brain. This technique is particularly helpful when evaluating the effect of blunt trauma injury that does not present with distinct evidence on regular imaging. DTI is capable of visualizing axonal damage in disorders such as concussions, therefore providing information about the pathophysiology underlying DAI. Studies have shown that alterations that were evident with the use of DTI correlate with outcomes, pointing towards its potential for use as a prognostic factor. With greater knowledge of the mechanisms of trauma, the use of DTI in diagnosis can potentially result in enhanced monitoring of recovery and represent a valuable component of treatment planning aimed at facilitating rehabilitation in patients with blunt force trauma. Additionally, imaging advancements extend to biomarkers as a complement to standard imaging techniques.

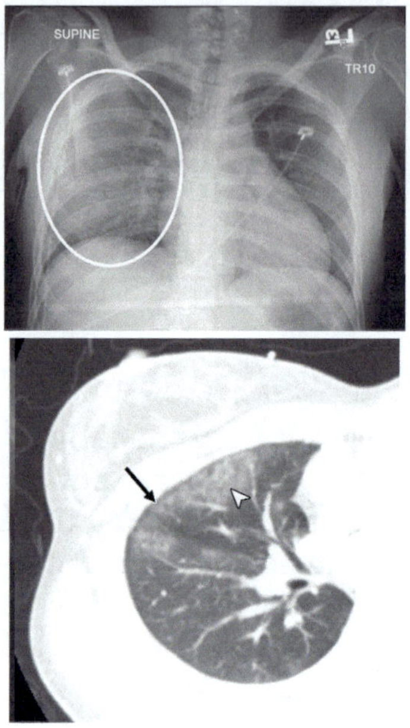

Figure 5.16. Pulmonary contusions in a 27-year-old woman following a motor vehicle collision (MVC). (a) Anteroposterior (AP) chest radiograph shows diffuse haziness over much of the right lung, with relative sparing of the right apex (oval). In the setting of blunt trauma, this is concerning for extensive pulmonary contusions. (b) Corresponding axial chest CT image obtained on the same day shows typical features of contusions, with regions of ground-glass attenuation (arrowhead) in the right upper and lower lobes, crossing the major fissure. Note the 2 mm of subpleural sparing (arrow) of the affected lung.

Source: https://pubs.rsna.org/cms/10.1148/rg.2021210042/asset/images/large/rg.2021210042.fig1a.jpeg.

For instance, researchers have examined the promise of serum biomarkers, such as SNTF, as indicators of DAI following traumatic brain injury, a form of injury most frequently induced by blunt trauma. Recent studies have indicated that the presence of SNTF is associated with poor clinical outcomes, implying its potential use as a complement to existing imaging assessments. Combining biomarker evaluation with imaging technologies can yield a truly multi-dimensional assault on diagnosis and monitoring of injury, which serves to emphasize the progression of the topic towards more focused and accurate patient management. The future of imaging for blunt force trauma will adopt such an integrated method, enabling improved diagnostic potential and eventually a deeper understanding of traumatic brain pathophysiology, as new research into DAI mechanisms and consequences following TBI (Cullen et al., 2015; Cerretani et al., 2017) was able to demonstrate (Figure 5.16).

5.4.3. Differential Diagnosis

For blunt force injuries, differential diagnosis is an essential process for determining the specific nature and degree of injury that a person has suffered. In such injuries, the nature of the injuries may range from minor trauma, such as contusions and lacerations, to severe trauma in the form of fractures or internal damage to organs. Effective differential diagnosis is facilitated by proper patient evaluation, such as a full physical examination and relevant imaging investigations. Such a multidisciplinary intervention will enable clinicians not only to identify emergent life-threatening conditions but also to differentiate between injuries with contrasting presentations. It is essential to differentiate these injuries for the sake of guiding proper management modalities and interventions that will ultimately contribute to better patient outcomes and efficient utilization of healthcare resources. One of the most important aspects of learning differential diagnosis for blunt force trauma is knowing the potential complications that will arise, which will make patient management difficult. For instance, when managing blunt head trauma, medical professionals should evaluate the risk for concomitant traumatic brain injury (TBI) or psychiatric disorders, such as posttraumatic stress disorder (PTSD). Studies have indicated that patients with clinician-assigned diagnoses of PTSD or mTBI demonstrate patterns of impairment that warrant careful consideration for appropriate assessment and treatment. Such complexity again underscores the need for clinical judgment in distinguishing concomitant symptoms of blunt trauma injuries and concomitant comorbidities. Failure to appropriately differentiate such conditions may lead to suboptimal care and impaired patient outcomes. Also, the role of an extensive history-taking cannot be overstated when distinguishing between blunt force injuries. Awareness of the context of an injury serves to streamline potential causes as well as treatment options. The study of historical cases, for example, such as the osteological remains from the Longobard necropolis of Povegliano Veronese, illuminates the nature of the injuries and potential survival reactions. By applying bioarchaeological methods, links between archaeology and biological data can show that people responded to traumatic events, and this has the potential to inform contemporary practice in the management of trauma. Such knowledge improves the concept of differential diagnosis by highlighting the varied presentations and coping responses people may demonstrate after suffering from blunt trauma, ultimately allowing for a more subtle examination of trauma in clinical practice.

Test Your Knowledge

1. What are the physical examination findings?
2. What is the process of Differential diagnosis?

5.5. Treatment Options

Learning Outcome

1. Understand the provision of immediate first aid.
2. Describe the role of surgical interventions in the management of blunt force injuries.
3. Describe the rehabilitation and recovery after blunt force injuries.

Effective treatment of blunt force injuries in humans varies in terms of their immediate care and subsequent recovery of victims. The first response is generally to encompass assessment of the severity of injuries through imaging techniques such as X-rays and CT scans, allowing medical practitioners to prioritize interventions. For instance, musculoskeletal injuries might involve immobilization and surgery, particularly when there is proof of fractures. Treatment for soft tissue injury is typically rest, ice, compression, and elevation (RICE) to allow swelling to decrease and healing to occur. Studies contrasting identical pathologies of dogs emphasize the importance of extensive anatomical information to treat the injury appropriately and highlight the parallels with human and animal injury. This case is notable for the value of individualized rehabilitation techniques consisting of physical therapy to restore function following blunt trauma, which produces optimal patient recovery (Franini et al., 2022). For extreme cases of blunt trauma, such as traumatic brain injury or internal organ damage, high-level surgical intervention is generally required. Treatment of traumatic intracranial aneurysms, for instance, comes with endovascular interventions, which are less invasive than the previously utilized open operations. Flow diversion and balloon-assisted coiling have shown promise, but efficacy is still inconsistent, necessitating patient selection and monitoring. Complications arising from the nature of the trauma, like a brain hemorrhage as a confirmatory diagnosis, need instant medical intervention. With advancing technology in imaging and surgery, trauma medicine is more directed towards minimally invasive techniques to encourage recovery at the cost of curtailing hospital stays. Knowledge of specific procedures depending on the nature and site of injury is necessary to achieve the optimum outcome (Lewis et al., 2021). Rehabilitation following the trauma is a critical component of overall treatment regimen aimed at returning physical function and emotional well-being. Physical therapy like strength training, balance, and range-of-motion exercises are incorporated into the patient-specific rehabilitation regimens depending on the requirements of the patient. Psychological counseling is also crucial as blunt trauma injury has the potential to induce extreme emotional distress in the form of anxiety and post-traumatic stress disorder.

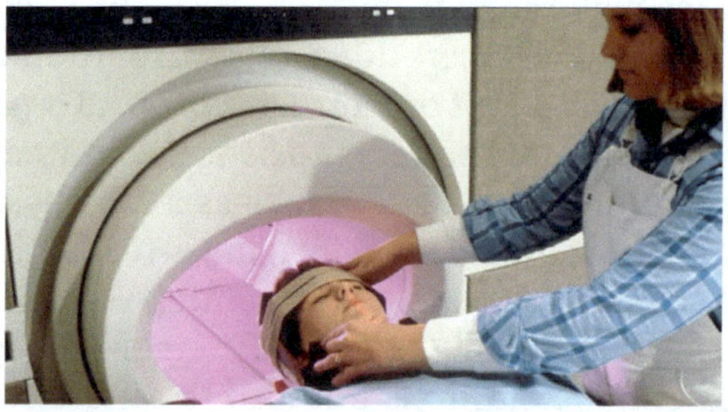

Figure 5.17. Blunt force trauma to the head.

Source: https://greenbergandstein.com/wp-content/uploads/2024/03/Blunt-Force-Trauma-to-The-Head-%E2%80%93-What-Is-It_-.webp.

Multidisciplinary approaches, involving physiotherapists, occupational therapists, and mental experts, offer comprehensive treatment for both physical and emotional recovery. Innovative methods such as tele-rehabilitation and virtual reality therapy are gaining momentum, raising patients' involvement and the effectiveness of the therapy. This integrated approach reflects the complexity of healing from blunt force trauma, highlighting that healing goes beyond the treatment of physical injury but also involves involvement in mental well-being throughout the recovery process (Franini et al., 2022) (Figure 5.17).

5.5.1. Immediate First Aid

The initial first aid intervention is paramount to the management of blunt force trauma because it may greatly influence the destiny of the traumatized patient. Early intervention can reduce the severity of the injury, decrease the complications, and increase the likelihood of recovery. The initial assessments are to evaluate the primary survey, checking the airway, breathing, and circulation (also known as the ABCs). In blunt trauma, this assessment is significant in diagnosing life-threatening conditions that are not apparent at first sight. It is significant to be aware of the nature and extent of injury sustained because blunt injury may also include not just external apparent wounds but also internal non-apparent injury, which may complicate the treatment process and require immediate medical attention to prevent further injury (Kennedy et al., 2015). Following the initial evaluation, providing appropriate interventions for injuries observed is crucial. For instance, if the patient demonstrates internal bleeding or shock due to blunt trauma, maintaining the patient in a supine position, elevating the legs, and oxygenation can be lifesaving measures that stabilize the patient's status. In situations where lacerations or contusions are involved, clean dressings and pressure can be used to halt bleeding. Ice application will also help in managing swelling and pain, which may prove to be extremely important in recovery from injuries due to blunt trauma. First responders will have an essential function in applying assessment and intervention modalities and keeping the casualty calm, which has direct impacts on their physiological recovery from trauma (Aoude et al., 2013). Lastly, effective communication with emergency medical services is required in order to deliver the patient timely and accurate higher-level care. The first responders' information should provide vital details like the mechanism of injury, all monitored vital signs, and relevant interventions administered. Rich communication facilitates medical staff to prepare for immediate patient needs upon arrival so as to maximize care pathways and accelerate further management plans. Initiating first aid not only serves the function of an initial defense for avoiding possible complications due to blunt force trauma but also forms a basis for subsequent treatment, healing, and eventually rehabilitation. Physical as well as psychological elements of blunt trauma must be cared for in curbing the long-term consequences of such injury, highlighting the significance of immediate first aid in the whole healthcare process (Kennedy et al., 2015) (Figure 5.18).

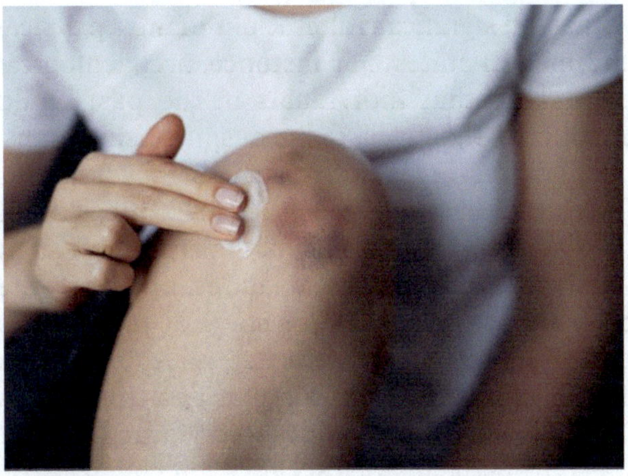

Figure 5.18. Treating a knee contusion.

Source: https://www.verywellhealth.com/thmb/UQPLmOZcCsTCbvx0bywnpfpBXGw=/600x450/filters:no_upscale():max_bytes(150000):strip_icc()/GettyImages-1325715530-8e418254b22e475086b268e82da2a970.jpg.

5.5.2. Surgical Interventions

Surgery plays a crucial role in the management of blunt trauma, often serving as a necessary component of both acute and rehabilitative care. Upon arrival at the emergency room following a motor vehicle accident or fall, the initial assessment and intervention can be life-saving. Surgical techniques—ranging from internal fixation to limb amputation—are critical in fracture, soft tissue damage, and vascular trauma treatment. In other circumstances, such as compound fractures, stabilization through orthopedic surgery can promote more rapid healing and restore function. Proper choice of surgery often is a function of the severity and nature of the injuries, along with the patient's overall health, necessitating a very skilled surgical team adept at having the ability to make rapid, informed decisions in the midst of high-stakes crises. Amputation is an extremely severe surgical intervention that may be called for in the case of irreparable damage to limbs due to blunt trauma. Previous and current studies reveal that amputated patients are able to withstand significant alterations in their physical and mental states. For instance, archaeological data show that individuals in the past could adapt very effectively to life despite losing limbs, through restoring function using prosthetics (Boggioni et al., 2018). The significance of this adaptation cannot be overstated, as it illustrates not only the adaptability of the body but also the role of surgical procedures in supporting adaptive strategies. Appreciation of the importance of surgical decisions is as fundamental in modern medical practice as it was during the historical climate of trauma care, wherein amputation decisions determined the patient's life course. Furthermore, enhanced decision-making both during surgery and during post-surgery care has yielded greater patient outcomes from blunt trauma injury. Production of precise surgical models, that is, the open femoral osteotomy, enables fracture healing and recovery from trauma to be better understood in detail (Akkus et al., 2020). Such models offer not only statistically significant findings on the healing process but also information that can be applied to enhance clinical protocols. In the past few years, integration of surgical practice with biomechanical testing and imaging technologies has revolutionized the field, enabling surgeons to refine their approach to managing complex injuries. Consequently, the field of surgical intervention evolves with increasing dependence on the need for ongoing research to improve techniques and improve recovery in blunt force injury victims (Figure 5.19).

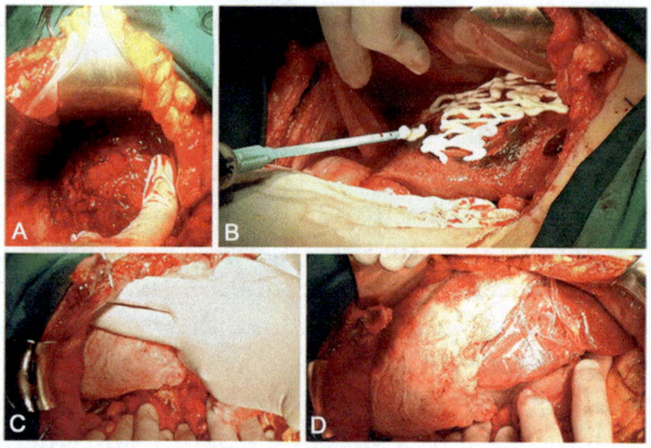

Figure 5.19. Damage control surgery in blunt liver trauma (DCS I –Initial laparotomy). A 41-year-old exsanguinating man with AAST grade V blunt liver injury (a). In order to control life-threatening hemorrhage, an emergency laparotomy was followed by direct liver vessel repair, with bleeding vessels sutured prior to liver packing and hemostatic fibrin gel on the liver surface (b). We performed liver packing with four abdominal swabs to provide liver compression (c, d).

Source: https://www.researchgate.net/profile/Aleksandar-Karamarkovic/publication/280629101/figure/fig1/AS:267391783403560@1440762577940/Damage-Control-Surgery-in-blunt-liver-trauma-DCS-I-Initial-laparotomy-A-41year-old.png.

5.5.3. Rehabilitation and Recovery

Recovery and rehabilitation from blunt trauma is a complex process that necessitates multidisciplinary team management tailored to the individual needs of the patient. Effective rehabilitation attempts to restore physical function without complication due to pain, stiffness, or the development of heterotopic ossification (HO). HO, or improper bone ossification in soft tissue sites, can substantially impair recovery by limiting the motion and function of joints. Notably, both those with previous high-energy trauma, such as those with blunt trauma, are at risk of developing HO due to the inflammatory responses created by their trauma. This dynamic between injury severity and the body's healing mechanisms is critical in the determination of recovery trajectory, necessitating intense physical therapy and targeted interventions with the aim of optimizing movement and functional independence while controlling secondary complications of the initial injury (Jessica et al., 2018). Physical rehab for blunt force trauma patients involves not just strength and mobility, but cognitive and emotional rehabilitation as well. Psychological problems are a great aspect of the healing process since patients tend to deal with frustration, depression, and anxiety due to their injuries. Intensive rehabilitation services should include psychological education and counseling, helping the patients set realistic goals, cope with lifestyle changes, and build resilience during the recovery phase. Intensive treatment can include family involvement, as a good support system enhances motivation and emotional well-being. Further, specially designed exercises considering the peculiar limitations of blunt force trauma can prompt gradual recovery without enhancing the risk of re-injury, which is significantly relevant in the case of HO-related injury since HO renders rehabilitation difficult (Adler et al., 2015). Additional studies suggest that optimal recovery from blunt force trauma can be facilitated by new approaches to therapy that integrate pharmacologic and non-pharmacologic interventions. Newer treatments, including the localized delivery of anti-inflammatory medications and targeted physical therapies, aim to reduce the formation of complications like HO while promoting maximal recovery. Even newer strategies, including the addition of gait retraining and neuromuscular stimulation, promise improved physical outcomes from injury. The goal of rehabilitation is not just to restore baseline capability but also to equip individuals with knowledge to manage their health on a long-term basis, adapting to any variations in physical capability. Ultimately, a good rehabilitation system acknowledges the intricacy of recovery that comprises physical, psychological, and social processes that are needed to optimize quality of life for individuals suffering from blunt force injuries (Jessica et al., 2018).

Test Your Knowledge

1. What is immediate first aid?
2. Which surgical techniques are commonly used to stabilize compound fractures?

5.6. Legal and Forensic Implications

Learning Outcome

1. Describe the role of forensic pathology.
2. Understand the legal definitions and classifications of blunt force injuries.
3. Know the impact of blunt force injuries on criminal investigations.

In blunt force trauma examination, the forensic and legal implications are of greatest significance, since they regulate both the assessment of injury and interpretation of evidence in a court of law. Accurate determination of the features and degree of blunt force trauma is paramount for forensic pathologists, since such diagnoses may seal or break criminal cases. For instance, the presence and condition of lacerations or contusions may hint at the severity level as well as the intent to inflict the injuries. In criminal cases, disputes in interpreting or documenting injuries may lead to various verdicts in court and subsequently impact the outcome of the trials. Hence, an accurate and unflinching forensic examination of blunt trauma is crucial not just to document victims' conditions but also to establish a tangible narrative that will stand up in court. Additionally, forensic data collected from blunt force trauma must be accurately documented and deciphered. This involves not just the trauma itself but also any available artifacts that can affect how the evidence can be interpreted in a court of law. For example, forensic investigation can be complicated by post-mortem procedures, such as those by arthropods, which alter the nature of the injury or remain undetected. Research has proven that alterations brought about by insects can mislead forensic pathologists and complicate interpretation regarding time and cause of death. Therefore, awareness of such processes is essential while compiling a credible forensic report. The overlap between legal processes and pathology demands that practitioners are perceptive in distinguishing between injury-related evidence and that which is affected by external factors, as this perceptiveness ensures the integrity of the legal process involved in the case. Last but not least, the validity of forensic technique assumes utmost significance with respect to blunt force injury, affecting both expert testimony and jurors' attitudes in the courtroom. Judicial professionals rely on evidence derived from forensic analysis, and hence the accuracy and reliability of these analyses assume pivotal importance in justice. As discussed in previous research, the effect of heat on bony injuries and marking patterns can influence the conclusions regarding the trauma inflicted on victims. In addition, cut mark analysis can provide critical information regarding the tools used during an incident (Aerssens et al., 2017). Therefore, encouraging proper knowledge of legal and forensic issues ensures that all data is appropriately scrutinized. Moreover, the development of careful procedural principles helps to avoid misinterpretations, presenting a robust approach to legal investigation and enhancing the credibility of the forensic field (Montisci et al., 2019).

5.6.1. Role of Forensic Pathology

Forensic pathology has an essential role to play in the investigation of blunt trauma injuries, delivering crucial insight into the mechanisms and circumstances of trauma. Forensic pathology is a specialty that combines the investigative aspects of pathology with the legal framework of death and injury issues. Through examination of autopsy results and use of advanced technologies, forensic pathologists are in a position to reconstruct the chain of events resulting in injury or death. Application of techniques such as post-mortem computed tomography (PMCT) enhances forensic pathologists' ability to visualize internal trauma, thereby facilitating better diagnosis and understanding of cranial and cervical trauma, as well as other injuries to the body. This technology incorporation is essential in situations of blunt force trauma, where the information of the extent of damage and timing would ascertain legal decisions and possible options of prosecution (Henningsen et al., 2024). Blunt force injury examination would use multi-disciplinary research in forensic pathology to address the various complexities, particularly in road traffic accident cases. Among the rising challenges of forensic analysis is the incidence of cervical spine distortions that are frequently seen together with soft tissue injuries and significantly complicate assessments for trauma. Forensic pathologists need to detect such accompanying injuries in order to provide full reports that are helpful to legal proceedings.

Through forensic medical report analysis and the application of neurosurgical principles, clinicians can make well-informed decisions about the seriousness of injury sets. This general strategy is required to determine causation and definiteness in the oft-muddled aftermath of violence or accidents, ultimately guiding prevention for future events (Travenko et al., 2022). The role of forensic pathology extends beyond mere determination of cause of death; it serves a broader role for society by contributing to the knowledge of blunt force trauma. By systematically documenting cases and analyzing patterns of injuries involving various mechanisms, forensic pathologists produce valuable information that can be applied to inform public policy and safety legislation. Not only does the data-driven process improve the resolution of individual cases, but it also informs the development of preventive strategies for common causes of blunt force trauma. Since the field continues to evolve, embracing new technologies and enhancing research culture can enhance forensic pathology's effectiveness in serving legal systems and public health (Henningsen et al., 2024) (Figure 5.20).

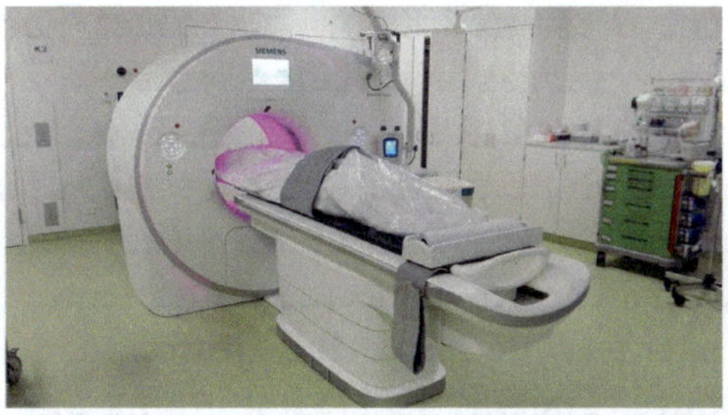

Figure 5.20. Scanning of the study body in a body bag on the Siemens SOMATOM force® dual source CT scanner.

Source: https://media.springernature.com/full/springer-static/image/art%3A10.1007%2Fs00414-019-02219-6/MediaObjects/414_2019_2219_Fig1_HTML.jpg?as=webp.

5.6.2. Legal Definitions and Classifications

In the context of definitions and classifications as understood in legal contexts, there is a need to conceptualize a clear typology of injury types. Legal definitions tend to classify blunt force injuries in terms of severity and type, from minor contusions to fatal trauma. These categories have substantial implications for legal constructions across cases of personal injury, assault, and homicide. In addition, the distinction between various forms of blunt force injury is important; for instance, injuries may be classified as those that resulted from accidents versus injuries that resulted from intent. The intent distinction and circumstances under which the injuries transpired are essential in the justice system as it decides criminal charges and civil liability. The formation of a sophisticated comprehension of such classifications educates legal professionals, medical examiners, and jurors in the consideration of cases involving blunt force trauma to the human body. The legalities involved in blunt force trauma necessitate a comprehensive understanding of contributing causes, origin, and resultant evidence presented before the court. Forensic pathology serves a priceless role, providing experts with the tool to accurately assess and categorize blunt force trauma in terms of intent and causation. For example, whether or not an injury results from an accident or an altercation can essentially change the direction of legal procedure. Specific legal definitions allow for the delineation of duties and liabilities through illustrative examples outlining how the physics of trauma is interpreted in the framework of jurisdictional law. Understanding these classifications allows legal professionals to guide complex cases of injury and opens the way for a fairer application of legal standards in the processing of personal injury claims and criminal cases of blunt force trauma, so proper penalties or rewards are given. Besides, the interrelation of medicine and law is evident in the medical-legal classification of blunt force trauma, as evidenced by legal definitions applied in forensic examination. The forensic pathology classifications elucidate the spectrum of blunt force trauma, including abrasions, contusions, and fractures, each attributed to distinct forensic and legal determinants. These classifications not only help in the accurate documentation of injuries in hospital records but also form the basis of legal cases heard in court trials. Forensic experts typically provide vital evidence that dictates the severity of injuries, which then forms the basis of decisions on culpability and negligence. The legal test of the reasonable person is also widely employed in such cases, again bridging the gap between the medical typologies and their employment within the courts, and so emphasizing the inbuilt interconnection between legal definitions and the typology of blunt force trauma (Corrigan, 2012; Granacher, 2003).

5.6.3. Impact on Criminal Investigations

The study of blunt force trauma in human beings is a significant field of criminal justice, particularly when determining intent, motive, and circumstances surrounding violent attacks. The application of forensic techniques to incidents that involve blunt force trauma can make significant enhancements to the obtained evidence and its reliability and quality. By analyzing patterns of injury, forensic scientists can establish whether the injuries resulted from an accident, a battle, or a planned attack. Also, the specifics of the injuries can assist law enforcement officials in narrowing down potential suspects by patterns of injury that may reflect known behavior or brawls. This not only helps to build an explanation for what occurred but also serves to help bring eventual convictions based on sound forensic evidence. The drug use implications in pregnancy are also true in the scenario of blunt trauma injuries and criminal investigations. There is worry about how substance-abusing mothers can be treated within the judicial system when their prenatal behavior is disclosed. As Stone (2015) indicates, pregnant women's perception of drug use—along with the risk of criminalization—can potentially camouflage their medical treatment needs, and can lead to delayed or inadequate responses from police and medical professionals alike. In cases of blunt injuries involving such women, the investigations can be rendered more complex by gender and class prejudices against the mothers, and the gathering of correct information can be impacted. This complexity poses a challenge for investigators to digest when dealing with the intersections of health, social policy, and criminal justice, and acknowledges the need to be responsive to the particular circumstances of each case. Furthermore, the historical context of legislation concerning pregnant women can complicate criminal investigations whenever blunt force trauma is present. As outlined in Lynn et al. (2012), cases where the pregnancy of an expectant mother directly affects the legal outcomes demonstrate a complex legal setting that inclines towards criminalizing maternal behaviors. Investigators must not only respond to the evident physical traumas but also be sensitive to the legal implications that can be activated in case the victim is pregnant. Thus, this can affect the presentation of the case, the perception of the victim's credibility, and the role of evidence. With these legal and ethical considerations in mind, law enforcement agencies can improve their investigative techniques and enable a fair examination of the facts of blunt force injuries, particularly in sensitive cases, toward a more balanced outcome (Figure 5.21).

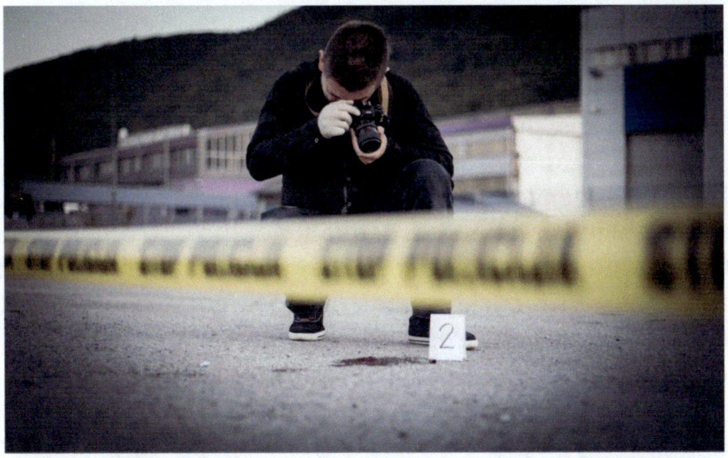

Figure 5.21. Criminal investigation.

Source: https://skillpointe.com/sites/default/files/styles/max_1300x1300/public/2020-08/Criminal%20investigator.jpg.webp?itok=q2DMjZOc.

Test Your Knowledge

1. What is the role of forensic pathology?
2. Which factor is most critical in distinguishing between accidental and intentional blunt force injuries in a legal context?

SUMMARY

In summary, the study of blunt force injury in humans is marked by the complex interaction between injury mechanisms and biomechanics because it also raises to the forefront the determinants of blunt force injuries. Understanding the impact of ground reaction forces (GRF) on the body can be of vital significance in injury prevention and rehabilitation activities, particularly in hazardous undertakings such as dance, sports, and military combat. Observation of frequent involvement of lower spine, knee, and ankle joints is a suggestion towards taking specific preventive measures in such vulnerable areas. Notably, the wide differences in maximum GRF among various dance disciplines indicate varying degrees of risk associated with different activities and imply the need for individualized injury prevention strategies accommodating each discipline's unique demands (Gorwa et al., 2024). The consequences of blunt force trauma go beyond immediate physical harm; they extend into mental well-being and long-term quality of life outcomes. Blunt force trauma injury is well known to have profound psychological effects, including stress and post-traumatic stress, most often amplified in victims with backgrounds of repeated harm or substandard post-incident treatment. It has been realized through research that an understanding of cavitation effects in blunt impacts can shed valuable light on brain injuries and their resulting implications, making impact monitoring of extreme importance (Eric et al., 2024). To solve the intricate nature of blunt force injuries, an interdisciplinary approach involving both physiological and psychological aspects is needed. Lastly, extending our understanding of blunt force injuries entails an interdisciplinary approach that involves biomechanics, psychology, and preventive medicine. As observed from the advances in the human phantom models to replicate real impact, additional research should be pursued to further improve protective equipment and injury assessment methods. With precise calibration of detection methods for mechanisms of injury, especially in the context of cavitation effects of brain injuries, we can better protect people from high-risk situations. Additionally, designing support systems that address the physical and psychological implications of such injuries is essential so that people who go through this kind of trauma get the comprehensive care they need to recover fully and live long and healthy lives (Eric et al., 2024).

In the study of the mechanics of human blunt force injuries, it should be highlighted that the mechanisms and the consequences of blunt force trauma. Blunt force injuries are often caused by forces that do not penetrate deep into the skin or underlying tissues, which may cause significant internal damage. The impacts of these types of injuries can be significantly different depending on the severity of forces, the involved body part, and the overall health of the victim. For instance, trauma to organs results in hemorrhage or contusion, while trauma to bones results in fractures or soft tissue injury. Understanding these mechanisms is important in creating successful treatment protocols and prevention methods in the clinic. Another essential factor to discuss is the role of nutrition in recovery from blunt force trauma. Body healing also requires adequate nutrient intake to support the repair of cells and the immune response. Inadequate protein intake, for example, has been found to have considerable influence on muscle repair and immune response. Moreover, micronutrient deficiencies, particularly vitamins A and C, and minerals such as zinc, have been associated with an increased risk of infection and retarded healing. With optimal nutritional profile optimization, inflammation and oxidative stress can be reduced, ultimately to healing from blunt trauma force, thereby enhancing patient outcomes as well as reducing healthcare costs due to complications arising from inappropriateness of diet (Iddir et al., 2020). Lastly, more recent studies have begun exploring how oxidative stress relates to blunt force injury, particularly in terms of cellular damage and the mechanisms of healing. The body's response to trauma is likely to be followed by a rise in reactive oxygen species (ROS), which, without proper regulation, could increase tissue damage. While physiological processes are mediated by low concentrations of ROS, there are toxic processes in the case of uncontrolled release, including cell death and limited recovery. Oxidative stress signaling pathways have been proposed to be a target for optimizing recovery after injury. This approach can unveil potential therapy interventions that can mitigate the harmful effects of blunt force trauma and enable a more effective recovery process (Bertero et al., 2018).

KEY TERMS FROM THIS CHAPTER

- Abrasions
- Assaults
- Bruises
- Depression
- Falls
- Neuroinflammation
- Swelling
- Anxiety
- Blunt force injury
- Contusions
- Epilepsy
- Fractures
- Post-traumatic stress disorder
- Traumatic brain injury

CRITICAL THINKING QUESTIONS

1. **What is the primary characteristic of a blunt force injury?**
   a. Penetration of the skin by a sharp object.
   b. Injuries caused by a blow or impact without skin penetration.
   c. Damage resulting from chemical exposure.
   d. Trauma caused by high temperatures.
2. **Which of the following is a typical manifestation of a blunt force injury?**
   a. Incised wound
   b. Laceration
   c. Puncture wound
   d. Burn
3. **What differentiates a contusion from other types of blunt force injuries?**
   a. It involves tearing of the skin.
   b. It is a deep tissue injury with minimal external signs.
   c. It results from blood vessel rupture, causing discoloration of the skin.
   d. It involves the penetration of foreign objects into the skin.
4. **Which of the following factors most influences the severity of a blunt force injury?**
   a. Type of clothing worn by the victim.
   b. The angle of the blow.
   c. The force of the impact and the surface area of the object.
   d. The presence of moisture at the site of injury.
5. **What is the defining characteristic of a laceration caused by blunt force trauma?**
   a. Clean edges with no tissue bridging.
   b. Irregular, torn edges with tissue bridging.
   c. Circular wound caused by a pointed object.
   d. A straight cut with minimal bruising.

Short Answer Questions

1. What is a blunt force injury?
2. List the types of blunt force injuries.
3. What is the mechanism of injury of blunt force trauma?
4. What are the common causes of blunt force injuries?
5. What is the treatment for blunt force trauma?

Answer to Critical Thinking Questions

1. (b); 2. (b); 3. (c); 4. (c); 5. (b)

REFERENCES

1. Adler, Y., Charron, P., Imazio, M., Badano, L. P., Barón-Esquivias, G., Bogaert, J., Brucato, A., et al. (2015). 2015 ESC guidelines for the diagnosis and management of pericardial diseases. *European Heart Journal, 36*, 2921–2964. https://doi.org/10.1093/eurheartj/ehv318 (accessed on 12th July 2025).
2. Aerssens, A., Allen, M., Alunni, L., Ambade, A., Ankersen, B., Banasr, M., Bartelink, H., et al. (2017). Effects of heat on cut mark characteristics. https://core.ac.uk/download/74204621.pdf (accessed on 12th July 2025).
3. Akkus, O., Anderson, J. M., Collier, C. D., Din, S., et al. (2020). Characterization of a reproducible model of fracture healing in mice using an open femoral osteotomy. https://core.ac.uk/download/288845958.pdf (accessed on 12th July 2025).
4. Aoude, G. Y. (2013). Mouthguards for contact sports: Current state of use. https://open.bu.edu/bitstream/2144/12045/6/Aoude_George_2013_nosig_nocv.pdf (accessed on 12th July 2025).
5. Asikainen, K., Bazarian, J. J., Bigler, E., Brain Trauma Foundation, Byrne, P., Chew, C., Englander, J., et al. (2014). Prognostic value of early magnetic resonance imaging in dogs after traumatic brain injury: 50 cases. https://core.ac.uk/download/157854824.pdf (accessed on 12th July 2025).
6. Azevedo, A., Binetti, A. C., Coelho, C., de Ridder, D., et al. (2012). Trauma-associated tinnitus: Audiological, demographic, and clinical characteristics. https://core.ac.uk/download/224999466.pdf (accessed on 12th July 2025).
7. Ball, N., Barnetson, V., Foster, B., Guy, A., et al. (2015). Fantastic plastic? Experimental evaluation of polyurethane bone substitutes as proxies for human bone in trauma simulations. https://core.ac.uk/download/42142579.pdf (accessed on 12th July 2025).
8. Bertero, E., & Maack, C. (2018). Calcium signaling and reactive oxygen species in mitochondria. *Circulation Research, 122*, 1460–1478. https://doi.org/10.1161/circresaha.118.310082 (accessed on 12th July 2025).
9. Bertilsson, J., Fransson, P. A., Fredriksson, P. J., Magnusson, M., et al. (2017). Use of pepper spray in policing: Retrospective study of situational characteristics and implications for violent situations. https://core.ac.uk/download/83793219.pdf (accessed on 12th July 2025).
10. Boggioni, M., Di Vincenzo, F., Giostra, C., Manzi, G., et al. (2018). Survival to amputation in the pre-antibiotic era: A case study from a Longobard necropolis (6th–8th centuries AD). https://core.ac.uk/download/159268258.pdf (accessed on 12th July 2025).
11. Boom, B., Daly, D., Daly, D., Dennis, F., European Food Safety Authority AHAW panel, Fackler, M., Finnie, P., et al. (2014). Evaluation of a spring-powered captive bolt gun for killing kangaroo pouch young. https://core.ac.uk/download/36778301.pdf (accessed on 12th July 2025).
12. Cerretani, D., Fiaschi, A. I., Fineschi, V., Fraschetti, A., et al. (2017). Diffuse axonal injury and oxidative stress: A comprehensive review. https://core.ac.uk/download/154289706.pdf (accessed on 12th July 2025).
13. Chait, A., & den Hartigh, L. J. (2020). Adipose tissue distribution, inflammation, and its metabolic consequences, including diabetes and cardiovascular disease. *Frontiers in Cardiovascular Medicine, 7*. https://doi.org/10.3389/fcvm.2020.00022 (accessed on 12th July 2025).

14. Chen, Y. (2023). Mechanism analysis of injury tools based on fracture mechanics model and collision dynamics model. *Proceedings of the 6th International Conference on Information Technologies and Electrical Engineering*. https://www.semanticscholar.org/paper/8345dc02a64f7b01fd3cf266906f5f86e384f148 (accessed on 12th July 2025).

15. Corrigan, G. (2012). Essential forensic pathology: Core studies and exercises. https://www.semanticscholar.org/paper/f21defbc9a68f3f4a8189df450b57f4202002541 (accessed on 12th July 2025).

16. Courtney, A., & Courtney, M. (2008). A thoracic mechanism of mild traumatic brain injury due to blast pressure waves. https://core.ac.uk/download/pdf/287975.pdf (accessed on 12th July 2025).

17. Cullen, D. K., Johnson, V. E., Siman, R., Smith, D. H., et al. (2015). SNTF immunostaining reveals previously undetected axonal pathology in traumatic brain injury. https://core.ac.uk/download/46165322.pdf (accessed on 12th July 2025).

18. DiSabato, D. J., Quan, N., & Godbout, J. P. (2016). Neuroinflammation: The devil is in the details. *Journal of Neurochemistry, 139*, 136–153. https://doi.org/10.1111/jnc.13607 (accessed on 12th July 2025).

19. Faizi, Z., Morales, J., Seng, S., Faizi, K., Simone, J., Geller, C., & Ratnasekera, A. M. (2023). Papillary muscle rupture of the mitral valve following blunt thoracic trauma. *Baylor University Medical Center Proceedings, 36*, 406–407. https://www.semanticscholar.org/paper/c8a4b7f2ff28e99d63b0bad2446d82d83b4320dc (accessed on 12th July 2025).

20. Fortier, C. B., Maksimovskiy, A. L., McGlinchey, R. E., Milberg, W. P., et al. (2014). Effects of OEF/OIF-related physical and emotional co-morbidities on associative learning: Concurrent delay and trace eyeblink classical conditioning. https://core.ac.uk/download/28948417.pdf (accessed on 12th July 2025).

21. Franini, A., & Entani, M. G. (2022). Common digital extensor tendon injury in three sporting dogs. *Animals: An Open Access Journal from MDPI, 12*. https://www.semanticscholar.org/paper/b29cf128c65d76972be4e52744fa6703c3a11a24 (accessed on 12th July 2025).

22. Fullerton, J. L., Kinch, K., & Stewart, W. (2018). One-hundred years (and counting) of blast-associated traumatic brain injury. https://core.ac.uk/download/141439713.pdf (accessed on 12th July 2025).

23. Galindo, E. J., Flores, R. R., Mejía-Alvarez, R., Willis, A. M., & Tartis, M. (2024). Simultaneous high-frame-rate acoustic plane-wave and optical imaging of intracranial cavitation in polyacrylamide brain phantoms during blunt force impact. *Bioengineering, 11*. https://www.semanticscholar.org/paper/c3864335d181b9c25a95c17f9ee92a510e244e4c (accessed on 12th July 2025).

24. Gorwa, J., Nowakowska-Lipiec, K., & Michnik, R. (2024). Ground reaction force as a factor responsible for the topography of injuries in professional dance: An analysis of three dance styles: Classical dance, modern dance, and folk dance. *Scandinavian Journal of Work, Environment & Health, 50*, 103–112. https://www.semanticscholar.org/paper/117dea82c0eb8ca25a5f62ecd86efa1986cf052c (accessed on 12th July 2025).

25. Granacher, R. (2003). Traumatic brain injury: Methods for clinical and forensic neuropsychiatric assessment. https://www.semanticscholar.org/paper/919ddf35b6cd7a5297ece65bd659a548e9b14058 (accessed on 12th July 2025).

26. Henningsen, M. J., Lindgren, N., Kleiven, S., Li, X., Jacobsen, C., & Villa, C. (2024). Subject-specific finite element head models for skull fracture evaluation—a new tool in forensic pathology. *International Journal of Legal Medicine, 138*, 1447–1458. https://www.semanticscholar.org/paper/a2fe57ea3ea561b4704e39c5168b8f0358e40ccf (accessed on 12th July 2025).
27. Hurwitz, S. (1984). The effects of indirect blunt trauma on adult canine articular cartilage. *The Journal of Bone and Joint Surgery. American Volume, 66*(1), 152. https://www.semanticscholar.org/paper/f027a3dd652a83874aa1181d433ef7afb2ccb27c (accessed on 12th July 2025).
28. Iddir, M., Brito, A., Dingeo, G., Sosa, S., Samouda, H., La Frano, M. R., & Bohn, T. (2020). Strengthening the immune system and reducing inflammation and oxidative stress through diet and nutrition: Considerations during the COVID-19 crisis. *Nutrients, 12*, 1562–1562. https://doi.org/10.3390/nu12061562 (accessed on 12th July 2025).
29. Izquierdo, M., Aziz Merchant, R., Morley, J. E., Anker, S. D., Aprahamian, I., Arai, H., Aubertin-Leheudre, M., et al. (2021). International exercise recommendations in older adults (ICFSR): Expert consensus guidelines. *The Journal of Nutrition, Health & Aging, 25*, 824–853. https://doi.org/10.1007/s12603-021-1665-8 (accessed on 12th July 2025).
30. Juarez, J. K., Wenke, J. C., & Rivera, J. C. (2018). Treatments and preventative measures for trauma-induced heterotopic ossification: A review. *Clinical and Translational Science, 11*, 365–370. https://doi.org/10.1111/cts.12552 (accessed on 12th July 2025).
31. Kennedy, I., Murray, V., Petley, D. N., et al. (2015). A systematic review of the health impacts of mass earth movements (landslides). https://core.ac.uk/download/41989325.pdf (accessed on 12th July 2025).
32. Knüsel, C. J., & Outram, A. K. (2013). Fragmentation of the body: Comestibles, compost, or customary rite? https://core.ac.uk/download/12825347.pdf (accessed on 12th July 2025).
33. Kroman, A. M. (2007). Fracture biomechanics of the human skeleton. https://core.ac.uk/download/268770463.pdf (accessed on 12th July 2025).
34. Lane, K. M. (2018). Fracture patterning and distribution in the appendicular skeleton of pigs resulting from explosions: Implications of blast trauma in forensic anthropological investigations of human rights abuses. https://core.ac.uk/download/215175756.pdf (accessed on 12th July 2025).
35. Lewis, K., Vigil, J., Norris, N., Merritt, W., & Becker, T. (2021). P-060 application of non-destructive mechanical characterization testing for creating *in vitro* vessel models with material properties similar to human neurovasculature. *Oral Poster Abstracts*. https://www.semanticscholar.org/paper/620f46c0d4d628d52ff9fd3f0e06febbab139beb (accessed on 12th July 2025).
36. Medaramatla, S. C., Samhitha, C. V., Pande, S., & Vinta, S. R. (2024). Detection of hand bone fractures in X-ray images using hybrid YOLO NAS. *IEEE Access, 12*, 57661–57673. https://www.semanticscholar.org/paper/41cece990ebddab6d7b6deb91c19ec25cda3f45f (accessed on 12th July 2025).
37. Montisci, M., Pelletti, G., Vanin, S., et al. (2019). Crime scene and body alterations caused by arthropods: Implications in death investigation. https://core.ac.uk/download/237175902.pdf (accessed on 12th July 2025).
38. MP, A., Courtney, A., Bruton, C., CDC, C., Cernak, I., Cernak, I., & Courtney, M. (2008). Links between traumatic brain injury and ballistic pressure waves originating in the thoracic cavity and extremities. http://arxiv.org/abs/0808.1443 (accessed on 12th July 2025).

39. Paltrow, L. M., & Flavin, J. (2012). Arrests of and forced interventions on pregnant women in the United States, 1973–2005: Implications for women's legal status and public health. *Journal of Health Politics, Policy and Law, 38*, 299–343. https://doi.org/10.1215/03616878-1966324 (accessed on 12th July 2025).

40. Pitsillides, A. A., Anderson, B. A., Armstrong, B. A., et al. (2015). Non-invasive mouse models of post-traumatic osteoarthritis. https://core.ac.uk/download/36778518.pdf (accessed on 12th July 2025).

41. Samudra, E., & Kusumaningrat, D. R. (2025). Fakta forensik yang mengungkapkan pembunuhan dalam kasus dugaan kecelakaan: Laporan kasus yang menguak kebenaran di balik pengakuan. *Indonesian Journal of Legal and Forensic Sciences (IJLFS).* https://www.semanticscholar.org/paper/a52f5a847bd89a10cb789d28e673c59925f65783 (accessed on 12th July 2025).

42. Schafer, M. J., White, T. A., Iijima, K., Haak, A. J., Ligresti, G., Atkinson, E. J., Oberg, A. L., et al. (2017). Cellular senescence mediates fibrotic pulmonary disease. *Nature Communications, 8.* https://doi.org/10.1038/ncomms14532 (accessed on 12th July 2025).

43. Shibuya, S., Yamamoto, T., & Itano, T. (2009). Glial and axonal regeneration following spinal cord injury. *Cell Adhesion & Migration, 3*, 106–99. https://www.semanticscholar.org/paper/4233131e3bb6acfc27ae2db3f654bdce95bbeb40 (accessed on 12th July 2025).

44. Stone, R. (2015). Pregnant women and substance use: Fear, stigma, and barriers to care. *Health & Justice, 3.* https://doi.org/10.1186/s40352-015-0015-5 (accessed on 12th July 2025).

45. Travenko, E., Porodenko, V., Anuprienko, S. A., Ashkhotov, A. V., & Penkin, A. S. (2022). Forensic evaluation of cervical spine distortion injuries in non-fatal road traffic accidents: An observational study. *Kuban Scientific Medical Bulletin.* https://www.semanticscholar.org/paper/0a7fab6515b1420752a2a3418f1b1d3aa8da508c (accessed on 12th July 2025).

46. Tyr, A., Heldring, N., & Zilg, B. (2024). Examining the use of alternative light sources in medico-legal assessments of blunt-force trauma: A systematic review. *International Journal of Legal Medicine, 138*, 1925–1938. https://www.semanticscholar.org/paper/42de5876022db6e2be2845583d743936171274bd (accessed on 12th July 2025).

47. Whelton, P. K., Carey, R. M., Aronow, W. S., Casey, D. E., Collins, K. J., Dennison Himmelfarb, C., DePalma, S. M., et al. (2017). 2017 ACC/AHA/AAPA/ABC/ACPM/AGS/APhA/ASH/ASPC/NMA/PCNA guideline for the prevention, detection, evaluation, and management of high blood pressure in adults: A report of the American College of Cardiology/American Heart Association Task Force on Clinical Practice Guidelines. *Hypertension, 71.* https://doi.org/10.1161/hyp.0000000000000065 (accessed on 12th July 2025).

48. Wiles, M. D. (2017). Blood pressure in trauma resuscitation: 'Pop the clot' vs. 'Drain the brain'? *Anesthesia, 72*, 1448–1455. https://doi.org/10.1111/anae.14042 (accessed on 12th July 2025).

SHARP FORCE INJURIES

6

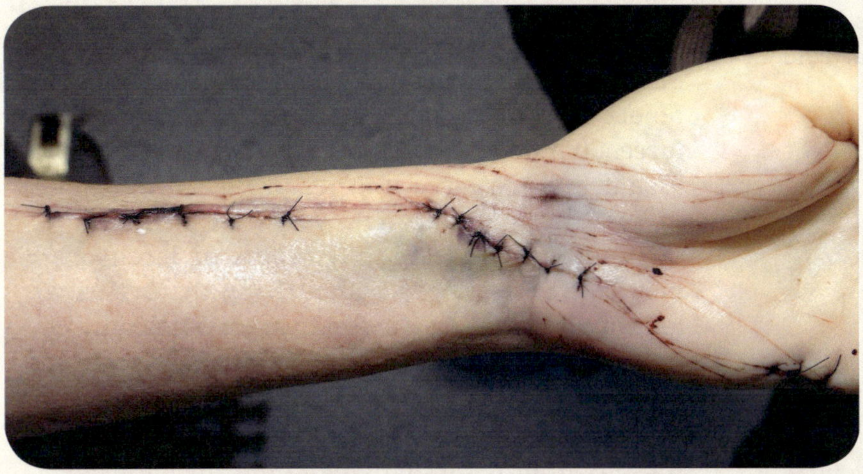

LEARNING OBJECTIVES

After studying this chapter, you will be able to:

1. Describe the types of sharp force injuries;
2. Understand the mechanisms of injury associated with sharp force incidents;
3. Understand the forensic analysis;
4. Know the psychological ramifications of sharp force injuries;
5. Describe the prevention and safety measures of sharp force injuries.

Introduction

In human beings, sharp force injuries must be studied in order to conduct comprehensive investigations into both their medical outcomes and social impacts. Sharp force injuries, by definition, are wounds inflicted using instruments or weapons with a cutting-edged surface, that is, knives or pieces of glass, that can range from minor lacerations to deadly stabbings. The incidence of such wounds is significant in contexts such as domestic violence, criminal activity, and accidents, and calls for multi-disciplinary analysis involving forensic, clinical, and psychological examination. Sharpened force injuries are witnessed through research with significant medical treatment implications to healthcare professionals, while the police and policymakers better understand how to approach the socio-physical underlying circumstances of such incidents. The clinical picture of sharp force injuries is highly variable based on the weapon used, wound location, and the general state of the victim's health. Some could be managed with minor wound care, while others may induce disastrous complications, including major blood loss, organ injury, or death. The Emergency Medical Services (EMS) are also often confronted with such cases, so they need rapid assessment and intervention steps depending on the nature of the injury. Also, differentiation between various sharp force injuries—lacerations, stab wounds, and punctures—is necessary to determine in order to develop an appropriate medical and legal response. Such understanding concurs with the emphasis on individual professional judgment of healthcare professionals in François Mach et al. (2019), as it points to their central role in managing sharp force injuries.

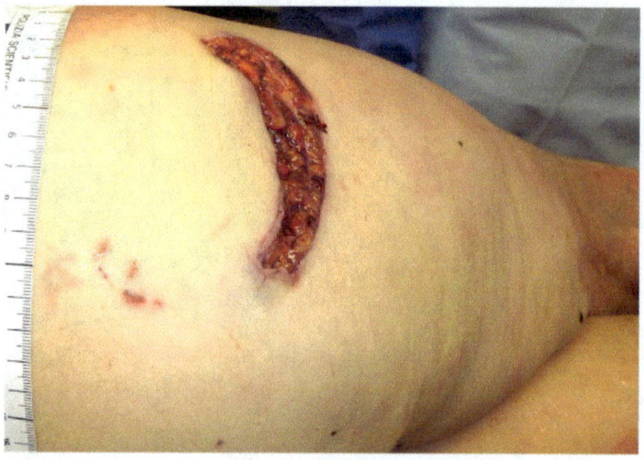

Figure 6.1. Sharp force injuries.

Source: https://www.pathologyoutlines.com/imgau/autopsysharpforceVarious17.jpg.

In addition, socio-economic determinants of sharp force injuries exemplify complex interlinks between health, education, and overall welfare. Research has found injury patterns are typically linked to broader concerns, such as poverty levels, educational attainment, and health resources. For instance, individuals from more socio-economically depressed groups can have higher rates of violence and ensuing injuries, which would mean growing health education and resources in the community would be a significant prevention factor. Moreover, the connectivity between education level and health level is highlighted in Grossman (2017), reinforcing the argument that increased access to education can guarantee better control and understanding of health. Addressing such multi-determinant factors may reduce sharp force injuries and promote a healthier population as a whole (Figure 6.1).

Definition of Sharp Force Injuries

Sharp force wounds describe wounds caused by the application of force with a sharp object, most commonly incised or penetrating injuries. Sharp force wounds can vary extensively with regard to both depth and severity, depending on the type of object, the manner in which the object is applied, and the amount of applied force. Commonly found to be involved in violent assaults, sharp force injuries are usually seen in assault or suicide. The very categorization of injuries is an essential aspect of forensic medicine as it helps in identifying the events leading to an event. Medical experts and police officers should learn about sharp force injuries because they allow them to determine the mechanism of injury, make an estimate of the potential for lethality, and aid in the legal process in cases related to violence. Also, sharp force injuries have power beyond the physical harm; they are sometimes a reflection of the hidden social problems or mental conditions of the sufferers. As depicted in some forensic writing, the prevalence of such injuries has the capacity to reflect the trend of violence in society and raise issues concerning mental health and support structures. The correlation between sharp force injuries and rigorous exercise, as recognized in some environments, suggests that physiological states may be the determining factor for vulnerability to injury in some situations (Abt et al., 2012). This connection highlights the importance of addressing not only the immediate effects of sharp force injuries but also the wider determinants of society that cause them to establish an integrated prevention and intervention strategy. Besides their social and physical effects, sharp force injuries are also rather problematic when it comes to medical treatment and recovery. The seriousness of these injuries normally demands complex surgical operations, ranging from suturing to more complicated procedures to manage potential complications such as infection or blood loss. The brutality that sharp force injuries impart can also impose long-term mental effects, hence the need for extensive treatment for mental health as part of the recovery. This cross-disciplinary approach is required in the promotion of patient outcomes as it bridges physical rehabilitation with psych support, an aspect that is critical to those who may undergo emotional trauma following injury (Williams et al., 2012). As such, a broad knowledge of sharp force injuries and their definitions and consequences is required in the implementation of effective treatment procedures and support networks for the affected (Figure 6.2).

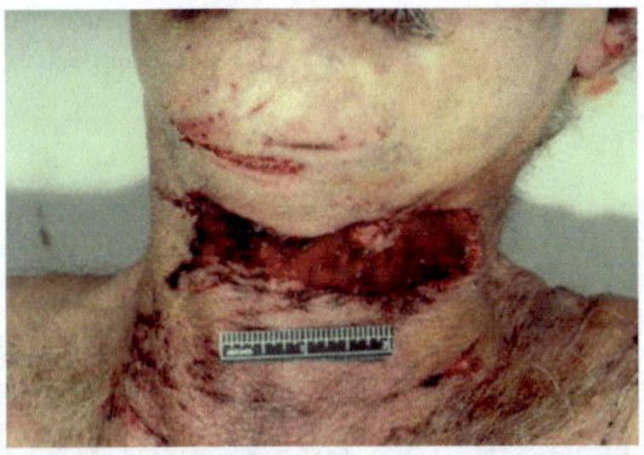

Figure 6.2. Sharp force injury deaths.

Source: https://media.springernature.com/lw685/springer-static/image/chp%3A10.1007%2F978-1-59745-404-9_14/MediaObjects/978-1-59745-404-9_14_Fig25_HTML.jpg.

Importance of Studying Sharp Force Injuries

The interest in learning sharp force injuries is not limited to clinical alone; it encompasses public health, legal, and psychological implications as well. Understanding the mechanism and outcome of such injuries can inform prevention, especially in societies where violence is prevalent. Detailed analysis of sharp force injuries helps develop sound public health policies towards violence prevention. Further, epidemiological data derived from such studies can guide healthcare workers regarding resource allocation and trauma preparation. Ultimately, the data acquired through the study of such injuries can reduce the incidence of violence cases and enhance community safety, a priority requirement for focused study. Research on sharp force injury is also significantly contributing to forensic medicine and legal processes. Accurate measurement of injury is essential in legal proceedings, where documentation and interpretation of wounds may decide the case direction. Forensic specialists utilize accurate descriptions of sharp force wounds to identify mechanisms of injury, manner of death, and even identification of weapons used. The data collected through meticulous investigations can be employed as strong evidence in criminal trials and could also provide an understanding of pathological behavior in relation to such injuries. This intersection of law and medicine makes it imperative to have a high-level strategy towards the examination of sharp force injuries that takes into consideration both medical and legal aspects, thus allowing for justice. Lastly, the psychological impact of sharp force injuries is another crucial element that must be studied. Sharp force injury victims usually experience lasting psychological illness issues, including post-traumatic stress disorder (PTSD), anxiety, and depression. Through the study of the psychological impacts of sharp force injuries, researchers will have a better understanding of the cognitive and emotional processes that affected victims experience during the recovery process. It is important for the development of targeted mental health interventions that target specific survivor needs. These studies also inform the overall social relevance of violence, stimulating community awareness and resilience. The analysis of sharp force injuries, thus, is not academic; it is an indispensable aspect in public health improvement, legal understanding, and psychological healing in victimized communities.

6.1. Types of Sharp Force Injuries

Learning Outcome

1. Learn about stab wounds.
2. Know the incised wounds.
3. Describe the lacerations.

Sharp force injuries classification is comprised of a broad category of injuries caused by the application of a sharp object, with this being usually classified based on the weapon's characteristics and the injury's morphology. Incised wounds, for example, are caused by cutting weapons, such as knives or broken glass, with the wound length being greater than the depth. These wounds will bleed since blood vessels were cut, providing a determining aspect in medical care. Stab wounds are created by cutting objects entering the body, typically creating deeper wounds that may cause little outward damage but large amounts of internal damage. These differences are crucial to understand in order to assess the severity of injury and the relevant medical treatment appropriately, which may vary significantly depending on the nature of the sharp force injury (Abt et al., 2012). Puncture wounds are another type of sharp force injury in which the skin is pierced by a sharp, pointed instrument, that is, a needle or a nail. These are smaller wounds than incised or stab wounds, but have higher risks of infection or complications due to the minimal opening provided by pathogens to enter the body. Incised or stab wounds do not typically cause internal damage, but punctures can produce serious internal damage since the depth of a puncture can result in extensive internal injuries, particularly when delicate organs, blood vessels, or nerves are affected. This emphasizes not only the external features of the injuries but also the psychological consequences of different classes of sharp force injuries since the victims may be injured differently depending on the context and severity of the injuries (Abuja et al., 2018). Also, the difference among these classes of injuries impacts forensic examination and the courts. All injuries possess specific characteristics that can produce significant evidence in the context of an assault, for example, weapon and assailant intent. The depth, length, and orientation of the wounds are commonly measured by forensic practitioners and compared with potential forms of weapons to enhance their ability to reconstruct events. Additionally, understanding these differences will help in creating proper treatment methods, particular to the nature of the injury. This will further improve outcomes for those affected by it. With more advances in research regarding sharp force injuries, clinicians will be able to treat both the physical and emotional damage resulting from such violent attacks (Abt et al., 2012).

6.1.1. Stab Wounds

A review of stab wounds reveals the complexity involved in sharp force trauma and its implications in trauma management. Stab wounds are produced by penetration of human tissue by a sharp weapon, resulting in different degrees of damage depending on variables like the weapon's properties, thrust angle, and site of injury in the anatomy. The depth and degree of such injuries are also complicated by clothing, which can influence the direction and depth of the cut. The friction of clothing, for instance, can alter the type of injury and, in fact, the diagnosis and therapeutic plan followed by physicians. This diversity highlights the need for proper evaluation, particularly in stab wound-associated trauma, with potential delayed recognition of injury being correlated with excessive morbidity or mortality. In the left thoracoabdominal (TA) stab wounds, awareness about the possibility of occult injuries, such as diaphragmatic ruptures, becomes necessary. Recent research at the Trauma Centre, Groote

Schuur Hospital, explored the management of asymptomatic patients presenting with left TA stab wounds, demonstrating the need for careful evaluation in trauma pathways. In a parallel-group trial, patients were randomized into two groups: one receiving diagnostic laparoscopy and the other receiving clinical and radiological follow-up. The findings revealed that while laparoscopic examination verified a 29% incidence of occult diaphragmatic injury, conservative treatment did not incur morbidity or mortality, indicating the potential safety of conservative intervention in some instances.

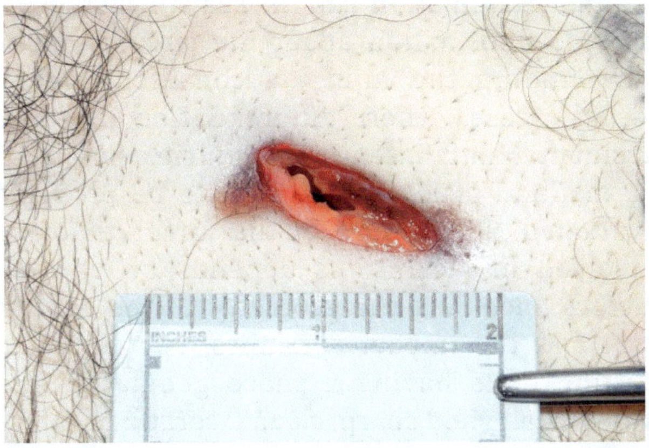

Figure 6.3. Stab wounds. These wounds are typically deeper than their cutaneous length. The wound track can be observed in the center of the wound.

Source: https://www.pathologyoutlines.com/imgau/autopsysharpforce_Various02.jpg.

The research verifies the concept that not all stab wounds need immediate surgery, thereby transforming patterns of trauma treatment for stab injuries. Knowledge of stab wounds extends beyond the acute medical effects to their forensic importance, particularly in criminal cases. Such is the case, as the increased occurrence of sharp force trauma as a feature of violent crimes, particularly in the United Kingdom, lends forensic study of stab wounds a significant role in determining criminal accountability. A broad disparity in correlating weapons used in stabbings to resulting skeletal injuries has been indicated by research, which makes life harder for forensic pathologists. Another study of fabric influences on stab cases also indicates the subtleties involved in the analysis of clothed victim wounds. The findings above confirm the need for proper forensic investigation through the interaction between fabric resistance and weapon characteristics to accurately determine stabbing outcomes. Therefore, such a multidimensional approach is essential to the process of evolving forensic practices and improving the knowledge about sharp force wounds in humans (Figure 6.3).

6.1.2. Incised Wounds

Incised wounds, with their clean edges and high likelihood of bleeding, represent a particular subset of sharp force injuries. They typically result from sharp-bladed weapons such as blades or knives that cut through tissue extensively when they strike it. The severity of the wound will often correlate with the sharpness of the weapon, the amount of force utilized in the attack, and the location of the body that was cut. Injuries to vital regions, such as the abdomen or neck, can be life-threatening due to the relationship with organs, arteries, and other critical structures. Understanding the presentation and character of incised wounds is important to analyze them in a forensic laboratory because it aids in classifying types of assault and reconstruction of events involving criminal acts. Forensic analysis of incised wounds also places emphasis on the offender's behavior and psychological personality. Research indicates that the weapon used and the patterns of injury it creates can reveal significant narratives about an attacker's motivation and preplanned victimology. These examinations can involve an assessment of whether an attacker selected a particular weapon opportunistically or with intent, which can influence the nature of the resulting injury. The distinction between planned and unplanned weapon utilization is significant in comprehending how the variables determine the causes of injuries on victims, highlighted in the literature of weapon choice and serial murders (Fletcher et al., 2022). Such comprehension not only helps advance legal cases but also contributes to more inclusive discourse regarding crime prevention and intervention. Additionally, incised wound investigations are also aided by forensic science technology, for instance, via alternative tissue models mimicking the pattern of wounds. Innovative techniques, such as the use of ballistic soap and other simulants, give researchers a platform to model and examine the mechanics of several types of injuries under a simulation environment. These methods provide beneficial information regarding penetration depth and morphology of the wound, enabling a straightforward correlation between the utilized weapon and resulting injury patterns (Steimle et al., 2020). This kind of research is important to enhance the efficacy of forensic interpretation as well as aid in criminal prosecution by providing overwhelming visual evidence on the formation of sharp force injuries. In conclusion, a detailed understanding of incised wounds provides an important contribution to interdisciplinary research of forensic science and fills knowledge gaps in a manner that enhances ties between empirical research and application in criminal justice (Figure 6.4).

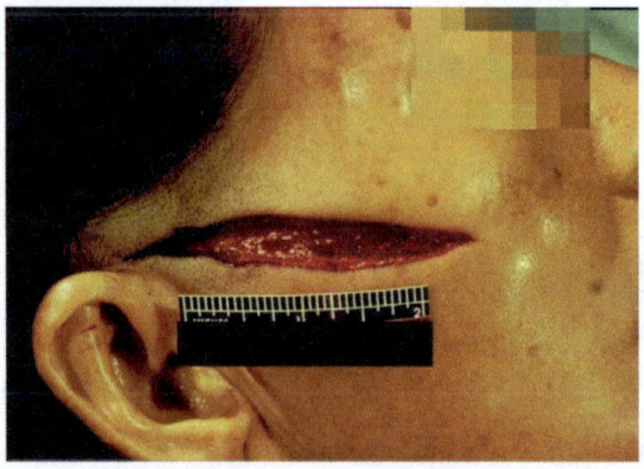

Figure 6.4. An incised wound of the face.

Source: https://img.medscapestatic.com/pi/meds/ckb/89/9689.jpg.

6.1.3. Lacerations

Lacerations are a common form of sharp force injury that can be described as a cut or tear in the skin as a result of the transmission of force through an object that is sharp. Lacerations may vary from minor abrasions to wounds that penetrate into deeper structures like muscles, nerves, and blood vessels. Laceration mechanisms are significant both clinically and in forensic investigations. The depth and direction of a laceration, and the instrument with which the cutting was done, all bear directly on healing and potential complications like scarring or infection. Wound examination can, in certain instances, provide information about the circumstances surrounding the injury, a consideration in forensic cases where differentiation between accidental and intentional injuries needs to be made in order for the case to be properly evaluated. The nature of the forces that are involved in lacerations depends on various factors, including the geometry of the cutting tool and the impact dynamics. For instance, cutting tools having a sharp geometry, like knives, will yield sharp, clean lacerations, while higher-order geometries will yield jagged and irregular wounds. The pathophysiology of trauma is pivotal in recognizing how different conditions can yield differing patterns of injury, thus gaining insight into the severity of lacerations sustained. Research indicates that surface area and manner of force application are two critical variables in determining the resultant patterns of injury. This is consistent with the new priorities of trauma examination, as highlighted in fracture pattern analysis and its interface with other types of trauma, such as sharp force trauma like lacerations, for which anatomical response to impact forces is to be appreciated (Kroman et al., 2007). Furthermore, the healing process of lacerations is also based on a number of variables, such as the wound depth and the contamination with foreign substances introduced during the trauma. It will be severely hampered in a deep or contaminated laceration;

hence, proper clinical evaluation and care must be undertaken. As medical science progresses with new developments, proficiency in assessing and treating lacerations has grown stronger, emphasizing the significance of wound treatment immediately to rule out any complications. An understanding of such injuries in the context of forensic examination can also be useful in reconstructing the chains of events to causation. The intersection of the engineering principles and the biological responses sheds light on the delicacy of lacerations as sharp force trauma and directs clinical and forensic practice (Bajd et al., 2015). The multidisciplinary approach is essential for a comprehensive understanding of lacerations in the broad context of sharp force trauma in humans (Figure 6.5).

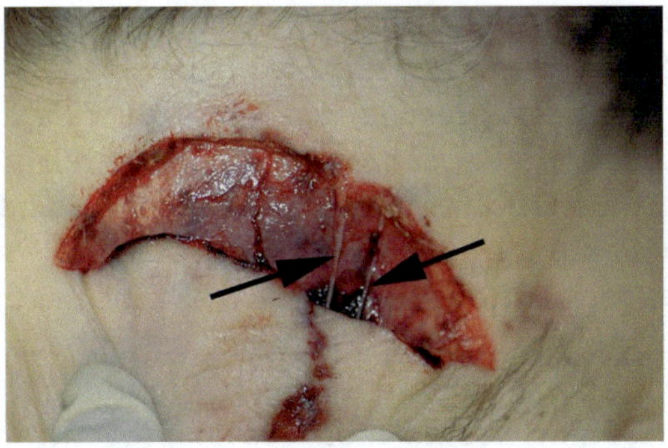

Figure 6.5. Laceration (caused by blunt force trauma) mimics a sharp force injury. The presence of "tissue bridging" (arrows) helps to differentiate a laceration from a sharp injury.

Source: https://img.medscapestatic.com/pi/meds/ckb/87/9687.jpg.

Test Your Knowledge

1. What is an incised wound?
2. What are lacerations?

6.2. Mechanisms of Injury

Learning Outcome

1. Describe the types of weapons used.
2. Understand the depth and angle of penetration.
3. Know the tissue damage and physiological response.

To be useful to forensic analysis and medical treatment, an understanding of sharp force trauma injury mechanisms is vital. Sharp force trauma injuries are known for their capability to cut through living tissue, with varying levels of trauma depending upon the magnitude of force exerted and the type of weapon utilized. Factors like the sharpness of the blade, angle of use, and the application rate of the instrument are what define the severity of the injury. This is especially when examining the manner in which sharp objects can inflict shallow and deep cuts that could aim at essential organs and structures of the body, and by doing so, it necessitates a thorough examination of each case. Through the comprehension of these disparate mechanisms, clinicians and forensic experts can better assess patterns of injury and outcome and, ultimately, treatment and legal strategy. Furthermore, analysis of sharp force injuries reveals intricate biomechanical interactions between the tissue and the weapon. With impact, the energy transferred by the cutting device can lead to local tissue harm, producing laceration or puncture wounds. The severity of such damage is based on various parameters, such as the velocity of impact and the location of the anatomy in which the injury is produced, which influences the type of tissues that are being penetrated. For example, an incision wound in soft tissue, such as in the abdomen, can have entirely different outcomes compared to cutting through more solid materials like bone or cartilage. This complexity serves to highlight the need to utilize different methodologies, including animal models, in order to model and study these interactions in an effective way. Through isolation of various parameters, scientists can learn about the mechanisms behind these injuries and create methods of prevention to reduce their occurrence in humans, particularly in settings where sharp force injuries are most common. Moreover, recent research into the effects of various mechanisms of injury, such as the effect of blast pressure waves, is of value in the conceptualization of sharp force injury within a broader context. Although conventionally associated with penetration trauma, investigation of concomitant injury, for instance, mild traumatic brain injury (mTBI), reveals complex interactions between various forces directed at the body. For instance, thoracic mechanisms studied in the context of blast wave research, as outlined in the body of trauma literature, also illustrate the way various injury dynamics can create multi-modal presentations of injury (Courtney et al., 2008). Similarly, studies of non-invasive models of the joint illuminate the significance of mechanical injuries and their value in enhancing an understanding of degenerative conditions potentially caused by or exacerbating sharp force injuries (Pitsillides et al., 2015). These interdisciplinary approaches are necessary to unravel the intricate processes of damage in order to guide both clinical practice and future research efforts in the field of human trauma.

6.2.1. Forms of Weaponry Used

Sharp force weapon classification used in sharp force injury is significant in the understanding of the nature and consequences of such injury. Sharp force weapons are categorically divided into two broad groups: bladed objects and pointed objects. Bladed weapons like swords and knives, through the cutting edge of the objects, produce injuries that typically result in incised or lacerated wounds. Conversely, pointed instruments like ice picks or even screws can reproduce stab wounds that penetrate underlying tissues. The distinction between these categories becomes vital in forensic contexts, as the injuries produced often differ significantly in severity and type. Consequently, the analysis of wound patterns can offer insights into the weapon employed, potentially aiding law enforcement in investigations related to violent crimes. The weapon of opportunity selected in sharp force attacks may also reflect the offender's personal circumstances and motivation. As identified in recent studies, certain weapons might be used as instruments of opportunity, that is, used spontaneously in the course of a violent altercation and not with prior premeditation. This is evident in cases where domestic or household items, for example, kitchen knives, are employed in domestic fights. Knowledge of this variable, especially how victimology factors in, can provide a fundamental understanding of the nature of crime, attacker psychology, and victim characteristics. Research involving variables of forensic literacy and weapon selection finds that choice often relies on circumstances rather than prior intentions, thereby influencing resulting sharp force injuries sustained by victims (Fletcher et al., 2022). Furthermore, forensic analysis of sharp force wounds demands a strong understanding of how weapon design attributes control the type of wounds created. Different design aspects of blades, including sharpness, length, and angle, have a strong bearing on the type of wounds created. A longer and more acute blade, for instance, is capable of creating deeper and more harmful wounds, whereas a shorter blade will create superficial or less harmful wounds. Such knowledge is not just essential for legal procedures but also enhances preventive measures in public health and safety. Understanding the various patterns of injury with the use of various weapons allows forensic scientists to make inferences about the character of an event, such as the premeditated or spontaneous nature of the action. These analyses assist in closing existing knowledge gaps in the area of sharp force trauma and its various implications for both victims and offenders (Bolton-King et al., 2016) (Figure 6.6).

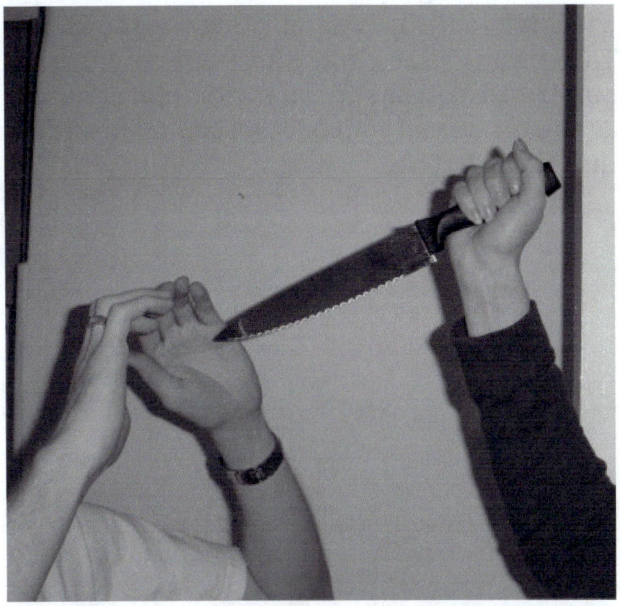

Figure 6.6. Mechanism of injury to hands/ arms defending an overarm knife attack.

Source: https://08f043fb5b.clvaw-cdnwnd.com/65cf06e22b1051f5df11dfe70b7dd6da/200000150-2600926fac/knife%20overhand%20attack.JPG.

6.2.2. Depth and Angle of Penetration

An understanding of sharp force injury demands a complete evaluation of depth and angle of penetration, two variables that dictate the character of the wound created. A wound's severity is significantly affected by the depth of a penetrating wound, and often equates with vital tissue compromise. Wounds penetrating deep into organs or major vessels, for instance, may create life-threatening circumstances justifying instant medical response. Analyzing bone cut marks facilitates forensic scientists to make deductions regarding the tools used and the way they were used, as described in various cut mark analysis research, although much more is to be learned about traumatized tissues depending on depth and heat (Aerssens et al., 2017). The angle of penetration also alters the path of sharp instruments, making it more difficult to analyze injuries. The victim's anatomical position during an attack also produces variations in depth and angle. Penetration angle is informative as it defines the type and the extent of tissue damage. Despite the obvious simplicity of a vertical stab, evidence indicates that even small deviations can affect the wound pattern, produce increased tissue disruption, and complicate healing. For instance, stabbings that are performed at an angle cause very distinct patterns of wounds, which forensic investigators examine in such cases to determine the type of assault and tools used. This effect highlights the significance of understanding the interaction between depth and angle, especially as these factors will tell us different things about the situations involving stabbing cases. Research has also established how the angle and depth of penetration can also yield crucial details as to the intent of the wound—whether it was an assault, self-defense, or a fatal accident (Boom et al., 2014). The deeper wounds and specific angles can also yield micro-traumas around the wound that sometimes might not be visibly detected, but are important in proper forensic examination. For instance, when knives are utilized as instruments, micro-fissures and cut mark development produced may significantly influence forensic investigation. Some of the methods applied in establishing such factors include micro-CT and digital microscopy, but variations in the precision of measurements underscore the need to apply caution when selecting a technique (Aerssens et al., 2017). Understanding how these factors of depth and angle relate to each other can guide researchers in the discrimination between mechanisms of sharp force injuries and the circumstances of sharp force incidents. Thus, the study of penetration depth and angle becomes a vital part of forensic investigation into sharp force injuries, offering valuable input into legal inquiries and clinical assessment.

6.2.3. Tissue Damage and Physiological Response

Sharp force injury in humans triggers a complex physiological reaction that includes both local and systemic effects. With cutting and stabbing injuries of tissues by cutting and stabbing objects, the first impact is tissue damage, disruptively impairing homeostasis and cellular integrity. This compromise triggers a cascade of biochemical responses known as the inflammatory response that targets containment and prevention of further injury. When they get hurt, white blood cells such as neutrophils and macrophages get activated and migrate to the site of injury, producing pro-inflammatory cytokines that contribute to healing and activating repair processes for tissues. The relationship between tissue damage and the metabolic response of the body is also important, as massive damage can lead to complications in the body's systems, such as shock or infection. For instance, the mechanisms by which a blast pressure wave can affect the brain ensure that the intricate interplay between gross physiological effects and localized trauma indicates just how tissue injury can provoke different responses at every level of the body (Courtney et al., 2008). Apart from the inflammatory response, tissue injury due to sharp force trauma significantly stimulates ~~the~~ body's coagulation cascade so as to maintain hemostasis. Following a primary trauma, platelet activation and aggregation as a result of vascular damage form a hemostatic plug, while coagulation factors are activated to enable the clot to become solid. It plays a crucial role in stopping hemorrhage and enabling the body to initiate healing. Such factors of vitamin K-dependent proteins play a significant role in the coagulation cascade, echoing the significance of nutritional factors in tissue repair. Particularly, certain amino acids and vitamins have been observed to influence healing processes at the cell level, with implications for supplementation potentially supporting tissue healing after trauma. Vitamin C and glycine have both been seen to impact tendon and muscle healing, for instance, though robust evidence from human trials is presently limited (Abuja et al., 2018). This means that while the body might have innate mechanisms to deal with injuries, there are also external influences, such as nutrition, that can influence healing.

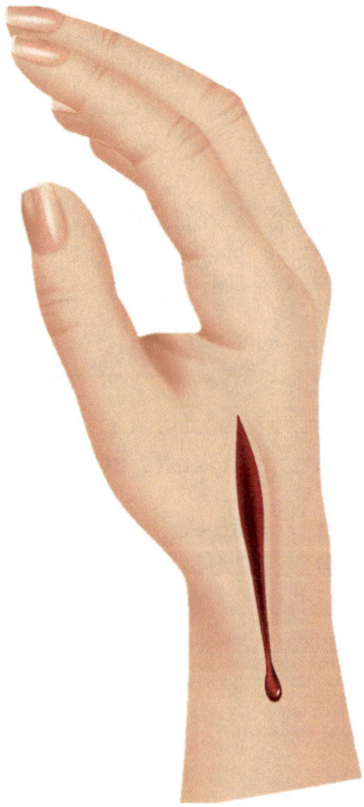

Figure 6.7. Tissue Damage.

Source: https://blogger.googleusercontent.com/img/b/R29vZ2xl/AVvXsEjrTP4jqIWtV_iVXYOF6VYHjDTdvABb8-p45evvcQBVQ5V47PTTxg6nsXFqFfS4eyp6Hdpch0Cy5Xm07WBaOGlliEjx2zM-xREYTBIKR79Gb3MO2FtjlnClQxqd93WkNkPGGo6FUvX96jMFMvj3UTgOB6JOC6u-RRYD-bSbosefKulWNsWzT67B1J3I/s960/Laceration.png.

Moreover, the physiological reaction to sharp force injuries is not just limited to the initial healing response but also has long-term implications on tissue function and morphology. The subsequent healing stage involves scar formation, whereby the fibroblasts deposit collagen to repair the damaged tissue. This causes tissue architecture changes, which can influence function, particularly if the involved portion impairs mobility or other body functions. The potential for improper healing, such as excess scar tissue or chronic pain, makes it critical to monitor and manage recovery effectively. The identification of musculotendinous healing factors, as identified in present research on amino acids and vitamins, attests to the urgency of multifaceted recovery. Through additional research, understanding of the physiological reactions that form the basis of these reactions will be critical in developing interventions that will optimize healing after sharp force injury with a view to maximizing patient outcomes and quality of life (Figure 6.7).

Test Your Knowledge

1. What are the 2 types of sharp force weapons?
2. Which factors are most critical in analyzing sharp force injuries?

6.3. Forensic Analysis

Learning Outcome

1. Understand the role of forensic pathology.
2. Collect and preserve the evidence.
3. Interpret the injury patterns.

This section discusses why forensic textile analysis is crucial to the interpretation of sharp force trauma. This specialized field examines the behavior of different materials when stabbed or cut and provides vital data regarding the circumstances of an injury. A pilot study demonstrated that not all knives create an identical damage pattern on fabrics, as the visual appearance of severance depends on weapon characteristics. The research involved simulated attacks with regular knives on a physical model and discovered that experienced operators produced disparate patterns that would complicate forensic analysis. Such evidence requires rethinking traditional forensic interpretations since they may fail to encompass all the nuances of damage produced by different sharp objects. The intricacy contributes to the need for forensic experts to include textile reactions to trauma to increase accuracy in case examination and ultimately result in better-informed judicial rulings (Carr et al., 2016). In forensic investigation, advanced documentation techniques are becoming commonly useful in decomposing scenarios of sharp force trauma. Recreation methods, hitherto bounded by their two-dimensional modality, give way to three-dimensional scanning technologies that enhance the accuracy of crime scene reconstructions. They are not just applied in crime scenes but also in the thorough probing of victims, and they offer a more advanced understanding of weapon-target interaction. For example, in the analysis of a vehicle-pedestrian accident, 3D scanning was applied to record the impact area and victim wounds, thus helping investigators comprehend the relationship between the dynamics of the vehicles and the victims' wounds. Such methodological refinement enhances a more sophisticated consideration of evidence essential in the development of a coherent event sequence leading to sharp force injuries (Dustin et al., 2020). To this effect, the convergence of multidisciplinary approaches to forensic analysis is evidence of the evolving face of criminal investigations, particularly that of sharp force trauma. Through converging approaches from multiple disciplines, forensic experts can have a better understanding of cases. For instance, the convergence of forensic radiology and three-dimensional imaging contributes to a greater level of transparency in the documentation of injuries and evaluation of the circumstances under which they were sustained.

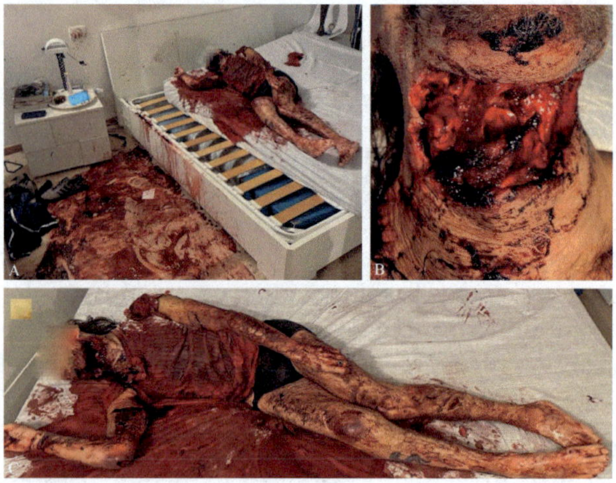

Figure 6.8. Death scene. A) The bedroom where the man was found lying on the right side in his blood-drenched bed; B) the large wound in the submandibular area with laceration of the internal airways; C) numerous deep cuts and bloodstains on the body were observed.

Source: https://www.minervamedica.it/upload_html/R11Y2022N04A0071/Figure%201_fmt.jpeg.

This broadened methodology enables the detection of injuries that could be missed by other autopsy methods, and thus sheds information on parts of cases otherwise lost. With ongoing advancement in forensic science, emphasis on precision and accuracy in the documentation of sharp force injuries remains most crucial. These advancements not only assist in crime scene reconstructions but also enable a better understanding of injury mechanism dynamics, ultimately enhancing the efficiency of forensic investigations and providing support for equitable decisions in the judicial system (Figure 6.8).

6.3.1. Role of Forensic Pathology

Forensic pathology is important in the investigation of sharp force trauma since it provides essential information about the events surrounding the incident. It is the role of the forensic pathologists to determine the cause and manner of death, where death occurs due to knife cuts or sharp injuries. By studying tissue trauma, blood loss, and wound features, they can identify if a wound is accidental, suicidal, or homicidal. The intricacy of sharp force trauma necessitates great insight into how different implements interact with human tissue, something best reviewed by forensic pathologists. It not only helps in the medical evaluation of the victim but also aids law enforcement in generating timelines and patterns that can be vital to criminal investigations. Moreover, a sharp object damaging the analysis of clothing is a significant factor in the forensic pathology discipline. The pilot study that the article writes about in the forensic textile science society shows how well-trained shooters with sharp weapons produce typical damage patterns on apparel that forensic pathologists must be able to identify and interpret. For instance, variation in severance patterns based on weapons used, as viewed by the many different kinds of knives producing various forms of damage, can prove to be critical in linking an assailant to a crime scene. Moreover, the presence of slash and stab severances on apparel can provide necessary background information as to the type of attack, indicating whether the attack was spontaneous or well-planned. These examinations contribute significantly to building the general image of sharp force cases. In addition to knife-caused injuries, forensic pathology also encompasses the examination of other weapons, such as arrows, in terms of sharp force injury. One study analyzed the penetration potential of aluminum arrows in soft tissue and the effect of clothing on these findings.

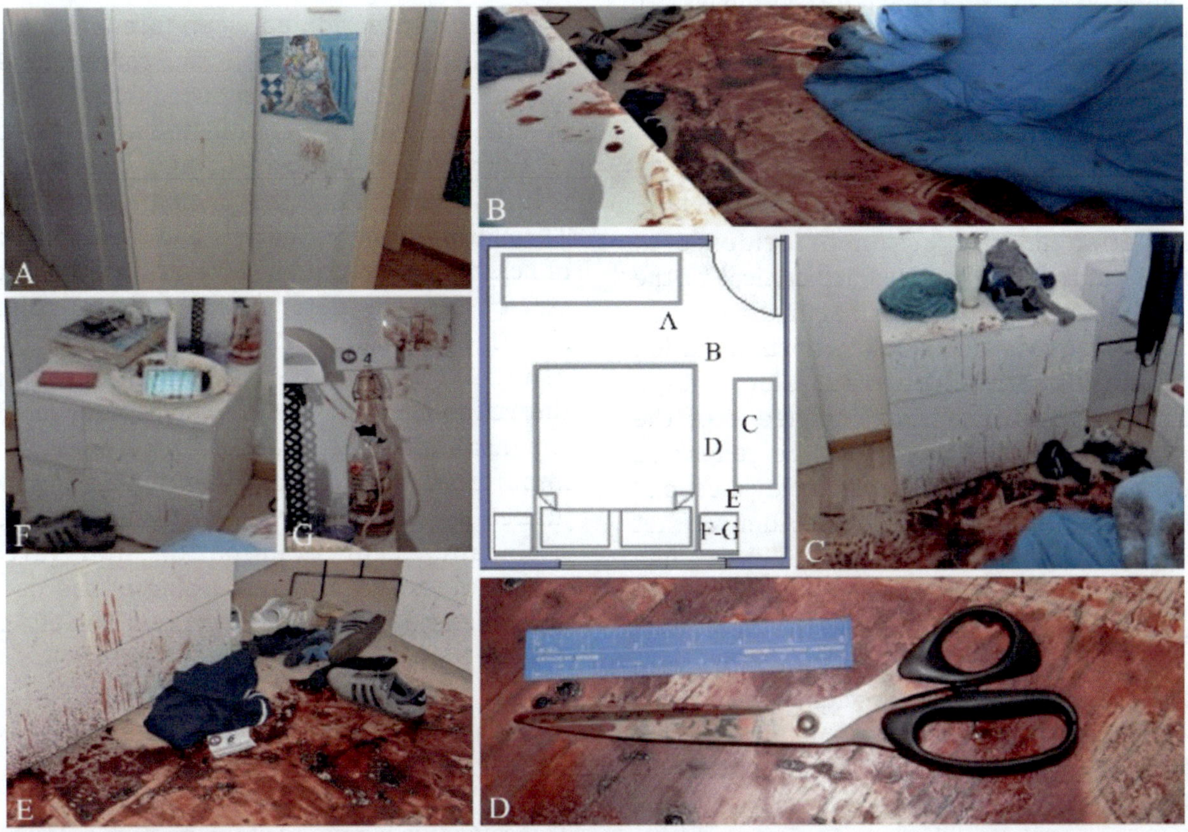

Figure 6.9. Map of the bedroom. A) Near the room's entry, the light switch has a blood transfer stain. On the lateral side of the closet, a transfer stain left by a hand and a drip stain (B). The floor was covered with a large pool of blood and a swipe pattern. The top surface of the chest of drawers has multiple drip stains. C) The anterior surface of the chest of drawers with multiple transfer and drip stains; D) the blood-drenched pair of scissors with evident traces of blood recovered a few centimeters from the bed and from the body; E) Blood-drenched pair of trousers with no lesions and a pair of shoes with spatter stains; F) mostly the anterior and superior surface of the bedside table with a drip pattern; G) the bottle on the bedside table with multiple transfer stains and the light switch, near the bottle, with a transfer stain left by a hand.

Source: https://www.minervamedica.it/upload_html/R11Y2022N04A0071/Figure%202_fmt.jpeg.

Forensic pathologists must consider the different types of projectiles and how they engage the human body in the course of investigations. Variable rates of penetration, depending on both arrowhead type and clothing fit, can have an impact on determining the intensity of injuries and purpose. This is crucial, since the dynamics may reveal something about the circumstances of the injury and even traces of the attacker's modus operandi. Forensic pathology is thus a salient discipline that demands continuous liaison with other forensic sciences to ensure that investigations into sharp force injuries are optimized in their validity and reliability (Figure 6.9).

6.3.2. Collection and Preservation of Evidence

Preservation and collection of evidence in cases of sharp force injuries are critical to the establishment of facts in criminal investigations. Not only is it a case of meticulous documentation and handling procedures, but also a high reliance on comprehensive knowledge of the many types of evidence that can be generated in such injuries. Forensic experts play a crucial role in collecting both physical evidence, that is, tissue and blood, and material evidence like weapons or clothing. The evidence needs to be collected from the crime scene to the laboratory to be admissible in court. The transition from theory to practice of forensic science is the most critical; the understanding of the nuances of how sharp force injury presents and the importance of such injuries can profoundly impact judicial processes, paralleling the saying that the dead do not speak when their stories are properly understood through scientific analysis (Black et al., 2017). In order to properly maintain the evidence collected at a crime scene, strict protocols must be followed. Contamination of samples can result in incorrect conclusions, compromising the integrity of judicial processes. Preservation involves keeping biological samples at particular temperatures and using proper storage techniques to avoid degradation. In addition, chain-of-custody procedures provide for all evidence to be traced and its handling to be recorded in minute detail. The necessity for maintaining a pure integrity of evidence is underscored by previous cases where mishandling resulted in wrongful convictions or acquittals of suspects. Through the use of advanced methods and strict standards, forensic specialists guarantee the lucidity and reliability of findings regarding sharp force injuries in order for courts to make informed decisions based on empirical data (Allison et al., 2007). Last but not least, the correlation between forensic analysis and evidence collection is the cornerstone of criminal justice. The procedure not only aids us in understanding the circumstances and setting of sharp force trauma but also plays a vital role in establishing the principles of justice. Through systematic analysis and the application of scientific techniques, victims' and offenders' stories emerge, determining judicial rulings. As forensic science evolves, further study of collection techniques will further enhance the reliability and precision of evidence. This expansion indicates a general awareness of the importance of evidence retention in pursuing justice so that the truth in a narrative may withstand legal examination and further contribute to the understanding of the nature of crime and the impact it has on society as a whole.

6.3.3. Interpretation of Injury Patterns

The causative elements of the pattern of injury in sharp force trauma must be studied thoroughly. Sharp force injuries, due to their characteristic of producing very distinct and typically lethal wounds, are exhaustively scrutinized by forensic science to establish the extent of damage caused. The nature of the weapon, manner of application of force, and angle of attack can significantly impact the resulting patterns of injury. An understanding of these variables allows forensic professionals to recreate what transpired prior to the injury being caused, thereby making clear the character of the conditions of violent encounters. Specific patterns, such as incised wounds versus stab wounds, can inform us about the intent behind the attack, with varying lengths and depths indicating variation in the level of aggression and forethought. Thus, expertise in the interpretation of these patterns is crucial for building a complete forensic narrative in sharp force injury cases. Demographic features and conditions have been identified in studies as valuable to know during interpreting sharp force injury patterns. For instance, age, gender, and socio-economic status have been found by different studies to influence the incidence of the injury. A study conducted at Muhimbili National Hospital set out the way young men were predominantly impacted by sharp force injuries, typically in terms of external causes such as road traffic accidents or inter-personal violence (Kileo et al., 2012). Such population trends not only assist in targeting preventive interventions but also guide resource allocation for health care systems managing trauma care. Accordingly, the incorporation of demographic analysis with the interpretation of injury patterns enhances the depth of understanding of sharp force injuries and enables evidence-based interventions that target the unique needs of the population. Additionally, advanced imaging modalities and forensic pathology have greatly enhanced the interpretation of sharp force injury patterns. Using radiological examinations in conjunction with clinical evaluations enables practitioners to achieve a more complete assessment of injury, which leads to accurate diagnosis and proper management plans. Notably, the findings of peri-mortem trauma, as brought out in the study of Verteba Cave, underscore the ways in which peri-mortem trauma can offer insights into activities of the past between persons and societal behavior over sharp force injury (Lillie et al., 2025). Combining historical input and present-day forensics gives experts a multi-disciplinary picture of injury patterns that enhances both investigation yield and scholarly debate on sharp force trauma. Accordingly, interdisciplinary approaches remain paramount to developing the forensic science field and effectively tackling acute force injuries in contemporary society (Figure 6.10).

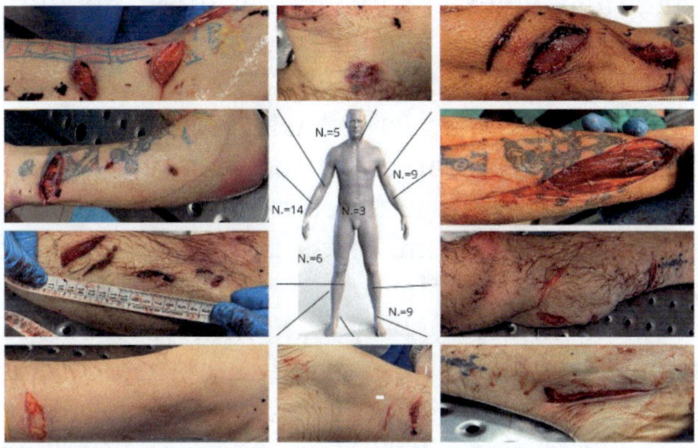

Figure 6.10. Distribution of the sharp force wounds is as follows, with some examples. N.=5 face and neck; N.=9 left upper limb; N.=14 right upper limb; N.=3 pelvic region; N.=9 left lower limb; N.=6 right lower limb.

Source: https://www.minervamedica.it/upload_html/R11Y2022N04A0071/Figure%203_fmt.jpeg.

Test Your Knowledge

1. What is the primary role of forensic pathologists in investigating sharp force injuries?
2. What is the primary goal of collecting and preserving evidence in cases of sharp force injuries?

6.4. Psychological Aspects

Learning Outcome

1. Know the motives behind sharp force injuries.
2. Describe the impact of sharp force injuries on victims and families.
3. Describe the psychological profiles of offenders.

The psychological effects of sharp force trauma extend much further than the physical pain that they invoke. The victims often develop long-term mental disturbances, including post-traumatic stress disorder (PTSD), anxiety, and depression, that utterly transform their lifestyle. The psychological effect of such traumatic events is also compounded by the vulnerability and fear that come with the experience of violence. As people cope with the aftermath of their injuries, they can find themselves struggling with intrusive memories and exaggerated arousal reactions, features typically associated with PTSD. In addition, violent injury stigma can further promote feelings of shame and isolation, discouraging victims from accessing needed psychological care. It is also essential to have an understanding of the psychological factors involved in developing integrated treatment plans that include mental health interventions and medical treatments for victims of sharp force injuries. It is also essential to understand how society and culture condition the psychological impact of sharp force injuries. Victimhood continues to carry a strong stigma in most cultures, particularly if violence is inflicted by someone with close personal relationships to the victim. As reported in research, the social dynamics may undermine open discourse on violence and its impacts, thus leading to underreported and poorly handled sharp force injury cases. This kind of cultural silence often isolates victims without support, further intensifying psychological trauma. The contribution of medical education towards addressing these issues seems to be central because it equips prospective medical professionals with the capacity to recognize and attend to psychological effects that accompany physical trauma. Through the integration of the instruction of trauma's psychological problems into medical schools, medical professionals can deliver effectively in service and contribute to an overall healing process. (Keygnaert et al., 2020) Furthermore, the relationship between psychological well-being and recovery from sharp force injury is a complicated process that involves a multidisciplinary intervention. Research has established that the mental state of a person after injury significantly influences their rehabilitation. Resilience, coping mechanisms, and support systems are some of the factors that play a significant role in determining how effectively a person will recover from physical as well as psychological injuries. It is only through a sophisticated understanding of these interconnections that healthcare professionals, as well as mental health practitioners, are empowered. For instance, rehabilitation staff may be assisted with expert therapeutic interventions that help both physical disabilities and psychological recovery processes. Implementing empowerment and resilience strategies among the wounded can partially dismantle negative psychological effects and facilitate overall recovery (Abt et al., 2012).

6.4.1. Causes of Sharp Force Injuries

The causes of sharp force injuries are multifaceted and can be deeply rooted in the psychological backgrounds of the offenders. Among the most studied causes are those involving interpersonal conflict and aggression, where sharp objects serve as weapons of violence during confrontation. Research has determined that homicide cases are mostly precipitated by personal conflicts that lead to spontaneous attacks resulting in severe injury or death. Sharp force trauma, particularly in serial murder, can exhibit patterns that show the offender's mindset and working style. These patterns are significant in separating the weapon of choice and nature of inflicted injuries, as varying environments can influence the degree to which attacks are planned or opportunistic, each situation having different injury-specific reactions (Fletcher et al., 2022). This, therefore, with the understanding of the motives, can enable an appreciation of the finer points involved in the complications of sharp force injury. The offender's psychological profile, particularly in terms of the Macdonald Triad of animal cruelty behavior, bedwetting, and fire setting behavior, is the second major etiological factor in sharp force injuries. The findings show that individuals who have experienced various forms of abuse—physical, sexual, or psychological—tend to exhibit traits of the Macdonald Triad and thereby are more at risk of committing violent crimes as adults (Zuniga et al., 2021). This pattern points towards an alarming association of childhood trauma and sharp force injuries, such that unresolved psychological issues could manifest in the form of violent crime. These findings are of valuable background information for forensic examiners, as they highlight the value of intervention at earlier phases in addressing the psychological variables underpinning violent behavior and, consequently, sharp force trauma. Lastly, the environment of the attack is significant, as one can ascertain the reasons for sharp force trauma through this. Victimology—the victim's response to the offender—is crucial in the investigation of such violent crimes. Researchers have noted that the selection of victims typically reflects the offender's psychological profile or specific targets based on past complaints or perceived complaints. This victim-offender dynamic can further identify whether the use of sharp force injuries is motivated by a need for power and control, retaliation, or thrill-seeking behavior. By studying the impetuses that drive people to perpetrate such brutal crimes, the picture becomes clearer regarding the forces behind these actions, uncovering the complexity of human behavior and the situations that lead to sharp force injuries (Fletcher et al., 2022). The motivations are critical to understand~~ing~~ in order to create appropriate prevention and intervention measures (Figure 6.11).

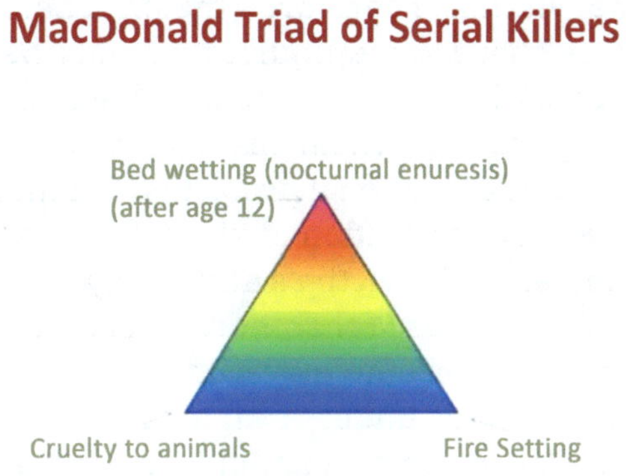

Figure 6.11. MacDonald's triad of serial killers.

Source: https://scontent-del1-2.xx.fbcdn.net/v/t1.6435-9/46667551_2241235989423837_891476668374 3191040_n.jpg?_ nc_cat=104&ccb=1-7&_nc_ sid=9eae26&_nc_ ohc=BlIPRgZ MTa8Q7kNvwFsi4dR&_nc_ oc=AdmvzBHdUNqwlllw8b FKpj4x QQgeU Z4Ao_ wBiQNyUUS 9pIP97jnpy- F3dbdRhXik iSU&_ nc_ zt=23&_nc_ht= scontent-del1-2.xx&_nc_gid=_ y11szDKf02OqT5kbyKclg&oh=00_AfTSiVhtWe_ R2fHKxEMEyZfO20RhTp_ qprOTy0COGfhTAQ&oe= 68904319.

6.4.2. Impact on Victims and Families

The impact of the sharp force injuries extends well beyond the immediate physical harm to victims, and they yield profound and often lasting effects on families. Victims of sharp force injuries endure much psychological trauma, and this resonates through family relationships. Families themselves can become strained and anxious as they experience the potential for losing a loved one or seeing them disabled for life. The psychological consequences are also extreme;

survivors will often have difficulty with post-traumatic stress disorder (PTSD), depression, or anxiety, changing family life and dynamics. As members of the victim's family take on the role of caregiver, their own psychological states could be adversely affected, creating a stress cycle that complicates the initial trauma suffered by the victim. Therefore, the psychological effect of sharp force injuries extends beyond the victims but reaches their families as well, and supportive mechanisms need to deal with such complex emotional problems. Additionally, the financial implication of sharp force injuries contributes to the victim's and family's burden. Medical expenses, rehabilitative charges, and potential lost income may add up rapidly and put the victims under a significant financial burden. The majority of families are unprepared for the initial influx of medical ailments and the potential need for continued care. This typically translates into an inability to meet fundamental living expenses, as the caregivers must reduce working hours or leave their jobs to attend to the injured individual. The financial consequences can be devastating, inducing mounting anxiety and stress in the family, leading ~~in turn~~ to aggravat~~ing~~ mental illness. Thus, the financial impact of sharp force injuries reiterates the paramount significance of institutional and social interventions to ensure that families are dealt with in the right manner at the time of need. Social impacts of sharp force injuries also illustrate the mass impact on victims and families. Where such injuries are the result of wrongful actions, families may find redress in legal avenues, which may be a lengthy and traumatic process. Social perception of violence, especially in the case of sharp force injury, can also affect the reputation and interpersonal relationships of the concerned families. Stigma can result from the nature of the events leading to the injury, and hence, social contact and welfare networks may become challenging. In addition, the broader population must confront the aftereffects of violence resulting in sharp force injuries, typically provoking debates on prevention and intervention strategies as well as safety issues. Interdependence of family life, individual trauma, and social reaction underscores the widespread nature of the effects of sharp force injuries, throwing light on the critical need for a holistic response to address the health, economic, and social consequences of such a devastating event.

6.4.3. Psychological Profiles of Offenders

Psychological profiling of criminals, particularly violent criminals, is significant in illustrating the rationale behind their crime and also the nature of injuries inflicted on victims. Research has proven that differences in lifestyle characteristics and psychological variables can significantly determine one's likelihood of being violent. For instance, Highlands' study of convicted murderers and nonviolent offenders established that the latter had lower social interest and more child hyperactivity symptoms, which indicates the association between psychological factors and violent behavior. These findings imply the possible contribution of psychological tests in shaping preventive and remedial policies in the management of offenders. Such differences not only contribute to the categorization of crime but also provide vital information that criminal justice professionals can use to develop targeted interventions and rehabilitation programs for violent offenders presenting acute force injury cases (Highland et al., 2008). Additionally, serial killers' psychological profiles must be thoroughly examined by considering the individual and situational factors influencing their criminal behavior. Serial killing, where the planned and recurring killing of individuals occurs, typically involves many aspects related to weapon preference as well as patterns of injury inflicted on victims. Research based on the motives and weapons of choice by serial killers indicates that victimology and forensic understanding may play a critical role in influencing the methods of infliction. Previous literature has posed observations about a broad disparity in the spontaneous use of weapons and the psychological foundation of such decisions. Based on the assessment of these elements, it is feasible to build on the understanding of the psychological models of offenders, thus predicting when it comes to sharp force injury and the enhancement of preventive policies (Fletcher et al., 2022). With criminologists and forensic psychologists increasingly seeking to bridge these gaps in their knowledge, the combination of psychological profiling and sharp force injuries becomes increasingly important. Describing the process by which offenders select weapons—either opportunistically or premeditatively—provides valuable information on the behavioral trajectories towards specific types of injury. Such a strategy promotes psychological assessment tools to be employed in criminal investigation to enable a holistic framework connecting offender typologies and modes of violence employed. By means of these interfaces, the discourse on sharp force injuries can change from the simple reporting of incidents to the evaluation of the psychological mechanisms that drive such behaviors. Thus, more advanced profiling techniques would lead to more effectiveness in criminal justice responses and improved public safety that would reduce violent crime (Highland et al., 2008; Fletcher et al., 2022) (Figure 6.12).

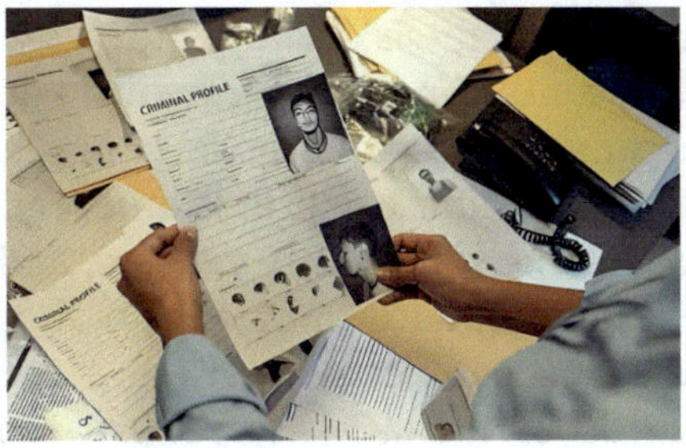

Figure 6.12. Psychological profiling of criminals.

Source: https://www.aryaman.co.in/wp-content/uploads/2024/01/Criminal-Profiling-Psychology-Identifying-Suspects-By-Aryaman-Detective.jpg.

Test Your Knowledge

1. What is the impact of sharp force injuries on victims and families?
2. What are the psychological profiles of offenders?

6.5. Prevention and Safety Measures

Learning Outcome

1. Describe the public awareness campaigns.
2. Understand the self-defense strategies.
3. Understand the role of law enforcement in addressing sharp force injuries.

Prevention of sharp force trauma in humans involves a multi-faceted approach, particularly in environments such as workplaces where risk is high. Employers need to put in place comprehensive safety programs that educate employees on the dangers of utilizing sharp tools and the precautions necessary to prevent them. This involves providing appropriate training for tool utilization and maintenance, with emphasis on design ergonomic strategies to reduce the possibility of accidents. By integrating a culture of safety within the company, early detection of possible hazards can lead to timely intervention, thus minimizing the chances of injury. Moreover, the application of safety technology, such as automatic shutdown devices, can be a significant factor in enhancing workplace security by limiting human failure in handling sharp objects. These robust prevention techniques are pillars to decreasing the incidence of sharp force injuries (Kriebel et al., 2011). Besides occupational safety, the prevention of sharp force injuries is necessary through awareness programs at the community level, especially in urban cities. Training workshops for high-risk groups such as children and adolescents can promote healthy behavior towards knives and other sharp implements. Awareness programs can utilize different media, such as schools, community centers, and social media, to disseminate information about how to handle sharp objects safely and recognize the hazards of misuse. Awareness programs can also emphasize first aid techniques for handling sharp force trauma, which can prove invaluable in mitigating long-term damage in the event of an accident. By creating safety culture consciousness within community settings, the rate of injuries can be further decreased, ultimately leading to improved populations and secure surroundings (N/A, 2005). In addition, the establishment and implementation of guidelines that address tool safety standards play an important role in averting sharp force injuries. Regulatory measures should require the fitting of safety devices in the design of sharp instruments, such as blades with shields or retractable blades, that can significantly minimize accident-caused injury risk. Moreover, regular workplace inspections and enforcement visits in workplaces where sharp tools are used can reinforce the importance of following established safety protocols. These regulatory mechanisms not only set minimum safety standards but also impose a constant drive for improvement in safety standards among employers and manufacturers. By emphasizing preventive action and adherence to strict safety standards, the incidence of sharp force injury can be dramatically decreased, making the environment safer for all (Kriebel et al., 2011) (Figure 6.13).

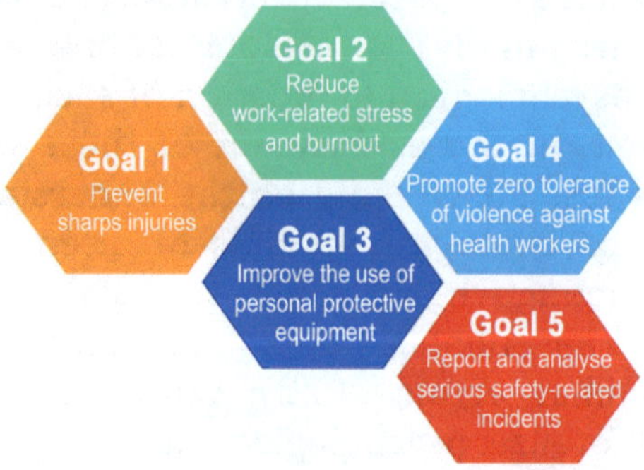

Figure 6.13. World Health Organization's number 1 goal: Prevent sharps injuries.

Source: https://www.qlicksmart.com/wp-content/uploads/2020/11/Qlicksmart-WHO.jpg.

6.5.1. Public Awareness Campaigns

Public information campaigns play a key role in the control of sharp force injuries, which usually follow traumatic events or accidents. Public information campaigns tend to increase awareness among the general population for the cause and risk factors of sharp force injuries, and also prevention methods. Public information campaigns can reduce the incidence of such injuries by making people aware of the risk of handling knives or other sharp instruments without caution. The effectiveness of such campaigns is often enhanced when the same is made to address focused communities through culturally relevant communications and local influencers in raising awareness. In addition, the inclusion of first aid response modules on sharp force injury is likely to empower individuals to act swiftly and effectively in the event of emergencies, thus decreasing morbidity and mortality from such accidents. Therefore, there needs to be a strategic focus on public education so that society is better adapted to deal with the implications of sharp force injuries. Central to the conduct of successful public awareness campaigns is the generation of a sense of concern about the prevalence of sharp force injuries. Campaigns that highlight the prevalence and severity of such injuries can start to generate a sense of shared understanding regarding the implications for community safety. For instance, statistics that reveal the frequency of such injuries among certain populations or socioeconomic strata can move policymakers and health officials to action. Secondly, campaigns can employ narrative imagery using personal stories, hence making the data personal and evoking empathy. For instance, N/A (2005) offers the requirement of standard message delivery in public health communications, reminding us that well-crafted campaigns can facilitate changes in behavior leading to dramatically reduced injury rates.

By the deployment of both statistical information and anecdotal narrative, public awareness campaigns can mobilize community involvement and stimulate an engaged reaction to the prevention of injury. It is also important that the partnership contributes to public awareness campaigns. When local agencies, health professionals, and schools collaborate, there is a synergistic effect that enhances outreach efforts. By the sharing of networks, resources, and information, such partnerships can enhance the overall effect of campaigns against sharp force injuries. The unification of various stakeholders ensures that campaigns are not only innovative but also based on the realities of the target population. As Magavern et al. (2017) have pointed out, what regional and local collaboration is required to respond to such urgent issues as preventing injury, with resulting far-reaching community effects. In such a situation, encouraging local heroes—individuals or organizations that are driving the process—can also contribute to further mobilizing, ultimately toward long-term cultural change in the safety of sharp instrument handling and, ultimately, in reducing sharp force injury occurrence.

6.5.2. Self-Defense Measures

It is necessary to understand self-defense techniques for individuals who wish to protect themselves against possible aggressors, particularly in attacks that may lead to sharp force injuries. These techniques can be physical techniques, training in awareness, and the utilization of defensive tools such as pepper spray. A notable one is pepper spray, or Oleoresin Capsicum (OC), which has been commonly used as a non-lethal defense. Its effectiveness in its operations has been reported in a series of studies, most notably by having a de-escalation of 93% for violent confrontations. However, the tactical use of OC is much reliant on the skill of the user to spray the same effectively at a close range, and this poses difficulties when encountering unstable or violent attackers (Bertilsson et al., 2017). Therefore, even though pepper spray might be an effective tool of personal protection, one must be adequately trained in its usage and aware of its limitations to use it most effectively in a crisis. Other than chemical deterrents, physical defense strategies are yet another fundamental element of personal protection. Studying martial arts or enrolling in self-defense courses can equip an individual with the needed skills to repel physical attacks successfully. Self-defense methods generally focus on pinning an attacker down using leverage, pressure points, or locks and thereby minimizing opportunities for severe injury. More importantly, self-defense training also emphasizes a strong stance on situational awareness or the capacity to recognize threats before they can escalate into physical confrontations. By building such skills, one learns to avoid dangerous situations in the first instance and lowers the possibility of having to deal with sharp force injuries. This holistic approach toward self-defense supports the learning of human behavior and threat assessment rather well, ultimately developing a proactive response towards protecting oneself. Additionally, the necessity of self-defense skills becomes most relevant in the case of sharp force injuries, for these are typically met in confrontational scenarios. Knowledge and readiness enable individuals to respond effectively when faced with threats to life. For example, employing defense gadgets like pepper spray will give us valuable seconds to escape from an attacker. However, users need to consider the potential risks as well, like exposure to collateral in case of misuse, particularly in crowded environments (Bertilsson et al., 2017). Being aware also of the legal implications of defensive action is important because excessive use of force might bring severe consequences to the defender. Therefore, an effective self-defense strategy involves not only the physical and psychological conditioning of the individual but also an informed knowledge of the legal frameworks that underpin self-defense processes, in such a manner that individuals can successfully face confrontational encounters with efficiency and responsibility (Figure 6.14).

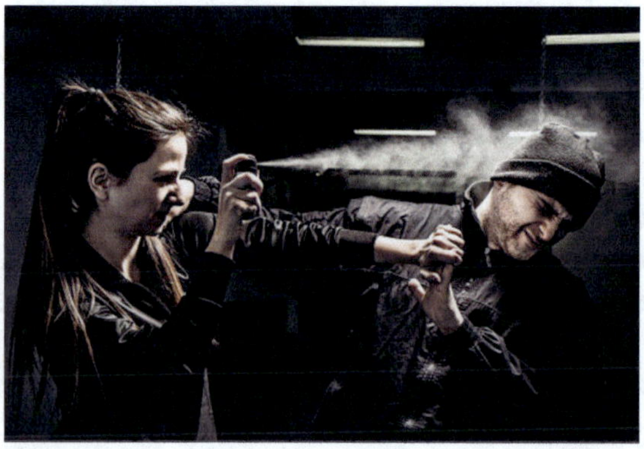

Figure 6.14. Pepper spray for self-defense.

Source: https://www.securityprousa.com/cdn/shop/articles/Screen_Shot_2023-02-21_at_9.09.17_AM.png?v=1745814252&width=1100.

6.5.3. Role of Law Enforcement

The role of law enforcement in responding to sharp force injuries extends beyond response to incidents to include prevention, investigations, and community engagement. Police are most likely the first responders to violent crimes, including those resulting in sharp force injuries. They have a critical function of securing the scene, collecting evidence, and providing emergency medical treatment. Also, officers are trained in the dynamics of such violent encounters so that they can effectively assess risks and interact with victims and suspects appropriately. Beyond their immediate functions, law enforcement officers conduct community outreach to educate the public on effective violence prevention strategies to foster a safe environment for safety and crime prevention. Engagement with community members facilitates building trust, which enables law enforcement to be part of the working team within public safety initiatives, thus assisting in containing risk linked to sharp force injuries. Policy and regulation are influenced by law enforcement activity, where agencies take part in making plans for reducing incidents of sharp force injuries. Through the recording and analysis of data on violent crime, such as offenses by sharp force, police can identify patterns to inform policy. Recommendations for enhancing safety procedures can come from this evidence-based approach, as is seen in case studies on occupational health hazards and enforcement reactions (Kriebel et al., 2011). These findings translate into broader implications for public safety, including the design of public spaces and ongoing officer training in threat assessment and de-escalation of conflict, all of which are critical in preventing situations that can lead to injury. The police thus function as both a reactive force, reacting to threats and abuses as they occur, and as a preventive force that is able to guide preventive measures with policy recommendations based on sound intelligence. Furthermore, the methods employed by police departments in dealing with threats of sharp force are critical to knowing their general role. Even though weapons like pepper spray are applied to subdue violent behavior without causing lasting harm, studies indicate their shortcomings in high-risk scenarios (Bertilsson et al., 2017). The effectiveness of such a weapon presents a call for thorough training to facilitate officers in responding appropriately to different situations. With a reported 93% success rate for eradicating violent acts, it is apparent that non-lethal options do work in addressing conflict. But the danger posed by the close calls, particularly with weapons, determines law enforcement to continually update its strategies. In addressing sharp force trauma, the agencies will need to balance the principles of good policing with the first priority of officer and public safety, prepared for any array of possible threats (Figure 6.15).

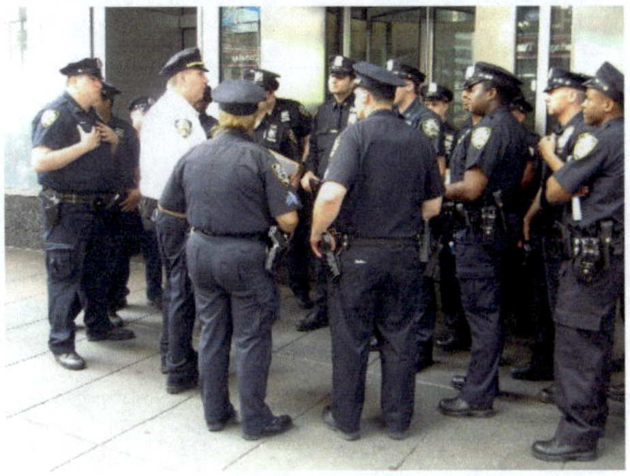

Figure 6.15. Law enforcement.

Source: https://upload.wikimedia.org/wikipedia/commons/2/28/5.29.10NYPDByLuigiNovi6.jpg.

Test Your Knowledge

1. What are the self-defense strategies?
2. What is the role of law enforcement?

SUMMARY

In summarizing the findings of sharp force injuries in human beings, it is critical to note the important implications the injuries bear on the health of individuals and overall societal structures. Sharp force injuries, which in most instances are associated with violence and crime, underscore the importance of greater prevention and medical intervention. The complexity of the etiology of these injuries requires an interdisciplinary approach involving the inputs of forensic science, psychology, and public health. A knowledge of the injury mechanisms, including the physiological response to trauma, enables healthcare providers to optimize treatment protocols while informing prevention efforts at a community level. Integrating these varied viewpoints ultimately yields better outcomes for victims of sharp force injury. Those trends that are observed in sharp force injuries, both their occurrence and accompanying demographics, speak to deeper facts about matters in society, such as violence and mental illness. Empirical findings point towards populations being disproportionately affected, suggestive of system issues like socioeconomic inequality and mental health care access. Addressing the root causes of violence, including drug addiction and denial of access to education, will be a preventive measure against sharp force injuries. Integrating mental health treatment with medical care for victims of injury gives a holistic approach, aiming not just to cure physical wounds but also to heal psychological traumas. This holistic approach is required to eliminate the long-term consequences of these traumatic injuries. Additional research is crucial in forming the knowledge regarding sharp force injuries and refining prevention and treatment guidelines. Past studies have been useful, but the dynamic nature of human activity and transformation in society necessitates continuous research. New approaches, such as the incorporation of technology in trauma and emergency management, can be breakthroughs in the treatment of sharp force injuries. In addition, enhanced sensitization and education regarding the effects of violence and injury can render communities proactive in taking preventive measures. On reflection of the key aspects of sharp force injuries, it is more apparent than ever that interdisciplinary discussion and commitment to research are building blocks in the combat against this extensive issue in society (Courtney et al., 2008; Abt et al., 2012).

In the analysis of sharp force injuries in humans, it is imperative to take into account the mechanisms of damage from such accidents. Sharp force injuries are a class of penetrating trauma caused by objects like knives or broken glass, leading to tissue injury of differing severity. Such injuries can potentially lead to severe morbidity and mortality, based on the wound location and depth, the weapon used, and the time of presentation. Understanding the pathophysiology of these types of injuries not only informs treatment algorithms but also assists in planning preventive strategies. For example, initiatives to combat knife crime have been put in place within some cities, a sign that there is a need for an interrelated approach to combat the trends of sharp force injury within society. Additionally, the psychological impact on victims and perpetrators of sharp force injuries should not be overlooked. Victims may experience long-term emotional trauma as a result, which may present itself as post-traumatic stress disorder (PTSD) or depression following violent assault. For criminals, the expense could include legal punishment and severe psychological repercussions stemming from their actions. Increased knowledge and awareness about the psychological dynamics of sharp force injuries can foster a more complete appreciation of their societal effects. As indicated in studies of occupational health hazards, there is an absolute necessity for regulatory actions that address not only physical safety but also incorporate mental health programs. By giving priority to these characteristics, communities can combat the incidence and effect of sharp force trauma, understanding the complexities of such violence (Kriebel et al., 2011). Moreover, early and proper medical care plays an important role in treating sharp force trauma. Treatment timeliness has a crucial role in determining outcomes, and it is therefore essential that emergency responders are equipped to deal with such attacks. Training of first responders and medical personnel in proper treatment of penetrating injuries can drastically reduce the likelihood of complications, for instance, infection or excessive blood loss. Ongoing revision of examination and treatment guidelines for sharp force injuries based on new research and case studies is necessary. Initiatives like these would not only inform clinical practice, but would also provide insight into broader public health interventions for injury prevention and control. These projects, which synthesize evidence from multiple sources regarding sharp force injuries, including insights from previous interventions, are vital to ensuring that healthcare procedures remain effective and current in addressing this ongoing issue (Courtney et al., 2008).

KEY TERMS FROM THIS CHAPTER

- Bladed weapons
- Criminal offenses
- Forensic medicine
- Lacerations
- Physical rehabilitation
- Puncture wounds
- Societal welfare
- Blood vessels
- Domestic violence
- Incised wounds
- Medical education
- Psychological support
- Sharp force injury
- Stab wounds

CRITICAL THINKING QUESTIONS

1. **What defines a sharp force injury?**
   a. Injury caused by a blow or impact with no skin penetration.
   b. Injury caused by a sharp-edged object penetrating the skin.
   c. Injury caused by chemical exposure.
   d. Injury caused by friction and scraping of the skin.
2. **Which of the following is NOT a type of sharp force injury?**
   a. Incised wound
   b. Stab wound
   c. Laceration
   d. Chop wound
3. **What is the primary characteristic of an incised wound?**
   a. Deep penetration with minimal external length.
   b. Tearing of the skin with tissue bridging.
   c. A wound longer than it is deep with clean edges.
   d. A wound caused by blunt force trauma.
4. **A stab wound is characterized by:**
   a. A superficial wound longer than it is deep.
   b. A deep wound caused by a pointed object and deeper than its length.
   c. A superficial scrape caused by friction.
   d. An irregular tear of the skin caused by blunt force.
5. **Which factor most affects the characteristics of a stab wound?**
   a. The angle and force of the stab.
   b. The amount of clothing worn by the victim.
   c. The environmental temperature.
   d. The weight of the victim.

Short Answer Questions

1. What are sharp force injuries primarily characterized by?
2. List the types of sharp force injuries.
3. Which factors most significantly influence the severity of sharp force injuries?
4. What are some common psychological challenges faced by victims of sharp force injuries?
5. What is a recommended safety technology for minimizing sharp force injuries in workplaces?

Answer to Critical Thinking Questions

1. (b); 2. (c); 3. (c); 4. (b); 5. (a)

REFERENCES

1. Abt, J. P., Fleishman, K. A., Crawford, K., et al. (2012). The relationship between musculoskeletal strength, physiological characteristics, and knee kinesthesia following fatiguing exercise. https://core.ac.uk/download/12212102.pdf (accessed on 12th July 2025).
2. Abuja, A., Akdemir, A., et al. (2018). The physiological mechanisms of effect of vitamins and amino acids on tendon and muscle healing: A systematic review. https://core.ac.uk/download/287581405.pdf (accessed on 12th July 2025).
3. Aerospace medicine and biology: A continuing bibliography with indexes (supplement 331). (2025). https://core.ac.uk/download/pdf/42824791.pdf (accessed on 12th July 2025).
4. Aerssens, A., Allen, M., Alunni, L., Ambade, A., Ankersen, B., Banasr, M., Bartelink, H., et al. (2017). Effects of heat on cut mark characteristics. https://core.ac.uk/download/74204621.pdf (accessed on 12th July 2025).
5. Allison, K. J., Bailey, G. B., Bartlett, J. E., Boylston, A., Briden, C., Buikstra, J., et al. (2007). An Anglo-Saxon execution cemetery at Walkington World, Yorkshire. https://core.ac.uk/download/52301.pdf (accessed on 12th July 2025).
6. Bajd, T., Belder, R., Haddadin, S., et al. (2015). A tool for the evaluation of human lower arm injury: Approach, experimental validation and application to safe robotics. https://core.ac.uk/download/132311760.pdf (accessed on 12th July 2025).
7. Beattie, E., Fraser, J., MacPhee, N., et al. (2018). A comparison of penetration and damage caused by different types of arrowheads on loose and tight fit clothing. https://core.ac.uk/download/228178194.pdf (accessed on 12th July 2025).
8. Bertilsson, J., Fransson, P. A., Fredriksson, P. J., Magnusson, M., et al. (2017). Use of pepper spray in policing: Retrospective study of situational characteristics and implications for violent situations. https://core.ac.uk/download/83793219.pdf (accessed on 12th July 2025).
9. Black, S., Hackman, L., Nic Daéid, N., et al. (2017). The role of forensic anthropology in cases of dismemberment. https://core.ac.uk/download/195287834.pdf (accessed on 12th July 2025).
10. Bolton-King, R., & Schulze, J. (2016). Firearms and ballistics. https://core.ac.uk/download/80691312.pdf (accessed on 12th July 2025).
11. Boom, B., Daly, D., Daly, D., Dennis, F., European Food Safety Authority AHAW panel, Fackler, M., Finnie, P., et al. (2014). Evaluation of a spring-powered captive bolt gun for killing kangaroo pouch young. https://core.ac.uk/download/36778301.pdf (accessed on 12th July 2025).
12. Carr, D. J., Cowper, E. J., Godhania, K., et al. (2016). A pilot study examining garment severance damage caused by a trained sharp-weapon user. https://core.ac.uk/download/42144462.pdf (accessed on 12th July 2025).
13. Courtney, A., & Courtney, M. (2008). A thoracic mechanism of mild traumatic brain injury due to blast pressure waves. https://core.ac.uk/download/pdf/287975.pdf (accessed on 12th July 2025).
14. Facco, E., Lucangeli, D., & Tressoldi, P. E. (2017). On the primacy and irreducible nature of first-person versus third-person information. https://core.ac.uk/download/84922410.pdf (accessed on 12th July 2025).

15. Feldman, A. (2015). From trauma to trial: Proposing new methods for examining the variability of sharp force trauma on bone. https://core.ac.uk/download/70426371.pdf (accessed on 12th July 2025).
16. Fletcher, E. (2022). Weapons of choice: A statistical comparison between different weapons and resulting injuries, opportunist weapon selection and forensic awareness. https://core.ac.uk/download/533941028.pdf (accessed on 12th July 2025).
17. Fröhlich, D. D., C., Hague, D., Williams, M. A., Payne, M., Matthews, T., Donnelly, M. J., et al. (2020). A holistic multi-scale approach to using 3D scanning technology in accident reconstruction. https://core.ac.uk/download/305119975.pdf (accessed on 12th July 2025).
18. Grossman, M. (2017). On the concept of health capital and the demand for health. *Columbia University Press eBooks*. https://doi.org/10.7312/gros17812-004 (accessed on 12th July 2025).
19. Highland, R. A. (2008). Murderers and nonviolent offenders: A comparison of lifestyle, pampering, and early recollections. https://core.ac.uk/download/71421631.pdf (accessed on 12th July 2025).
20. Iowa Health Focus. (2005). *Iowa Health Focus*, December 2005. https://core.ac.uk/download/11346248.pdf (accessed on 12th July 2025).
21. Keygnaert, I., Manuel, B., Roelens, K., Tiago, M., et al. (2020). Medical curricula on intimate partner violence in Mozambique. https://core.ac.uk/download/286086429.pdf (accessed on 12th July 2025).
22. Kileo, B. F. (2012). The pattern of oral and maxillofacial injuries among patients attending Muhimbili National Hospital, Dar es Salaam, Tanzania. https://core.ac.uk/download/pdf/11307821.pdf (accessed on 12th July 2025).
23. Kriebel, D., Tickner, J., Jacobs, M., & Markkanen, P. (2011). Lessons learned: Solutions for workplace safety and health. https://core.ac.uk/download/71352756.pdf (accessed on 12th July 2025).
24. Kroman, A. M. (2007). Fracture biomechanics of the human skeleton. https://core.ac.uk/download/268770463.pdf (accessed on 12th July 2025).
25. Lammasniemi, L. (2020). "Precocious girls": Age of consent, class, and family in late nineteenth-century England. https://core.ac.uk/download/287606177.pdf (accessed on 12th July 2025).
26. Lillie, M., Nikitin, A., Potiekhina, I. D., Sokhatsky, V., et al. (2025). First evidence for interpersonal violence in Ukraine's Trypillian farming culture: Individual 3 from Verteba Cave, Bilche Zolote. https://core.ac.uk/download/151159376.pdf (accessed on 12th July 2025).
27. Mach, F., Baigent, C., Catapano, A. L., Koskinas, K. C., Casula, M., Badimón, L., Chapman, M. J., et al. (2019). 2019 ESC/EAS guidelines for the management of dyslipidemias: Lipid modification to reduce cardiovascular risk. *European Heart Journal, 41*, 111–188. https://doi.org/10.1093/eurheartj/ehz455 (accessed on 12th July 2025).
28. Magavern, S., & Schneekloth, L. (2017). The climate justice movement in Western New York. https://core.ac.uk/download/233839622.pdf (accessed on 12th July 2025).
29. Malherbe, G. F. (2015). Laparoscopy (to detect occult diaphragm injury) versus clinical and radiological follow-up to detect diaphragm injury and herniation, in patients with asymptomatic left thoracoabdominal stab wounds: A prospective randomized controlled study. https://core.ac.uk/download/185400832.pdf (accessed on 12th July 2025).

30. Pitsillides, A. A., Anderson, B. A., Armstrong, B. A., et al. (2015). Non-Invasive Mouse Models of Post-Traumatic Osteoarthritis. https://core.ac.uk/download/36778518.pdf (accessed on 12th July 2025).

31. Steimle, B. (2020). The recreation of wound patterns using various tissue simulants for crime scene reconstruction. https://core.ac.uk/download/386366625.pdf (accessed on 12th July 2025).

32. Thor, C., Lo, M., Baumann, M. C., & Cowles, N. A. (2016). Furniture stability: A review of data and testing results. https://core.ac.uk/download/75785791.pdf (accessed on 12th July 2025).

33. Williams, J. (2012). The scientific disciplines: What comes first among equals? https://core.ac.uk/download/9836283.pdf (accessed on 12th July 2025).

34. Zuniga, V. A. (2021). A descriptive study of serial killers and the presence of Macdonald triad symptoms. https://core.ac.uk/download/482688844.pdf (accessed on 12th July 2025).

7

GUNSHOT WOUNDS AND BALLISTICS

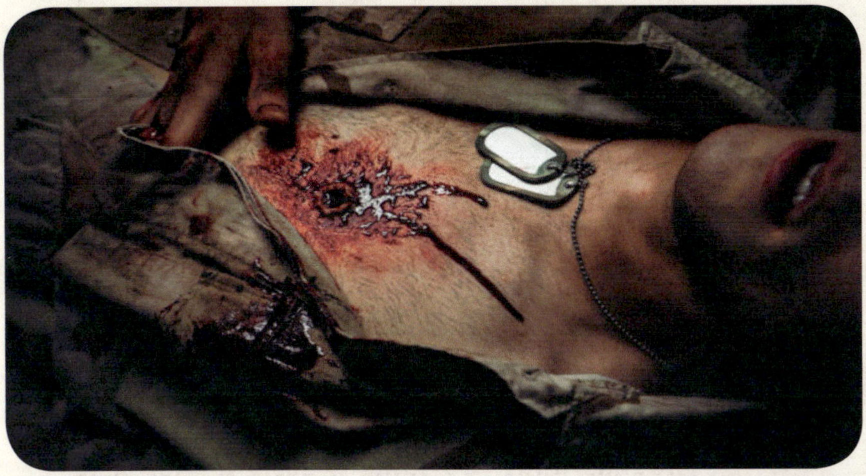

LEARNING OBJECTIVES

After studying this chapter, you will be able to:

1. Describe the types of gunshot wounds;
2. Understand the mechanisms of injury resulting from gunshot wounds;
3. Know the fundamentals of ballistics;
4. Understand the forensic ballistics;
5. Describe the medical management of gunshot wounds;
6. Know the legal and ethical considerations in the examination of gunshot wounds and ballistics.

Introduction

The study of gunshot wounds and ballistics in the human body is a multidisciplinary science that intersects medicine, forensic science, and engineering. Knowledge of projectile behavior and firearm injury's biological effects is necessary for a variety of applications, from legal investigation to trauma care to protective device design. Firearms have become a prominent characteristic of violence in society and have fueled an epidemic of gunshot wounds and homicides. Thus, it is important to study how the laws of ballistics affect human biology for the sake of determining gunshot wound severity, treatment, and prevention. Furthermore, it is essential to keep on enhancing forensic ballistics techniques, particularly shooting incident reconstruction, for enhancing the efficiency of criminal investigation and court proceedings (Humphrey et al., 2017). Ballistics encompasses the examination of projectiles from the moment of their first discharge to the moment of impact, comprising the first discharge, trajectory, and impact effects. The physical characteristics of cartridges and guns play a very significant role in energy delivery to human tissue upon impact. High-velocity projectiles produce more destructive wounds compared to projectiles with slower velocities due to the shockwave and cavitation phenomena, which significantly increase the wound cavity and affect surrounding organs. Latest research has indicated intricate information about the mechanisms of penetration of the projectiles in the various tissues, confirming that the nature of the wounds depends on a multitude of factors varying from the ammunition type and firing distance to the target zone anatomical structure (Humphrey et al., 2017). In such a manner, detailed knowledge of these interactions is pivotal for accurate assessment of the damage and formulation of appropriate medical interventions.

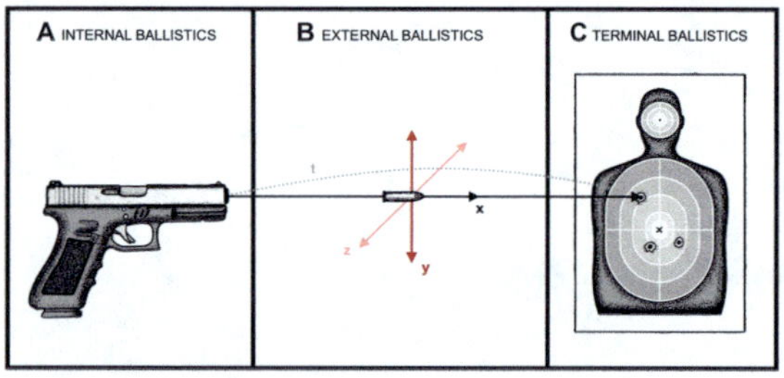

Figure 7.1. Phases of ballistics.

Source: https://www.dovepress.com/article/fulltext_file/378278/aW1n/ORR_A_378278_O_F0001g.jpg.

Moreover, forensic examination is necessary to understand the effects of gunshot injuries beyond immediate health problems. Employing techniques from diverse scientific disciplines like chemistry, physics, and computational modeling, examiners reconstruct the incidents of shooting and analyze GSR patterns to determine shooting distances and mechanisms (Brooke et al., 2020). The combination of advanced technologies, such as radiography, raises the precision of such analyses, facilitating more detailed examination of both GSR dispersal and the resulting tissue damage of gunshot wounds. In the long term, integration of knowledge from these interdisciplinary areas helps to counteract the broader impact of gun violence on public health and safety by influencing practice in medical care and policing strategy (Figure 7.1).

Definition of Gunshot Wounds

Gunshot wounds, by definition, are caused by a projectile, in most instances a bullet, entering the human body due to the firing of a gun. The character of such an injury is greatly influenced by an array of factors, including the type of firearm used, the caliber of ammunition used, and the range of fire. Familiarity with these factors is important as they influence wound factors and potential outcomes. For example, high-velocity rounds will impact and cause a lot of tissue damage and cavitation, leading to more serious injuries than low-velocity rounds. The study of wound ballistics—a branch of terminal ballistics—gives important information about the way the different parameters interact with each other in order to create different gunshot wounds, thus providing a basis for forensic examination as well as medical intervention (Bolton-King et al., 2016). The classification of gunshot wounds is primarily interested in the path, velocity, and force of the bullet. These three are accountable for the formation of various types of injuries, ranging from penetrating to perforating wounds. A penetrating gunshot wound will have an entry but no exit wound, which means that the bullet has gotten lodged within the body and can cause severe internal damage. Conversely, a perforating wound shows entry and exit points, suggesting greater tissue disruption. The nature of the injury sustained also typically relies on the ballistic properties of the weapon and bullet; for example, a study utilizing synthetic models demonstrated contrasting effects of 7.62 x 39 mm ammunition on tangential and contact wounds, highlighting the importance of discovering the intricacy of producing wounds (Mahoney et al., 2018). Moreover, clinical and forensic aspects of gunshot injuries deserve comprehensive knowledge of their definition and classification. Their accurate assessment and management are important in both clinical practice and in the legal setting. Discrimination among wound types in forensic examinations is useful in reconstructing the conditions of a shooting occurrence and can exert a profound influence on legal findings. With advances in the field of forensic science, the integration of ballistic theory into the analysis of gunshot wounds enhances a better understanding of mechanisms of injury. The application of multiple disciplines, in addition to enriching trauma care, also enhances means of forensic analysis, enabling practitioners to better understand ballistic evidence (Bolton-King et al., 2016) (Figure 7.2).

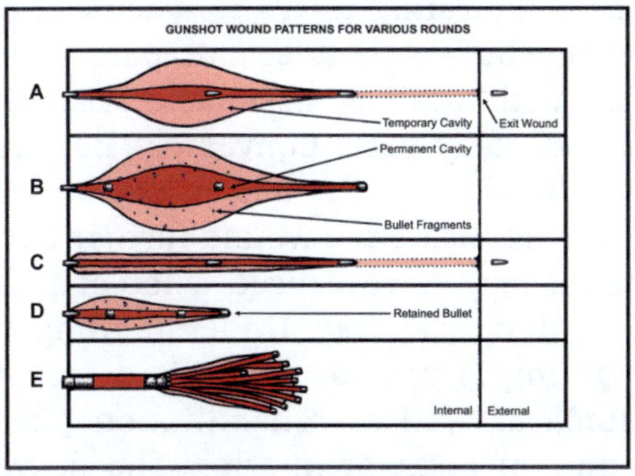

Figure 7.2. Gunshot wound patterns for various rounds. (A) High-energy wound from a non-deforming round. (B) High-energy wound from a deforming round. (C) Low-energy wound from a non-deforming round. (D) Low-energy wound from a deforming round. (E) Low-energy wound from a shotgun shell (deforming round).

Source: https://www.dovepress.com/article/fulltext_file/378278/aW1n/ORR_A_378278_O_F0003g.jpg.

Importance of Studying Ballistics in Relation to Gunshot Wounds

Ballistic analysis is essential in the understanding of gunshot wounds due to its intricate relationship with the physical nature of projectiles and how they interact within human tissue. Ballistics exists in three forms: internal, external, and terminal ballistics, and each of them plays an important role in the analysis of the wound~~ing~~ mechanism. Terminal ballistics, in particular, deals with how the bullet interacts with the tissue when it hits and, therefore, how different ammunition causes different amounts of damage. Individuals who know the scientific foundations of these principles can better assess the kind and severity of wounds and subsequently guide more productive medical interventions and forensic analysis. The conclusions from ballistic studies advance the knowledge of wound ballistics, the discipline that investigates the process of forming wounds and their use, thus allowing forensic experts to possess the much-needed information that can aid in investigations and treatment of patients (Bolton-King et al., 2016). Of interest in ballistics is its application in determining the performance of different types of ammunition, more so their influence on wound patterns and tissue damage. For instance, contemporary wars often entail the use of advanced ammunition technology, such as hollow-point and expanding bullets, specifically designed to achieve maximum wound effects. Awareness of their characteristics, particularly from a terminal ballistics viewpoint, enables medical professionals and forensic experts to predict potential effects in terms of their velocity and design. Research that has proven hollow-point ammunition to more than double the area over which an injury will be created compared to non-hollow-point equivalents emphasizes the importance of being capable of discerning variations between ammunition. Through applying this knowledge to clinical practice, doctors are able to guide treatment decisions and provide better prognoses for gunshot victims (Dubenko et al., 2021). Moreover, the advances in ballistic science facilitate easier development of quality training programs for medical and forensic specialists. Incorporating ballistics into medical school curricula allows clinicians to become proficient at recognizing some wound features typical of certain types of cartridges. This basic knowledge enhances correct diagnosis and helps in the formulation of treatment protocols in line with the injury. Additionally, awareness of the biomechanical forces involved in a ballistic event fosters collaboration among emergency medical responders, forensic experts, and legal experts. Lastly, while gun violence persists worldwide, with an emphasis on the importance of ballistics in gunshot wound investigation that not only enhances medical treatment but also assists in criminal investigations, thereby maintaining its invaluable role in the criminal justice and public health fields (Bolton-King et al., 2016; Dubenko et al., 2021) (Figure 7.3).

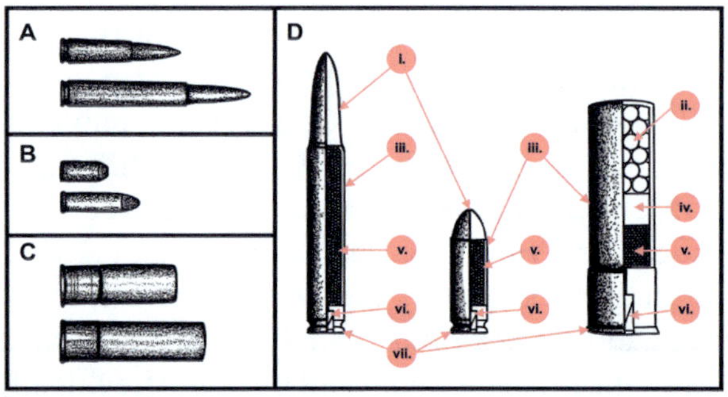

Figure 7.3. Ammunition anatomy. (A) High velocity/energy cartridges, typically fired from rifles, are designed for long-range use for hunting or armed conflict. (B) Low velocity/energy rounds, typically used in handguns. The sketches depict one round with a hollow point and one with a round point. (C) Shotgun ammunition, typically used in muzzle-loading rifles, is designed for short-range targets. (D) Ammunition generally consists of the following: (i) Bullet (projectile); (iii) Casing; (v) Propellant; (vi) Primer; (vii) Rim. Uniquely, shotgun shells contain (ii) Pellets (projectiles) and (iv) Wadding.

Source: https://www.dovepress.com/article/fulltext_file/378278/aW1n/ORR_A_378278_O_F0002g.jpg.

7.1. Types of Gunshot Wounds

Learning Outcome

1. Understand the distinction between penetrating and perforating wounds.
2. Describe the types of firearms and their impact on wounds.
3. Know the common injuries associated with gunshot wounds.

The classification of gunshot injuries is instrumental to learning about how they impact human anatomy and the subsequent medical intervention required. Gunshot injuries are typically classified into three types: penetrating, perforating, and blunt trauma injuries. Penetrating refers to when the bullet enters the body but does not pass through, typically with localized tissue and organ injury in the trajectory path. Conversely, perforating wounds do have an entry and an exit, and this is going to complicate the wound further because the bullet may have caused a lot of internal damage along the way. Understanding these types is important for both field treatment of trauma as well as rehabilitation planning in victims of gunshot injuries. The degree of tissue destruction from gunshot injuries varies significantly based on the caliber of the bullet and range of fire, highlighting the significance of proper diagnostic protocols in the clinical setup. Different types of gunshot wounds have varying presentations clinically, risks, and modes of treatment. As an illustration, low-velocity gunshot wounds, typically from handguns or shotguns, are more tissue destructive and produce more cavitation than are high-velocity rifle injuries, creating a transient cavity extending to adjacent organs considerably by shock waves. This difference becomes crucial in the evaluation of trauma because the risk for secondary injury may significantly influence immediate and late outcomes. Moreover, the presence of clothing during a shooting incident can also determine the extent and characteristics of wounds sustained. Science demonstrated that the types of clothing could produce effects on bullet penetration, suggesting that practitioners should not only look at the wound but also extrinsic variables governing injury severity to better guide treatment (Beattie et al., 2018). Improvement in the forensic analysis of gunshot wounds is also possible with information about the mechanical response of various materials simulating human tissue and bone in ballistic testing. Synthetics like polyurethane have come into use as surrogates to model human skeletal response to gunshot impacts. These are models made artificially that allow scientists to conduct controlled experiments, more comprehensively grasping the behavior of different projectiles upon contact with biological tissues without the concerns of utilizing human cadavers. Even though these materials show overall similarity in response to ballistic trauma, they are limited in their ability to accurately simulate the complexities of human bone when subjected to such trauma, indicating the requirement for judicious application of these findings to real cases (Ball et al., 2015). Lastly, ongoing research into patterns of gunshot wounds and relevance continues not only to inform medical professionals but to advance the efficacy of forensic investigations (Figure 7.4).

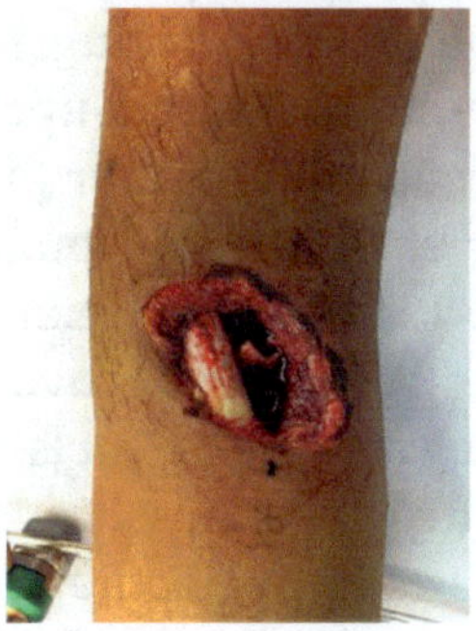

Figure 7.4. Gunshot wounds.

Source: https://upload.orthobullets.com/topic/1059/images/weatherford_110829_25.jpg.

7.1.1. Penetrating Versus Perforating Wounds

It is crucial that forensic and medical experts recognize the distinction between perforating and penetrating wounds to assess gunshot wounds. A penetrating wound occurs when the bullet enters the body but does not exit, inflicting injury to the tissue in localized areas near the point of entry. The injury varies in severity based on circumstances like the caliber and range of the bullet. Penetrating injuries may also present with minimal obvious external damage compared to perforating wounds but still possess a risk of extensive internal damage, complications, and infection unless managed accordingly. Identification of the type of injury will play a significant role in impacting the clinical management and surgical operation in managing the patient, particularly in emergency situations where immediate intervention is critical. In contrast, perforating wounds are defined by the course of the bullets within the body that create an entry and an exit wound. The harm is that which entails a greater extent of damage since the missile may cause extensive tissue disruption in its path. The two orifices that are present in perforating wounds complicate the picture clinically because they can offer pathways for contamination as well as increased hemorrhaging. Moreover, the patients with perforating wounds usually receive more trauma and shock since the wound possesses a double nature. Such added complexity is required to comprehend fully ballistic effects and patterns of tissue damage of both types of wounds in order to execute effective triage and treatment (Mabbott et al., 2016). The clinical implications of penetration rather than perforation wounds extend beyond immediate care; they can also affect long-term recovery and rehabilitation. For instance, the tissue damage from a perforating wound can require more surgical intervention and longer recovery times, and can lead to complications like chronic pain or loss of mobility. Also, improvements in ammunition technology, with the development of new tungsten-tin bullets (Anderson et al., 2000), further complicate matters by altering energy transfer at impact and the ensuing wounding ability. It is necessary to comprehend these variations in ballistic research because they affect body armor design and medical response strategies to gunshot trauma. Essentially, differentiation between penetrating and perforating injuries is important not only for treatment of acute trauma, but also for optimizing the outcome from gunshot wound in long-term care (Figure 7.5).

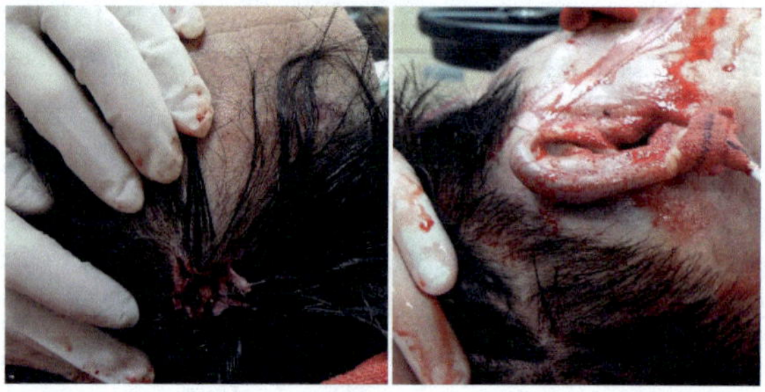

Figure 7.5. The bullet penetrated the left parietal region and stopped at the posterior auricular area.

Source: https://www.jtraumainj.org/upload/thumbnails/jti-31-082f1.jpg.

7.1.2. Types of Firearms and Their Impact on Wounds

The classification of firearms is of importance in identifying the nature and degree of injuries sustained by victims. Firearms are broadly categorizable into handguns, rifles, and shotguns, each of which is designed based on various operating mechanisms and projectile designs. Handguns, such as revolvers and semi-automatics, typically discharge medium-velocity projectiles that produce localized tissue destruction, leading to contusions and lacerations surrounding the wound zone. Conversely, rifles fire high-velocity projectiles that can cause extensive tissue damage and cavitation effects when penetrating the body. Such injuries typically yield poor outcomes, including severe damage to organs and increased chances of death. Shotguns, in their dispersal of numerous small projectiles, can produce atypical patterns of wounds, such as large, irregular holes, with destructive damage to soft tissue and bone, profoundly affecting the medical management of gunshot injuries (Humphrey et al., 2017). Kinetic energy transfer and velocity of a projectile have a key impact on the lethal effect of gunshot injuries. As the projectile travels through tissue, its kinetic energy is converted to tissue damage depending on the type of weapon. Studies have demonstrated that the high-velocity rifle bullets create an initial cavity larger than the bullet with extensive tissue destruction, shock waves, and secondary damage to surrounding structures. Handguns cause smaller, contained wounds with less damage to the peripheral wound. It is critical to know these dynamics for the medical professionals who are responsible for the examination and treatment of injuries. Furthermore, forensic ballistics compares these differences to properly reconstruct shooting incidents, a requirement in the legal proceedings and devising prevention measures (Brooke et al., 2020). Moreover, the design and makeup of ammunition utilized in firearms add further complexity to the injury pattern observed in gunshot wounds. Hollow-point and FMJ rounds, for instance, react in differing manners upon impact. Hollow-points expand upon their impact on soft tissue, becoming larger in diameter and creating wider channels of wounds, equivalent to more tissue loss and internal bleeding. FMJ bullets, conversely, may travel farther but leave narrower wound channels that may have survivable injury if vital organs are not hit. Research into these projectile trajectories, for example, how they affect different organs of the body as described in research, is important to make appropriate medical treatment plans and surgical procedures in case of gunshot wounds (Humphrey et al., 2017). Understanding these nuances also informs the production of bullet-resistant materials and protective vests, improving protective equipment from gunshot injuries (Figure 7.6).

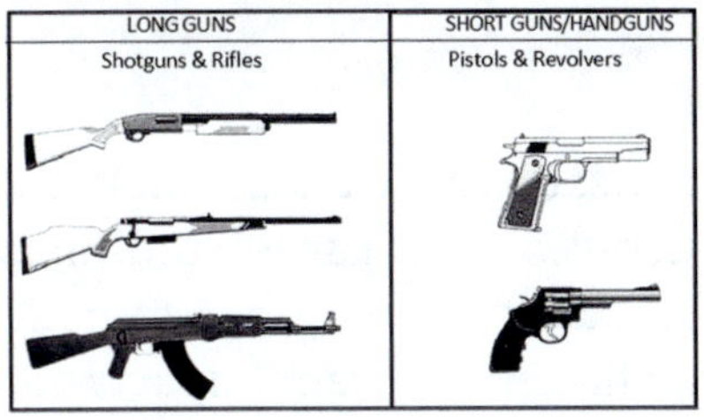

Figure 7.6. Types of firearms.

Source: https://wholeeartheducation.com/wp-content/uploads/2023/07/Long-guns-vs-short-guns.jpg.

7.1.3. Common Injuries Associated with Gunshot Wounds

Gunshot injuries are a critical public health problem, typically causing multiple injuries that inflict severe physical and psychological trauma. Prevalent injuries of such wounds include soft tissue damage, bone fractures, and organ perforation. Soft tissue damage dominates due to the rapid speed of projectiles, leading to laceration and contusion that both compromise the skin as well as the musculature. Apart from that, they induce massive bleeding, which provides the foundation for urgent life-threatening complications requiring expedited medical attention. Alongside the physical injuries, the psychological impacts of gunshot survival are post-traumatic stress disorder (PTSD), depression, and anxiety, which illustrate the multifaceted aspect of gun injury trauma. Trauma to the bones is the most frequent occurrence in patients presenting with gunshot wounds, particularly if the bullet strikes at point-blank range. Hitting bullets with high speed has the resultant effect of fracturing bone and imparting complex fractures that make healing and surgical interventions complicated. Mechanisms of such effects are crucial for medical doctors to understand, as they inform interventions and rehabilitation (Ball et al., 2015).

Researchers have noted that despite ballistic trauma being studied using animal surrogates, the effect may not be a true reflection of how bones in humans react to bullets (Ball et al., 2015). As a consequence, anatomical and physiological differences are to be considered during the evaluation of specific injuries, bringing into perspective the importance of detailed investigations in health institutions. In addition to soft tissue damage and bone damage, gunshot injuries also frequently result in internal damage that becomes fatal. These injuries usually involve vital organs such as the lungs, heart, and liver, whose severity depends on the caliber and velocity of the bullet. For instance, a chest gunshot wound may result in a pneumothorax, which is where air enters between the lung and chest wall, a condition that can prove fatal if treatment is not administered promptly. Furthermore, the interaction between the weapon and ammunition shot has a direct impact on the character of the wound and associated injuries, demonstrating the principles of wound ballistics (Bolton-King et al., 2016). The complexity of such intracorporeal injuries demonstrates the pressing need for medical and forensic professionals to consult in addressing the effect of gunshot wounds in practice (Figure 7.7).

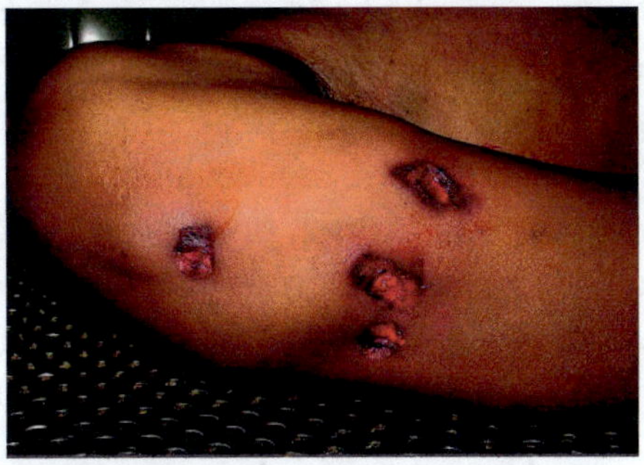

Figure 7.7. Gunshot injury.

Source: https://ars.els-cdn.com/content/image/3-s2.0-B0123693993002147-gr9.jpg.

Test Your Knowledge

1. What is the difference between a perforating and penetrating wound?
2. What are the types of firearms?

7.2. Mechanisms of Injury

Learning Outcome

1. Describe the tissue damage caused by bullets.
2. Understand the role of velocity and energy in injury severity.
3. Know the secondary injuries from bone fragments and debris.

Understanding the mechanisms of gunshot injury demands an awareness of the ballistic parameters that control the trajectory of projectiles under impact. Wound ballistics, a significant area of terminal ballistics, offers knowledge on the physical and chemical phenomena that establish patterns of injury in the human body. The speed, weight, and shape of bullets largely influence the extent and nature of the injury inflicted. For instance, high-velocity projectiles initiate temporary cavitation, which creates a large-diameter wound channel larger than the bullet's trajectory.

This results in extensive tissue damage, not confined to the bullet's trajectory, thus complicating surgical treatment and recovery. Knowledge of such dynamics offers important information to both medical physicians and forensic specialists who must evaluate the impact of gunshot wounds and provide appropriate treatments. Firearm caliber and ammunition type also play a crucial part in determining mechanisms of injury, and a thorough analysis becomes of paramount importance in forensic cases. Different guns, ranging from handguns to rifles, possess distinct ballistic properties that determine the manner of penetration of bullets in tissue, as well as their impact on bone structures. The use of full-metal jacket bullets, for example, compared to hollow-point bullets, can have significant impacts on lethality and severity of injury. Expanding bullets when they hit are going to create bigger channels of harm, aggravating tissue damage and increasing the potential for negative effects such as infection or organ failure. In addition, certain ammunition produces injury patterns that are unique in character, such as fragmentations that are depressing to tissue injury and inhibiting healing, and hence it is necessary for clinicians to understand these variations in designing treatment and for forensic personnel to collect appropriate evidence. Last but not least, clothing interaction with bullets has a significant role in the mechanisms of injury from gunshot wounds. Studies affirm that clothing not only influences penetration depth but also the overall wound profile, highlighting the interactive relationship of outer variables and ballistic performance. Loose garments, for instance, can restrain penetration capability, potentially altering the course and impact of the bullet when it enters the underlying tissue.

Alternatively, tight-fitting or multi-layer garments can enhance absorption effects by causing greater tissue distortion and penetration. Evidence from such studies points to the importance of noting clothes debris at the crime scene, as it could provide forensic examiners with important information regarding the mechanism of injury and even assist in reconstructing the events surrounding the shooting incident. Such aspects are important in understanding the broader implications of gunshot injuries both in medical and legal environments (Figure 7.8).

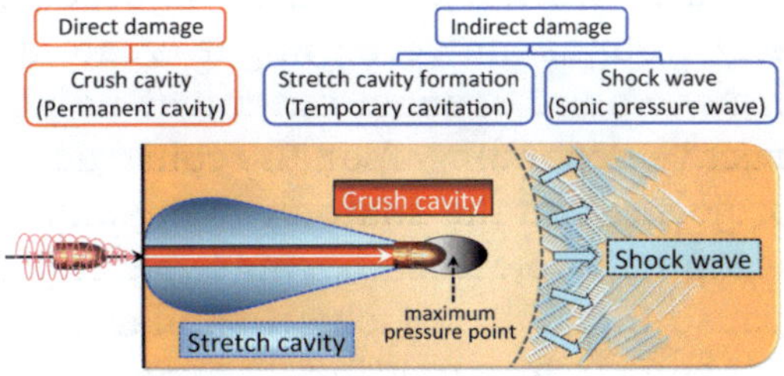

Figure 7.8. A diagram illustrating the mechanisms underlying gunshot wounds.

Source: https://www.researchgate.net/publication/348888433/figure/fig4/AS:985910309048320@1612070743363/A-diagram-illustrating-the-mechanisms-underlying-gunshot-wounds-Direct-damage-occurs-as.png.

7.2.1. Tissue Damage Caused by Bullets

Effects of bullets upon soft biological tissue create complex and often catastrophic damage that is largely due to high velocity and energy transfer on impact. Upon penetrating human tissue, a projectile creates a temporary and a permanent wound channel. The temporary cavity may create widespread disruption of the surrounding tissue, often leading to extensive vascular damage and bleeding. The extent of tissue damage depends on the bullet's velocity, mass, or construction. High-velocity rounds, for example, create extensive secondary damage via cavitation effects, in which the shockwave propagates beyond the immediate impact zone and damages critical structures and organs even if these are not directly hit. Research has also shown that the dynamics can alter the trajectory of blood vessels and nerves and, therefore, make diagnosis and treatment after gunshots more complicated (Humphrey et al., 2017). Furthermore, the type of injury is mostly dependent on the type of tissue the bullet encounters. With soft tissues like muscles and organs, the degree of damage is mostly dependent on the energy transfer of the projectile and how it acts on contact with the tissue. High-energy bullets can create larger wound cavities and more severe contusions, and low-energy ammunition can create smaller wounds. The variation in the response of various tissues to penetration by gunshot is to highlight the necessity of a broad investigation of tissue types and interactions with projectiles. For instance, organs such as the heart and lungs are particularly vulnerable; damage to them can lead to immediate death through hemorrhage or respiratory failure. Understanding these mechanisms is of immense importance for forensic investigation, treatment protocols, and creating modes of prevention of these injuries (Brooke et al., 2020).

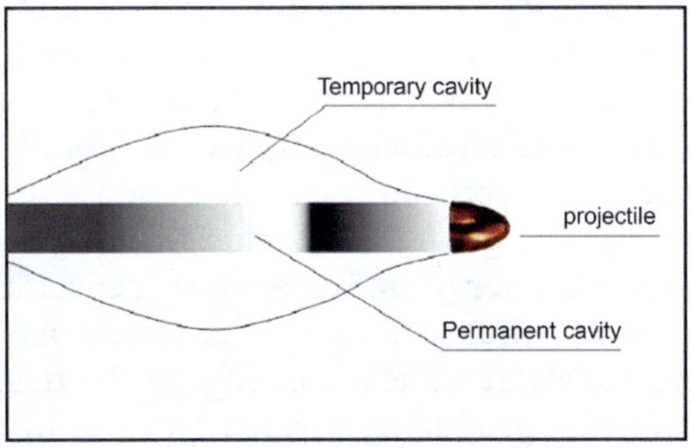

Figure 7.9. The mechanism of cavitation can cause tissue destruction along the bullet diameter.

Source: https://www.researchgate.net/profile/Hans-Pape/publication/44690314/figure/fig1/AS:216371033055232@1428598282553/The-mechanism-of-cavitation-can-cause-tissue-destruction-along-the-bullet-diameter.png.

Critical examination of ballistic trauma to bone structures also indicates the intricacy of tissue damage by shooting. Bullets may cause various types of bone fractures, ranging from small nicks to complex shattering, based on the velocity and the bullet design. For example, bullets shot at high velocity have been found to cause comminuted fractures of the vertebrae, making them particularly disabling or lethal. Injury patterns not only assist in uncovering the forces at work but also assist in reconstructing gun accidents for forensic purposes. Injury patterns are critical for medical professionals to understand when treating such wounds, as the location and extent of skeletal damage determine the decision-making process during surgical procedures and enable predictions. Consequently, the intersection of ballistics science with medical care strategy is paramount in averting the impact of gunshot wounds (Humphrey et al., 2017) (Figure 7.9).

7.2.2. The Role of Velocity and Energy in Injury Severity

It is necessary to know how velocity impacts energy so that the severity of gunshot wounds can be explored. When entering the human body, the projectile's velocity impacts not only the penetration depth but also the tissue damage intensity. The greater the velocity, the greater the kinetic energy and the more devastating the impact when colliding with tissue. As the bullet travels, it transfers energy to the tissues it traverses, producing various types of injury, such as fractures, contusions, and lacerations. Furthermore, the distinction between low-velocity weapons such as bows and arrows and high-velocity guns is essential, since low-velocity weapons can create different patterns of injury that are potentially very severe under certain circumstances. Understandings of ballistic mechanics impact perceptions of severity of injury in forensic analysis, and what is learned supports the importance of velocity when evaluating the outcome of gunshot wounds. Kinetic energy of a projectile in relation to both mass and velocity is a significant consideration in establishing the nature of gunshot wounds. A high-velocity bullet (over 1000 feet per second) can cause explosive tissue damage due to the energy transfer when impacting, leading to extensive cavitation—an effect that creates secondary trauma to surrounding tissues that are not necessarily injured. Low-velocity wounds, however, might create a less extensive wound channel but might be just as destructive depending upon the construction of the projectile and the anatomy being impacted. For example, projectiles having a blunt profile can cause injury in a fashion similar to blunt force trauma, highlighting the requirement for thorough ballistic examination in forensic environments.

As such, the kinetic energy transferred to body tissues upon impact is a critical factor in determining injury severity in gunshot casualties, further emphasizing the need for thorough forensic examinations. Apart from initial penetration and tissue damage, the velocity of the projectile also controls the likelihood of secondary injuries, complicating the determination of the wound severity. Factors such as bullet design, muzzle velocity, and the presence of clothing or other obstructions alter injury severity and complicate medical interventions. For instance, studies on arrows demonstrate how speed, as well as clothing fit, can greatly affect penetration and resultant injuries; loose or tight clothing can decrease or increase the effectiveness of arrow penetration, respectively (Beattie et al., 2018). The analogy is transferable to bullets, in which clothing can affect energy dissipation in penetrating the body. Understanding these interactions not only assists medical personnel in predicting the results of injuries but also assists forensic experts in reconstructing shooting accidents and evaluating the circumstances under which gun-related injuries are sustained (Bolton-King et al., 2016). The complexity of such factors underscores the significance of both velocity and energy in pronouncing the gravity of gunshot injuries.

7.2.3. Secondary Injuries from Bone Fragments and Debris

The trajectory of a bullet, upon penetration into the human body, does not just make entry and exit wounds. Instead, the kinetic force of the projectile is likely to cause secondary damage caused by bone shrapnel and debris. Bullets, during passage through bone, release the energy imparted by their travel, which causes shrapnel to displace fragments in the surrounding tissue. This is particularly so in high-velocity rounds, where the immense force applied can significantly comminute the bone structure. The comminuted bone fragments not only enhance direct tissue damage, but also infection, healing time, and even chronic pain could result as complications. Knowledge regarding the physics behind such injuries is crucial for treating physicians handling victims of gunshot wounds, as proper wound management must take into consideration the total extent of damage caused by the bullet and fragmentation of the surrounding bones (Bolton-King et al., 2016). Secondary bone fragmentation injuries in forensic analysis are extremely significant when reconstructing a shooting crime scenario. Through an analysis of the path of bone fragments and related soft tissue damage, forensic specialists are able to make conclusions about the caliber and type of firearm used and the distance at which the weapon was fired. Developments in imaging technology in the past few years, such as Micro-CT scanning, have enabled more detailed knowledge of on how different ammunition affects bony structures. Studies also show that differences in bullet design result in differing patterns of impact damage, and forensic experts can utilize this to have a better idea not only of the victim's main injury but also of the secondary injuries resulting from the shrapnel that is created (Coupar et al., 2020). This information can be utilized to make more accurate findings in legal proceedings, where the specifics of the injury have significant legal ramifications. Secondary injuries from bone spurs caused by gunshot wounds also pose substantial concerns in the rehabilitation and treatment of the victim.

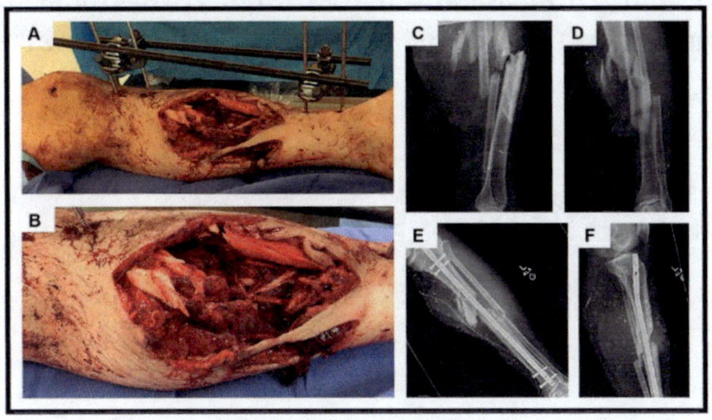

Figure 7.10. Gunshot injury to the lower extremity from a high-powered assault rifle. Clinical photographs show a traumatic wound measuring 16×16 cm with significant muscular, fascial, nervous, and vascular injury (A and B). Comminuted and markedly displaced fractures through the mid-diaphysis of the tibia and fibula with extensive shrapnel are evident on initial radiographs (C and D). A total of 16 operations were performed for this injury. During the initial operation, small pieces of fabric, bone, and metallic objects were removed, the tibial nerve was repaired, ligation of posterior tibial artery and vein was performed, and a tibial external fixator was placed. Five repeat I&D procedures were performed before the tibia was fixated with an intramedullary nail and a latissimus dorsi free flap was placed and then skin grafted (E and F). Later operations included repeat I&D and treatment of the tibial nonunion with bone grafting.

Source: https://www.dovepress.com/article/fulltext_file/378278/aW1n/ORR_A_378278_O_F0007g.jpg.

Aside from the initial risk caused by the trajectory of the bullet, the residue of the injury may consist of complex complications like non-union of fractured bones and osteomyelitis formation by debris embedding in tissue.

Doctors must thus employ a multidisciplinary strategy in treating gunshot wounds, synthesizing surgical intervention, pain control, and physical rehabilitation tailored to deal with primary and secondary trauma. Awareness of such complications not only governs short-term medical care but can guide longer-term rehabilitation strategies as well, resulting in an integrated process of recovery for gunshot victims. By recognizing the intricacy of such injuries, healthcare provision enhances patient outcomes and remains professional (Bolton-King et al., 2016) (Figure 7.10).

Test Your Knowledge

1. What type of projectile is most likely to produce extensive secondary damage in biological tissue?
2. What is the role of velocity and energy in injury severity?

7.3. Ballistics Fundamentals

Learning Outcome

1. Define the ballistics and its branches.
2. Describe the internal ballistics and external ballistics.

Ballistics is a fundamental science that explains the mechanisms of gunshot wounds and their impact on the human body. Ballistics involves the behavior of the projectile upon discharge from a weapon, for example, flight characteristics, impact dynamics, and resulting tissue damage. Guns produce bullets of varied velocity, and this parameter decides the extent of injury. For instance, high-speed bullets can produce extensive tissue disruption and cavitation effects that lead to severe organ damage, as noted in a study that analyzed the impact of high and medium velocity bullets on pig organs (Humphrey et al., 2017). Forensic experts use this data to reconstruct shooting mishaps, identify the type and extent of injury, and establish the path and force of a bullet. Further, the development of proper storage tissue simulants has expanded the range of ballistics research, enabling improved understanding of gunshot wound patterns. Use of simulants such as ballistic soap and ordnance gelatin enables researchers to simulate and examine wound patterns without the ethical concerns associated with the use of live tissues (Steimle et al., 2020). These simulants are almost exact replicas of the human organs and skin, and through their use, forensic scientists can compute penetration depth and examine the effects of different forms of ammunition. This is crucial in establishing correlations between bullet characteristics and resulting tissue injury. These experiments are documented with meticulous care by forensic specialists to obtain evidence supporting crime scene reconstructions and provide critical information during legal cases. The interplay between tissue damage, projectile energy, and wound characteristics reflects the relevance of ballistics to medical and forensic medicine. The different manifestations of ballistic injuries present with varying characteristics based on bullet type, velocity, and the angle of entry (Humphrey et al., 2017). The forensic analysis not only reveals the physical evidence observed with gunshot injuries but is also useful in lighting up the events that occurred in the course of the shooting incident. With good knowledge of the fundamental principles of ballistics, experts are able to analyze and investigate injuries more effectively, ascertain the cause of death, and eventually have a better understanding of firearm-related incidents.

This blend of science and legal investigation emphasizes the need for ongoing research and the adaptation of techniques used in ballistics analysis to improve the accuracy and reliability of forensic findings (Figure 7.11).

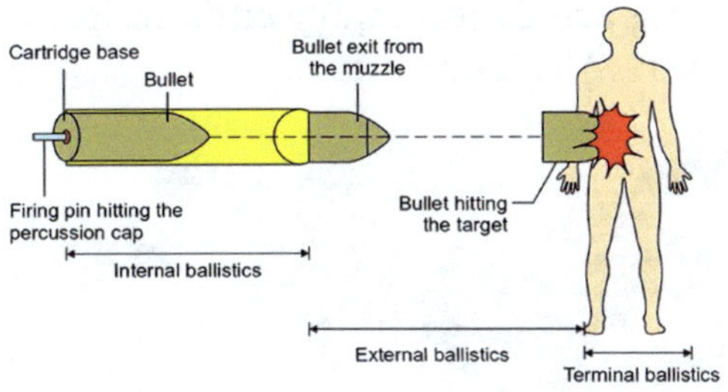

Figure 7.11. Wound ballistics.

Source: https://radiologykey.com/wp-content/uploads/2024/03/01146.jpeg.

7.3.1. Definition of Ballistics and Its Branches

Ballistics, a crucial discipline in the field of firearms and projectile dynamics, is the science of projectile flight, that is, bullets, when discharged through the air and subsequently striking targets. It is a science that comes under a variety of different branches, although these are commonly referred to as internal, external, and terminal ballistics. Internal ballistics investigates the events that take place inside a firearm from the time it is ignited through the exit of the projectiles from the barrel, including pressure, temperature, and chemical reactions involved in the process. External ballistics, on the other hand, investigates the flight of projectiles, taking into account factors like drag, wind resistance, and gravity as it moves towards its destination. Terminal ballistics provides a study of the effects of the projectile upon striking the target, an important component for understanding the nature of gun wounds in a human being, thereby helping forensic investigations within criminal justice settings. Forensic ballistics is a specialized discipline within a broad setting, applying the principles of ballistics for crime investigation involving firearms. This branch is generally focused on the projectile dynamics and how projectiles interact with targets, enabling specialists to replicate shooting mishaps. A key part of forensic ballistics is the analysis of gunshot residues (GSR), providing invaluable evidence for a firearm discharge. The examination of patterns of GSR and the extent of their spread can yield useful information about the distance from where a shot has been fired and the nature of the firearm involved, thereby assisting in linking suspects with crime scenes. Brooke et al. (2020) point out the multidisciplinary nature of forensic ballistics through the integration of chemistry, physics, and even computer science to better tackle the potential for an increase in accuracy and reliability in the reconstruction of crimes, thereby building upon current knowledge of GSW damage. In addition to the scientific research that is inherent with ballistics, the applied use is further extended into high-stress fields such as military and humanitarian work. Awareness of the principles of ballistics also profoundly affects decision-making in prefrontline cases, since rapid and timely intervention for gunshot wounds frequently becomes the decider for survival. Watching projectile behavior and consequent injury carefully helps medical practitioners to solve the puzzle of trauma care under resource-constrained settings. (N/A) highlights the importance of delivering concise, actionable information to professionals in such scenarios. By combining ballistics with clinical practice, the field can significantly contribute to the therapy of gunshot injuries, influencing both acute medical treatment and subsequent legal examination.

7.3.2. Internal Ballistics: Bullet Performance Within the Firearm

Internal ballistics is a critical study area to learn how bullets travel within the gun. Internal ballistics examines what goes on within the firearm upon firing the round, primarily focusing on the dynamics between the cartridge, the firing pin, and the inner mechanism of the firearm. Here, the gunpowder burns to create high-pressure gases that propel the bullet. The efficiency of this drive is based on factors such as the type of firearm, configuration of the cartridge, and barrel length. An understanding of these dynamics is not only crucial to the optimization of firearm design but also for the prediction of the bullet's performance upon firing, which has direct input to the subsequent impact injuries in human physiology cited in Humphrey et al. (2017). As the bullet travels down the barrel, the stability of the bullet and the forces on it are essential aspects of internal ballistics. The stability of the bullet is achieved through gyroscopic stability, facilitated through the rifling within the barrel, to guarantee the bullet is on a stable path through the airspace. A maximally optimized stable bullet trajectory results in maximum accuracy and consistency, critical in sport shooting as well as forensic science. Furthermore, bullet internal ballistics can influence the terminal performance of the bullet when entering human tissue. The impact energy transferred can be utilized to produce varied wound features, which can be quantified to analyze the dynamics of gunshot wounds cited in Brooke et al. (2020). All of these results are important in forensic analysis, where the chronology of operations during the shooting incident is dependent on the behavior of bullets upon exit from the gun. Moreover, the effects of internal ballistics on the bullet are also transferred to its interaction with different tissues upon penetration. The bullet's structure and materials can determine the level of energy transfer and conversion upon impact, generating various wound patterns that are analyzed by forensic specialists once the event has occurred. High-speed projectiles may generate deep cavitation effects on soft tissues, causing extensive damage that is proportional to the energy imparted upon impact. Besides, learning about the energy transfer dynamics of the bullet to tissue biology highlights the interactivity of internal ballistics and forensic medicine. The interaction influences not only best practices optimums for evidence collection and examination but also enhances the design of safer firearms and ammunition categories for mitigating accidental injury cited in Humphrey et al. (2017) (Figure 7.12).

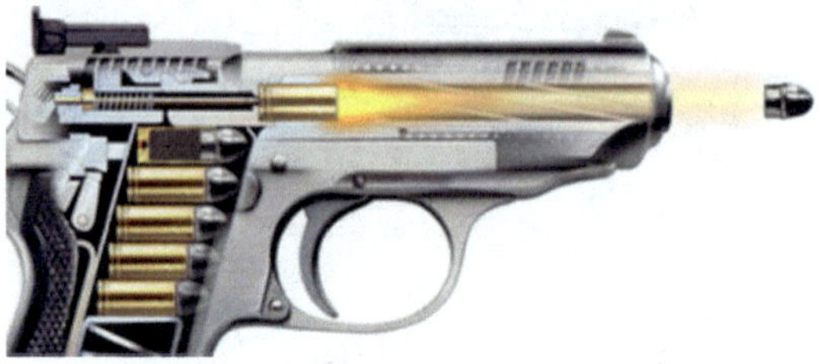

Figure 7.12. Internal ballistics.

Source: https://aegisacademy.com/cdn/shop/articles/internal-ballistics-aegis-academy-firearms-instructor-485x190_600x.jpg?v=1573324355.

7.3.3. External Ballistics: Bullet Trajectory and Environmental Factors

External ballistics is an important branch of study for understanding the trajectory and behavior of bullets while in flight, following their release from a weapon, since it combines all types of factors influencing the bullet trajectory and performance. The length of the barrel, type of bullet, and muzzle speed all play important roles in establishing the initial trajectory. However, when the bullet is airborne, external environmental factors are also very crucial. Weather factors such as wind, temperature, and humidity can potentially alter the path of the bullets, thus leading to deviation from their intended target. The factor plays a significant role in applications ranging from hunting to police use, where accuracy has extreme consequences. Significant discrepancies are likely to occur, and an understanding of such physical concepts is required to prevent potential discrepancies in the probability of hits, thus enhancing safety and efficacy in fire use (Bolton-King et al., 2016). In addition to environmental considerations, the interaction between the composition of a bullet and travel through different media also affects its terminal performance. Bullets are constructed of different materials and designs, which influence their stability and aerodynamic properties when in flight. Drag is a function of the build-up of bullets as they resist air drag, which has the tendency to reduce velocity and kinetic energy. These changes in dynamics are particularly crucial in forensic investigations, where the conditions involved in a shooting scenario could significantly impact the type and extent of injuries sustained. For instance, a tumble, yaw, or fragmentation of the bullet upon impact with target tissue can similarly extend the injury caused, proving that there is a strong connection between external ballistics and wound ballistics and that the latter is crucial in determining the consequences of gunshot wounds (Dinets et al., 2023). External ballistics enhances not just the performance of practical shooting but also gunshot wound examination in forensic science. Investigations also employ principles of external ballistics in reconstructing shootings, analyzing trajectories to determine both the shooter's and the victim's location. From the trajectory of bullets, they can make inferences of detail concerning the mechanics and dynamics of a shooting, enabling more informed findings on intent and circumstances. Accuracy in trajectory modeling continues to be subject to weather conditions and informs medical personnel on the potential methodology of resultant injuries. External ballistics research is thus priceless in its contribution to marksmanship excellence as well as legal liability in the case of gun crime, ultimately highlighting its relevance in the broader context of ballistics and forensic science (Bolton-King et al., 2016) (Figure 7.13).

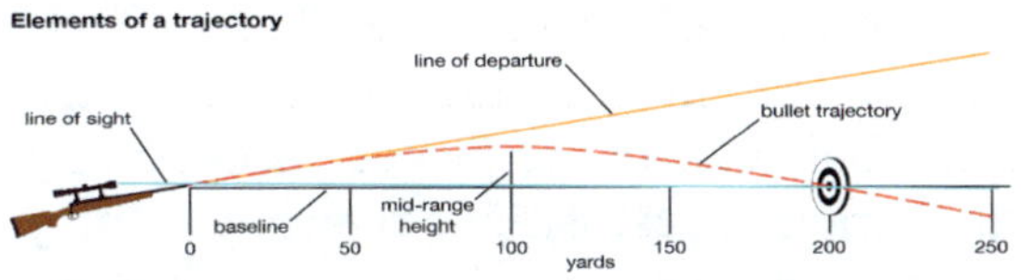

Figure 7.13. Trajectory of a bullet. A bullet fired from a rifle follows a parabolic trajectory because it is subject to the effects of gravity. Other forces, such as drag and lift, also affect the bullet's path.

Source: https://cdn.britannica.com/30/178630-050-D12B8390/bullet-rifle-trajectory-effects-gravity-forces-path.jpg.

Test Your Knowledge

1. What are the branches of ballistics?
2. What are the internal ballistics of a gun?

7.4. Forensic Ballistics

Learning Outcome

1. Understand the role of forensic ballistics in crime scene investigation.
2. Describe the techniques for matching bullets to firearms.
3. Understand the importance of ballistic evidence in legal proceedings.

The field of forensic ballistics is core to the understanding of the impact of gunshot wounds on human physiology and potential long-term impacts. Forensic ballistics refers to the analysis of firearms, cartridges, and their effect on targets, primarily the study of ballistic traces and the behavior of the projectile upon impact with a target. Investigations typically employ an array of methodologies from historic gunshot residue analysis to advanced imaging techniques tracing the path of a bullet through body tissue. This analysis not only reconstructs a crime but also introduces a fuller understanding of how different calibers and types of ammunition interact with the human body. Furthermore, since the interpretation of gunshot trauma is dynamic, forensic specialists today are more likely to consider the impact of pressure waves of bullets, which have the potential to cause unexpected injuries outside the projectile's direct path. The physiological effects of gunshot injuries extend beyond immediate tissue damage, necessitating further research into secondary effects, such as traumatic brain injury (TBI). Research has established that pressure waves from a bullet strike can travel through the body, causing neurological damage even without direct cranial cavity contact by the bullet. Exactly, research indicates that remote impacts to areas of the brain can produce pressure waves that can cause mild to moderate TBI, which refers to the complexities of ballistic trauma. For instance, 15–30 psi pressure pulses have been found to induce TBI in model animals, while similar findings have been observed in living organisms exposed to equivalent forces. This association reinforces the importance of understanding ballistic dynamics, since proponents of such a hypothesis challenge epidemiological research to explore further the connection between gunshot wounds and subsequent neurological disorders, such as epilepsy, particularly in those victims of shooting in the thoracic region (MP et al., 2008). Technological developments in forensic ballistics also extend to the methods of examining trauma in skeletal remains with associations to firearms. The recognition and interpretation of violence-related injuries increasingly rely on comparative analysis involving recorded case studies and experimental work.

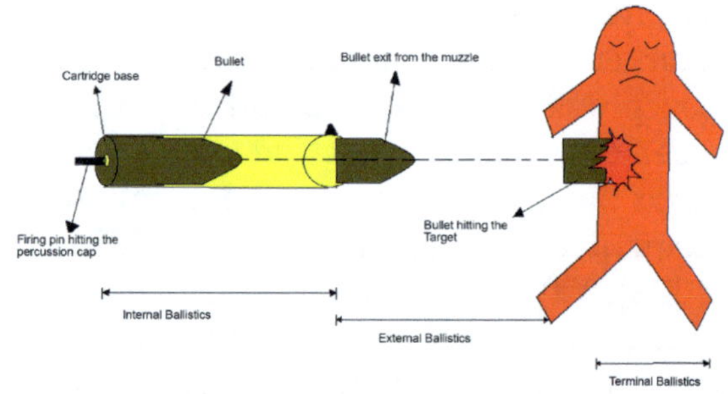

Figure 7.14. Forensic ballistics.

Source: https://blogger.googleusercontent.com/img/b/R29vZ2xl/AVvXsEjMCIsSnL8_x6tvvC6QYEfauIceI6emCxwYLjYxH58mj6Dw7bhoVCfyepk8sYI49aYGIRkRi07kny-1CXXDZ5fFSNYTLevgIzThINci-1b1iwJOR-IL1f2cgBjQyMpRpWOpVzwRMT7i-TE/s1600/Picture1.png.

Standard procedures typically prove to be ineffective when an evident instance of trauma does not exist, thus forcing researchers to look for other models upon which ballistic impact can be examined. Current developments have put polyurethane materials in the spotlight as substitutes for human bone, demonstrating how they can undergo various kinds of projectile testing. While preliminary findings suggest that these artificial materials will respond in a similar manner to human bone on a general level, careful analysis points to discrepancies that ensure prudence. The intricacies of these results call for caution in extrapolating experimental model data to human cases, emphasizing the progressive development of forensic ballistics research (Ball et al., 2015) (Figure 7.14).

7.4.1. Role of Forensic Ballistics in Crime Scene Investigation

Forensic ballistics is an essential component of criminal investigations, particularly in gunshot cases. Forensic ballistics is intended to establish the manner in which bullets and other ammunition travel through various stages of their flight, providing law enforcers with valuable information about a shooting. By analyzing the ballistic features of firearms, researchers can determine what firearm was used, at what distance a shot was fired, and what unique characteristics the projectile possesses. These pieces of information not only assist in recreating the scenario surrounding a shooting but can also help differentiate between homicide, suicide, and accidental discharge of the weapon. The application of wound ballistics, which is an area of forensic ballistics, is also supportive of this investigative process since it indicates how different ammunition types produce different patterns of wounds, which can assist the forensic analyst in identifying the gun's lethality potential (Bolton-King et al., 2016). Apart from the identification of the type of weapon and the patterns of usage, forensic ballistics assists in the identification of gunshot residues (GSR) in various contexts. Detection of GSR will confirm a suspect's involvement in a shooting or provide significant pointers that chart the course of an investigation. For instance, analysis of GSR, specifically its presence at bullet entry wounds, can offer significant information with respect to the dynamics of a shooting. A case report of a suicidal headshot explained how grains of unburned powder were observed within the muzzle and alongside the exit wound. This finding validated the significance of extensive proof examination of such evidence. This finding suggests that GSR analysis not only documents the technical characteristics of the incident but also adds additional layers to the narrative of the investigation through extensive analysis of the crime scene (Kneubühl et al., 2022). Forensic ballistics as part of the proof of crime scene research must be comprehensive and involve the collection, preservation, and analysis of ballistic evidence. Ballistic specialists are further tasked with deformed bullet and fired cartridge analysis, and any recovered ballistic materials at the crime scene. Their findings usually construct the majority of the evidence in a courtroom, which determines judicial rulings. Forensic ballistics, also being an interdisciplinary field, requires collaboration among professionals, including forensic pathologists, chemists, and investigators. This collaboration enhances the accuracy and credibility of evidence that ultimately contributes to solving the crimes. By deploying scientific techniques and abilities, forensic ballistics does not only provide critical information about particular cases but also helps in advancing the comprehension of trends of gun violence, hence informing preventive interventions and policy-making in relation to firearms (Bolton-King et al., 2016) (Figure 7.15).

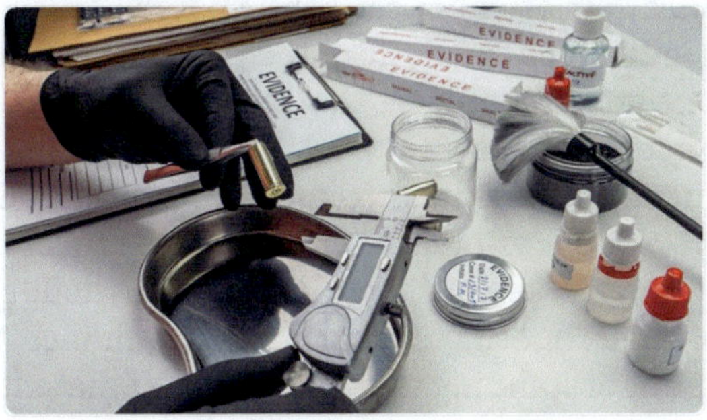

Figure 7.15. Role of forensic ballistics in crime scene investigation.

Source: https://www.azolifesciences.com/image-handler/picture/2021/7/shutterstock_1963488109.jpg.

7.4.2. Techniques for Matching Bullets to Firearms

The examination of gunshot wounds and the subsequent process of gun-to-bullet matching is an underlying aspect of forensic ballistics. The process is basically a question of meticulous analysis techniques that can potentially determine or exclude specific guns as the source of bullets recovered from crime scenes. A common one that is applied extensively is the comparison of striations, or very small markings created on bullets as they move through the barrel of the gun. Special patterns of striation result from the manufacturing process of the barrels, aging, and wear and tear, among other things, thereby providing forensic ballistics experts with a means of determining that a specific bullet comes from a specific gun. This comparison often requires specialized equipment, such as comparison microscopes, which allow forensic examiners to study the minute variations in bullets to establish a definite link between the projectile and the firearm from which it was launched. In addition, gunshot residue (GSR) analysis also constitutes an essential component of the forensic investigation of gun incidents, complementing bullet matching procedures. GSR, composed of tiny particles released from a gun when fired, both constitute trace evidence and suggest recent firing of a gun. With the application of chemical confirmatory methods and advanced analytical techniques, forensic scientists are able to determine if suspects or victims wore GSR and therefore assist in connecting individuals to specific shootings. GSR dispersal experiments at varying distances are particularly key, as they inform knowledge of potential shooting scenarios and enhance the root understanding that allows bullet matching. Insufficient literature on GSR dispersion over extended distances further indicates the necessity for ongoing research in this area since data can significantly refine the predictive models used in forensic examination (Brooke et al., 2020). Furthermore, the development of artificial models replicating human tissue and bone is revolutionizing the evaluation of gunshot wounds by forensic analysts. These models provide researchers with a platform to examine ballistic injury patterns of various ammunition types and their reactions with human tissues. For instance, impact tests of varying calibers, such as the 7.62 x 39 mm bullet, produce valuable data on wound parameters and trajectories that will direct further study. Apart from this, the models can also facilitate the analysis of the impact of external media, such as glass and other materials, on the behavior of bullets upon collision, thereby ensuring greater accuracy in case preparation. As a result, they not only assist in improving existing firearm-to-bullet matching methodologies but also enlighten the overall understanding of gunshot wounds and their implications in forensic science (Mahoney et al., 2018).

7.4.3. Importance of Ballistic Evidence in Legal Proceedings

The use of ballistic evidence in courts of law is of a consequential nature, particularly in shoot-outs. The correct analysis of ballistic evidence can establish decisive connections between a gun and the incident at hand, thus aiding prosecution and defense cases. The characteristics of a projectile, such as its trajectory, point of impact, and deformation when penetrating a target, hold deep insight into the occurrence of a shooting incident. Such data can support witness testimony or bring meaning that may exculpate a suspect. Besides, the extensive examination of ballistic patterns normally provides conclusive findings on the range from which a firearm was discharged, illuminating the intentionality or accidentality of the discharge. In addition, ballistic evidence is also significant in that it is utilized for crime scene reconstruction, which is essential in establishing the sequence of events in a shooting episode. Analyzing the physical evidence deposited at the scene, such as bullet casings and entry and exit wounds on the victim, through forensic studies, experts are able to determine if specific types of ammunition were used. For instance, detailed examinations determine the nature of the damage brought about by varying bullet velocities and their interaction with body tissue, giving significant indications of the nature of the attack (Humphrey et al., 2017). These results, along with interpreting the dynamics of the injury, help develop a clear account of the incident, and hence support the court's understanding of the incident's dynamics. Lastly, the legal implications of ballistic evidence are widespread since it plays a role in establishing culpability and intent. The ability to demonstrate the caliber of weapon utilized and the precise method of injury can carry significant weight in charging, including first-degree murder or manslaughter. Although the presence of ballistic evidence can strengthen a case, it also requires careful scrutiny to eliminate bias and present objectivity (Beattie et al., 2018). In court, the evidence must be presented in a manner that is easily comprehensible to juries who lack a scientific background, and the expert testimony becomes even more crucial. Finally, the integrity of ballistic evidence can have profound impacts on trial outcomes, cementing its position as an essential component in the pursuit of justice (Figure 7.16).

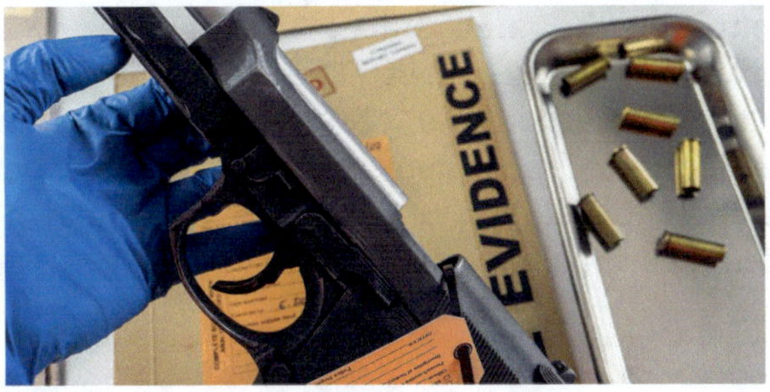

Figure 7.16. Importance of Ballistic Evidence.

Source: https://microscopes.unitronusa.com/wp/wp-content/uploads/2021/08/forensics-feature-image.jpg.

Test Your Knowledge

1. What is the role of forensic ballistics in crime scene investigation?
2. What is the importance of ballistic evidence in legal proceedings?

7.5. Medical Management of Gunshot Wounds

Learning Outcome

1. Know the immediate first aid and stabilization.
2. Describe the surgical interventions and techniques for gunshot wounds.
3. Understand the long-term rehabilitation and psychological impact.

Effective management of gunshot injury depends on a comprehensive approach that begins with the initial trauma care and stabilization of the patient. The first evaluation typically consists of the ABCs of trauma—Airway, Breathing, and Circulation—and rapid evaluation to ascertain the extent and site of injury. Early treatment is crucial; research has proven that high-velocity bullets can potentially inflict a lot of damage to vital organs, leading to catastrophic hemorrhagic shock or respiratory distress if not treated immediately (Humphrey et al., 2017). Trauma professionals should be properly trained to handle such complications in the manner of pulmonary contusions or liver lacerations because such issues could become fatal at any moment. Use of advanced imaging enables a precise understanding of the ballistic path and consequent injury, enabling directed interventions to optimize patient survival. As stabilization of the patient progresses, focus is given to definitive therapy, which can involve surgical repair to fix damaged organs and preserve vascular patency. Operative methods can vary considerably based on projectile type and path. For instance, abdominal trauma may be followed by exploratory laparotomy, while craniofacial injury can involve reconstructive surgery with finite element modeling to simulate the mechanical loading on bone structures (Quintero et al., 2020). Knowledge of the biomechanics of projectile impact allows surgeons to choose appropriate repair methods in order to enable functional recovery and avoid complications.

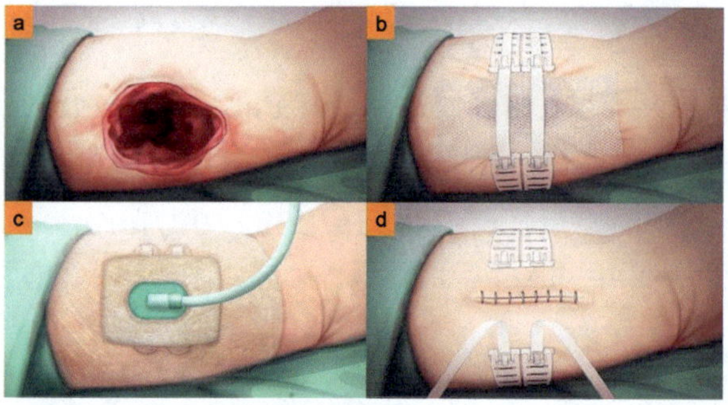

Figure 7.17. Schematic picture showing management of gunshot wound of the arm of patient 1. (a) Wound after initial debridement; (b) immediate approximation of wound edges; (c) skin approximation by tension relief system and wound coverage by regulated negative pressure-assisted wound therapy; (d) complete wound closure by mechanical creep at day 12.

Source: https://www.researchgate.net/profile/Itamar-Ashkenazi-2/publication/351900407/figure/fig2/AS:1033808962936833@1623490672368/Schematic-picture-showing-management-of-gunshot-wound-of-the-arm-of-patient-1-a-Wound.jpg.

Moreover, enforcement of wound care regimens, for example, appropriate debridement and antibiotics, is necessary in order to prevent infection, particularly in the case of an open fracture or extensive damage to soft tissue. Care of gunshot patients after surgery has its own set of challenges. Continued observation for signs of infection, organ failure, or complications such as compartment syndrome is necessary during the first few days after surgery.

Rehabilitation must be a component of the recovery process, including physical rehabilitation, in order to regain mobility and function, especially for the extremities that are subjected to gunshot injuries. Multidisciplinary intervention through pain management, psychiatric care, and occupational therapy is required to facilitate overall recovery. Also, with the improvement in survival rates, ongoing research in the long-term fate of ballistic injury will guide future medical management to improve outcomes in gunshot injury survivors (Humphrey et al., 2017; Quintero et al., 2020) (Figure 7.17).

7.5.1. Immediate First Aid and Stabilization

Early stabilization and first aid are also important features in gunshot wound treatment, as early intervention can significantly impact patient outcomes. The immediate response to a gunshot wound entails scene security first, before any care is given, to avoid endangerment to the victim and also the rescuer. Once the situation has been assessed, first aid attendants should quickly assess the character and site of the wound. Gunshot wounds most commonly result in massive blood loss, and consequently, hypovolemic shock can occur. Therefore, the most critical aspect of stabilizing the patient is to manage the hemorrhage through direct pressure, tourniquet application, or hemostatic agents if required. Early intervention not only arrests further physiological compromise but also provides the foundation for greater medical intervention when emergency personnel arrive on the scene. Following the initial assessment and stabilization of the wounded patient, the management of the specific aspects of the injury is attended to. Familiarity with the mechanisms of injury, based on the principles of ballistics, becomes necessary for proper immediate management. Different calibers of firearm ammunition and different weapons produce different profiles of wounds, which need customized first-aid management. For example, high-velocity bullets can lead to extensive damage to internal structures remote from the point of entry, making treatment challenging. As explained in literature, attaining knowledge of the implications of wound ballistics—how, for example, there can be cavitation effects—allows first responders to predict complications arising during the process of stabilization (Bolton-King et al., 2016). This data aids in the order of interventions and ensures adequate care is routed to reverse life-threatening situations in the crucial minutes subsequent to the wound. In addition, the psychological impact of gunshot wounds on the victim needs consideration within initial care. Victims may experience acute stress reactions or trauma aside from physical injury. The psychological and emotional components are now a part of first aid. Reassuring and supportive communication can de-escalate bewilderment and anxiety in the presence of a very traumatic event. As evidence from supporting research illustrates, traumatic animal injury in law enforcement contexts provides emphasis on the point that a well-rounded understanding of the full gamut of trauma, both physical and psychological, is invaluable (Stojsih et al., 2015). Therefore, giving immediate first aid and stabilization following a gunshot injury is not merely addressing the physical injury but also involves respect for the psychological well-being of the individual, emphasizing the holistic nature of trauma care.

7.5.2. Surgical Procedures and Methods

Surgical management of gunshot wounds (GSWs) is an important approach in treating the immediate physical injury from weapons. The management of such injury typically involves multi-disciplinary management, integrating trauma surgery, orthopedics, and, in the majority of cases, vascular surgery due to the severity of the injuries. Hemorrhage control, fracture stabilization, and healing of the wound are the primary goals. Surgical procedures may entail debridement of necrotic tissue, closure of soft tissue wounds, and reduction of fractured bones. In addition, familiarity with the ballistic profile of the engaged projectile is relevant, as it dictates the possible course of injury and degree of tissue compromise. As soft tissue injury and bone fracture are prevalent in GSW patients, surgical repairs are engineered to address the unique complications of such wounds, particularly in the lower extremities, where the restoration of function is critical to patient rehabilitation and recovery (Belli et al., 2021). Understanding ballistic trauma extends beyond the initial surgical treatment; it becomes significant in deciding postoperative management and rehabilitation protocols. Following surgery, the patients usually have complications in muscle regeneration and functional recovery. Skeletal muscle injury caused by ballistic trauma remains a subject of active investigation because such injuries can be associated with long-term consequences like wasting of muscle tissue and vascular dysfunction. Successful rehabilitation regimens usually involve physiotherapy for promoting recovery with both strength and mobility improvement. Moreover, progress in recent surgical procedures is aimed at reducing muscle damage but enhancing its regeneration. This holistic approach towards treatment emphasizes the importance of complementing surgical and rehabilitative interventions to achieve the best outcomes for GSW victims (Belli et al., 2021). Moreover, sufficient knowledge of the impact of clothing on the GSW pattern has emerged as a significant consideration in surgical intervention and planning. It has long been proven by research that the attire that one has on when injured can significantly alter the nature and extent of the resultant injuries. Military attire, for example, can destabilize or deflect the impact of a projectile and hence cause varying degrees of injury. Synthetic limb model experiments have proven that in full clothing conditions, the severity of the damage to the tissue as well as the complexity of the surgical intervention increases. Such an understanding indicates the necessity for tailored surgical approaches based on the specific situation of the shooting case and the physical characteristics of the patient. Enhanced surgical techniques are thus critical in treating the diverse presentations of GSWs and thereby improving patient outcomes and best practice guidelines in the treatment of trauma (Figure 7.18).

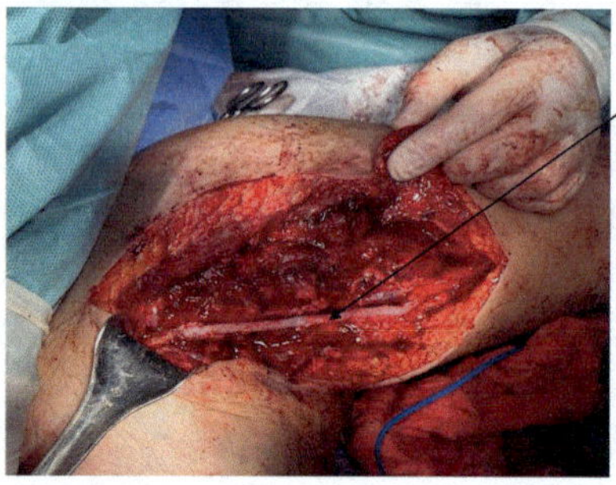

Figure 7.18. Surgical interventions for gunshot wounds.

Source: https://media.springernature.com/lw1200/springer-static/image/art%3A10.1007%2Fs00268-022-06577-y/MediaObjects/268_2022_6577_Fig3_HTML.jpg.

7.5.3. Long-Term Rehabilitation and Psychological Impact

Long-term rehabilitation following gunshot injuries is a multifaceted process that not only incorporates physical recovery but also psychological and emotional recovery. Victims typically experience severe physical disability, chronic pain, and impairments in functions, which significantly impair their quality of life. In addition, the process of rehabilitation is prolonged and complex, with patients often receiving multiple operations, physical therapy, and occupational therapy. The demand for adaptive equipment or daily living changes means that their recovery is further complicated. Piled onto the physical burden are the numerous psychological effects, with the individuals confronting the harsh reality of their injuries and requiring extensive mental health services to establish resilience and adaptation to their new reality. Unless they are given proper rehabilitation, both mental and physical, victims risk having a lowered capacity to re-enter society and fulfill life's aspirations. The mental impacts of gunshot wounds extend far beyond the immediate shock of the injury. Survivors tend to exhibit symptoms for which terms synonymous with post-traumatic stress disorder (PTSD), depression, and anxiety are employed, which manifest long after the acute physical wounds heal. Trauma of the experience, coupled with the difficulties of adapting to life post-injury, can reinforce the sensations of loneliness, helplessness, and despair. Moreover, social stigma surrounding gun violence can induce shame, further stunting emotional healing. The integrated process that includes counseling, group therapy, and community assistance, therefore, becomes essential. Involvement in supportive environments can allow survivors to work through their trauma, acquire coping mechanisms, and ultimately reclaim their self-esteem and social connections, further advancing their overall rehabilitation. Moreover, attention to psychological recovery underscores the need for intensive intervention strategies sensitive to gunshot survivors' unique experiences. Specialized programs sensitive to the mental health needs, including cognitive-behavioral therapy and trauma-informed care, can have a significant effect. These treatments not only mitigate the adverse effects of trauma but also promote resilience and personal development among survivors. Early recognition of mental illness cannot be overemphasized because early intervention can deter the formation of chronic psychological conditions. Literature states that successful rehabilitation programs incorporate physical recovery alongside mental health interventions to enable an overall recovery strategy of gunshot casualties, thereby enhancing their long-term quality of life and functional autonomy (Magalhães et al., 2013; Mäkitie et al., 2006) (Figure 7.19).

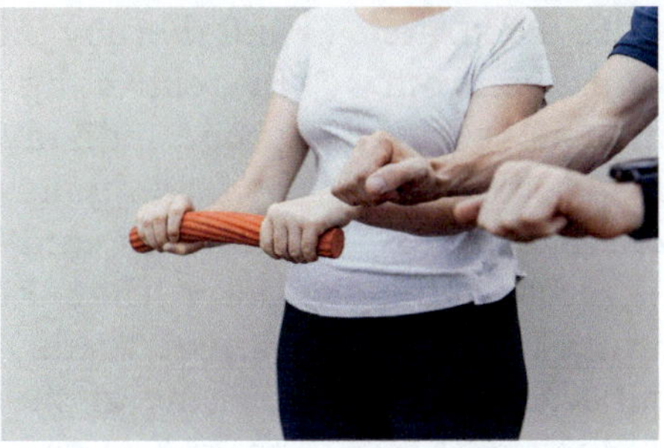

Figure 7.19. Rehabilitation steps for gunshot injury recovery.

Source: https://lh7-rt.googleusercontent.com/docsz/AD_4nXcYSXBx4aP7LLp97ytypnpxi96RH7c0faddVtMlHrxx2o2p_lVUT1wDXK4b-76pR00J_9tNy9xD2f7YY8qgqzjFghUQxoraiqKQQcoiJQ2QX5M-1U8YIZ4QTS2Am7tpkuz20Os1SWxi4CrdofWc3g?key=kL98t4U0mkMdHijILuBxTF2N.

Test Your Knowledge

1. What is a common cause of physiological decline in gunshot wound victims?
2. What is a hemostatic agent used to control bleeding?

7.6. Legal and Ethical Considerations

Learning Outcome

1. Know the gun control laws and their implications.
2. Describe the ethical dilemmas in treating gunshot victims.
3. Understand the role of healthcare professionals in violence prevention.

Legal and forensic issues in the treatment of gunshot wounds and ballistics extend beyond clinical spheres, being central to legal and forensic systems. Legal issues primarily occur in criminal cases of gunshot injuries, in the middle of determining culpability, or in understanding the injury mechanism. Both of these experts have a double role: to provide good scientific analysis and to remain objective as witnesses. The accuracy of their findings has the potential to greatly affect legal conclusions, with strict adherence to protocols in ballistic analysis that have been established. Ethical standards are most important in research environments, especially when handling sensitive issues involving human misery. Researchers are left to tread the fine line of advancing scientific knowledge and preserving the dignity and rights of victims and their families regarding the investigative process, with the emotional and social stakes involved in gun violence. Additionally, the study of past and contemporary firearms, as illustrated in seminal research such as that utilizing Civil War-era weapons, illustrates the importance of ethical historical inquiry. Examinations of how ancient weapons interacted with human bodies not only add to forensic understanding of gunshot trauma but also create ethical issues about representation and descendant communities' influence. An example is archival studies revealing the violence inflicted by such weapons, which can be utilized in informing current forensic anthropology and enhancing more accurate field methods. But such research must confront sensitive historical testimony cautiously, so that the pain of people and individuals is accurately represented and not sensationalized. The ethical responsibility to be respectful of the record of the victimized communities has to continue to be the pivot around which both historical scholarship and forensic science today turn, linking past to present implications. Lastly, gunshot injury and their evaluation raise immediate ethical issues around gun control and public health policy. As research unearths the horrendous impact of gunshot injuries on victims and the community, ethical implications extend to promoting well-informed legislative movements towards reducing gun violence. Public health research has to deal with the intricacies of gun trauma, such as statistical analysis of injury patterns and determinants. While dissemination of this knowledge can bring about legislative change, it must also be accompanied by responsible discussion of the social, cultural, and economic factors being weighed regarding access to and use of firearms. It is the balance between ethics and science that will assist in shaping a balanced understanding of gunshot wounds so that research findings are converted into actionable steps that can ultimately result in a safer world, as supported by the huge body of evidence from research like that referred to in (Humphrey et al., 2017) and (Reeder et al., 2025).

7.6.1. Gun Control Laws and Their Impact

The controversy about gun control laws is inextricably linked with research into gunshot wounds and their ballistic effects. Legislative measures for regulating access to firearms are often justified in terms of a requirement to limit the occurrence of firearms injuries and fatalities. More rigorous controls, as gun control proponents act out, have the potential to reduce substantially the risk that firearms will end up in the possession of aspiring violent offenders and thereby influence resultant injury patterns. By restricting the availability of guns to risk-prone individuals, chances are that there will be fewer gunshot injuries and hence fewer gun fatalities and ballistic injuries. Experiments show that because prospective criminals cannot readily obtain weapons, the resultant slowing of shooting incidents not only reflects on public safety but also upon the nature of injury presented to hospitals that treat gun trauma patients (Humphrey et al., 2017).

Further, the effects of gun control laws extend beyond raw statistics for firearm fatalities; they have significant impacts on the nature of injury presented to emergency medicine. Studies have shown a correlation between high-velocity projectiles and extensive body damage, particularly to large organs. For instance, studies into the impact of varying projectile velocities on porcine tissue have shown considerable differences in the nature and seriousness of injuries incurred. High-velocity projectiles are likely to produce complex ballistic trauma, which is correlated with advanced surgery and prolonged recovery times. Thus, the imposition of strict gun controls can lower not just the rate of gunshot injuries but also the health care workload caused by treating traumatic gunshot wounds from violence (Humphrey et al., 2017). The interrelatedness of gun controls with public health is also shed light upon through offenders' patterns of gun purchases. Research into sources of guns for violent attackers in cities emphasized that the majority of respondents got their guns from personal networks and not from retail spaces or by theft. This indicates a default problem in addressing gun violence, that even when there are tight gun control laws, social networks and criminal organizations can evade control mechanisms. Gun control policies, thus, to tackle gun control holistically, should consider such social structures and their effects on public safety. The focus on cutback in the supply of guns to high-risk communities, besides having promise in stemming gunshot injuries, also needs a multi-dimensional approach that includes community education, targeted enforcement, and rehabilitation programs (Harold et al., 2015) (Figure 7.20).

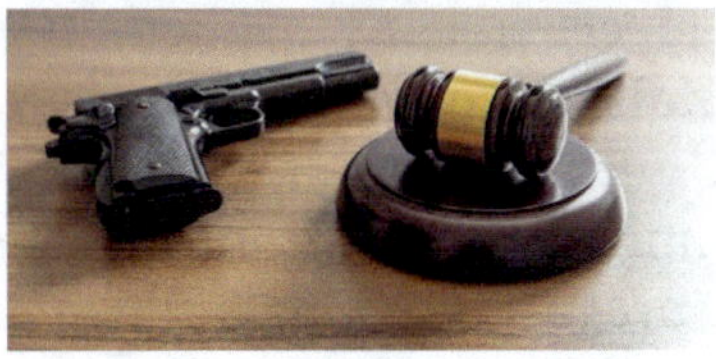

Figure 7.20. Gun control laws.

Source: https://cdn.lawdistrict.com/images/d/a/6/6/b/da66b0ac11a71c5ba65b26fcb941c2839a48fef9-gun-control-laws.jpg.

7.6.2. Ethical Dilemmas in Treating Gunshot Victims

Ethical dilemmas abound in the treatment of gunshot casualties, particularly where medical professionals are compelled to weigh their professional obligations and ethics. One of the key problems is the provision of immediate life-saving interventions against the complexity of the cause of the injury. This is particularly pertinent where such treatment risks feeding a vicious cycle of violence, where situations involve suspected offenders or gang violence. Physicians can be grappling with what it means to care for individuals whose behavior in the short term has the potential to inflict harm on others, such that they are wondering how much medical care providers must value a patient's autonomy or look at the broader social implications of their medical practice (Gitonga et al., 2024). Such dilemmas push the foundations of medical ethics, including beneficence, nonmaleficence, and justice, ultimately shaping the course of not only individual patient care but also public health outcomes for victims of gun violence communities. The prevalence of extrajudicial killings and cultural perceptions of gun violence also affect the ethical climate of healthcare professionals. When gunshot victims are viewed in criminal or ethical terms, medical professionals must contend with their own biases while trying to uphold equitable treatment. The way that media present cases of gun violence has a significant influence on public perceptions, and these can in turn create pressure on healthcare facilities and workers to conform to societal norms surrounding accountability and justice (Gitonga et al., 2024). Reporters tasked with coverage of these events also have their part to play in building narratives, with ethical considerations of the role of sensationalism in shaping opinion. Medical professionals must then subsequently cope with pressures external to the profession, with the potential to skew their choices and compel them towards behaviors that contravene their ethical responsibilities of patient care and confidentiality. Advancement in forensic technologies adds a new level to the ethical challenges encountered in the handling of gunshot casualties. Application of sophisticated devices for data gathering and scene analysis offers improved precision and efficiency in forensic analysis, but also raises privacy and informed consent concerns. For instance, the technology supporting remote analysis or live assessment can develop heightened awareness regarding the treatment techniques applied, contaminating the confidence among medical practitioners and patients. Secondly, the application of technological advancements in the case of emergency treatment presents ethical concerns in the context of how much the advancements will benefit the patient without invading personal space. Thus, a balance must be struck between the application of technology to benefit patients and the resolution of the natural ethical challenges posed in order to protect the integrity of the healing process from erosion whenever biomedical capabilities evolve.

7.6.3. Role of Health Workers in Preventing Violence

Healthcare providers are also important actors in preventing violence, especially in the case of gunshot injuries and their concomitant health consequences. Medical workers can take preventive actions by understanding the risk factors of firearm violence. They can advise patients against the risks posed by firearms, especially from families with a history of mental illness or drug abuse. Furthermore, healthcare professionals are in an ideal position to recognize signs of potential violence, either by counseling individuals at risk or their families. Through facilitating frank discussion about the injury gun violence causes, health professionals can play a useful role in promoting a broader cultural shift towards non-violence and safety in communities, and hence affect rates of gun injury and mortality. Furthermore, healthcare professionals must be at the forefront in advocating for public policies that address and curb gun violence. Their experience working on the ground gives them a special knowledge of the impact of gunshot injuries and of the systemic failures that permit such violence to thrive. Groups like Amnesty International point out that medical professionals have the expertise to advocate for less lethal gun laws and policies aimed at reducing gun deaths and injuries among the population. For instance, recommendations set forth in reports laying down needed changes in legislation can be followed by health workers who can offer evidence of the destructive nature of gun violence from experience. By collaborating with public health officials and policymakers, doctors can ensure that a strategy that is multifaceted in scope, with an interest in human rights as well as firearms safety, will emerge. This will then create a better society. Medical professionals' work also entails the treatment and rehabilitation of victims who have been shot, with the emphasis on a holistic approach to the prevention of violence. In crisis situations, clinicians are charged not only with delivering initial treatment but also with addressing the long-term physical and psychological effects of gun violence on their patients. This dual response is crucial, as argued in texts like Fundamentals of Frontline Surgery, which is concerned with best practice in conditions of resource limitation. Medical professionals can implement programs that focus on mental health treatment and counseling, which are essential for victims of shootings. By developing an environment for recovery through psychological evaluation and community systems, medical practitioners empower victims and families, ending the cycle of violence and fostering resilience in gun-violence-inflicted communities (Figure 7.21).

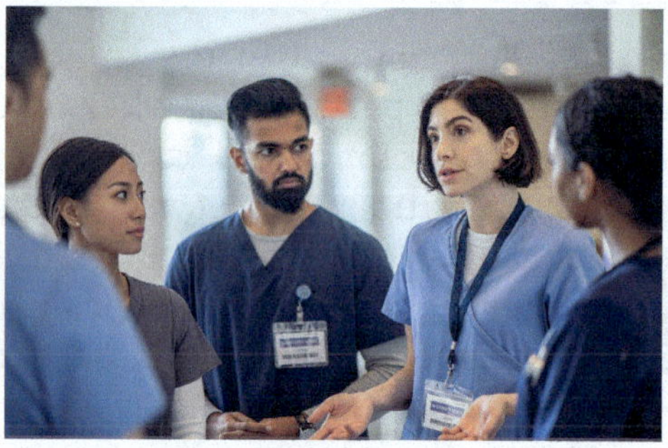

Figure 7.21. Role of Health Workers in Preventing Violence.

Source: https://blogs.cdc.gov/niosh-science-blog/wp-content/uploads/sites/22/2024/05/HeartEKG_000-002.jpg.

Test Your Knowledge

1. What are the gun control laws?
2. What is the role of healthcare professionals in violence prevention?

SUMMARY

In the context of the complex interaction between ballistics and gunshot wounds in humans, a multidisciplinary process is clearly necessary for effective forensic investigation. Ballistic injury is not merely a matter of wound description; it is a matter of understanding the mechanisms of producing them. Forensic examiners must consider the weapon type, ammunition used, and the physics of ballistics to reconstruct shooting incidents in the right order. Also, methodological improvements have increasingly enabled practitioners to link contemporary findings to historical instances, to inform and augment the forensic database, and to enhance the profession's ability to make meaningful inferences from skeletal evidence and injury patterns. As hypothesized in biological anthropologists' research, developments in the identification of trauma associated with violence are contingent on a greater knowledge of laboratory as well as applied environments, indicating a firm existing debate in the field (Ball et al., 2015). Ballistics' nuances also reveal central issues regarding the material effects of different types of ammunition on human tissue. An understanding of these ballistic properties is critical to the assessment of the potential for lethality of trauma. A close understanding of wound ballistics, a part of terminal ballistics, forms the basis of appreciating the dynamics of a shot. Not only does it lend insight into the immediate effect of gunshot wounds, but it also allows for subsequent discussion of the collection and analysis of forensic evidence. Having proper protocols for the retrieval of ballistic evidence from crime scenes, whether human subjects or forensic animal models, has a critical bearing on the direction of investigations. This is so meticulous, given that the intricacies of firearm-related trauma necessitate a scrupulous, methodical effort by law enforcers and forensic experts as well (Bolton-King et al., 2016). Lastly, the scientific principles involved in ballistics inform not only forensic strategies but also gun violence public health policies. By exploring the trends indicated by gunshot injury analysis, stakeholders can advocate for preventive interventions beyond the direct clinical intent. As the field evolves, further interactions between forensic specialists, anthropologists, and law enforcers will yield greater insight, enhancing investigative techniques and legal processes on gun incidents. Overall, as the discourse on gunshot injuries and their implications becomes more complex, ongoing research and development on forensic processes will remain key to controlling the social impact of gun-related violence and providing a safer future society.

The study of gunshot wounds and their effects transcends the physical injury inflicted to encompass the scientific principles that play a role in ballistics. Complete comprehension of the different guns and cartridges is required for forensic examination because various combinations leave individual patterns and effects on wounds. Ballistics has numerous divisions, primarily internal, intermediate, external, and terminal ballistics. Wound ballistics, the most critical component of terminal ballistics, addresses only the impact projectiles have on human tissue. This data not only assists in medical treatment but also aids forensic scientists in reconstructing the shooting episodes and, ultimately, assists the justice system. By describing the mechanics of wound formation, professionals can better make sense of the conditions surrounding firearm-related injuries and deaths and thus emphasize the importance of good and knowledgeable evaluation in forensic practice (Bolton-King et al., 2016). Lastly, the interplay between projectile dynamics and the human body is a complex one, as illustrated by the investigation of traumatic brain injury resulting from ballistic or blast pressure waves. Research has shown that mechanisms such as acceleration of the head and direct pressure wave loading can induce mild to moderate traumatic brain injury (mTBI).

Most notably, research on the passage of ballistic pressure waves through the body underscores the need for immediate examination of cranial as well as thoracic mechanisms in causality. It is revealed through this study that effects on the brain may occur even when cranial trauma does not, so increased awareness of how gunshot injuries affect neurological health is ever more pertinent. This kind of information is important not only for medical treatment but also for the design of protection against such catastrophic injury (Courtney et al., 2008). Overall, the interface of guns, ballistics, and the human body supplies valuable information about the severe effects of gunshot wounds. The different aspects of evaluating gunshot wounds involve the mechanisms of injury to forensic relevance, emphasizing the necessity for proper comprehension of the related scientific concepts. As forensic science continues to advance, the incorporation of data on wound ballistics and traumatic brain injury will enhance medical response as well as forensic examination. Integration will enable professionals to more effectively assess gunshot injury impacts, affirming that investigation and instruction remain key to effectively curtailing firearm trauma within society. The continued pursuit of information in these domains is essential to enhancing public safety and health measures regarding gun violence.

KEY TERMS FROM THIS CHAPTER

- Ballistics
- Bullets velocity
- Gunshot wounds
- Impaired mobility
- Organ perforation
- Perforating wounds
- Societal violence
- Bone fractures
- Chronic pain
- High-velocity projectiles
- Muzzle velocity
- Penetrating wounds
- Radiography
- Soft tissue injuries

CRITICAL THINKING QUESTIONS

1. What is the primary factor that determines the severity of a gunshot wound?

a. The type of firearm used.

b. The distance between the firearm and the target.

c. The angle at which the bullet strikes the body.

d. The weight of the victim.

2. What is the defining feature of an entrance wound?

a. Irregular, jagged edges with tissue bridging.

b. Clean, circular or oval edges, often surrounded by an abrasion collar.

c. Larger than the bullet diameter with no soot or stippling.

d. Always accompanied by an exit wound.

3. Which of the following is typically observed in close-range gunshot wounds?

a. Abrasion collar only.

b. Tattooing or stippling due to gunpowder particles.

c. Stellate-shaped wound with no soot.

d. Absence of soot and powder burns.

4. What distinguishes an exit wound from an entrance wound?

a. Exit wounds are smaller than entrance wounds.

b. Exit wounds lack tissue bridging and are irregular.

c. Exit wounds always have soot and tattooing.

d. Exit wounds are always circular with an abrasion collar.

5. What is the term used for the study of the motion and effects of projectiles?

a. Ballistics

b. Forensic pathology

c. Criminology

d. Traumatology

Short Answer Questions

1. What is a gunshot wound?
2. List the types of gunshot wounds.
3. What subset of ballistics focuses on the study of how projectiles interact with biological tissues?
4. What factor significantly influences the extent of damage caused by a bullet?
5. What is forensic ballistics?

Answer to Critical Thinking Questions

1. (b); 2. (b); 3. (b); 4. (b); 5. (a)

REFERENCES

1. Alexander, M. P., Courtney, A., Bruton, C., Center for Disease Control and Prevention (CDC), Cernak, I., Cernak, I., Courtney, M., et al. (2008). Links between traumatic brain injury and ballistic pressure waves originating in the thoracic cavity and extremities. http://arxiv.org/abs/0808.1443 (accessed on 12th July 2025).
2. Anderson, B. O. (2000). Evaluation of tungsten tin and lead projectiles against real and synthetic bones encased in ballistic gelatin. https://core.ac.uk/download/578419752.pdf (accessed on 12th July 2025).
3. Ball, N., Barnetson, V., Foster, B., et al. (2015). Fantastic plastic? Experimental evaluation of polyurethane bone substitutes as proxies for human bone in trauma simulations. https://core.ac.uk/download/42142579.pdf (accessed on 12th July 2025).
4. Beattie, E., Fraser, J., MacPhee, N., et al. (2018). A comparison of penetration and damage caused by different types of arrowheads on loose and tight fit clothing. https://core.ac.uk/download/228178194.pdf (accessed on 12th July 2025).
5. Belli, A., Bowen, T. S., Egginton, S., et al. (2021). Firearms-related skeletal muscle trauma: Pathophysiology and novel approaches for regeneration. https://core.ac.uk/download/424771193.pdf (accessed on 12th July 2025).
6. Bolton-King, R., & Schulze, J. (2016). Firearms and ballistics. https://core.ac.uk/download/80691312.pdf (accessed on 12th July 2025).
7. Brooke, N., & Brooke, N. (2020). Correlation of distance and damage in a ballistic setting. https://core.ac.uk/download/492114142.pdf (accessed on 12th July 2025).
8. Chango Llerena, X., Flor Unda, O., Gil Jiménez, P., et al. (2024). Technology in forensic sciences: Innovation and precision. https://core.ac.uk/download/622341556.pdf (accessed on 12th July 2025).
9. Coupar, N., Fraser, J., Newton, J., et al. (2020). Preliminary investigation into the use of Micro-CT scanning on impact damage to fabric, tissue, and bone caused by both round and flat nosed bullets. https://core.ac.uk/download/337602419.pdf (accessed on 12th July 2025).
10. Courtney, A., & Courtney, M. (2008). A thoracic mechanism of mild traumatic brain injury due to blast pressure waves. https://core.ac.uk/download/pdf/287975.pdf (accessed on 12th July 2025).
11. Dinets, A., Furkalo, S., Gorobeiko, M., et al. (2023). Modeling of wound ballistics in biological tissue simulators. https://core.ac.uk/download/588445116.pdf (accessed on 12th July 2025).
12. Dubenko, D., Gryshchenko, O., Gumeniuk, K., et al. (2021). Woundary ballistics of biological tissue's plastic deformation on the model of ballistic plasteline using hollow point and shape-stable bullets. https://core.ac.uk/download/587245320.pdf (accessed on 12th July 2025).
13. Fundamentals of frontline surgery. (2025). https://core.ac.uk/download/637931189.pdf (accessed on 12th July 2025).
14. Gitonga, S. K. (2024). Journalists understanding and coverage of extrajudicial killings in Kenya. https://core.ac.uk/download/613050885.pdf (accessed on 12th July 2025).
15. Humphrey, C. L. (2017). Characterization of soft tissue and skeletal bullet wound trauma

and three-dimensional anatomical modelling. https://core.ac.uk/download/159130738.pdf (accessed on 12th July 2025).

16. In the line of fire: Human rights and the US gun violence crisis. (2018). Amnesty International: In the Line of Fire. https://core.ac.uk/download/539979831.pdf (accessed on 12th July 2025).
17. Kneubühl, B. P., Rabl, W., & Weber, A. (2022). Gunshot residues found at the exit wound: A case report. https://core.ac.uk/download/527937623.pdf (accessed on 12th July 2025).
18. Quintero Lopez, Y. A. (2020). Influence of the cortical bone characterization in computer simulation of short-range shots in two regions on the human mandible. https://core.ac.uk/download/326804195.pdf (accessed on 12th July 2025).
19. Mabbott, A. J. (2016). The overmatching of UK police body armor. https://core.ac.uk/download/74410011.pdf (accessed on 12th July 2025).
20. Magalhães, T., Pereira, A. R., & Vieira, D. N. (2013). Fatal intimate partner violence against women in Portugal: A forensic medical national study. https://core.ac.uk/download/19731733.pdf (accessed on 12th July 2025).
21. Mahoney, P. F. (2018). Development of a synthetic bone and tissue model to simulate overmatch military ballistic head injury. https://core.ac.uk/download/188365120.pdf (accessed on 12th July 2025).
22. Mäkitie, I. (2006). Epidemiologinen ja kliininen tutkimus ampuma- ja räjähdysvammoista Suomessa. https://core.ac.uk/download/14917994.pdf (accessed on 12th July 2025).
23. Pollack, H. A., Cook, P. J., & Parker, S. T. (2015). Sources of guns to dangerous people: What we learn by asking them. https://core.ac.uk/download/75782570.pdf (accessed on 12th July 2025).
24. Reeder, M. K. (2025). Firearm trauma across time: Investigating civil war gunshot trauma and their impact on modern forensic analysis. https://core.ac.uk/download/655998250.pdf (accessed on 12th July 2025).
25. Steimle, B. (2020). The recreation of wound patterns using various tissue simulants for crime scene reconstruction. https://core.ac.uk/download/386366625.pdf (accessed on 12th July 2025).
26. Stevenson, T. (2018). Ballistic extremity wounding: Quantifying tissue damage associated with military firearms. https://core.ac.uk/download/374287668.pdf (accessed on 12th July 2025).
27. Stojsih, S. (2015). A biomechanical assessment of canine body armor. https://core.ac.uk/download/56687452.pdf (accessed on 12th July 2025).

ASPHYXIAL DEATHS

8

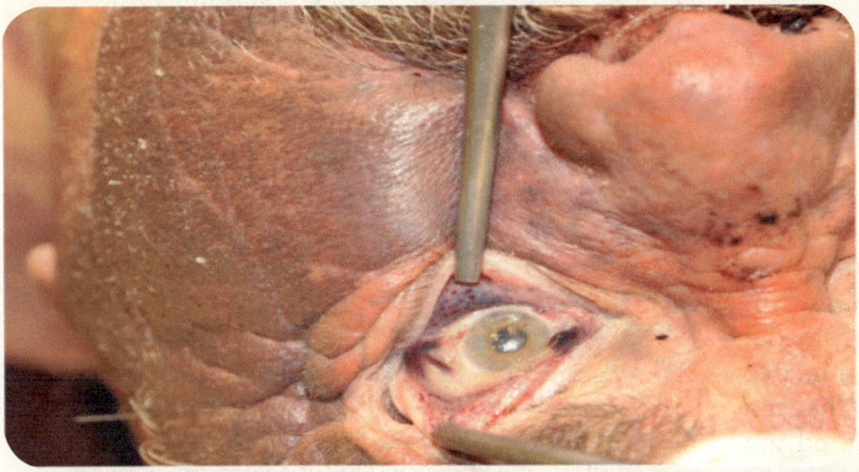

LEARNING OBJECTIVES

After studying this chapter, you will be able to:

1. Describe the types of Asphyxial deaths;
2. Understand the mechanisms of asphyxia;
3. Know the causes of asphyxial deaths;
4. Examine the risk factors contributing to asphyxial deaths;
5. Know the prevention strategies in addressing the issue of asphyxial deaths;
6. Describe the legal and ethical considerations surrounding asphyxial deaths.

Introduction

The mechanism of asphyxia is an important field of study under the general domain of human death since it entails various forms of loss of oxygen leading to severe neurological deficits or death. Asphyxial deaths are observed in different groups of people, including infants and adults, typically as a result of multiple causative factors like drowning, choking, and medical illnesses like cardiac arrest. Knowledge of the mechanisms of asphyxial death is necessary to avoid these unfortunate circumstances, especially in susceptible groups such as infants undergoing perinatal asphyxia. Scientific studies show that oxygen deficit during delivery may lead to long-term severe consequences like neurodegenerative disease, intellectual disability, and permanent functional psychotic syndromes (Cebioglu et al., 2011). Thus, the relevance of early intervention and problem-focused prevention cannot be overstressed. They can mitigate the catastrophic impact of asphyxia on personal health trajectories. Asphyxial deaths also highlight the significance of early medical intervention in sudden emergencies like cardiac arrest, which is an illness that claims an unprecedented number of people annually. Because over 300,000 Americans experience cardiac arrest every year, the consequent brain damage poses formidable challenges, including extensive memory loss, impaired motor function, and, worst of all, death due to a failure to recover (Combs et al., 2013). Physiological response to asphyxia involves complex neurobiological processes, including the excessive activation of glutamatergic N-methyl-D-aspartate receptors (NMDAR) that amplify neuronal death through excitotoxic cascades. As a result, the understanding of these mechanisms is key to the development of effective treatment strategies. Studies indicate that modulating the activity of NMDARs strategically following arrest can be more effective, which also points to the importance of furthering medical knowledge in asphyxial emergencies. In the context of the multifaceted repercussions of asphyxial deaths, research still attempts to improve therapeutic approaches and prevention that can radically alter mortality narratives behind the events. Because asphyxia not only represents an impairment of the individual's health but also a serious burden on health systems, it is also important to consider the socio-economic consequences of the introduction of advanced diagnostic equipment and personalized treatments (Cebioglu et al., 2011).

Moreover, a complete understanding of the neurodegenerative sequences initiated by asphyxial events could give precise ways of prevention in neonatal and pediatric populations. With the development of a framework for individualized medicine focusing on individual molecular targets and potential biomarkers, eventually healthcare professionals can be made capable of counteracting the long-term consequences of asphyxia in a manner that better treats the tragic outcomes of these accidents (Figure 8.1).

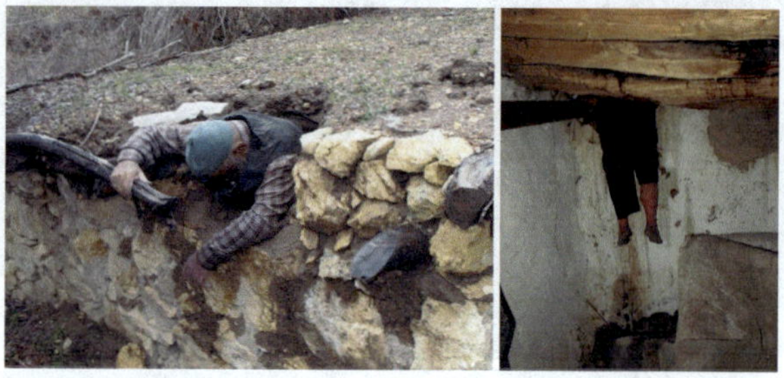

Figure 8.1. Seventy-two-year-old man had lost the key of the door of his house in his vineyard and he tried to go in from a small hole which he made on the roof. He was stuck and found dead in the hole due to positional asphyxia.

Source: https://cdnintech.com/media/chapter/19160/1512345123/media/image2.jpeg.

Definition of Asphyxial Deaths

Asphyxial deaths constitute an emergent area of study in forensic pathology characterized by the absence of oxygen caused by various forms of asphyxia. These comprise deaths due to mechanisms of suffocation, drowning, strangulation, and obstruction that all lead to acute hypoxia. The pathophysiologic process involves interference with normal respiration, resulting in insufficient oxygenation of alveolar blood and ultimately the brain and vital organs. The effects of asphyxia can have an abrupt onset, typically leading to death and irreversible injury within minutes if not promptly treated. Owing to the many etiologies of asphyxial death, forensic investigation has a vital role in determining cases as separate from other causes of death, which sometimes require identification of the precise situation of each case. Clinically, asphyxia can be classified based on underlying mechanisms, which may either be intrinsic or extrinsic. Intrinsic mechanisms might be in the guise of medical disorders that interfere with normal respiratory function, for example, anaphylactic shock or severe asthma, whereas extrinsic mechanisms are usually more environmental in nature, for example, accidents of smothering or drowning. The very definition of asphyxia is the inability of the body to deliver tissue and organ systems a sufficient quantity of oxygen. In certain cases, asphyxia leads to a state of asphyxial death, which means the deprivation of oxygen is so severe that it leads to cardiac arrest. Awareness of these types allows more effective prevention measures and interventions, which ultimately reduce the incidence of such tragic incidents. The implications of asphyxial deaths are not restricted to short-term clinical consequences but also expose severe public health problems as well. These deaths indiscriminately victimize vulnerable groups like children and individuals with medical conditions, necessitating widespread awareness and preventive interventions. The role of educational interventions in the areas of drowning awareness, safe sleeping practices for infants, and first aid cannot be overstated in further improving results.

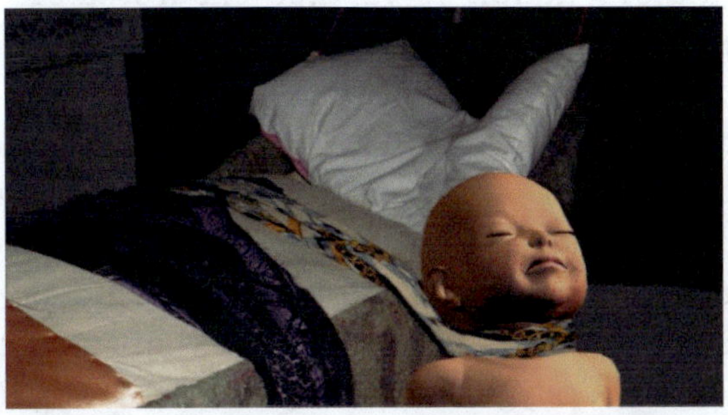

Figure 8.2. The position of the dead infant in the swing-like cradle. As the victim leaned out of the cradle, the ligature that was tied around the swing-like cradle wrapped around the child's neck, resulting in asphyxia.

Source: https://cdnintech.com/media/chapter/19160/1512345123/media/image34.jpeg.

Furthermore, refinement in emergency response protocols, for example, by emergency cardiovascular care agencies, demonstrates ongoing endeavors to minimize asphyxia-related mortality. With these intricacies, a broader comprehension of asphyxial death remains pivotal to better preventive strategies and responsive capability in healthcare and community centers, unscrambling the multifaceted nature of the problem (Gurung et al., 2013; Aickin et al., 2019) (Figure 8.2).

Importance of Studying Asphyxial Deaths

The importance of asphyxial deaths must be understood in forensic medicine because it has a direct bearing on the validity of death investigation and legal proceedings. Asphyxial death is an umbrella term for a wide variety of circumstances, and each one poses a different diagnostic challenge. It is often the precise distinction between drowning and other types of asphyxia that depends on certain signs that are not always demonstrable during autopsy. For instance, the presence of strategic internal hemorrhage, such as intra-pyramidal hemorrhage, may be used to confirm drowning diagnoses, while findings like diatoms in the lungs can be used to corroborate water inhalation (Alhemyari et al., 1988). Thus, building a robust body of knowledge in asphyxial phenomena not only improves forensic reliability but also sheds light on preventive interventions that help reduce the risks associated with drowning and other events related to asphyxia. Furthermore, asphyxial death research has important implications for public health, namely in the case of predisposing factors to such events. Studies on respiratory disease like obstructive sleep apnea (OSA) have shown arousal deficits in such patients as a predisposition to sudden deaths during sleep (Tinworth et al., 2003). From the study of physiological pathways, caregivers may plan interventions that minimize associated risks. In this context, the study of asphyxial deaths transcends the field of forensic interest and becomes a part of public health, where awareness and education can influence community safety and determinants of health. Secondly, research on asphyxial deaths expands our understanding of trauma and the human body's response to loss of oxygen. Systematic review of various mechanisms of asphyxia, including hypercapnic hypoxia, offers insightful information on the body's maladaptive and adaptive responses to dangerous circumstances (Tinworth et al., 2003). Such knowledge regarding the biological events is necessary in developing effective treatment strategies in emergency medicine and enhancing preventive interventions in high-risk populations. Lastly, this body of research is in a position to contribute to enhanced clinical practice and inform legislation aimed at reducing asphyxial death, thereby underpinning the multidimensional importance of research into asphyxial death in a broader social context.

8.1. Types of Asphyxial Deaths

Learning Outcome

1. Understand drowning and suffocation.
2. Describe the choking incidents.

Asphyxial deaths can be subdivided into several distinct categories, each having particular physiological and environmental contributions. One of the predominant types arises through mechanical obstruction, in which an individual's airway is physically blocked, either by a foreign substance or swelling of the encircling tissue. Choking accidents, particularly in vulnerable populations such as children and the elderly, exemplify this form of asphyxiation. Moreover, strangulation and positional asphyxiation incidents, wherein the body position of a person prevents airflow, may result in death. Of these incidents, knowledge of the anatomical and situational factors is important in the prevention and intervention of such incidents. The traumatic nature of these incidents makes it critical that people receive proper public education on choking risks and the effective first aid measures that can prevent deaths. In contrast to asphyxia by mechanisms, chemical asphyxia involves inhalation or absorption of substances that interfere with oxygen utilization or transport. One widespread example of this mechanism is carbon monoxide poisoning, where the gas binds more easily to hemoglobin in the blood than oxygen to create systemic hypoxia. In situations where levels are elevated for industrial chemicals or in which underventilation is occurring, exposures may be increased, particularly for those working in confined areas.

The long-term effects of exposure to specific chemicals are yet an active area of research, as in the case of Persian Gulf Veterans' Illnesses, where occupational chemicals led to chronic illness, perhaps including asphyxial mechanisms. These intricacies call for rigorous scrutiny and regulatory action to further ensure safety in the workplace. Finally, a less discussed method of asphyxial death is hypoxic asphyxia, which occurs in situations where there is a diminution of the total oxygen supply. Drowning, exposure at high altitudes, or atmospheres lacking proper atmospheric oxygen are typical examples. In this instance, the body is deprived of sufficient amounts of oxygen necessary for sustaining life, resulting in irreparable organ damage and death unless treated immediately. The physiological response of the body in such instances could be quite different based on the health of the person and the ambient conditions. Once again, like in the case of mechanical and chemical asphyxia, safety and caution are extremely important to avert hypoxic asphyxia accidents. Safety precautions that aim to alert individuals about hazards in low-oxygen environments can avert such avoidable fatalities. Having knowledge of the diversified types of asphyxial deaths allows a more integrated strategy for prevention and intervention techniques in human deaths (Figure 8.3).

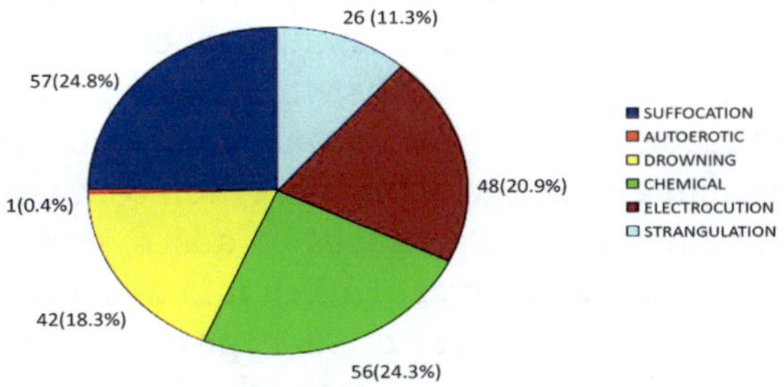

Figure 8.3. Classes of asphyxial death.

Source: https://www.researchgate.net/publication/335672678/figure/fig1/AS:867620421120002@1583868236409/Classes-of-asphyxial-death.png.

8.1.1. Suffocation

Suffocation is among the primary problems in the broad context of asphyxial death in man. It occurs when an individual fails to receive sufficient oxygen due to blockage of the airway. The blockage could be from a foreign body, foodstuffs, or even the surroundings. Notably, toddlers are particularly vulnerable to suffocation, often because of their inquisitiveness and tendency to insert foreign objects into their mouths. The adverse effects of such mishaps are often aggravated by the lack of adult supervision during playtime or feeding time. In foreign body aspiration, prompt action is critical; nevertheless, inadequate training on maneuvers like the Heimlich maneuver can yield cataclysmic results. As illustrated in studies, fatalities caused by food obstruction due to food material, such as mozzarella cheese or raw beans, emphasize the imperative necessity of effective preventive strategies and caregiver education (Asmundo et al., 2020). Examination of suffocation in terms of sleep-related accidents, namely Sudden Infant Death Syndrome (SIDS), reveals a more serious facet of asphyxial mortality. SIDS hypotheses often specify positional asphyxia as a condition where the sleeping position of an infant leads to airway patency restriction. Research on SIDS epidemiological risk factors has led to more safety recommendations on sleeping habits, such as placing infants on their backs during sleeping hours and preventing co-sleeping in bedrooms filled with soft bedding. Such interventions target the reduction of suffocation risk, hence fewer unexplained infant death cases. However, with still ongoing debates over what causes SIDS, doubts have been cast on the adequacy of available hypotheses. Full understanding of these factors is essential to improve infant security mechanisms and reduce asphyxiation risks during unsafe sleeping periods (Malamitsi-Puchner et al., 2011).

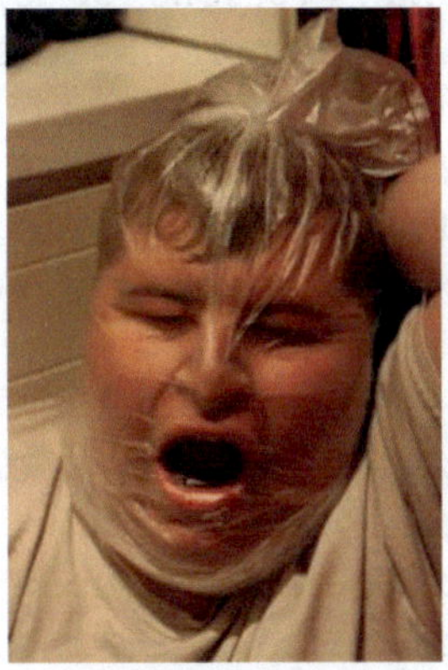

Figure 8.4. Suffocation deaths.

Source: https://imageserver.ebscohost.com/img/embimages/ers/sp/embedded/89312379-74084.jpg?ephost1=dGJyMNHX8kSepq84xNvgOLCmsE2epq5Srqa4SK6WxWXS.

In order to effectively counter the risks of suffocation, there is a need for public health education and health awareness interventions. Such interventions have to stress identification and identification of potential hazards at home and in the community setting. In addition, training parents, caregivers, and teachers can prepare them with the appropriate skills to manage choking effectively. Educated caregivers who are able to recognize the signs of suffocation due to airway obstruction and execute the appropriate responses have been found to significantly prevent suffocation complications. In addition, reminding parents about safe feeding, for instance, watching children and avoiding high-risk foods, can be a breakthrough in preventing catastrophes. By integrating preventive practices into standard care and educating caregivers, we can work towards reducing the incidence of asphyxial suffocation-related deaths and ultimately safeguard vulnerable populations (Asmundo et al., 2020) (Figure 8.4).

8.1.2. Drowning

One of the primary reasons for asphyxial death is drowning, where a person gets submerged in water or any other fluid that cannot be inhaled as part of normal breathing. The physiological processes that lead to death due to drowning are both hypoxia and hypercapnia, both resulting from dilution of the blood's oxygen content. When water enters the lungs, it pushes away air and reduces blood oxygenating capacity, ultimately leading to loss of consciousness and eventual death unless acted upon immediately. Drowning can lead to numerous circumstances, particularly among vulnerable populations, for example, children and individuals with limited swimming ability, hence the critical need for public sensitization and countermeasures aimed at minimizing risks associated with the use of water. The sequence of events following immersion also plays a crucial role in deciding the outcome of drowning cases. Involuntary gasp reflex due to compromise of the airway of the swimmers is the initial event that results in aspiration of water. The aspiration can produce a cascade of physiological events, including surfactant release and ensuing pulmonary edema, for which it becomes arduous to continue respiration. Pre-existing medical conditions, such as cardiac disease or respiratory disease, place a person at a higher risk of drowning and thus of death. It is through these compounding issues that the need for prompt intervention and high-level life support in drowning becomes clear, dictating to a large extent the survival rate and neurological recovery in the long term. Current studies have examined the potential neurological impact of drowning, and this has introduced insight into the mechanism behind brain damage due to asphyxia. When compared with other asphyxial causes of death, such as asphyxial cardiac arrest (ACA), it is observable that both diseases result in hypoxic-ischemic damage, although the nature of the damage may be varied. Research highlights the outcomes of excitotoxic processes caused by oxygen deprivation, which lead to lasting cognitive and motor deficits following resuscitation. Further, interventions aimed at reversing the effects of asphyxia, for example, through the use of agents like D-cycplements, are investigated for their potential efficacy in fostering recovery from neuronal damage. With the complexity of drowning and its impact, further evaluation of therapeutic treatments and prevention strategies is still essential in the management of asphyxial deaths in humans, as indicated by previous studies (Combs et al., 2013; Dickinson et al., 2014) (Figure 8.5).

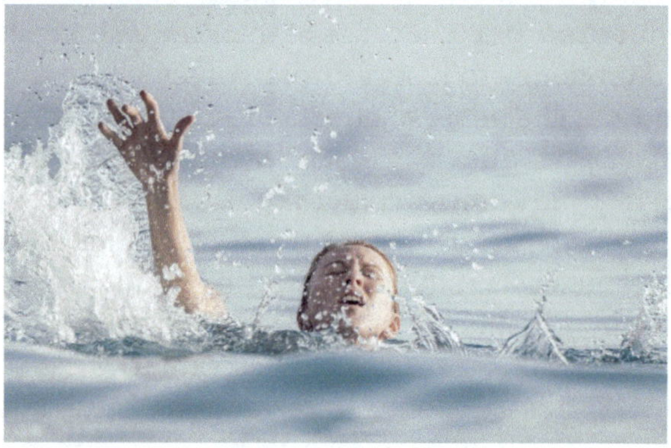

Figure 8.5. Drowning.

Source: https://www.helpinginjuredpeople.com/wp-content/uploads/2021/10/Drowning-Accident.jpg.

8.1.3. Choking

Choking, a critical public health matter, significantly contributes to asphyxial deaths in human beings, particularly among vulnerable groups like the elderly and children. The pathophysiology of choking most often occurs when foreign material obstructs the airway, closing normal respiration. The obstruction in the majority of cases consists of organic material, specifically within the population of children, where toddlers are prone to aspiration accidents. For instance, research has indicated that foreign body aspiration (FBA) is quite common as a result of ingestion of certain food items like grapes or hot dogs, and this can lead to death if left untreated. Education of the caregivers and parents is of paramount importance in order to lower the risks of choking. Such programs would be required to emphasize appropriate supervision during meals and the appropriate use of emergency procedures such as the Heimlich maneuver, as observed in the review of four FBA-related fatalities (Asmundo et al., 2020). The consequences of choking extend beyond momentary respiratory collapse; they have the potential to become larger-scale systemic health issues. Studies prove that the reflexive choking mechanism may lead to asphyxial cardiac arrest, a condition in which the heart becomes ineffective due to a lack of oxygen. Asphyxial cardiac arrest is, therefore, a critical medical emergency requiring immediate intervention in order to prevent irreversible damage to the brain and other complications. Surprisingly, long-duration asphyxia has been found to cause deep excitotoxic processes leading to neuronal injury, a mechanism described in neurological investigations of asphyxial cardiac arrest models (Combs et al., 2013). Clarification of the physiological cascade after an asphyxia event supports the immediacy of treatment and implementing prevention measures in vulnerable populations. Preventive strategies to reduce instances of choking comprise multi-faceted interventions that involve healthcare providers, educators, and families. Interventions to raise awareness should be focused on the identification of high-risk foods that are likely to lead to choking and sensitizing custodians on how to critically monitor eating habits. Additionally, as part of regular childhood education, first aid and resuscitation technique training can be incorporated so that custodians are more ready to address such incidents, thereby reducing asphyxial deaths caused by choking. Current research has raised to the surface that an educated populace, supplied with the potential to react in critical situations, can successfully curtail the number of deadly consequences attributed to cases of choking. Therefore, the promotion of holistic learning and education in these areas will certainly be pivotal in solving the ongoing issue of choking as viewed through the scope of asphyxial mortalities in humans, creating better health outcomes within all age categories (Asmundo et al., 2020) (Figure 8.6).

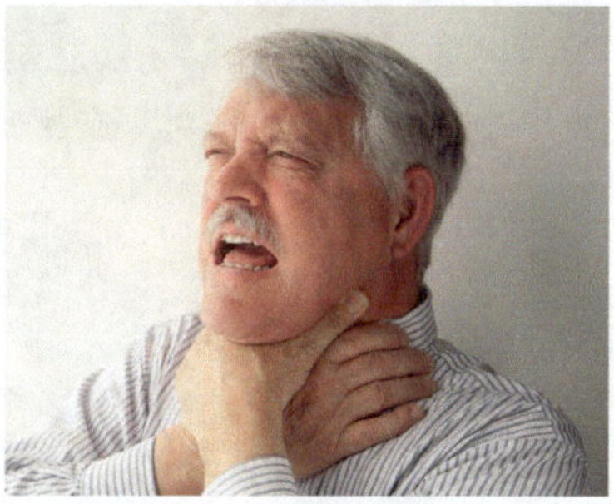

Figure 8.6. Choking.

Source: https://cprcare.com/wp-content/uploads/2018/03/choking-adult-CPR.jpg.

Test Your Knowledge

1. What is suffocation?
2. What is choking?

8.2. Mechanisms of Asphyxia

Learning Outcome

1. Understand the oxygen deprivation.
2. Know the carbon dioxide buildup.
3. Describe the physiological responses to asphyxia.

An understanding of the mechanisms of asphyxia is crucial in deciphering its impact on human physiology, particularly in appreciating the pathophysiological changes in an asphyxial episode. Asphyxia is basically a disruption of oxygen supply with an increase in carbon dioxide, which has the potential to lead to hypoxia and ultimately result in cell death. The foundation of the mechanisms is further categorized into mechanical suffocation, chemical asphyxia, and drowning, each with its specific challenge in clinical assessment and post-mortem examination. Mechanical suffocation, for instance, occludes the airway and interrupts effective gas exchange, while chemical asphyxia inhibits the body's ability to use oxygen, for example, in cases of carbon monoxide poisoning. It is important for forensic pathologists to understand these distinctions when they need to utilize circumstantial evidence since there are no specific diagnostic indicators in asphyxial deaths (Baldi et al., 2021).

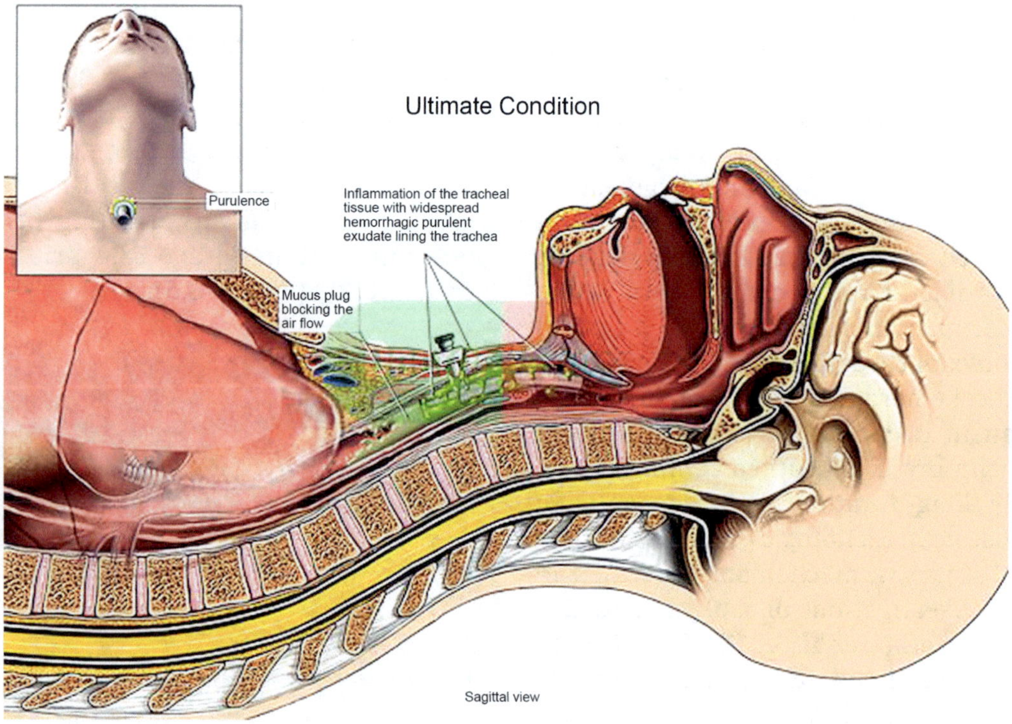

Figure 8.7. Mechanisms of asphyxia.

Source: https://www.doctorstock.com/img-get/I0000YPjOM1QrDzg/s/600/600/85958DS.jpg.

Furthermore, the physiological consequences of asphyxia extend beyond the lack of immediate oxygen; they trigger complex biochemical cascades within the body. Elevated levels of lactic acid may arise due to anaerobic metabolism, disrupting cellular function and causing metabolic acidosis. This condition not only impacts essential organs but may also lead to a cascade of neurodegenerative diseases in survivors of asphyxial events. For example, perinatal asphyxia has been reported to lead to permanent cognitive impairment through hypoxic-ischemic damage, resulting in substantial neurodevelopmental impairment later in life. It is also argued in the literature that asphyxia with subsequent re-oxygenation can be linked to a variety of chronic pathologies, including diabetes and cancer, thereby necessitating the need for ongoing monitoring and intervention among the survivors (Cebioglu et al., 2011). The results are important in highlighting the paramount importance of realizing that asphyxia not only is an immediate fatal threat but also an inducing agent of long-term health issues. Additionally, the improvement of diagnostic modalities has significantly facilitated the understanding of asphyxia's mechanism and its effects. The traditional histological examination provides fundamental information on the injury incurred at cardiac arrest due to asphyxia; however, novel techniques such as metabolomics have begun bridging the gap in discrimination between different causes of cardiac arrest. Through metabolic profiling, scientists have also identified some biochemical markers that are specific for asphyxia relative to other causes of cardiac arrest (Baldi et al., 2021). This discrimination is important in forensic pathology since it is generally hard to specify the exact cause of death (Baldi et al., 2021). With increased research, integration of such diagnostic techniques can provide a window to better individualized treatment protocols and prevention efforts and thereby improve outcomes for participating subjects. Understanding these mechanisms gives a comprehensive picture of asphyxial deaths and their far-reaching implications on human health (Figure 8.7).

8.2.1. Oxygen Deprivation

Oxygen deficiency, or hypoxia, is a serious pathological condition that can lead to asphyxial death among human beings. The condition occurs when the body or a single tissue does not get enough oxygen supply and subsequently experiences malfunction and cell death. The prevalence of oxygen deficiency is most worrying among certain groups of individuals, such as newborns, where data indicate that approximately 4 million infants have birth asphyxia annually. Of these patients, about 25% succumb to the condition, with an equal proportion having neurological sequelae such as cardiopulmonary encephalopathy (HIE) (Frøyland et al., 2008). It is crucial to appreciate the mechanism of the conditions in that early intervention within the window of therapy can significantly enhance the prognosis and decrease asphyxial event mortality. Among the critical factors in oxygen deficiency is the cascade of biochemical events that follow. When tissues are oxygen-deprived, they become acidotic, triggering a complex response that has effects on mitochondrial function and inflammatory processes. Recent research points out that acidosis is both beneficial and pathologic, depending on the timing relative to reoxygenation. Initial decreases in mitochondrial function and triggering of inflammatory cells may enhance neuronal injury, indicating that hypoxia's effects can persist even once oxygen is replenished. This latent cell death extends the therapeutic window of critical treatment with a view to minimizing damage from oxygen deficiency, thus emphasizing the importance of early clinical treatment and the construction of targeted interventions in affected patients, particularly in neonates (Frøyland et al., 2008). In forensic pathology, oxygen deficiency also poses serious diagnostic challenges, primarily due to the lack of available specific biomarkers for cardiac arrest due to asphyxia. The art of distinguishing mechanical asphyxia from the other causes of cardiac arrest involves judicious appreciation of circumstantial data and the skill of the pathologist. Histological examinations have been employed traditionally to confirm tissue injury, but they are not effective in differentiating the causes of asphyxial death.

New diagnostic technologies, such as 1H nuclear magnetic resonance (NMR) metabolomics, are providing valuable information regarding metabolic changes with asphyxia and towards a greater understanding of cell effects evoked by oxygen lack. Such technologies highlight the need for new diagnostic technologies to improve accuracy in diagnosing asphyxial death and raise overall comprehension of the underlying mechanisms (Figure 8.8).

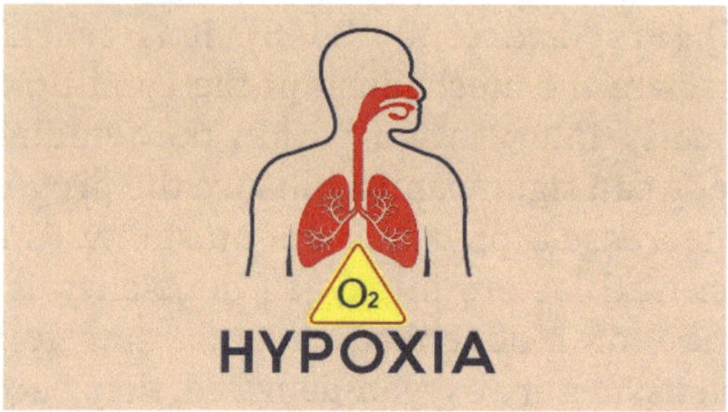

Figure 8.8. Hypoxia: when the brain is deprived of oxygen.

Source: https://www.happiesthealth.com/wp-content/uploads/2025/04/Hypoxia-Amar-P-scaled.jpg.

8.2.2. Carbon Dioxide Buildup

Carbon dioxide (CO_2) accumulation in the atmosphere is highly hazardous to human security and environmental well-being, primarily in the context of asphyxial death. As CO_2 rises, it becomes challenging for the body to expel this gas effectively, resulting in a lethal process of metabolic acidosis due to hypoxia and hypercapnia. When individuals are exposed to high concentrations of CO_2, their ability to exchange oxygen is diminished, leading to incapacitation or insensibility and ultimately resulting in asphyxia. This decline is heightened when they are confined in small areas where ventilation is poor; therefore, the identification of CO_2 thresholds that are safe becomes a priority. The potential for such buildups ~~to~~ lead to significant health effects necessitates monitoring and intervention, particularly in the workplace or during natural disasters when ventilation might be compromised. The process of evaluating carbon dioxide buildup is closely allied with forensic medicine, a scientific discipline that seeks to demystify the complexity associated with asphyxial death. Empirical data and emerging technologies can be used by forensic scientists to quantify environmental conditions at the time of death, for example, CO_2 levels. These quantifications not only indicate the immediate cause of death, but also overall trends for safety standards in industries. For instance, NIOSH standards emphasize the need to maintain control over exposure to harmful substances within the work environment, ensuring that CO_2 levels do not exceed critical levels so that health-related issues and deaths can be prevented. By integrating forensic medicine and environmental science, the risk factors for carbon dioxide exposure can be understood more accurately, and better safety methods and prevention can be achieved. Furthermore, advances in forensic science are enhancing our capacity to investigate asphyxial deaths due to carbon dioxide buildup. Advances in forensic medicine, while addressing the immediate causes of death, are concurrently addressing the social and legal aspects related to the occurrence of such fatalities. The integration of fresh findings within the various disciplines contributes to the approaches adopted during forensic investigations, thereby augmenting our understanding of the potentiality and constraints of carbon dioxide-related fatalities. Continued development in the field enables specialists to respond more competently to emergent threats caused by the environment, for instance, rising CO_2 levels. The contribution of carbon dioxide buildup in such a situation extends beyond the well-being of people and subsequently impacts policy and legislative measures applied to the purpose of maintaining public safety and environmental quality, noted in contemporary forensic practice and literature (N/A, 2021) (Figure 8.9).

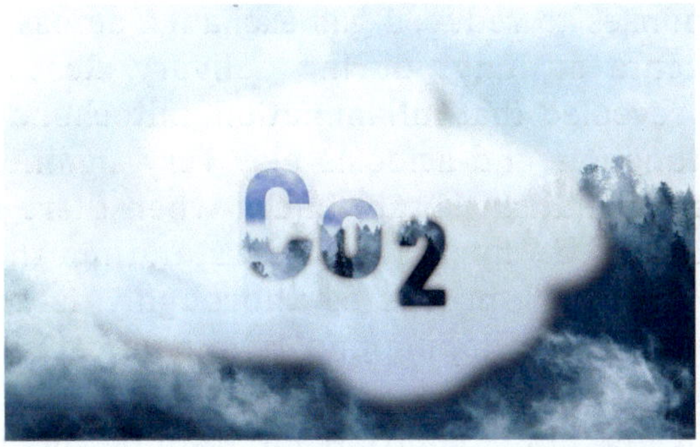

Figure 8.9. Household CO_2: What causes high carbon dioxide levels.

Source: https://www.youngshomecomfort.com/blog/wp-content/uploads/2022/07/carbon-dioxide-7123532_1920-1400x896.jpg?x69554.

8.2.3. Physiological Responses to Asphyxia

Asphyxia, with a deficiency of oxygen supply, provokes a series of subtle physiological compensations ultimately impacting multiple organ systems. An early response to asphyxia is the occurrence of hypoxia and decreased tissue availability of oxygen. Anaerobic metabolism follows, leading to lactic acid production and associated metabolic acidosis that may result in cellular dysfunction and death. As cellular stores of energy decline, organ systems such as the brain and the heart experience severe ischemic damage. It is worth acquiring knowledge of these early changes in physiology because they define an essential window of opportunity for potential therapeutic interventions to prevent asphyxia-induced permanent damage (Frøyland et al., 2008). Perinatal asphyxia in neonates is very dangerous and usually results in hypoxic-ischemic encephalopathy (HIE). The physiological alterations seen in newborns can develop into serious neurodevelopmental complications or even death. The pathophysiological processes involved are those of inflammation, mitochondrial damage, and delayed neuronal damage. Studies have shown that acidosis during the hypoxic period has a protective effect, but reoxygenation can lead to added injury through oxidative stress and inflammatory mediators (Cebioglu et al., 2011). The recognition and management of such physiological responses are important for the identification of effective therapeutic modalities to oppose the long-term adverse effects of asphyxia. Apart from immediate physiological responses, broad consequences of asphyxia involve risk for long-term disability in terms of cognitive impairment and neurodegenerative disease. Subtle asphyxic insults may be manifest as minimal brain injury leading to disorders of attention or hyperactivity. Conversely, severe asphyxia may result in severe neurological impairment or death. The socio-economic burden of such complications necessitates that it be addressed on a multi-faceted level in pediatrics and neonatology via predictive interventions, targeted therapy, and educational maneuvers aimed at the underlying molecular mechanisms of asphyxia (Frøyland et al., 2008). Sophisticated diagnostic devices and customized treatment programs hold promise to reduce the incidence of chronic ailments brought about by asphyxia, ultimately resulting in improved survival and health for individuals suffering from it.

Test Your Knowledge

1. What is oxygen depletion also known as?
2. What physiological condition results from the accumulation of CO2 in the body?

8.3. Causes of Asphyxial Deaths

Learning Outcome

1. Understand the accidental causes of asphyxial deaths.
2. Describe the intentional causes of asphyxial deaths.
3. Describe the medical conditions contributing to asphyxia.

Asphyxial death results due to a variety of conditions, including mechanical obstruction, environmental conditions, and medical illnesses. Mechanical asphyxia is seen when airflow to the lungs is prevented, similar to food or other matter getting stuck in the throat. This leads to ongoing hypoxia, as the oxygen cannot pass into the blood. Apart from this, environmental conditions like drowning and smothering are also leading causes of asphyxial death. In all these scenarios, there are certain barriers to resuscitation and rescue, and an immediate intervention is required. Sometimes, an early intervention may even restore the asphyxial process, but prolonged absence of oxygen always results in irreversible brain damage and death unless treated immediately. To avoid such events and to provide adequate training to recognize signs of asphyxia under various circumstances, it is important to learn these mechanical and environmental causes. The other important cause of asphyxial fatalities is attributed to the complications of natural childbirth, that is, birth asphyxia. Globally, approximately 4 million babies are affected by the condition in the form of restricted oxygen supply during delivery, leading to immediate and severe effects on infants. Approximately 25% of such affected babies are estimated to die of the condition, while many others suffer from long-term neurological damage such as hypoxic-ischemic encephalopathy (HIE). The mechanisms involved in this process are intricate, such as physiological responses to reduced gas exchange across the placenta or lungs during delivery. Research has revealed that inflammation, mitochondrial dysfunction, and acidosis play very significant roles in inducing brain injury when there are episodes of hypoxia. Understanding these physiological processes thoroughly is thus critical to developing and refining treatments that can avert the dangers of asphyxia at birth (Frøyland et al., 2008). Aside from mechanical and birth-related reasons, asphyxial deaths may also ensue in other medical situations, such as during the progression of a disease or prior conditions.

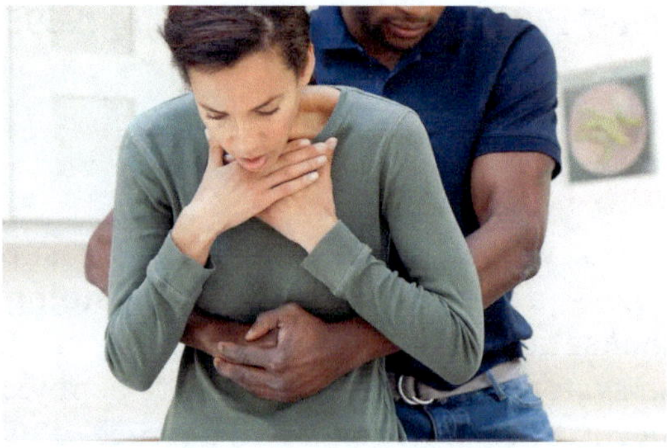

Figure 8.10. Choking is one cause of asphyxia and can prevent your body from taking in enough oxygen.

Source: https://img.lb.wbmdstatic.com/vim/live/webmd/consumer_assets/site_images/article_thumbnails/BigBead/asphyxia_bigbead/1800x1200_asphyxia_bigbead.jpg?resize=750px:*&output-quality=75.

During cardiac arrest or respiratory diseases such as chronic obstructive pulmonary disease (COPD), the body's ability to exchange gases may be severely impaired, thus resulting in asphyxia. In such cases, the very first priority would be the restoration of airway patency and effective ventilation. Furthermore, advances in clinical science, as the use of metabolomics to differentiate between the etiology of cardiac arrest, offer a potential avenue for investigation of the asphyxial process. For example, it has been found that certain metabolic patterns may occur in subjects undergoing asphyxia in cardiac arrest, shedding light on potential treatments (Baldi et al., 2021). These findings indicate the complexity of asphyxial death and the need for an interdisciplinary approach to prevention and management (Figure 8.10).

8.3.1. Accidental Causes

Incidental asphyxial causes contribute to a significant proportion of deaths and hold significant public health implications. It is necessary to know these causes so that preventative measures can be formulated. Environmental risks, that is, aspiration of food, drowning, and inhalation of gases, are some of the leading causes of accidental asphyxia. It should be noted that conditions related to the inhalation of toxic substances, that is, nitrous oxide, can lead to severe outcomes. Nitrous oxide is usually used recreationally, and its abuse results in death through acute asphyxiation and cardiac arrhythmias. It thus becomes an issue of immediate necessity to create awareness of the risks of abuse of inhalants and to introduce effective regulation to minimize such risks (Luigi et al., 2022). Aside from chemical poisoning, accidental asphyxia fatalities are also induced by unintentional episodes of choking among vulnerable individuals like the elderly and children. The Heimlich maneuver and first-aid response are of utmost significance during instances of choking accidents. Nonetheless, familiarity with proper procedures remains low. Moreover, the establishment of specific federal regulations to educate caregivers, parents, and individuals on choking prevention may significantly reduce cases. This prevention is essential, as choking attempts often go unreported but are a critical risk factor for asphyxial fatalities. Special efforts must be directed towards emphasizing education and rapid response training in public and private spheres for effectively tackling this growing problem. The joint impact of accidental asphyxial deaths, either related to environmental or human causes, emphasizes the need for a joint effort at public health education. The recent studies have highlighted the need for medical intervention following incidents of cardiac arrest caused by asphyxia. As noted in research targeting asphyxial cardiac arrest models, neurological recovery following resuscitation is significant in determining the long-term implications of such an incident (Combs et al., 2013). Through the support of public health initiatives targeted at prevention and response, society can minimize the occurrence of accidental asphyxia. Besides, there should be more investigation of the mechanisms and ramifications involved in these deaths in order to develop evidence-based policy and effective healthcare interventions that can reduce the resulting fatalities from asphyxial events (Figure 8.11).

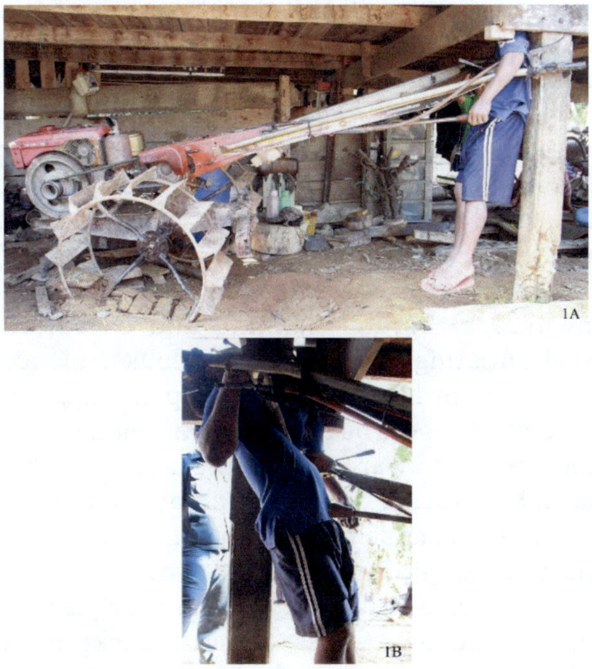

Figure 8.11. 1A and 1B: Victim compressed by handlebar of twowheel walking behind a tractor with a pillar of the basement.

Source: https://www.asianarchpath.com/storage/media_articles/20_files/20_1.jpeg.

8.3.2. Intentional Causes (Suicide/Homicide)

Human asphyxial death syndrome comprises a number of intentional causes, primarily suicide and murder. Individuals resort to such extreme measures for a range of psychological, social, and environmental problems. In suicides, particularly in the suicide cases of individuals who have horrible mental illnesses, individuals believe asphyxiation by methods such as hanging or strangulation is the sole means of ending their suffering. The urgent necessity for suicide prevention strategies cannot be overstated, as establishing motives for such actions is critical to intervention. Empirical evidence has established that socio-economic pressure, trauma history, and mental health service inaccessibility can exponentially escalate the risks of suicidal behavior. Thus, suicide as a voluntary means of asphyxial death calls into doubt the importance of treating mental health comprehensively in society. Homicide, an intentional cause of asphyxial, provides a highly dynamic interaction of motives like revenge, jealousy, and power. Typologies of homicide, that is, mass, spree, and serial homicides, explain various patterns of offender behavior. Serial homicide, by itself, deserves special consideration since it typically involves elaborate planning and execution, differentiating it from spontaneous violence. As quoted in literature, the weapon employed in homicide could be decided by the victimology and forensic awareness of the offender. This allows for varied degrees of premeditation for violent offenses so that an unplanned asphyxial method, like strangulation, could be a result of an impulsive emotional stimulus and not a planned effort. The awareness of such background dynamics goes into building prevention and intervention measures. Constant evolution of forensic medicine holds a central place in unraveling the complexities of voluntary death, like suicide and homicide. The field increasingly uses new techniques and interdisciplinary approaches to address conventional as well as new challenges to mortality investigation. According to scholastic literature, the intersection of technology innovation and professional interventions carries significant implications for understanding mechanisms of death, such as asphyxia. In addition, the link between forensic evidence and homicide motivation illuminates how perpetrator behavior is shaped by social and psychological determinants. Thus, future studies need to fill gaps in current knowledge, namely, how offender characteristics shape the manner in which asphyxial death is implemented, providing insights that could encourage preventive measures and legal strategies in forensic practice (Fletcher et al., 2022; N/A, 2021) (Figure 8.12).

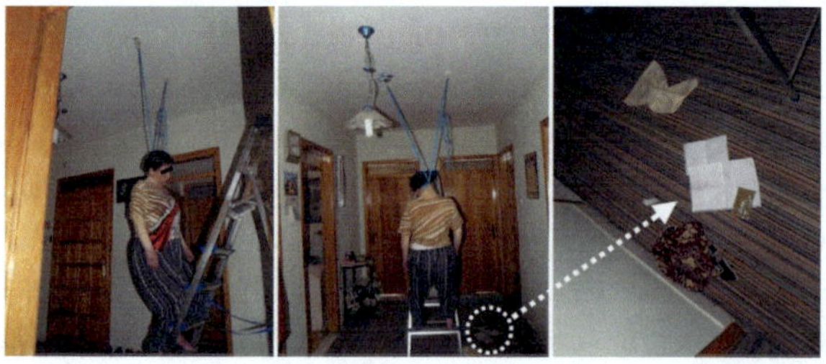

Figure 8.12. Thirty-seven-year-old woman hanged herself in her house. There was a farewell letter on the floor.

Source: https://cdnintech.com/media/chapter/19160/1512345123/media/image11.jpeg.

8.3.3. Medical Conditions Contributing to Asphyxia

Asphyxia, or deprivation of oxygenation of the tissues, can be produced by many clinical conditions impairing respiratory function. Underlying pulmonary disease, such as COPD, asthma, and pneumonia, makes asphyxial events highly probable. These diseases impair the mechanism of respiration or gas exchange and therefore create hypoxia that can very quickly lead to clinical emergencies. Even minor respiratory infections or other stressors in such individuals have the capacity to exacerbate their condition, magnifying their risk for asphyxia.

The etiologic complexity of asphyxia in these circumstances is a reflection of the fine balance between the baseline pathologies and the acute physiologic demands placed on the respiratory system, necessitating prompt intervention to avoid morbidity and mortality. The other significant etiology of asphyxia is neurological impairment, which disrupts the capability of the brain to control breathing. Conditions like stroke, traumatic brain injury, or neurological disorders like amyotrophic lateral sclerosis (ALS) disrupt the usual respiratory drive or disrupt the coordination required for effective ventilation. This impairment causes ineffective airway protection and defective gas exchange. Most strikingly, the effects of hypoxic-ischemic encephalopathy (HIE) in the newborn provide a vivid illustration of this interaction. In the neonate, compromised perinatal circulation or oxygenation can cause lethal brain injury that negatively affects the respiratory control centers. There are approximately 4 million instances of birth asphyxia annually, and a significant portion of them experience permanent neurological damage or death, which illustrates the complex relationship between neurological condition and asphyxial mortality in human beings (Frøyland et al., 2008). The cardiac factors are also of specific interest in the mechanism of asphyxia. When the heart fails to circulate blood adequately, hypoperfusion resulting from it may lead to insufficient delivery of oxygen to the vital organs, an effect that is akin to asphyxia. Cardiac arrest due to arrhythmias or other cardiovascular illnesses follows a rapid course, leading to unconsciousness and cessation of respiration. Such events are hard to differentiate from mechanical asphyxia without rigorous forensic examination, based on existing literature comparing histological examination with advanced techniques like metabolomics (Baldi et al., 2021). Understanding the overlap among cardiac disorders and asphyxia opens up the possibility of improved emergency action and interventions for prevention, emphasizing the importance of targeted research into how to reduce the risk burden associated with such overlapping medical conditions.

Test Your Knowledge

1. What causes accidental asphyxiation?
2. Which pre-existing condition commonly contributes to the risk of asphyxia?

8.4. Risk Factors

Learning Outcome

1. Understand the concept of age-related vulnerabilities.
2. Describe the role of environmental factors in the occurrence of asphyxial deaths.
3. Describe the role of behavioral factors in asphyxial deaths.

The risk factor analysis of asphyxial deaths among human beings reflects that many preconditions have the capability to significantly augment vulnerability at various phases of life. To illustrate, obstetric cholestasis during pregnancy has been demonstrated, wherein interventions are able to affect fetal outcomes and hence asphyxial events. Specifically, while therapies such as ursodeoxycholic acid (UDCA) have been found effective in relieving pruritus and even appear to be correlated with fewer instances of fetal distress, the cumulative evidence base remains inconclusive for their asphyxia-protective effects in the neonate. This highlights the complexities of risk factors among pregnant women, wherein fetal and maternal well-being can be determinants of delivery and post-delivery outcomes, pointing to a critical niche to investigate further the association between maternal and asphyxial occurrences in infants (Gurung et al., 2013). Perinatal asphyxia is also an emergent problem given its far-reaching implications for neonatal health. According to recent estimates, perinatal asphyxia caused by oxygen shortage at birth can result in irreversible hypoxic ischemic organ damage, leading to long-term complications such as neurodegenerative diseases or intellectual disability. The permanence of the effects underscores the importance of defining certain risk factors of perinatal asphyxia because they can significantly disrupt developmental processes. Pre-existing conditions, maternal age, and complications of labor management are just some of the numerous variables responsible for determining the likelihood of asphyxic events. This is why concerted effort involving intensified prenatal monitoring and care actions is instrumental in preventing asphyxial mortality in human beings (Cebioglu et al., 2011). Finally, socio-economic factors involved in asphyxial fatalities cannot be overlooked, as they bear a critical interrelationship with the identified risk factors. Marginalized groups, with reduced access to quality medical care, are typically disproportionately saddled with perinatal asphyxia complications. The interaction between educational and healthcare disparities contributes to the failures involved in the prevention of these risk factors, requiring educational interventions and strict diagnostic procedures. By focusing on community health programs and targeted intervention programs, the healthcare system can attempt to counteract the risk factors of asphyxial death. In effect, an interrelated strategy that encompasses research, community, and healthcare reform is crucial in preventing asphyxial occurrences and improving outcomes among vulnerable populations (Figure 8.13).

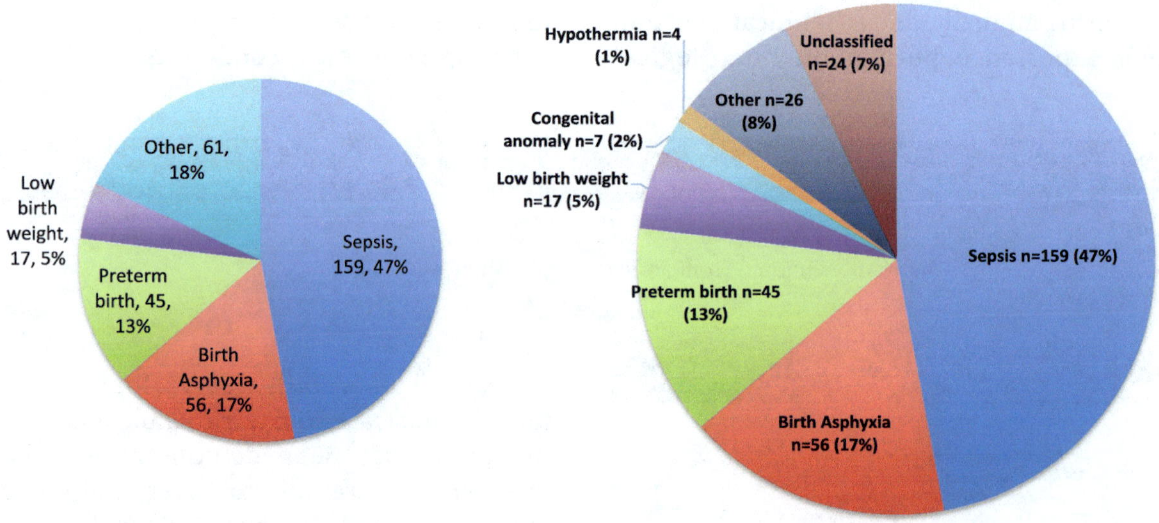

Figure 8.13. Cause of death distribution for newborns ($n = 338$) in six districts of Nepal from April 2012 to April 2013. Number and percent of deaths by cause for newborns ($n = 338$) in six districts of Nepal from April 2012 to April 2013. The other category included respiratory distress syndrome ($n = 6$, 1.8%), meconium aspiration syndrome ($n = 5$, 1.5%), birth injury ($n = 2$, 0.6%), severe jaundice ($n = 1$, 0.3%), and others ($n = 12$, 3.6%).

Source: https://media.springernature.com/full/springer-static/image/art%3A10.1186%2Fs13690-021-00771-5/MediaObjects/13690_2021_771_Fig1_HTML.png?as=webp.

8.4.1. Age-Related Vulnerabilities

The concern for age-related vulnerabilities deeply impacts our understanding of asphyxial deaths in human individuals, particularly in populations such as infants and the elderly. Neonates, for instance, possess various physiological impairments that make them more vulnerable to asphyxia. Their immature respiratory systems expose them to obstructive events such as diminished air flow or compromised airway integrity. Such susceptibility is not just a product of anatomical differences; it is further enhanced by factors such as the sleeping conditions of the infants, which have been linked to sudden infant death syndrome (SIDS) (N/A, 2021). As more research is conducted, the identification of the interaction of evolutionary biology, developmental maturity, and environmental hazard becomes critical in establishing causative mechanisms for asphyxial death in this vulnerable group (N/A, 2021). On the other hand, the elderly population also has unique vulnerabilities that result in asphyxial incidents. As age progresses, physiological alterations like reduced muscle strength, reduced lung capacity, and less effective reflexes, impairing airway protection and breathing critically, can occur. These are all added to by comorbid illnesses like chronic obstructive pulmonary disease (COPD) or neurological disease, further impairing an individual's response to asphyxiating conditions.

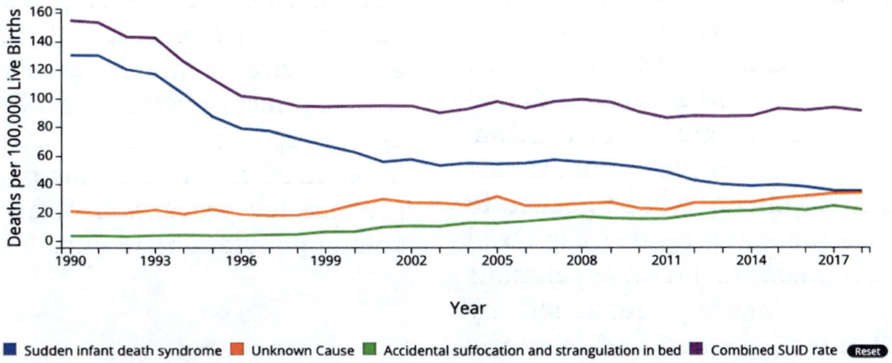

Figure 8.14. Mortality due to sudden infant death syndrome (SIDS) and other causes.

Source: https://cdn.lecturio.com/assets/SUID-1990-2018.jpg.

The confluence of these factors underscores the urgency of a coordinated response, both in clinical care and public health programs, to stem death by asphyxia among the aged. Further, the progress of research in forensic medicine continually re-evaluates the relevance of these vulnerabilities, encouraging enhanced understanding of how age affects causes of death and survival (N/A, 2021). Understanding age-related vulnerabilities is essential for preventing asphyxial deaths across the human lifespan. Protective measures should be tailored to the distinct needs of different age groups, emphasizing education, environmental modifications, and timely interventions. For infants, safe sleep practices must be prioritized to create an environment that minimizes risks associated with obstructive sleep apnea and SIDS. In the aged, community support and medical interventions can make a big difference in increasing their resistance to asphyxial risk. Since vulnerabilities superimpose over social, biological, and environmental factors, the multidisciplinary approach better accounts for asphyxial death. With enhanced awareness and differential intervention, it is achievable to decrease the risks caused by vulnerabilities with aging, ultimately resulting in the decrease of asphyxial death in human beings (Ball et al., 2024) (Figure 8.14).

8.4.2. Environmental Factors

Environmental factors play an important part in the creation of asphyxial death, particularly in conditions were insufficient air is compounded by external body circumstances. Poor air quality, for example, significantly plays a part in respiratory problems that can lead to asphyxia. Dense particles and harmful substances in urban atmospheres have the potential to obstruct channels and thereby decrease gas exchange effectiveness in vulnerable groups such as infants and the elderly. Furthermore, temperatures at extremes can consolidate underlying medical illness to induce spells like cardiac arrest and subsequent neurologic deterioration. Understanding how conditions in the air interact with biological susceptibility will be needed to design preventive measures against asphyxial death, particularly among high-risk populations who are disproportionately burdened by environmental contaminants and climatic extremes. In addition to air quality, socioeconomic status is also a significant environmental factor that could predispose individuals to asphyxial deaths. Individuals living in inferior living conditions have poor access to medical care and preventive interventions, whose lack can increase the effects of asphyxiation. Residents of substandard homes may be exposed to indoor toxics or suboptimal ventilation systems, thereby increasing the chances of such accidents as fires or gas leaks, leading to asphyxia. Additionally, infants and children are most vulnerable to such conditions, as clinical evidence in studies depicts arousal deficits associated with disorders like Obstructive Sleep Apnea (OSA) that could be compounded by environmental factors. A clear understanding of the convergence of social determinants with environmental risks is needed to design efficient public health strategies to mitigate asphyxial mortality among high-risk populations. The synergy between the environment and physiological pathways supports a multi-determined nature of risk in asphyxial death. Research with animal models has helped to elucidate the way in which exposure to hypoxia leads to extreme derangement of mechanisms of arousal necessary for survival. In younger groups, such as piglets, repeated exposure to the condition through intermittent hypercapnic hypoxia shows that the natural arousal responses needed for recovery can be impaired. These impairments can then remain latent with no further stimuli, presenting a confounding factor in assessing chronic exposures' impact on both acute and long-term effects. These results emphasize the need for comprehensive measures that not only address acute environmental hazards but also consider the long-term effects of exposure in different age groups. It is a complicated strategy that is required to direct public policy and medical practice for prevention of asphyxial fatalities among populations (Figure 8.15).

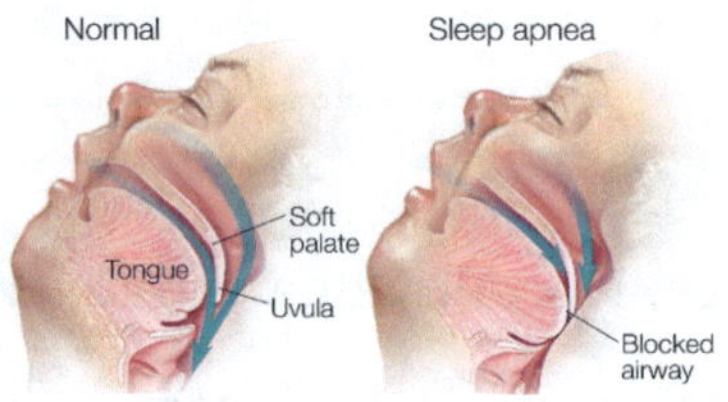

Figure 8.15. Obstructive sleep apnea.

Source: https://www.russellandbodedentistry.com/files/2019/06/OSAphoto.jpg.

8.4.3. Behavioral Factors

Behavioral causes play a tremendous role in causing asphyxial death, particularly through environmental and situational factors that manage individuals' activity and decision-making patterns. Risk-taking activities such as swimming without any appropriate supervision, engaging in risky activities in close proximity to water bodies, or the use of drugs that impair judgment can heighten the risk of asphyxia. For instance, in low- and middle-income countries (LMICs), high rates of drowning are often linked with socio-economic status and unawareness of safety. The presence of individuals who are less aware of swimming safety can be one of the contributing factors to such incidents, thereby creating a need for targeted educational interventions to minimize such risks. These preventive efforts need to address not only individual knowledge but also create social responsibility in water-risk environments and promote a deeper understanding of care processes, especially among children, to further reduce the incidence of unintentional asphyxial death. Another aspect of essential behavior leading to asphyxial deaths relates to the physiological and psychological response during emergencies. Panic can also be exhibited in disorganized behavior, and this has a tendency to make worsening of asphyxia or drowning more likely. Individuals can thrash about underwater and expend energy very rapidly, increasing the likelihood of drowning if they are unable to manage their responses effectively. This behavioral factor emphasizes the need for well-established situational awareness training, particularly in water environments. Evidence implies that teaching basic survival from water and emergency response to individuals, especially children, can influence asphyxial accident prevention to a significant extent. The introduction of systematic programs to enhance coping ability in emergencies, especially among LMICs, can lead to sharp reductions in asphyxial deaths, as it indicates the interaction between training behavior and survival (Combs et al., 2013). The functioning of behavior processes in asphyxial death is also evident in alcohol and drug consumption and the dangers that accompany such activities. Consuming alcohol or drugs can interfere with consciousness functions and reduce physical coordination, thereby increasing vulnerability to asphyxia, especially in aquatic environments. In most cases, individuals who drink and are near water are less likely to have in place the necessary safety precautions, thereby being susceptible to drowning incidents. Harm reduction interventions, which manage the interplay between substance use and behavior, are therefore important in limiting such preventable deaths. Public education campaigns that enlighten young adults regarding the danger of drug usage in water sources can foster behavioral changes that strive to prioritize safety and awareness. Public engagement for the establishment of responsible behavior in water safety is central to avoiding occurrences of asphyxiation through substance use (Combs et al., 2013).

Test Your Knowledge

1. What condition is closely associated with asphyxial deaths in infants?
2. Which behavioral response is most likely to exacerbate asphyxial situations in emergencies?

8.5. Prevention Strategies

Learning Outcome

1. Understand the importance of education and awareness in preventing asphyxial deaths.
2. Describe the safety measures in high-risk environments.
3. Understand the emergency response training.

In the prevention of asphyxial deaths among human beings, the measures should focus on both the immediate interventions and management strategies for the long term. Identification and prevention of risks related to perinatal asphyxia remain an important aspect. For example, through the promotion of sophisticated obstetric practice and close monitoring, the health providers can lessen the occurrence of oxygen deprivation at birth to a great extent. The emphasis on early diagnosis and the use of powerful diagnostic tools to identify susceptible newborns leads to timely interventions that preclude severe consequences, thereby reducing lifelong disabilities caused by asphyxia. These preventive interventions save not only the health of the individual but also curb the socio-economic costs associated with chronic diseases caused by perinatal asphyxia, thus establishing the multi-faceted benefits of preventive mechanisms for such a parameter (Cebioglu et al., 2011). Aside from perinatal issues, the application of preventive measures in the adult population is also crucial. Acute ischemia–reperfusion injury (IRI) is an important mechanism by which asphyxial death may happen as a result of oxygen deficiency in different clinical conditions. As such, the discovery and utilization of novel therapeutic methods, including remote ischemic conditioning (RIC), have been identified as effective measures to mitigate the occurrence of IRI. RIC's ability to safeguard various organs by employing uncomplicated, noninvasive methods underlines its own potential strength in safeguarding individuals exposed to high-risk conditions such as surgery or critical injuries. The incorporation of RIC into practice enables professionals to formulate a model of prevention aimed at counteracting the impact of sudden oxygen deficiency, thus lowering rates of asphyxial mortality and improving patient outcomes (Candilio et al., 2013). Furthermore, education and community mobilization are important elements of evidence-based prevention programs. Programs of public health that establish awareness of the risk of asphyxia among vulnerable groups, such as infants and people with existing medical conditions, can enable communities to take preventative measures.

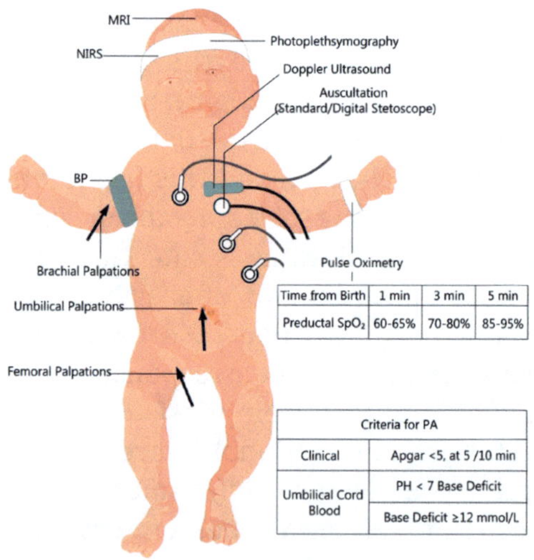

Figure 8.16. Clinical and paraclinical evaluation of the newborn with perinatal asphyxia.

Source: https://www.frontiersin.org/files/Articles/513880/fped-08-00068-HTML-r1/image_m/fped-08-00068-g001.jpg.

Educative interventions must focus on disseminating information regarding safe infant sleeping practices to reduce the risks of asphyxiation and suffocation. Similarly, providing first aid and CPR training can equip caregivers with the skills to respond effectively during emergencies, avoiding life-threatening situations. Collaborations between medical practitioners, teachers, and community organizations can enhance such initiatives, fostering a culture of safety and awareness that significantly reduces asphyxial deaths among different populations. Through such multimodal prevention strategies, the purpose of reducing asphyxial death in humans can be achieved with more ease (Figure 8.16).

8.5.1. Education and Awareness

The pivotal position of education and knowledge in preventing asphyxial deaths cannot be overstated, particularly among vulnerable groups such as children. Most of the incidents occur due to aspiration of foreign objects, which primarily occur in young children who are less responsive to obstruction of the airway. Education interventions founded on effective care for children during meals can go a great way in safeguarding against such incidents. For instance, education of caregivers and educators regarding the application of the Heimlich maneuver and cardiopulmonary resuscitation is important. A study highlights that inexperienced caregivers have a higher likelihood of such accidents occurring, which calls for exhaustive training programs in schools and homes (Asmundo et al., 2020). By supporting a system where the caregivers are well-educated and proficient, the number of asphyxial deaths can see a dramatic decline. For low- and middle-income countries (LMICs), there is a huge demand for targeted education programs in water safety and drowning prevention. Statistics show that 91% of drowning deaths occur in LMICs, and the disparity in health training and preventive methods becomes visible (Cenderadewi et al., 2020). Such situations call for the socio-economic status of families to generally result in ignorance regarding methods of safety. Therefore, targeted education campaigns aimed at remediating a particular cultural environment can increase participation and involvement of communities in safety practices. It is important to note that individuals living in close proximity to water bodies have a higher risk, and education must be directed at measures that promote safe swimming practices and surveillance. Arousing public awareness towards the correlation between socio-economic situations and cases of drowning accidents is crucial in designing effective prevention strategies. Enhancing educational interventions must, in turn, mean the development of robust community awareness towards asphyxial risks as a whole, encompassing both cases of choking and drowning incidents. Schools, health personnel, and community-based groups need to collaborate to develop an overall approach to risk reduction. These group activities should be in the form of workshops, seminars, and information dissemination campaigns focusing on the risk factors and prevention of asphyxial deaths. Research would also have to be directed towards developing accessible educational material that is acceptable for a large variety of people. Through proactive engagement of people in prevention in the form of awareness campaigns, general knowledge regarding asphyxial deaths can be enhanced. This combined push towards awareness and education will ultimately lead to the creation of safer environments for vulnerable populations and reduce the frequency of such tragedies in different communities.

8.5.2. Safety Measures in High-Risk Environments

In dangerous environments, especially where asphyxial hazards are significant, such as bodies of water and other confined spaces, there has to be the installation of far-reaching safety measures to negate hazards. Effective drowning prevention is critical, especially in low- and middle-income nations (LMICs) where the majority of drowning incidents occur. Safety conditions in these environments have severe effects on safety. For instance, crowding, nearness to water bodies, and family socio-economic status are all important predictors of high risks of drowning. In a bid to contain these risks, interventions for specific targeting of education in the community, availability of swimming classes, and the provision of safe spaces for play around water can be implemented. Strengthening data collection in LMICs is also important in the planning and evaluation of these prevention activities because data assures the development of causes for drowning and the effectiveness of safety interventions implemented (Cenderadewi et al., 2020). Further, asphyxial risks occur in various occupations, including emergency medical services. A practical example is the Search and Rescue (SAR) helicopter mission, where safety protocols must integrate effective medical practice with operational impact. Research on manual versus mechanical chest compressions during winching has demonstrated that the use of a mechanical device, like the Schiller Easy Pulse, significantly improves the compression fraction, resulting in less time lost during critical resuscitation attempts. This helps to highlight the use of advanced technology in dangerous settings to enable life-saving actions to be performed effectively, thereby reducing the occurrence of asphyxial event-related fatalities. Additionally, the findings attempt to emphasize the importance of ongoing training and testing of safety measures during response emergencies to match rising demands and refine protocols in place (Wild et al., 2023). Incorporating preventive education and expertise training into the culture of safety within high-risk environments is essential in limiting asphyxial deaths. All parties, including community leaders, government, and medical professionals, must collaborate and develop and implement measures geared towards instilling awareness and response capabilities for vulnerable populations. Identification programs for drowning risk, first aid, and emergency response procedures can prepare communities to respond appropriately in instances of asphyxia. In addition, regular simulation and drilling in emergency agencies can reinforce retention of skill competence and knowledge, thereby enabling a swift, knowing response to real emergencies. Lastly, establishing a culture of safety in such environments will go a long way towards eliminating asphyxial deaths, so preventive measures will be an integral part of addressing this significant public health issue.

8.5.3. Emergency Response Training

Effective emergency response training is also critical in minimizing risks associated with asphyxial death in humans, which is so regretfully prevalent in various situations such as drowning, choking, and suffocation. Training for both professionals and non-professionals aims to enhance the preparedness and competence of individuals for emergency responses. The International Liaison Committee on Resuscitation has also emphasized the importance of continuous education, and this calls for training to be evidence-based and up-to-date. This continuous update ensures first responders are well versed with the latest guidelines, including dispatcher-assisted cardiopulmonary resuscitation and advanced airway interventions. This preparedness not only makes it possible for a person to behave courageously in life-and-death situations but also significantly improves survival rates in asphyxial accidents, where speed is the determining factor between life and death (Aickin et al., 2019). The inclusion of realistic simulation-based training has also been identified as being instrumental in emergency response programs. Simulation-based training that simulates asphyxial conditions provides trainees with valuable decision-making skills during critical moments. This hands-on approach improves learning of the physiological and psychological aspects of resuscitation because students are able to engage with several emergency response techniques. For instance, conducting practice drills that mimic real choking emergencies allows learners to practice the Heimlich maneuver and other life-saving procedures in a simulated environment, hence increasing their confidence and skill levels. Also, constant monitoring and revisions in training methods are essential with every new research, pointing towards curriculum updates in order to keep up with developments in resuscitation science, such as researching therapeutic intervention efficacy in preventing brain injuries following cardiac arrests (Combs et al., 2013). Finally, grassroots emergency response training programs can significantly compound the impact of individual preparedness. By creating a culture of awareness and response, communities can unite to reduce rates of asphyxial death. First aid and resuscitation training for citizens makes citizens capable of acting in the event of emergencies, transforming passive bystanders into rescue actors. Programs such as CPR in Schools do more than add ranks of trained personnel; they also educate civic responsibility. As communities become better trained, the overall survival rate from asphyxial mishaps rises, testifying to the profound influence of extensive emergency response training. The collective knowledge acquired through such training not only enhances personal trauma but also makes communities stronger when faced with public health emergencies, such as asphyxia or equivalent emergencies (Aickin et al., 2019) (Figure 8.17).

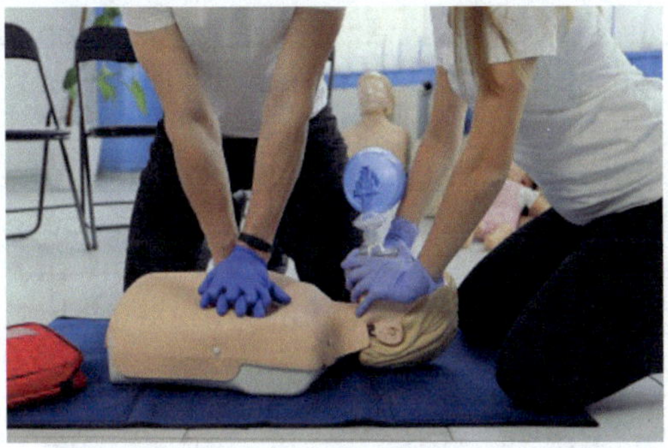

Figure 8.17. Emergency response training.

Source: https://cmscdn.nsc.org/cms/nsc.org/media/site-media/images/first-aid/cta/fa-cpr400px.jpg.

Test Your Knowledge

1. What is a critical approach to reducing drowning incidents in LMICs?
2. What technique is emphasized in training programs to address choking emergencies?

8.6. Legal and Ethical Considerations

Learning Outcome

1. Know the forensic implications of asphyxial deaths.
2. Describe the ethical dilemmas in reporting and investigation.
3. Know the legal ramifications for negligence.

The ethico-legal elements of asphyxial deaths in man offer complex challenges that intersect forensic science, medical ethics, and the law. The etiology of death during asphyxiation has been ascertained through meticulous inquiries to verify whether the accident was unintentional, deliberate, or due to negligence. Criminal laws necessitate forensic scientists to provide precise and unbiased testimony that bears significant meaning for criminal and civil lawsuits. In turn, the integrity of the forensic process must be highest and require strict adherence to protocols in the investigation and autopsy procedures. The effects of misinterpretation or tampering of evidence can lead to false accusations or inability to bring criminals to justice, raising serious ethical concerns about justice and victim advocacy regarding asphyxial death. Besides, the identification of new advanced forensic technology, such as NMR metabolomics, increases our understanding of asphyxial death and relevant metabolic changes. This sophisticated method yields valuable information regarding metabolic signatures that may indicate ante-mortem or post-mortem conditions, offering possible biomarkers for forensic investigation. However, inclusion of such technology presents ethical issues with respect to privacy, consent, and potential abuse of scientific discovery. As highlighted by research based on NMR metabolomics, the moral application of such machinery must strike a balance between seeking truth in forensic science on the one hand and safeguarding individual rights and dignity on the other (Chighine et al., 2020).

In doing this, it is imperative that professionals are open and ethical in their work so that advancement in forensic science may serve to enhance, and not weaken, justice. Finally, the ethical considerations extend to the medical field, more particularly to situations with neonates or vulnerable populations. The linkage of antenatal brain damage and asphyxial events points to the need for health providers to implement rigorous prenatal observation and treatment practices. Ethics involved here are quantifying the risk indicators of conditions like cerebral palsy because of asphyxia during birth, according to recent studies detecting signs of major neurological disabilities associated with in-utero trauma (Becher et al., 2006). It is an appeal by the medical profession to fulfill its duty of preventing such tragedies through education, distribution of resources, and policy formation. In short, the encounter of legal, ethical, and medicolegal issues in asphyxial deaths necessitates an overall, empathetic approach that prioritizes not only understanding the implication of death but also ensuring that such incidents are avoided in the future based on what is known (Figure 8.18).

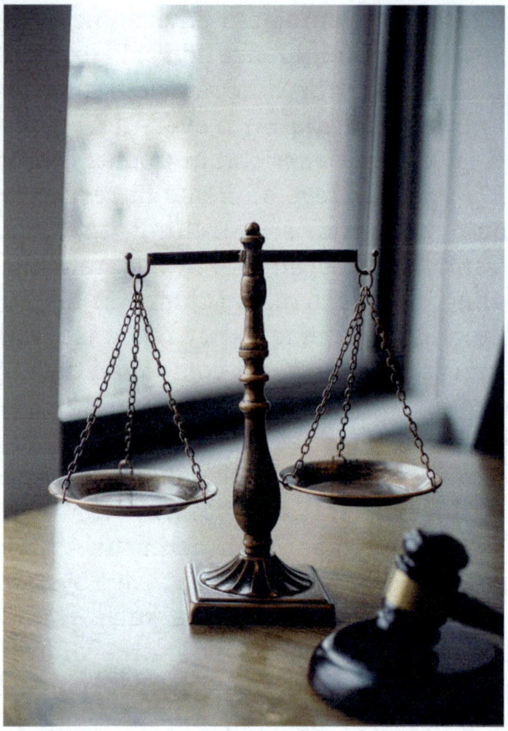

Figure 8.18. Legal and ethical considerations of asphyxial deaths.

Source: https://juriscentre.com/wp-content/uploads/2023/01/pexels-photo-5669602.jpeg.

8.6.1. Forensic Implications of Asphyxial Deaths

The forensic implications of asphyxial death are wide, particularly in the challenge of establishing the cause of death. Asphyxia could be due to various mechanisms, including suffocation, strangulation, and drowning, all requiring a comprehensive forensic investigation to establish the cause of death. In drowning, for instance, there could be no post-mortem indication of asphyxia, and thus forensic experts must conduct an in-depth investigation. The absence of pathognomonic features requires the use of a number of diagnostic tools, such as diatom analysis, which assists in identifying the medium of drowning and tracing a more precise timeline of the event (Badu et al., 2014). Finally, the intricacies involved in asphyxial deaths reinforce the need for careful forensic procedure in ensuring proper diagnosis and justice for the victims and their relatives. Furthermore, asphyxial deaths present unique challenges when trying to distinguish between intentional homicide and accidental death. The variable nature of asphyxia can lead to conditions where the mode of death cannot be determined, thereby complicating legal proceedings and the consequent investigations. Forensic specialists typically need to rely on a combination of autopsy findings, circumstantial evidence, and toxicological analysis in an attempt to make a determination of the mode of death. The emergence of advanced techniques such as NMR metabolomics has further enhanced the capability of detecting metabolic profiles in different forms of asphyxia with potential drug interference (Chighine et al., 2020). Through the generation of metabolic signatures due to some causes of asphyxia, forensic specialists can render a more accurate image and validate or invalidate hypotheses concerning the mode of death, thereby assisting legal processes. Moreover, proper detection of asphyxial deaths has important public safety and health implications. Understanding the patterns and causes of asphyxial deaths allows forensic scientists and law enforcement authorities to devise preventive measures for reducing asphyxia cases in various environments. As an example, insights gleaned from any form of study of drowning incidents can open the way towards greater safety regulations for swimming pools, aquatic safety instruction, and even legislation that restricts access to potentially lethal situations. Besides that, awareness of the signs and symptoms of asphyxia can enhance readiness for medical and police emergency response. Thus, not only does the forensic examination of asphyxial death serve the immediate purpose of determining causation, but it also provides significant contributions to broader societal efforts at preventing future occurrences.

8.6.2. Ethical Issues in Investigation and Reporting

The ethical dilemmas in asphyxial death reporting and investigation exhibit keen contradictions between public interest and the privacy of the families. While reporters cover such sensitive data, they must weigh between releasing correct and timely information and sensitivity to the loss of the bereaved families. Coverage in most instances is likely to be sensationalized, particularly if deaths occur suddenly and unexpectedly, and families have already experienced trauma. The joint agency approach (JAA) to investigating deaths from asphyxia, just like sudden unexpected death in infancy (SUDI), emphasizes these. The families have also complained concerning the emotional care provided during the investigations and how their suffering is aggravated by the involvement of the police and other professional agencies. This implies a major demand on the part of reporters to report such news with care, so that they are not contributing to the emotional burden already borne by grieving families. Further, correct classification and comprehension of asphyxial death raise a complex ethical issue having an impact on reporting and investigative processes. As is evident in the JAA for SUDI, inquiries have a tendency to complicate when multiple stakeholders, like police agencies, health professionals, and social services, come into play (Höök et al., 2021). Variations in the information reported between these stakeholders have a likelihood of triggering misreporting or underreporting of crucial results, undermining public awareness of the risk factors and etiology of asphyxial deaths. Journalists have to be careful not to swallow too much reliance on first reports or sensationalized but uninformed accounts, since this will incline towards misinformation. Instead, there must be an effort of concerted understanding of the investigative practices in order to present the depth of such tragic incidents correctly and to bring about the demands of families for transparency as well as bereavement guidance. Also, in asphyxial death documentation, moral dimensions encompass implications concerning technological innovations in investigation and their manifestation in media reports. Innovations such as the NeoTap Life Support application, which is designed to facilitate improved neonatal resuscitation in resource-constrained environments, emphasize the significance of innovative interventions in the ability to prevent subsequent deaths from asphyxia (Höök et al., 2021). The difficulty, though, lies in ensuring such technological interventions are properly and accurately portrayed in media coverage without overstating their effectiveness or downplaying underlying systemic issues.

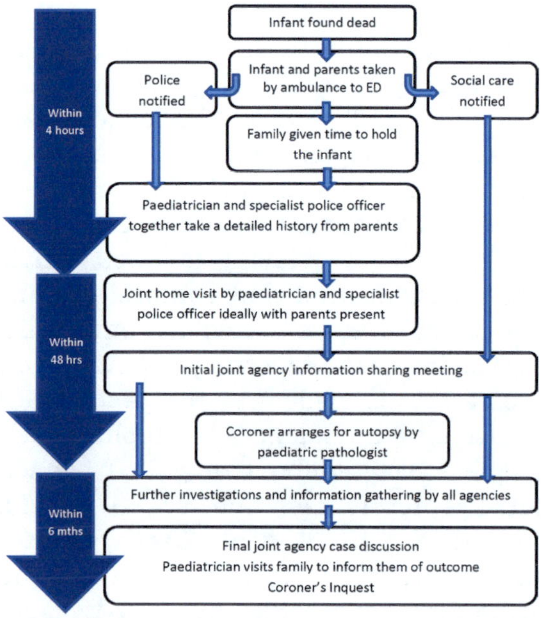

Figure 8.19. Flow chart of JAA investigation.

Source: https://media.springernature.com/full/springer-static/image/art%3A10.1186%2Fs12887-017-0803-2/MediaObjects/12887_2017_803_Fig1_HTML.gif?as=webp.

Media reporting has to reflect the nature of resource disparities while communicating greater comprehension of how such innovations may affect real-world effects in asphyxial incidents. Lastly, ethical reporting of asphyxial needs to be practiced in compliance with honest, sensitive account that honors the lives concerned and upholds the worth of well-informed public debate (Figure 8.19).

8.6.3. Legal Ramifications for Negligence

The law of negligence is involved in handling asphyxial deaths, accidents that are otherwise triggered by inaction or response to dangerous circumstances. In asphyxial deaths due to choking, suffocation, or carbon monoxide poisoning, proving negligence is a question of determining the action—or lack thereof—of individuals or groups of individuals who had a duty of care to them. For instance, physicians, attendants, or house owners may breach their statutory duties by neglecting to exercise reasonable care to protect individuals from asphyxiation hazards. Such negligence not only leads to horrific outcomes but also opens the practice to actions in civil law, where the victims' families sue for wrongful death damages. This model of law aims to hold responsible individuals accountable, and where there are no clear premises of negligence, ultimately encourage a culture of safety and vigilance in situations with potential danger. The interplay between asphyxial deaths and laws of negligence also raises important ethical questions of consent and responsibility. Cases involving individuals voluntarily engaging in risk-taking activities, such as some sadomasochistic activities, may complicate this legal framework of negligence. While others would argue that consent may excuse individuals from liability, the credibility of such a defense has been disputed. The argument is that despite consent being volunteered, it is not sufficient to fully justify harm, especially where the dangers involve drastic outcomes such as asphyxia. Such an argument follows the argument that consent narratives can minimize the seriousness of neglectful conduct and lower accountability. Thus, demarcating a clear line between valid consent and careless conduct is the core issue in legal thinking on asphyxial death. Ultimately, the legal implications of asphyxial death due to negligence pinpoint the necessity to strictly adhere to safety measures and comprehend the duty of care in various settings. Legal precedents show that if negligence is established, the courts can order serious penalties, which are a reflection of the societal requirement for individuals to be prudent and cautious. Within the context of asphyxiation, such negligence can arise from different areas, ranging from healthcare and childcare to domestic relationships. The broader implication of these legal precedents is not just at the level of individual cases but also on policy-making and public health strategies designed to minimize asphyxial episodes. Through the examination of these dynamics, the judicial system not only attempts to provide justice for the victimized families but also attempts to prevent such future occurrences of such incidents by promoting responsible behavior in such potentially deadly events (Figure 8.20).

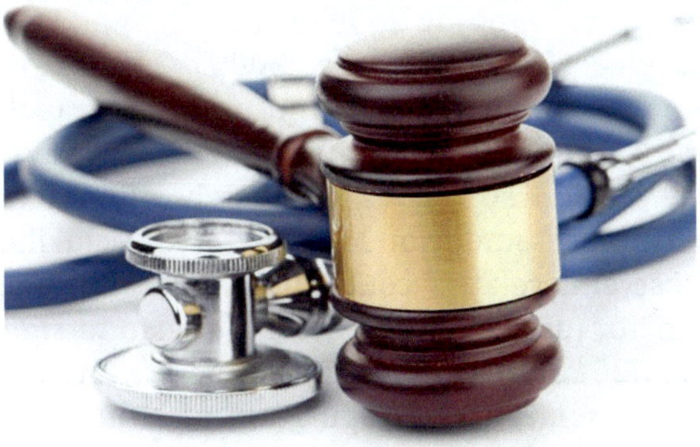

Figure 8.20. Legal ramifications for negligence.

Source: https://cdn.prod.website-files.com/5c9afb07feba5a3a9a87cc93/5ca582e3640690799618cddc_9t2jQZYcyHCnTBotj-icon.jpg.

Test Your Knowledge

1. What is a key challenge in establishing a definitive cause of death in asphyxial deaths?
2. Who can be held legally accountable for negligence leading to asphyxial deaths?

SUMMARY

In summary, asphyxial fatalities in man are a grave public health problem calling for wide-ranging knowledge and targeted interventions. Mechanisms by which asphyxia results in death or significant neurological injury, such as hypoxic-ischemic encephalopathy (HIE), are multifactorial and complex. According to the available data, approximately 4 million infants suffer from birth asphyxia annually, with an astounding 25% of these being fatal and another 25% producing permanent neurological sequelae (Frøyland et al., 2008). The statistics underscore the imperative for improvement in neonatal care processes and prevention techniques that will reduce the incidence of asphyxia at birth. Progress in identifying the pathophysiological mechanisms involved will lead to improved intervention strategies, ultimately minimizing the catastrophic effects conveyed by this form of death. Assessment of asphyxial death clarifies the neurologic consequences ensuing from cardiac arrest and related conditions. Studies indicate cardiac arrest in over 300,000 Americans every year, not just leading to death but also to significant brain injury and cognitive impairment (Combs et al., 2013). The combination of excitotoxicity and neuronal death is further exacerbated by the post-ischemic down-regulation of N-methyl-D-aspartate receptors (NMDAR). These mechanisms shed light on current therapeutic windows for treatment and rehabilitation in the affected patients. Through the application of such knowledge, clinicians can improve planning interventions to avoid neuronal damage and improve recovery in victims of asphyxial incidents and therefore treat acute and chronic consequences. Finally, the management of asphyxial death in humans is a multi-dimensional approach, which includes prevention, intervention, and rehabilitation. Research into the physiological responses to asphyxia will continue to be important in developing effective treatments and ultimately reducing mortality rates. As an illustration, acknowledgment of acidosis as a protective factor and an injurious effect of inflammation during hypoxic events can allow targeted therapy for limiting brain damage (Frøyland et al., 2008). In addition, redefining asphyxial cardiac arrest recovery by examining NMDA receptor mechanisms promises areas of investigation for improved patient care (Combs et al., 2013). With each mounting body of evidence, it is important to distill these results into practice, thus developing an interprofessional strategy for controlling the prevalent issue of asphyxial death.

It is crucial to understand asphyxial death in humans through a comprehensive study of various significant factors, ranging from physiological mechanisms to extrinsic factors. Asphyxia can be caused by a lack of oxygen supply to the tissues, which could be secondary to various conditions, like drowning, strangulation, and suffocation. Loss of consciousness could be rapid, typically within seconds after hypoxic brain damage, leading to permanent brain damage or death within minutes. Critical writing has demonstrated that asphyxia's reaction to the body is variable and depends upon several mechanisms of a biological nature, which, in critical situations, can break down. The necessity of treating asphyxia as soon as possible indicates the imperceptiveness to realize rapid intervention and good resuscitation techniques to improve survival and quality, which is affirmed in today's medical practice. One of the most important aspects of asphyxial death is the classification of such events, since they can happen through accidental as well as intentional actions. For instance, pathways for asphyxia are significantly different in instances of unintentional accidents, such as choking in children, versus intentional accidents, such as suicide by suffocation. An analysis of these accidents gives an insight into the behavior and social conditions resulting in asphyxial accidents. Also, forensic analysis tends to inquire into the context of asphyxial fatalities in establishing legal significance and preventive strategies. With knowledge of motives and environments in which such tragedies occur, public health interventions can be tailored to reduce the frequency of asphyxial fatalities in vulnerable populations. Moreover, investigation of body reactions in asphyxia has provided significant information towards therapeutic interventions. Studies in animal models illustrate the effect of asphyxial cardiac arrest and ensuing neurological effects after hypoxia, illustrated by the study on excitotoxicity and N-methyl-D-aspartate receptors (Combs et al., 2013). Therapeutic application of such agents that target these receptors is an emerging front in treating occurrences after asphyxial events. Beyond this, real-world uses, such as the effectiveness of interventions in prenatal and pediatric care, justify additional research and additional development of targeted treatments (Gurung et al., 2013). Ultimately, knowledge of asphyxial death from a holistic view establishes understanding of the interaction between biological, environmental, and behavioral factors, presenting an opportunity for prevention and improved outcomes in those affected.

KEY TERMS FROM THIS CHAPTER

- Acute hypoxia
- Cardiac arrest
- D-cycloserine
- Heimlich maneuver
- Intra-pyramidal hemorrhage
- Obstructive sleep apnea
- Personalized medicine
- Asphyxia
- Choking
- Drowning
- Hypoxic-ischemic encephalopathy
- Memory loss
- Oxygen deprivation
- Sudden infant death syndrome

CRITICAL THINKING QUESTIONS

1. **What is the primary cause of asphyxial deaths?**
   a. Trauma to internal organs.
   b. Deprivation of oxygen to vital tissues.
   c. Excessive loss of blood.
   d. Sudden cardiac arrest.
2. **Which of the following is a feature of mechanical asphyxia?**
   a. Respiratory depression due to poisoning.
   b. Blockage of the airways by a foreign object.
   c. Lack of oxygen due to reduced atmospheric oxygen levels.
   d. Pressure applied externally, restricting breathing.
3. **Which type of asphyxia is characterized by obstruction of the airway due to external compression of the neck?**
   a. Drowning
   b. Hanging
   c. Strangulation
   d. Smothering
4. **Which physical finding is considered a hallmark of hanging?**
   a. Horizontal ligature mark around the neck.
   b. Fracture of the hyoid bone.
   c. Petechial hemorrhages in the eyes.
   d. Presence of water in the lungs.
5. **What is the term for the pinpoint hemorrhages often seen in asphyxial deaths?**
   a. Cyanosis
   b. Ecchymosis
   c. Petechiae
   d. Abrasions

Short Answer Questions

1. What are asphyxial deaths?
2. List the types of asphyxial deaths.
3. What is the mechanism of asphyxia?
4. What are the causes of asphyxial deaths?
5. What therapy is mentioned as potentially reducing pruritus in obstetric cholestasis?

Answer to Critical Thinking Questions

1. (b); 2. (d); 3. (c); 4. (b); 5. (c)

REFERENCES

1. Aickin, R., Andersen, L. W., Atkins, D. L., et al. (2019). 2019 international consensus on cardiopulmonary resuscitation and emergency cardiovascular care science with treatment recommendations: Summary from the basic life support; advanced life support; pediatric life support; neonatal life support; education, implementation, and teams; and first aid task forces.
2. Alberto Chighine, E., Locci, E., d'Aloja, E., Ferraro, E., Locco, F., Bazzano, G., & Demontis, R. (2020). Forensic NMR metabolomics: One more arrow in the quiver. https://core.ac.uk/download/541243010.pdf (accessed on 12th July 2025).
3. Alhemyari, E. A. A. (1988). Drowning: A study of temporal bone hemorrhage and an analysis of vitreous humour. https://core.ac.uk/download/286352152.pdf (accessed on 12th July 2025).
4. Asmundo, A., Casella, F., Colosimo, F., Di Mizio, G., Di Nunno, N., Feola, A., Manno, E., et al. (2020). Risk management and recommendations for the prevention of fatal foreign body aspiration: Four cases aged 1.5 to 3 years and mini-review of the literature. https://core.ac.uk/download/521183164.pdf (accessed on 12th July 2025).
5. Badu, I. K., Beltrán Aroca, C. M., Girela López, E., et al. (2014). Diatoms in forensic analysis: A practical approach in rats. https://core.ac.uk/download/614632658.pdf (accessed on 12th July 2025).
6. Baldi, A., Chighine, A., d'Aloja, E., De-Giorgio, F., Ferino, G., Locci, E., Noto, A., et al. (2021). Metabolomics improves the histopathological diagnosis of asphyxial deaths: An animal proof-of-concept model. https://core.ac.uk/download/541244817.pdf (accessed on 12th July 2025).
7. Ball, H. L., Blair, P. S., De Bock, F., et al. (2024). Death from failed protection? An evolutionary-developmental theory of sudden infant death syndrome. https://core.ac.uk/download/614766576.pdf (accessed on 12th July 2025).
8. Becher, J. C. (2006). Epidemiological and pathological correlates of early neonatal mortality. https://core.ac.uk/download/429702244.pdf (accessed on 12th July 2025).
9. Candilio, L., Hausenloy, D. J., & Malik, A. (2013). Protection of organs other than the heart by remote ischemic conditioning. https://core.ac.uk/download/16245948.pdf (accessed on 12th July 2025).
10. Cebioglu, M., Golubnitschaja, O., Herrera-Marschitz, M., Morelli, M., & Yeghiazaryan, K. (2011). Birth asphyxia as the major complication in newborns: Moving towards improved individual outcomes by prediction, targeted prevention and tailored medical care. https://core.ac.uk/download/pdf/54569476.pdf (accessed on 12th July 2025).
11. Cenderadewi, M., Devine, S., & Franklin, R. C. (2020). Socio-ecological nature of drowning in low- and middle-income countries: A review to inform health promotion approaches. https://core.ac.uk/download/327170509.pdf (accessed on 12th July 2025).
12. Cipolloni, L., & De Simone, S. (2022). Nitrous oxide intoxication: Systematic literature review and proposal of new diagnostic possibilities. https://core.ac.uk/download/589969956.pdf (accessed on 12th July 2025).
13. Combs, V. M. (2013). Study of brain injury and neurodegenerative effects of D-cyclomerize using an asphyxial cardiac arrest rat model. https://core.ac.uk/download/162579518.pdf (accessed on 12th July 2025).

14. Dickinson, H., Ellery, S., Ireland, Z., et al. (2014). Creatine supplementation during pregnancy: Summary of experimental studies suggesting a treatment to improve fetal and neonatal morbidity and reduce mortality in high-risk human pregnancy. https://core.ac.uk/download/pdf/81094022.pdf (accessed on 12th July 2025).
15. Fletcher, E. (2022). Weapons of choice: A statistical comparison between different weapons and resulting injuries, opportunist weapon selection and forensic awareness. https://core.ac.uk/download/533941028.pdf (accessed on 12th July 2025).
16. Frøyland, E. (2008). Hypoxia in human NT2-N neurons: The role of acidosis, mitochondria, and inflammation. https://core.ac.uk/download/30860448.pdf (accessed on 12th July 2025).
17. Garstang, J. (2025). Why did my baby die? An evaluation of parental and professional experiences of joint agency investigations following sudden unexpected death in infancy. https://core.ac.uk/download/42609043.pdf (accessed on 12th July 2025).
18. Gill, M. A. (2002). Perinatal and late neonatal mortality in the dog. https://core.ac.uk/download/41232423.pdf (accessed on 12th July 2025).
19. Gurung, V., Hague, W., Middleton, P., et al. (2013). Interventions for treating cholestasis in pregnancy (Review). https://core.ac.uk/download/42508066.pdf (accessed on 12th July 2025).
20. Höök, S. M. (2021). Supporting neonatal resuscitation in low-resource settings: Innovations and new strategies. https://core.ac.uk/download/479090276.pdf (accessed on 12th July 2025).
21. Malamitsi-Puchner, A., Panigrahy, A., Panigrahy, A., Shatz, A., Bergman, A. B., Ponsonby, A. L., Williams, A. L., et al. (2011). A perspective on SIDS pathogenesis. The hypotheses: Plausibility and evidence. https://core.ac.uk/download/pdf/8589102.pdf (accessed on 12th July 2025).
22. Masterson, J. (2023). The ethics of kink. https://core.ac.uk/download/591440819.pdf (accessed on 12th July 2025).
23. N/A. (2021). Forensic medicine. https://core.ac.uk/download/478143372.pdf (accessed on 12th July 2025).
24. N/A. (2025). Occupational exposure to hydrazine's. https://core.ac.uk/download/144163578.pdf (accessed on 12th July 2025).
25. Nelson, R. A. (1995). Determining types of health effects to Persian Gulf veterans due to exposure to occupational hazards. https://core.ac.uk/download/588297558.pdf (accessed on 12th July 2025).
26. Tinworth, K. (2003). Arousal, sleep and cardiovascular responses to intermittent hypercapnic hypoxia in piglets. https://core.ac.uk/download/41230090.pdf (accessed on 12th July 2025).
27. Wild, A. (2023). Helicopter winching: Time off chest when performing CPR, manual compressions versus mechanical. https://core.ac.uk/download/588315493.pdf (accessed on 12th July 2025).

TOXICOLOGY IN FORENSIC PATHOLOGY

9

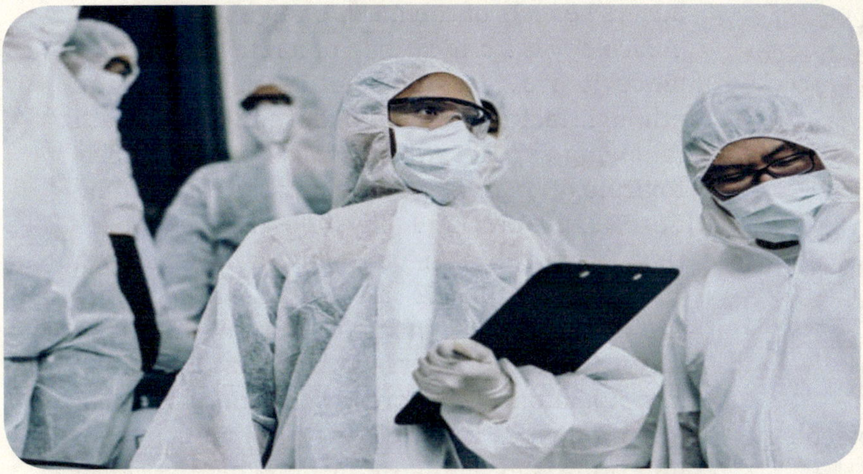

LEARNING OBJECTIVES

After studying this chapter, you will be able to:

1. Understand the various types of toxic substances;
2. Know the methods of toxicological analysis;
3. Understand the toxicology in death investigations;
4. Describe the challenges in forensic toxicology;
5. Describe the advances in forensic toxicology.

Introduction

The crossroad of toxicology and forensic pathology is essential in comprehending the meaning of exposure to substances in death and injury cases. Forensic analysis by toxicology, the science of poisons and drugs that examines the nature, action, and detection of drugs and poisons, is a key contributor in forensic investigations as it identifies toxic compounds that have caused or are causative factors in unexplained deaths. This interdisciplinary process combines pharmacology, chemistry, and pathology to account for the cause and manner of death. A broad introduction to forensic toxicology helps in defining the model analyses necessary for the identification of various toxins, assessment of their biological effects, and determination of relevance in forensic inquiry. For instance, the detection of drugs like zolpidem in postmortem samples can reveal toxicological profiles of death, indicating the importance of toxicological analysis during death investigations (Inés Sánchez-Sellero et al., 2024). Forensic toxicology mostly involves applying toxicological principles and methods of analysis in investigating criminal cases, sudden death, and overdose. It employs advanced techniques such as high-performance liquid chromatography (HPLC) to identify and quantify poisonous substances in biological samples, with vital information for forensic investigation. Verification of these techniques ensures that they are precise and reliable for both clinical and forensic purposes. For instance, there has been the establishment of a highly advanced HPLC-PDA technique for the determination of zolpidem concentrations in postmortem plasma, which shows extensive correlations with deaths when there are co-ingestions involving alcohol or other drugs (Inés Sánchez-Sellero et al., 2024).

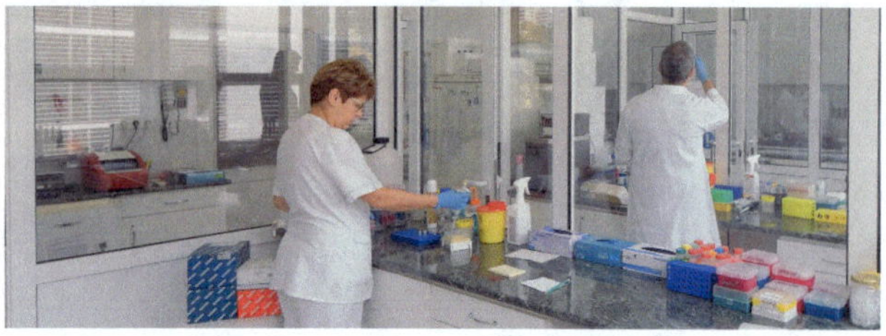

Figure 9.1. Forensic pathology and toxicology.

Source: https://aok.pte.hu/storage/menukep/110/0110_Igazsagugy_HDfejlec.jpg.

This analytical capability is all-important as it helps forensic pathologists deliver medically and legally valid opinions and also enhances public security by comprehending the risks inherent in particular toxins. The insertion of artificial intelligence into toxicology and forensic pathology brings new opportunities as well as challenges to the practice. Automated systems can potentially enhance data analysis and aid in the processing of large amounts of data, potentially increasing the validity of toxicological determinations. As stressed in current studies, AI tools in forensic use can assist post-mortem diagnosis and toxicological examinations, bringing significant advances in thanatology and forensic traumatology. Based on these benefits, however, legal responsibility issues and the implementation of AI in diagnostic processes must be thoroughly assessed. Forensic scientists should view AI as an auxiliary tool rather than a replacement for expertise, retaining final conclusions dependent on empirical evidence and professional judgment in the complexity of toxicological analysis (Figure 9.1).

Definition of Toxicology

Toxicology is a science that deals with the adverse effects of chemicals on living organisms. Toxicology is a critical area of forensic pathology since it provides information regarding the etiologic factors leading to morbidity and death following exposure to toxic agents. At its core, toxicology examines the relationships among dose, exposure, and physiological responses that chemicals can cause in living systems. This philosophy is also used in learning the mechanisms of toxic action, allowing forensic toxicologists to correlate victims' symptomatology with presumed toxins. In human pathology, the knowledge of individual toxin identities is essential ~~to~~ for knowing the cause of death in suspicious or unexplained deaths, and this information is of vital importance that can guide legal investigation and contribute to public health understanding on a broader scale. As toxicology science advances, its application in forensic pathology has also increased significantly, with ever-growing focus placed on the identification and analysis of specific toxins, particularly when dealing with emerging drugs. For instance, reliance on synthetic opioids such as fentanyl reflects the challenges facing forensic toxicologists today. Fentanyl is known to be highly potent—50 to 100 times more potent than morphine and traditionally associated with an emergent pattern of overdose death. The rapid onset and versatility of administration routes of fentanyl make the forensic toxicology scenario challenging, demanding sensitive detection and quantification in biological samples (Adley et al., 2017). This points to the value of toxicology in establishing the existence of specific substances and determining their potential involvement in death, thereby maintaining the field's value in forensic investigations. Besides chemicals and drugs, toxicology encompasses a broader field of biological interactions like the involvement of parasites in forensic examination. Whereas traditional toxicology is focused on chemical substances, the inclusion of forensic parasitology opens up new opportunities for analysis at crime scenes. Parasites can be utilized to provide insightful details about what transpired during a crime and can be utilized by forensic experts to evaluate sources of toxic exposure. For example, certain parasites have specific host behavior or environments that can indicate malice or add further information about a victim's circumstances (Alves et al., 2017). This cross-fertilization between parasitology and toxicology adds a plus to forensic pathology, enabling practitioners to reenact complex stories of death and providing critical facts for court cases (Figure 9.2).

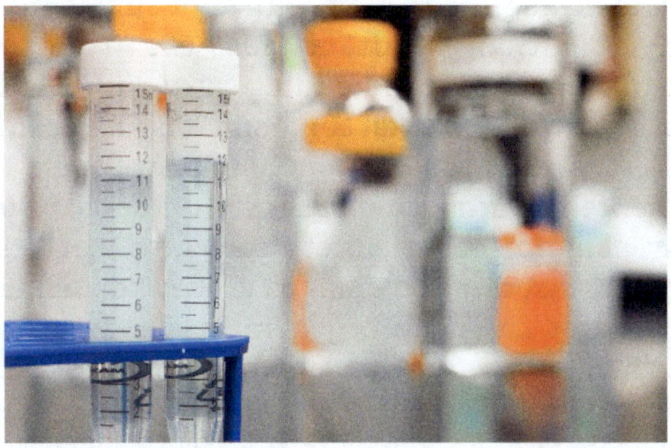

Figure 9.2. Toxicology.

Source: https://forensicresources.org/wp-content/uploads/2019/05/biology-blur-blurred-background-954585.jpg.

Role of Forensic Pathology

Forensic pathology is a pillar in pursuing justice in criminal proceedings, particularly where toxicological data is pivotal in determining the cause of death. As a subspecialty in medicine, forensic pathology entails the investigation of deceased persons to uncover the causes of their deaths. This discipline is especially valuable in cases where suspected poisoning from drugs, alcohol, or even environmental toxins is thought to have been a factor in death. By employing rigorous autopsy techniques and toxicology tests, forensic pathologists can provide useful information that helps guide law enforcement and court proceedings. The integration of toxicology into forensic pathology not only educates on individual cases further but also contributes more profoundly to heightened public awareness regarding substance abuse and environmental poisons. It is through such precise processes that forensic pathology retains its role in serving justice and ensuring public safety. The collaboration between toxicology and forensic pathology also has important public health implications, which are emphasized in contemporary forensic practice. An understanding of the interface of dangerous substances and health consequences enables forensic pathologists to guide concerned parties, including policymakers and public health officials. To this extent, comprehensive toxicological reports can provide illumination on patterns in death caused by substances, directing preventive efforts and public sensitization of the dangers of drug abuse and poisoning. Forensic examinations, for instance, typically demonstrate patterns in the use of illicit drugs that correspond with particular demographic variables. Such data not only contribute to the resolution of individual cases but also generate a perception of awareness for the wide social impacts of drug abuse, thereby requiring interventions in public health. Similar to other sections of forensic science, constant development of advanced toxicological techniques is essential to improve the accuracy of diagnoses within forensic pathology, thereby improving community health outcomes in general. Moreover, forensic pathology developments confirm the necessity for interdisciplinary collaboration to overcome the special difficulties of toxicological investigations. Due to developing technologies and methods, forensic pathologists have to cooperate in their work with toxicologists, clinical pharmacists, and jurists to become familiar in-depth with the toxic effects on human health. Through such unification of competencies, forensic investigations can be more efficient. For instance, new methods like molecular autopsy and digital pathology are transforming the level of capability that forensic pathologists have, allowing for greater precision in identifying toxins and what they do. Furthermore, compensating for difficulties experienced in low-resource areas like those described in Zambia's forensic system highlights the need to implement standardized protocols and educational channels. Lastly, the role of forensic pathology—particularly that of toxicology—requires a commitment to continuing improvement and the sharing of information with the broader forensics community so that justice is served fairly and equitably (Figure 9.3).

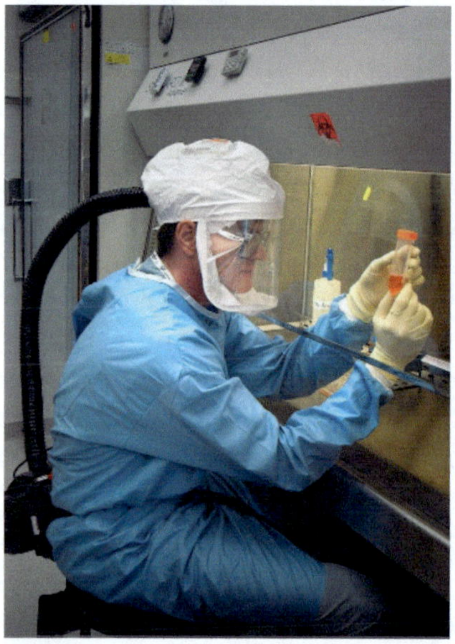

Figure 9.3. Role of a forensic pathologist.

Source: https://www.crimemuseum.org/wp-content/uploads/2023/08/Forensic-Pathologist.jpg.

Importance of Toxicology in Legal Investigations

Toxicology is at the heart of forensic investigations of poisoning, drug overdose death, and exposure to environmental toxins. Through analysis of biological fluids such as blood, urine, or tissue, toxicologists can detect and quantify the amount of toxic substances in order for investigators to determine how these factors contributed to the death of an individual. Forensic toxicology, aside from helping to determine cause and manner of death, is also helpful in identifying intent, such as drug-related homicides or suicides. Such large-scale analysis enhances the efficiency of the legal process via scientifically valid evidence, hence helping in the determination of culpability or innocence of suspects. The most cautious character of toxicological investigations also channels into general public health data, underlining the need for strict regulatory procedures in preventing exposure to injurious substances in society. Moreover, the merging of toxicological results with epidemiological investigation substantiates the role of toxicology in understanding systemic health issues. Environmental contaminants and health effects are increasingly ~~firmly~~ acknowledged, as science has attributed causality to exposure to air pollution for a variety of central nervous system diseases, including neurodevelopmental disorders and neurodegenerative diseases like Alzheimer's and Parkinson's disease. Increased awareness of these associations means that toxicology is no longer in the form of isolated instances, impacting broader public health policy and the legal system. Therefore, forensic toxicology results not only aid specific legal inquiries but also highlight the importance of comprehensive environmental health strategies with a focus on prevention and not response. By capturing these correlations, toxicologists are able to assist in setting regulatory measures that safeguard community health from toxic environmental exposures. In addition to serving as imperative evidence in criminal trials, the importance of toxicology can be observed in quality control and public safety. Toxicological measurements are more commonly utilized by regulatory bodies to inform levels of materials in consumer goods and the public environment that are safe, exemplified in the widespread scope of sources like Sweden's register of deaths, linking environmental health measures to death rates. Such datasets enhance the understanding of the effects of toxic exposures on altering health consequences over time and across groups, thus informing legislation to minimize risk. Toxicology also serves as an important bridge between scientific investigation and legal standards, emphasizing interdisciplinary interaction as vital in addressing toxic exposures to realize significant progress. This alliance not only aids defense and prosecution during litigation but also fosters a better-informed public discourse on the issues related to health policies and environmental regulations so that living habitats are made safer for communities.

9.1. Types of Toxic Substances

Learning Outcome

1. Examine the natural toxins.
2. Describe the synthetic drugs.
3. Describe the presence of heavy metals in the environment.

Understanding the various types of poisonous materials is very important in forensic pathology, particularly when experts are attempting to identify the cause of death in enigmatic cases. Toxic agents may generally be classified as chemical, biological, or physical agents. Chemical agents like heavy metals, pesticides, and drugs are harmful by ingestion, inhalation, or through dermal absorption. Moreover, the versatility of biological toxins, ranging from bacteria and their toxins to natural peptides, is extremely significant in toxicological examinations. Each type of toxic substance possesses its unique behavior in the human system, demanding a complete understanding of its effect and mode of action in order to have accurate forensic analysis. Toxic substance complexities are also heightened by the reality of drug interactions and the resulting challenges in terms of determining toxicity thresholds. An example is that in the case of multiple substances, post-mortem drug concentrations are very important but are marred by challenges as they rely on factors such as the timing of sampling and intersubject variability in metabolism. Researchers have noted that existing databases that began as data aggregates have since been augmented to cover sophistications such as sample origin and the co-prescription of multiple drugs. This sophistication is demonstrated by a Bayesian network model developed to quantify the chances of fatal outcomes due to drug levels, as evident in Bolton et al. (2015). These trends highlight the requirement for forensic toxicologists to approach each case both in terms of known information and case-specific factors. Caffeine, an omnipresent but potent drug, illustrates the dualistic quality of toxic substances, displaying both favorable and adverse consequences based upon levels of usage. While caffeine is mostly employed for its stimulating property, enabling concentration and physical performance, abuse has far-reaching health consequences, from toxicity to early death. Caffeine has been shown to react unfavorably with other substances, thus offering enhanced risks that complicate the forensic analysis. Defined by Aromatario et al. (2015), the comparative toxicity of caffeine shows that even non-toxic amounts can be involved in fatal outcomes when combined with a pre-existing medication or condition. Such complicating factors can indicate the need for a sophisticated appreciation of toxic agents in forensic pathology, especially as experts navigate the interrelated issues of consumption, addiction, and fatal consequence (Figure 9.4).

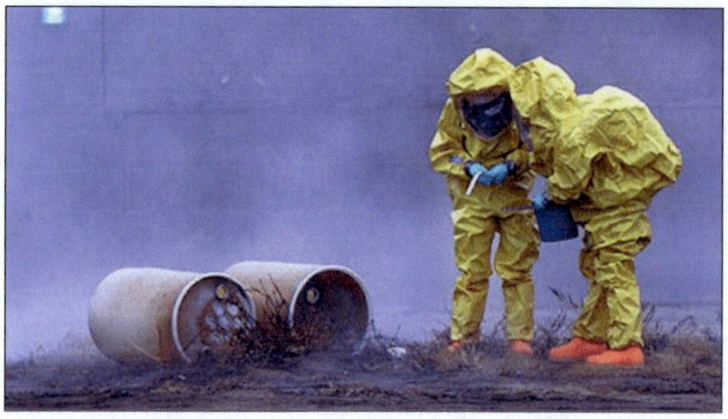

Figure 9.4. Toxic substances.

Source: https://healthybuildingscience.com/wp-content/uploads/2014/11/Toxic-Substances-Its-not-always-this-obvious.png.

9.1.1. Natural Toxins

Natural toxin analysis is among the most critical fields of toxicology in forensic pathology, particularly when determining their participation in cases of poisoning or sudden death. Natural toxins are chemical substances produced by living organisms, including plants, animals, and microbes, with the ability to negatively affect human health. They occur in various forms with varying impacts on biological systems. Forensic pathologists are constantly confronted with cases where victims consume toxic plants or become poisoned by poisonous species and need to have advanced knowledge of their biochemical interactions with the human body. Quantitation and determination of such toxins could be problematic, yet it is crucial to establish causal correlations in toxicology cases since the detection of a specific natural toxin can be a decisive piece of evidence in forensic examinations. In addition, advances in analytical techniques have significantly enhanced the identification and analysis of natural toxins in biological samples. Techniques such as liquid chromatography-mass spectrometry (LC-MS) have revolutionized forensic toxicology by enabling the detection of multiple toxins from various sources simultaneously. This method is amenable to combining various sample clean-up techniques, such as the "dilute-and-shoot" process, which makes the extraction process easier and allows complex biological matrices to be analyzed. The sensitivity and flexibility of these new analytical methods have provided forensic pathologists with the capability to decisively respond to the threat of natural poisons, particularly in polytoxic exposure. Increased analysis capacity also means that forensic scientists can better comprehend how these chemicals lead to death, resulting in improved toxicological analysis accuracy and support to legal cases (Greer et al., 2021). Finally, an understanding of the role played by natural toxins in forensic analysis is not merely identification.

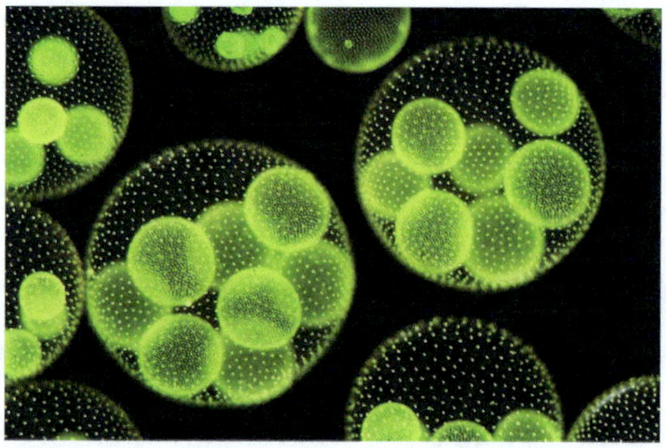

Figure 9.5. Natural toxins.

Source: https://media.springernature.com/lw725/springer-cms/rest/v1/content/17730384/data/v1.

It is a broader realization of the socio-cultural and environmental contexts in which such toxins are present. Natural toxins can be applied to medication or ritual practice in some societies, making their classification intricate and, consequently, the interpretation of results in forensic analysis. Plant poisons such as aconite or castor beans are not only potent but are often buried in historical-cultural contexts that require careful interpretation. In forensic investigations, it is crucial to determine whether the exposure was accidental, intentional, or socio-cultural practice related. This tacit appreciation enhances the pursuit of justice and proper understanding of circumstances near death associated with natural toxins, thus enhancing the debate in forensic pathology (Poalelungi et al., 2023) (Figure 9.5).

9.1.2. Synthetic Drugs

Synthetic drugs have been posing significant challenges to forensic toxicology, and new methods of analysis are needed to detect such drugs. Synthetic cannabinoids and synthetic opioids are designed to mimic the effects of traditional illicit drugs but avoid controls. Synthetic drugs are more potent, and hence more cases of overdose and death occur. An example was a recent case where a 30-year-old man died after consuming synthetic drugs, including U-47700, an opioid that is said to be 7.5 times more potent than morphine. This shows how dangerous synthetic drugs are because the extent of their effects tends to be underestimated by consumers who don't know they are highly toxic (Blanckaert et al., 2016). Therefore, forensic pathologists have to adopt advanced methods for systematic toxicological analysis of biological samples to detect and quantify these highly complex substances. Synthetic cannabinoids are also a wide category of synthetic drugs that have gained attention in the area of forensic pathology, along with opioids.

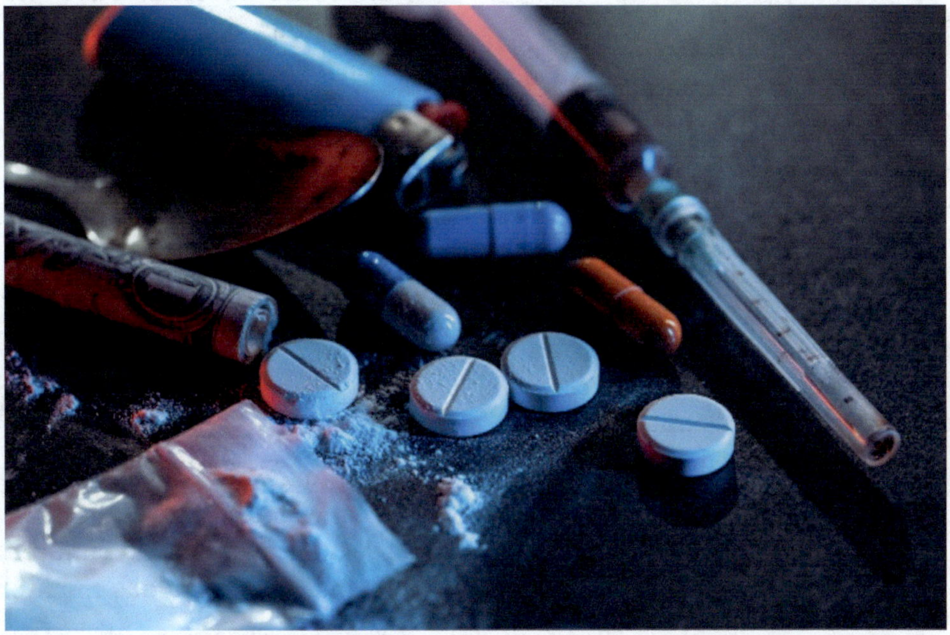

Figure 9.6. Synthetic drugs.

Source: https://www.cdc.gov/chemical-threats-and-toxins-laboratory/media/images/2024/05/synthetic-drugs-G.jpg.

These drugs are chemically diverse and are full agonists at the receptors of the endocannabinoid systems, producing effects that generally surpass those of natural cannabis in intensity. Side effects of their consumption can be effects that appear similar to extreme psychological disorders like agitation, psychosis, and compromised cognitive function, that mimic aspects of schizophrenia. The higher risk of cardiotoxicity among consumers of synthetic cannabinoids contributes to the threat they pose because reports of acute medical emergencies have been overwhelmingly prevalent (Corazza et al., 2017). With continually evolving legislation on cannabis and its analogs, forensic experts should be vigilant and aware of what the consequences of synthetic types entail, particularly because they raise serious issues regarding public safety and public health. The toxicological examination of novel drugs is intricate, involving pharmacological profiling and legal considerations. Forensic toxicologists must confront the daunting task of performing comprehensive examinations to establish causality in probable overdose situations in a setting where the legality and availability of drugs are subject to perpetual change.

This demands the analysis of new trends in drug use and the development of tailored analytical strategies capable of detecting new psychoactive drugs. Prevention and education are immediately necessary, as the forensic community of pathologists strives to remain up to date on synthetic drug design innovations (Corazza et al., 2017). Not only are laboratory techniques to be improved, but also cooperation between law enforcement, physicians, and toxicologists must be boosted in order to create an integrated approach towards mitigating the public health crisis precipitated by these new synthetic drugs (Figure 9.6).

9.1.3. Heavy Metals and Environmental Toxins

Heavy metal environmental occurrence poses a severe risk to human health, a situation that has been long-standing in toxicology and forensic pathology. In fact, metals such as arsenic, lead, and mercury have become powerful environmental poisons, yet they have critical functions in human physiology. Arsenic, frequently found in water supply contamination and produce, is widely recognized for its potential to induce malignancies and skin disease. Through investigative toxicology, forensic pathologists can analyze tissue samples to quantify levels of such heavy metals, thereby ascertaining sources of exposure and potential health risks. The ongoing industrialization further exacerbates the issue, necessitating increased awareness and regulatory measures to guard against exposure to such harmful substances. Hence, it is imperative to understand heavy metal biochemical processes in order to remedy public health issues resulting from environmental toxins, hence informing forensic examination and legal accountability (Achparaki et al., 2012). Moreover, the diverse origins of heavy metals underscore the complexity of environmental toxicology.

Exposure to lead, once prevalent with its ubiquitous use in paint and motor fuel, continues to be a concern in inner cities as well as among workers in certain occupations. Blood and organ tissue tests used in forensic pathology can yield important information about lead toxicity, especially dangerous to developing children, disabling intellectual capacity, and growth. Mercury, another very effective environmental poison, is also amplified up the food chain—especially ocean food chains—yielding higher concentrations in fish and other animals. Forensic examination of mercury toxicity can help illuminate exposure patterns, especially in vulnerable populations, like pregnant women and children, thus adding importance to meticulous monitoring.

Through examining the patterns of heavy metal accumulation, forensic pathologists are able to provide significant data to public health initiatives (Achparaki et al., 2012). Industry processes and environmental contamination overlap, making cadmium exposure even more complex. Shared application in batteries and certain agricultural fertilizers, cadmium presents itself as a carcinogenic hazard. Forensic toxicology measures cadmium levels in biological samples to aid in the investigation of intentional poisoning or occupational exposure. The impact of cadmium exposure goes beyond acute toxicity to encourage chronic health impairment, including kidney damage and bone demineralization. It is thus essential for forensic toxicologists to update their methods to adequately quantify the heavy metals and assess their toxic effects. In addition, enforcement of public health programs that would restrict exposure to such environmental toxins remains paramount. With interdisciplinary interaction among toxicologists, public health officials, and policy makers, society can institute effective prevention strategies for heavy metal-induced health crises and design a safer environment for all (Figure 9.7).

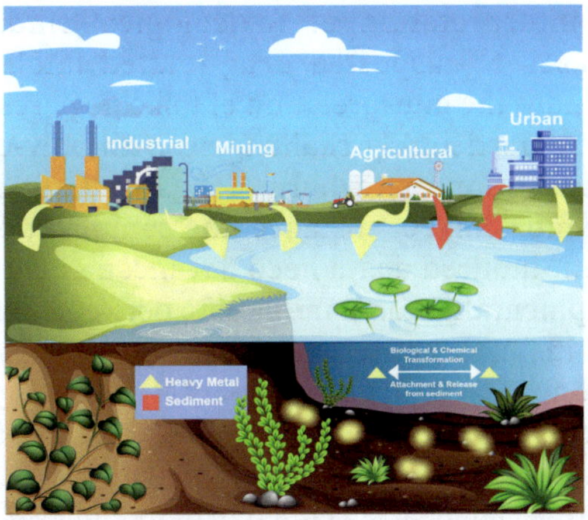

Figure 9.7. Diagrammatic explanation of heavy metals in the environment.

Source: https://ars.els-cdn.com/content/image/1-s2.0-S1018364722000465-gr1_lrg.jpg.

Test Your Knowledge

1. What are natural toxins?
2. What are synthetic drugs?

9.2. Methods of Toxicological Analysis

Learning Outcome

1. Know the process of sample collection and preservation.
2. Describe the analytical techniques.
3. Interpret the toxicological results.

In the field of forensic pathology, toxicological analysis methods are invaluable tools in the detection of the presence of drugs and poisons in post-mortem tests. One such ubiquitous method is liquid chromatography coupled with mass spectrometry (LC-MS/MS), which facilitates precise quantitation of various substances in biological matrices. This technique is highly sensitive and specific, hence allowing forensic scientists to detect trace amounts of drugs in matrices such as brain, liver, and blood tissues. Because toxicological analysis is complicated, the accuracy of findings relies on proper sample collection and preparation since any deviation may lead to inaccurate conclusions about the cause of death. An important aspect of this work is the understanding of the metabolic pathways of drugs, which can directly affect the interpretation of toxicological findings in cases of suspected drug-related fatalities. Secondly, the interpretation of toxicology results can be particularly challenging with poly-drug consumption or where drugs redistribute post-mortem. For instance, the complexities of heroin-induced death need advanced analytical equipment that can differentiate between heroin and its metabolites, such as morphine and 6-monoacetylmorphine (6-MAM). A study of toxicology results of 44 heroin-induced deaths highlighted the importance of using vitreous humor as an ideal specimen in detecting 6-MAM, which is crucial in proving heroin use. The presence of other drugs, such as codeine and papaverine, complicates the interpretation, given that they are indicative of illicit drug preparations. This points to the significance of meticulous toxicological analyses, given the level of detail involved in post-mortem analyses, which must be rigorously scrutinized to ascertain cause and mode of death (Beer et al., 2018). The incorporation of a Bayesian network model can introduce interpretive strength to toxicological information in forensic pathology by facilitating a more integrated assessment of drug levels against pathological endpoints. Such an approach is instrumental in assigning probabilities to the likelihood of fatality due to the presence of drugs, with consideration of the complex interaction between the substances involved in overdose cases. These systems complement the analytical process but also provide a methodological tool for the prediction of outcomes in cases where drugs are a causative factor, enhancing the accuracy of death certification. It gives forensic practitioners an idiomatic tool against conventional toxicological examination, enabling them to better assess the components leading to drug-related deaths (Bolton et al., 2015). With these advances, toxicological analysis remains an essential element in the forensic process, seeking to elucidate the often murky circumstances of human death (Figure 9.8).

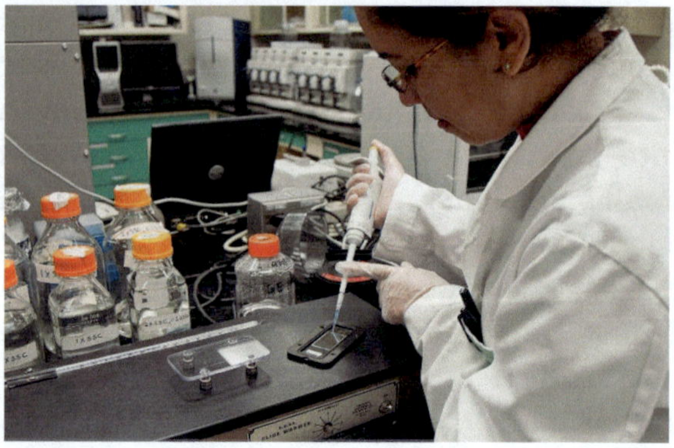

Figure 9.8. A toxicologist working in a lab.

Source: https://upload.wikimedia.org/wikipedia/commons/0/03/Toxicology_Research_at_FDA_%28NCTR_1193%29_%286009043040%29.jpg.

The process of sample collection and preservation is critical in toxicology, particularly in forensic pathology. Forensic pathologists must ensure that biological samples are collected in a manner that maintains their integrity throughout the investigation. This entails proper procedures in collecting specimens such as blood, urine, or tissue samples because any form of contamination or degradation would lead to false conclusions. Protocols that guarantee the proper use of aseptic techniques and environmental controls must be followed under such circumstances. Placing sound sample collection at the top can help forensic pathologists ensure maximum reliability in toxicological examinations subsequently conducted in laboratories. Enforcing a strict standard of sample preservation guarantees evidence presented is capable of standing up to the scrutiny of the courts and can be attributed to the final causes of death when evaluating potential toxic exposures, utmost in pursuing public health objectives and legal justice. Proper preservation methods are as critical as collection methods. Forensic samples can be susceptible to degradation due to temperature variation, exposure to light, or chemical reaction. Thus, adequate preservatives or storage, for instance, refrigeration or freezing, should be utilized, depending on the type of sample and the expected holding period before analysis. Abiding by set protocols allows forensic toxicologists to ensure chemical equilibria are maintained for sound toxicological analysis. Moreover, sample type classification, such as the distinction between antemortem and postmortem samples, is of paramount importance in establishing the physiological condition of the subjects under scientific investigation. Such classification can guide the interpretation of toxicological results, enhancing the clarity of correlations established in cases where exposure to the substances is suspected, and the legal implications of forensic evidence. Due to the multidisciplinary nature of forensic analysis, coordination among several diverse forensic professionals is usually necessary to ensure appropriate assessments. Proper sample collection and preservation procedures are more than just simple toxicologists; they intersect with veterinarians, pathologists, and law enforcement officers who may be responding to a crime scene. The suggested formats that enable documentation of field evidence are essential elements in this interdisciplinary work, enabling free communication across disciplines without compromising the dignity and integrity of the gathered evidence. Documentation cannot be overstressed; it provides vital background that can inform subsequent analyses. Adequate training of forensic and first responders in collection and preservation protocols, coupled with careful documentation methods, enhances the effectiveness of the forensic process from the time of discovery through its presentation at trial, ultimately improving toxicology as a science within forensic pathology (Cecchi et al., 2023; Barrett et al., 2015) (Figure 9.9).

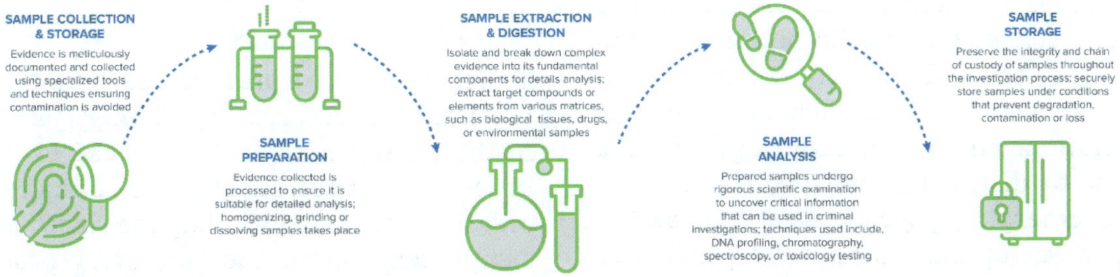

Figure 9.9. The forensic evidence collection and management process.

Source: https://cms-resources.coleparmer.com/a/Forensics-Hero2.jpg.

9.2.1. Analytical Techniques (e.g., Chromatography, Mass Spectrometry)

Forensic toxicology relies heavily on advanced analytical techniques for the identification and quantification of chemicals in biological specimens, which is crucial in the investigation of cases of poisoning. Chromatography, including gas chromatography (GC) and high-performance liquid chromatography (HPLC), underpins the analytical process. These approaches allow for the separation of complex mixtures into distinct elements and are tractable to careful analysis. For instance, GC is most appropriate for volatile materials, whereas HPLC is best used for non-volatile compounds that might be derivatizable. By employing these methods, forensic toxicologists are capable of preparing samples such as blood and urine for subsequent analysis to provide more accurate toxicological findings. For example, in a case of fatal overdose involving fentanyl and U-47700, gas chromatography mass spectrometry (GC-MS) was instrumental in the quantitative determination of the levels of these drugs, describing the circumstances around the death of the victim (Blanckaert et al., 2016). Mass spectrometry (MS) complements the forensic toxicology capabilities further by providing accurate molecular details about the analytes. Coupled with chromatography, MS is capable of identifying and quantifying complex analytes with high specificity and sensitivity. This is particularly important in the case of poisoning because traditional procedures may not be advanced enough to differentiate between structurally related compounds. Advancements in liquid chromatography tandem mass spectrometry (LC-MS/MS) have enormously improved the sensitivity of detection of various toxins so that forensic pathologists can screen for microgram or even nanogram quantities present in tissue or fluid. In recent studies of orrelanine (OR) toxicity, novel LC-MS/MS methods demonstrated the potential for detection of OR in kidney tissue at a low limit of detection of only 20 ng/g, demonstrating the potential of such methods to improve diagnosis accuracy in forensic evidence of mushroom intoxication (Anantharam et al., 2016). The amalgamation of mass spectrometry and chromatography has revolutionized forensic toxicology with the capability to distinguish not just established but also emerging psychoactive substances. With synthetic opioids and novel psychoactive substances appearing on the scene, sensitive and encompassing analytical techniques are increasingly essential. By adjusting techniques to target new compounds, forensic toxicologists can remain ahead of shifting drug patterns and provide law enforcers with significant evidence. When victims may have consumed new psychoactive substances but with no clear indications in post-mortem examination, tools like the detection of U-47700 have been of great importance. The ever-evolving nature of these analytical technologies not only enhances the effectiveness of toxicological analysis but also plays an important role in the orientation of drug-related incidents within public health interventions, making it a perfect marriage between forensic science and community safety initiatives (Figure 9.10).

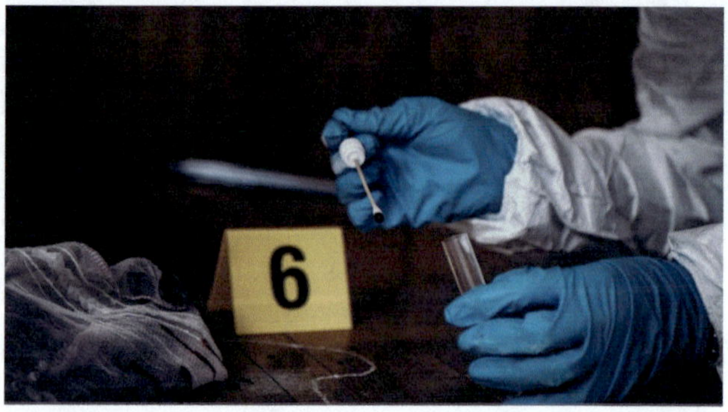

Figure 9.10. Spectroscopy techniques are most useful in forensics.

Source: https://www.azooptics.com/image-handler/ts/20230720041830/ri/950/src/images/Article_Images/ImageForArticle_2456_16898411093734469.jpg.

9.2.2. Interpretation of Toxicological Results

Toxicological interpretation is a complex but essential part of forensic pathology, particularly in the determination of the cause of death in drug-related cases. Effective interpretation relies on various factors, including the rigorousness of sample acquisition and laboratory processing, knowledge of the medical history of the victim, and the specific circumstances of every case. Post-mortem drug concentrations are most probably misleading; that is, drug redistribution may produce fluctuations in drug levels after death. Forensic practitioners must therefore be cautious in their methodology, using databases and pre-set reference tables, and placing in the background individual case vulnerabilities in order to present contextualized results. These are supplemented by expert systems, such as a Bayesian network system, to help apply a probability of death through the assistance of drug concentrations in pathological observations, thereby complementing the need for an interpretation of toxicological results at more than one level in forensic cases (Bolton et al., 2015). Heroin deaths are a complex case in the interpretation of toxicological findings based on their complex pharmacodynamics and all the metabolites that indicate use. 6-Monoacetylmorphine (6-MAM) is a key marker for heroin use, but with limited postmortem samples, the interpretation becomes complicated. In morphine and metabolite studies, the identification of morphine, morphine-3-glucuronide, and morphine-6-glucuronide in other biological matrices has helped a lot in providing insightful recommendations to forensic scientists. Regardless of this, it should be noted that detection variations may occur in other tissues, which complicates the development of an extensive toxicological profile. Thus, full comprehension of the action of such metabolites within post-mortem environments is of paramount importance in enabling solid interpretation and is a critical component in unveiling the dynamics of heroin use deaths (Beer et al., 2018). Aside from technical challenges created by toxicological analysis, efficient interpretation is reliant on the integration of toxicological data into forensic pathology contexts. This entails understanding the effect of various factors, such as time since death and other chemicals present, on drug clearance and drug metabolism. Interplay between pathological findings and toxicological evidence enhances the validity of conclusions arrived at from the investigation. Forensic pathologists must also merge this information judiciously, as misinterpretation can lead to severe legal consequences. Hence, a convergence of the field of toxicology with the general topic of the forensic case not only enhances the quality of examination but also guarantees that the findings serve to inform appropriate legal conclusions. Through interdisciplinary effort, forensic investigators can leverage toxicological results in informing their understanding of behavioral trends, effects of substance abuse, and ultimately the intricate causations of drug-related fatalities (Bolton et al., 2015; Beer et al., 2018).

Test Your Knowledge

1. What is the process of sample collection?
2. What are the analytical techniques?

9.3. Toxicology in Death Investigations

Learning Outcome

1. Determine the cause of death.
2. Distinguish between accidental and intentional poisoning.
3. Explore the role of case studies in toxicology.

Toxicology is an essential tool in death cases in forensic pathology since it provides valuable information regarding the cause of death from exposure to chemicals. Toxicological analysis is done for the detection of the presence and quantification of drugs, alcohol, and other poisons in body fluids. These analyses are important not just to decide the mode of death—whether accidental, suicidal, or homicidal—but also to establish the likely impact of drugs on the deceased's behavior that led to death. With improving techniques, forensic toxicologists can manage challenges like the discrimination of antemortem and postmortem chemical alterations that might complicate death investigation conclusions. The increasing sophistication of chemicals implicated in fatalities has prompted forensic toxicologists to extend their analytical techniques. Traditional immunoassay methods, though highly sensitive and convenient, are not good at distinguishing between closely similar chemical compounds. As recent publications amply illustrate, liquid chromatography coupled with mass spectrometry has emerged as an indispensable tool in forensic use. This sophisticated technique enhances selectivity by the power to distinguish between various types of insulin and its breakdown products, which is vital in cases of suspected insulin-related death, as noted in emphasizing the importance of precise toxicological examination (Bottinelli et al., 2020).

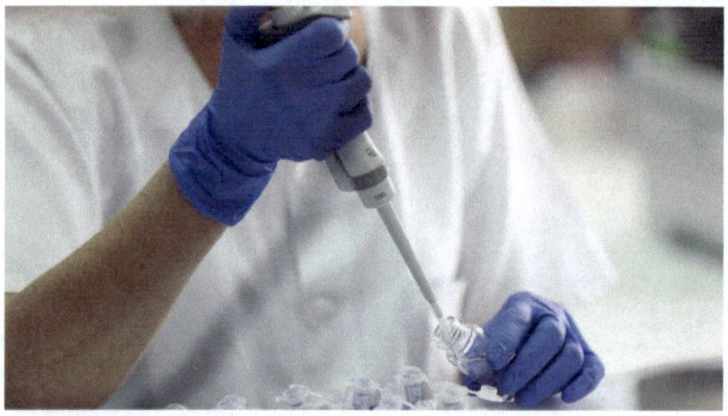

Figure 9.11. Toxicology tests in death investigations.

Source: https://images.foxtv.com/static.fox10phoenix.com/www.fox10phoenix.com/content/uploads/2023/11/1280/720/GETTY-Toxicology-Test-111523.jpg?ve=1&tl=1.

Hence, the choice of the analytic technique has significant implications for the outcome of death investigations since misinterpretation can lead to misleading findings about the cause of an individual's death. Moreover, the examination of various biological matrices has widened the scope of toxicological tests. While blood remains the initial sample to be tested, examination of various alternative matrices, for example, vitreous humor and tissue samples, also yields information of some utility supportive of toxicological findings. As an example, detection of drugs in muscle or in renal cortex can yield evidence of prior drug administration not detected in blood samples. Understanding the intricacies of how drugs metabolize upon death and the influence of factors on concentration levels is significant (Yuan et al., 2025). Finally, the interdisciplinary nature of toxicology in death investigation not only lends credibility to forensic pathology but is also required to achieve justice and understand the complex relationship between substance and death (Figure 9.11).

9.3.1. Role in Determining Cause of Death

Determination of the cause of death is an important function of forensic pathology, particularly where there is a toxicological implication. Autopsies are typically performed to ascertain the presence of toxins in body fluids and tissues and can provide information on potential causes of death that are not immediately obvious. Forensic toxicology, being a branch of forensic science, is concerned with microscopic examination of body fluids to identify drugs, alcohol, toxins, and other chemical compounds responsible for death. With the integration of toxicological findings with medico-legal autopsies, pathologists are able to provide detailed information about the cause of death. These studies not only assist criminal prosecution but also contribute to public health knowledge through patterns of drug use or exposure, ultimately informing preventive interventions for populations at risk. Sweden, for instance, the systematic recording of cause of death through the Swedish cause of death register illustrates how toxicology influences broad research agendas. Established in 1952, this register is a rich collection in which one can perform in-depth analysis of mortality data by groups and periods. From the analysis of this large data set, researchers will be able to establish trends in causes of death, including deaths caused by toxicological agents. By comparing mortality data with social and health data, the register provides vital background to gauge the impact of environmental forces on mortality rates. It is necessary for researchers and public health specialists to determine the strengths and limitations of such registries in a bid to optimize the impact of toxicological data on mortality research and health policy development (Hannah et al., 2017). The role of toxicology in forensic pathology becomes exceedingly obvious in cases of sudden and unanticipated death, for instance, those that are investigated among youths and children. Sudden cardiac death, for example, may be linked to unexpected toxicological causes, and forensic toxicology is therefore most important in these cases. The integration of clinical data with toxicological analysis yields a clearer image of the physiological status of the body at the time of death. Detailed investigations that analyze genetic and toxicological backgrounds are of the utmost significance and provide us with critical information that has the potential to reshape our understanding of the risk factors associated with sudden death among young persons (Richard et al., 2016). Therefore, starting an efficient toxicological inquiry system within forensic pathology not only increases cause of death certification precision but is also a beneficial contribution to current medical research as well as public health data.

9.3.2. Differentiating Between Accidental and Intentional Poisoning

The distinction between intentional and accidental poisoning is a critical area of research in forensic pathology due to its legal and public health significance. Accidental poisoning is most often the outcome of ignorance or negligence concerning chemicals, particularly in household settings where individuals may handle chemicals improperly or ingest poisons unintentionally. Various epidemiological studies estimate the patterns of accidental poisoning, underlining the need for specific preventive measures according to population subgroups. For instance, Fakiha (2024) points out that adults aged 20–39 years in Makkah constitute a key population affected by accidental poisoning, which occurs predominantly as a result of exposure to liquid substances. Such trends inform forensic scientists on interventions that reduce the chances of their occurrence, thereby enhancing safety and health in society.

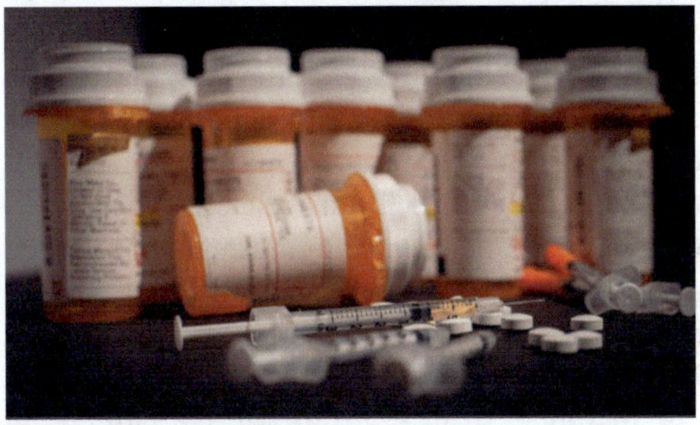

Figure 9.12. Accidental and intentional poisoning.

Source: https://cdn.emergencydispatch.org/IAED-JOURNAL/Resources/2019/04/shutterstock_1138870511.jpg.

Conversely, intentional poisoning entails the deliberate administration of noxious drugs with the objective of causing harm or killing. Intentional poisoning is characterized by enormous challenges and difficulties for forensic pathologists, given that this form of poisoning necessitates an in-depth investigative strategy and analysis in order to identify the underlying motives and circumstances. Forensic toxicologists will have to determine not only the presence of toxins but also intent from other fragments of evidence, such as the mode of delivery of the poison, the history of the victim and contacts with probable culprits, and the chain of events leading to toxicity. The findings of the investigations should be well documented so that they can help the courts, so that the distinction between murder, attempted murder, and suicide is clearly defined. The techniques used in such cases reflect an emergent crossroads for forensic toxicology and pathology, highlighting the importance of expert opinion in reaching legal conclusions. Also, the use of advanced toxicological analytical techniques is important to differentiate between both types of poisoning.

Forensic laboratories in the modern age make use of high-throughput screening technology, mass spectrometry, and gas chromatography for detecting and quantifying drugs from biological samples. These technologies enable forensic scientists to make clear links between the materials involved and exposure conditions. Whether or not an ingestion was intentional or accidental can be a huge factor in terms of case direction. For instance, from examination of patterns of toxicity, it is possible for forensic pathologists to identify irregularities that signify foul play over accidental exposure. As in Almakrami et al. (2024) suggested, the advancements in forensic toxicology keep closing loopholes in the process of death investigations with emphasis on the necessity of using standardized procedures and methodologies in determining the type of poisoning cases (Figure 9.12).

9.3.3. Case Studies Illustrating Toxicological Findings

Toxicology has made an excellent contribution to the field of understanding the connection between exposure to chemicals and pathological effects within forensic pathology by researching the use of case studies. For instance, research on Aconitum Sinomontanum Nakai (ASN) has indicated potential therapeutic applications in connection with its analgesic activity and raises an issue regarding its toxicity. A detailed study demonstrated that subsequent to single and repeated administration of ASN, there were no clear-cut acute toxic effects in BALB/c mice, such as markers of behavioral changes, weight variations, or blood profile changes. The absence of long-term toxicity studies calls for caution in clinical application, underscoring the necessity for in-depth toxicological studies to evaluate possible harms in herbal drug treatments (Woo et al., 2021). This case marks the critical juncture of traditional medicine and toxicology since it brings forth the complexities in determining the safe and effective therapeutic practice. The toxicity of nanoparticles is another sector wherein case studies have yielded significant results concerning toxicology in forensic pathology. Experiments with agglomerated/aggregated titanium dioxide (TiO_2 P_{25}) confirmed that even at higher doses of up to 1000 mg/kg for 90 days, there were no adverse systemic toxicological outcomes in Sprague-Dawley rats, and a no observed adverse effect level (NOAEL) could be determined. This finding is important in view of the increasing use of nanoparticles in cosmetics and the pharmaceutical industries. The study's detailed evaluation of organ weights, histopathology, and clinical pathology corroborates the need for rigorous toxicological control to analyze public health risks, as nanoparticles might be absorbed by biological systems and potentially induce non-specified toxic impacts (Heo et al., 2020). These studies form a foundation for development guidelines on nanotechnology use. As these case histories demonstrate, toxicology's role in forensic pathology extends beyond the mere identification of substances; it is crucial so that the broader implications of how a series of substances may affect human health and well-being can be understood. By summarizing findings of a range of toxicological tests, forensic pathologists are better placed to establish cause where poisoning or overdose is suspected and to provide crucial information in legal proceedings. The active interplay between evidence garnered from experiments in animals and clinical observations supports an understanding of the potential for harm by ubiquitous substances, both naturally and synthetically derived. Lastly, through case studies, forensic toxicology is a key nexus in meeting public health, regulatory, and justice requirements for toxic exposure cases.

Test Your Knowledge

1. What is used in determining the cause of death?
2. What is the difference between accidental and intentional poisoning?

9.4. Challenges in Forensic Toxicology

Learning Outcome

1. Understand the limitations of current testing methods.
2. Describe the issues with sample contamination.
3. Know the legal and ethical considerations of forensic toxicology.

One of the main challenges in the practice of forensic toxicology is the accurate identification and quantification of drugs in biological samples. There are a number of factors that explain this challenge, including the intricacy of human biochemistry and the variety of substances that may be encountered in forensic cases. For instance, the matrix effect, the impact from other substances in a sample on analysis of the target substance, can have the ability to significantly alter the accuracy of the results. Furthermore, compound degradation with time poses another problem, particularly in postmortem analysis, where sample collection timing is vital. While forensic toxicologists overcome these challenges, reliance on proven techniques such as gas chromatography and mass spectrometry remains first, but these are typically required to be tightly validated to ensure courtroom worthiness. Another challenge for forensic toxicology is in interpreting test results, especially from fatalities involving polydrug use. The patients might have multiple drugs present in the body, making it difficult to establish the causative factors of death. Interactions between drugs may produce unforeseen synergies or antagonisms, thus making it difficult to establish definite causality between a drug and its effect on the body. Furthermore, there exists a difference in body metabolism rates among humans, a sign that the same quantity of a substance may have different effects based on the individual. This questionably elaborate test demands forensic toxicologists to actively grasp pharmacokinetics and toxicodynamics in an effort to facilitate clear-cut interpretation. Additionally, recognition of the appropriate reference ranges for fatal intoxication complicates the assessment, necessitating continuous research to ascertain acceptable standards. The identification of new synthetic substances and constantly changing patterns in drug use present an ever-present challenge in forensic toxicology. Drugs like novel psychoactive substances and synthetic cannabinoids tend to go undetected initially because current screening techniques are limited.

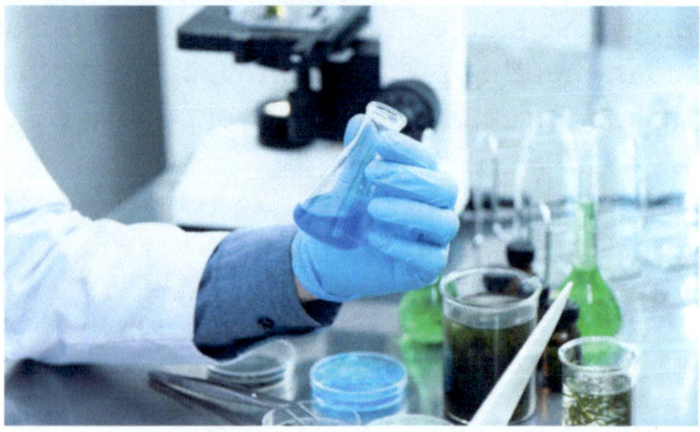

Figure 9.13. Challenges in forensic toxicology.

Source: https://lebeau-toxicology.com/wp-content/uploads/2023/09/1-2-1-1170x710.jpg.

These drugs contain intricate chemical structures that are quite different from classic drugs, so there is a need for ongoing evolution and creation of newer analytical tools in order to identify them properly. With the changing nature of drug abuse, forensic toxicologists have to focus on evolving methodologies in order to keep pace with new threats. Other matrices, such as bile, are also beneficial when standard blood samples are unavailable or deteriorated, as recent publications show the application of bile in forensic analysis. This flexibility not only benefits comprehensive inquiries but also ensures that forensic toxicologists are best placed to address mounting challenges and complexity in this area (Capiau et al., 2016; Bottinelli et al., 2016) (Figure 9.13).

9.4.1. Limitations of Current Testing Methods

Inadequacy in current testing protocols in forensic toxicology primarily impacts the validity and reliability of court evidence. The adulteration of urine samples is one of the most important problems due to its potential to modify the interpretation of toxicological test results. Research has indicated that chemicals like Zinc Sulfate can contaminate routine testing protocols such as the Enzyme Multiplied Immunoassay Technique (EMIT) and Enzyme-Linked Immunosorbent Assay (ELISA). In particular, the presence of Zinc Sulfate in urine specimens has been reported to interfere with the detection of certain drugs, including cannabinoids and opiates, complicating the process of forensic analysis (Cawley et al., 2016). Such interferences lower the reliability of toxicology reports and threaten the integrity of samples being analyzed. Also, existing testing procedures heavily depend on particular biomarkers, which may lead to partial evaluations of a person's use of substances. For example, Ethyl glucuronide (EtG) has come to be recognized as a consistent indicator of previous alcohol use but is not infallible. Although the detection of EtG is able to establish alcohol use between 80 hours following use, the application of this biomarker alone may miss cases where metabolites break down differently in different individuals and hence cause inconsistency in results. The Zinc Sulfate presence hypothesis is that it will not only affect alcohol levels, but it will also cause inconsistency in detecting EtG (Cawley et al., 2016). Therefore, differences in biomarker stability and risks of false positive or false negative results reflect significant deficiencies in current toxicological testing. Furthermore, the durability of biological samples and storage conditions represent additional toxicological testing challenges. Forensic samples are often required to be preserved and stored for several weeks or longer prior to analysis; however, factors such as temperature fluctuations or prolonged refrigeration can result in degradation or changes to the analytes. Experiments have shown that mishandling of samples can distort the results of tests, complicating the assessment of secure timelines of drug exposure or use. The validity of tests largely relies on sample preservation, which can be sacrificed in transit or storage. Hence, such restrictions call for continuous improvement in testing methods, that is, making them more standardized and robust protocols to warrant that forensic toxicology is a sound avenue to investigative accuracy (Figure 9.14).

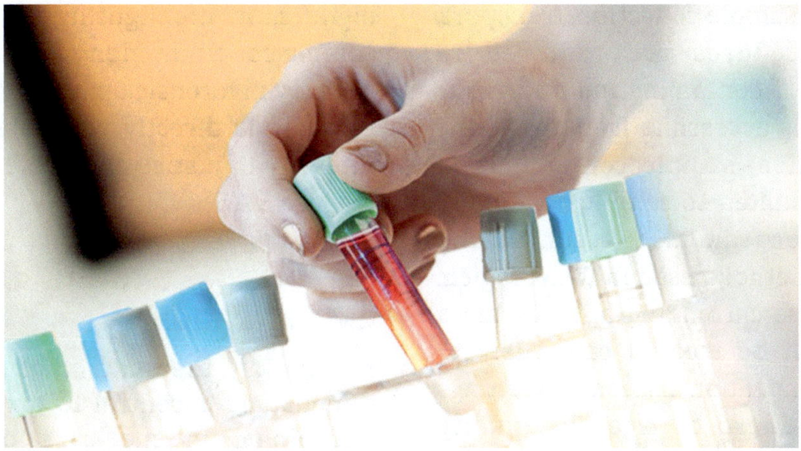

Figure 9.14. Pushing the limits of forensic toxicology.

Source: https://cdn.labmanager.com/assets/articleNo/2359/iImg/5029/c38ea7d4-0f14-4aee-bb92-1f16203f4d1f-mar18-tech-forensictoxicology-640x360.jpg.

9.4.2. Issues with Sample Contamination

Sample contamination is a critical issue in toxicology, particularly forensic pathology. Biological sample integrity is most important since forensic toxicologists have to make inferences based on true results of analysis of exposure of human remains to toxic substances. Contaminated samples may lead to erroneous conclusions regarding cause of death, poisoning, or drug abuse, ultimately impacting legal decisions and public safety. For example, contamination can be acquired from environmental sources, such as heavy metals in aquatic environments, which can unwittingly contaminate samples taken during post-mortem examination. Contamination not only makes forensic examination difficult, but it can also become harmful to the integrity of expert witness testimonies based on defective evidence.

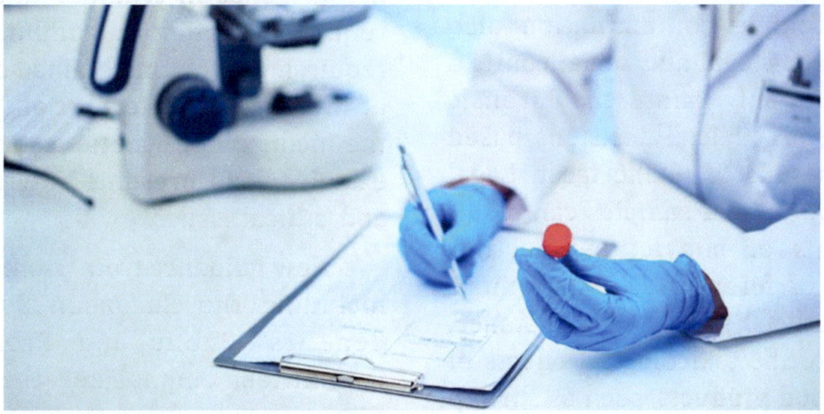

Figure 9.15. Sample preparation in forensic toxicological analysis.

Source: https://cdn.labmanager.com/assets/articleNo/26255/aImg/48393/sample-preparation-in-forensic-toxicological-analysis-may-have-huge-impacts-m.jpg.

Thus, rigorous sample collection, transport, and storage procedures are required to minimize the risk of contamination and make forensic conclusions accessible from authentic evidence. In addition, sample contamination problems are not limited to sample collection; cross-contamination can also occur during analysis. Analysis methods used in toxicological analysis, such as gas chromatography or mass spectrometry, must be treated cautiously to prevent cross-contamination. Laboratory settings are required to adhere to rigorous quality control procedures to prevent contamination from reagents, instruments, or even personnel. Forensic laboratories should also have standard operating procedures that emphasize cleanliness and proper controls to determine whether there is any contamination present. This is particularly crucial where several samples are investigated simultaneously because a single trace of contamination could produce false results. As stated, the ability to properly identify toxicants is crucial to delivering ethically correct medico-legal opinions and therefore prevention of contamination risk is of extreme significance in forensic examinations (Michał Szeremeta et al., 2024).

Apart from procedural controls, the implications of sample contamination also extend to the broader legal and social context. Contamination not only taints the forensic process but also robs judicial decisions based on toxicological results of public trust. Legal hearings resting on tainted samples can result in false acquittals or convictions, further making the task of forensic scientists more daunting in the judicial process. For instance, the investigation of the toxicological effects of heavy metals on food products, such as shrimp treated with industrial pollutants, reflects the need for robust assessment methods to avoid misinterpretation regarding human health risks (Nneoyi-Egbe, 2024). The implications are significant, highlighting the need to address sample contamination as a matter of immediate urgency in forensic toxicology, where the validity of analysis directly correlates to ensuring the integrity of justice and protecting public health (Figure 9.15).

9.4.3. Legal and Ethical Considerations

Navigating the matrix of legal and ethical dimensions is central to toxicology in forensic pathology. In the case of sudden death, particularly among youth, the forensic scientists have to pay close attention to the potential role of substances such as anabolic androgenic steroids (AAS). When AAS abuse is suspected, like in the recent case of a 24-year-old man who had a cardiorespiratory arrest, it is even more important that the forensic pathologists consider the ramifications of their findings.

This includes the methods used, such as the chemicotoxicological tests, which are not only used to reveal toxicological substances present in the body but also to prove a potential link between the use of the substance and death. In addition, these results can also impact legal proceedings since they can be used as key evidence in criminal and civil legal cases, requiring caution in handling so that ethical requirements are maintained during the process of investigation (Hern et al., 2019). Moreover, the inclusion of genetic testing in postmortem examinations presents a wide range of legal and ethical issues.

New guidance from prominent institutions, including the European Society of Human Genetics' Public and Professional Policy Committee, emphasizes the role of genetic testing in accounting for SCD events. Collecting genetic information not only makes identifying inherited conditions that may have caused a death possible but also raises issues of consent, disclosure, and future impact on surviving relatives. Ethical concerns are involved in the way such sensitive details are communicated and the duties of professionals in forensic pathology towards individuals and families who are likely to be endangered because of genetic risks. These are addressed through intense professional training and dedication toward upholding ethical principles that respect individual rights along with public health interests (Fellmann et al., 2019). Finally, the legal implications of toxicological findings extend beyond individual cases and include broader public interests as well. Forensic pathologists are often confronted with juggling exhaustive evidence collection with the possibility that their findings have on policy and legislative processes affecting drug abuse. Since the relevance of AAS and other substances is increasingly obvious in the public health forum, toxicological experts and forensic pathologists must call for continuous funding and supplies to enable apt research and education. This enables improved understanding of the consequences of the toxicants and facilitates interdisciplinary awareness, which is critical in addressing the multifaceted aspect of toxicological cases. Through their activities in legal and ethical matters, forensic pathologists are not just very relevant to specific cases but are also primary actors in coming up with more comprehensive methods that cater to issues related to public health and substance use (Fellmann et al., 2019) (Figure 9.16).

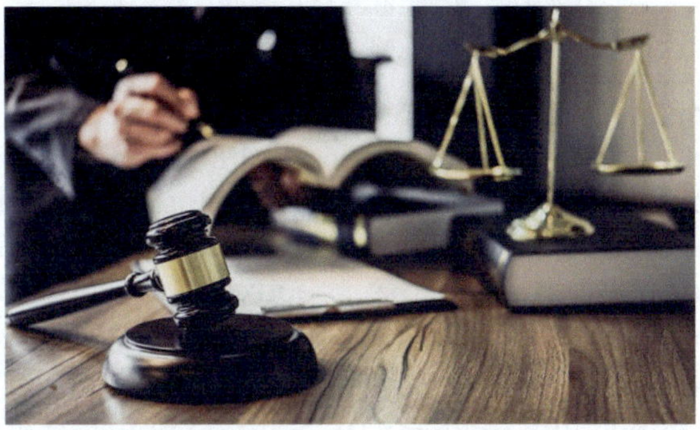

Figure 9.16. Legal and ethical considerations in forensic toxicology.

Source: https://lebeau-toxicology.com/wp-content/uploads/2021/09/p1-2-1170x710.jpg.

Test Your Knowledge

1. What are the limitations of current testing methods?
2. What are the ethical considerations in forensic toxicology?

9.5. Advances in Forensic Toxicology

Learning Outcome

1. Describe the emerging technologies and methodologies.
2. Integrate the toxicology with other forensic disciplines.
3. Describe the future directions and research opportunities.

Advancements in forensic toxicology have a primary role in deciphering the complexity of toxic substances in human pathology. Advances in analytical technologies, such as liquid chromatography-mass spectrometry (LC-MS), have increased the sensitivity and specificity of toxicological analyses, allowing forensic experts to detect and quantify trace levels of drugs and poisons in biological samples. This improvement in accuracy not only strengthens the validity of toxicological findings but also assists in the development of clearer narratives in trials in a courtroom. For instance, the ability to distinguish between toxic and therapeutic concentrations of drugs can be the deciding factor in proving culpability in cases of overdose or poisoning. With the multidisciplinary nature of forensic toxicology, chemists, forensic scientists, and law enforcement agencies working together have become increasingly important, resulting in more integrated investigations and an enhanced general effectiveness of forensic pathology of human death. Schools around the world have begun to provide their forensic science courses more expansively as a result of the increasing complexity and popularity of forensic toxicology. As the interest in solving crime has increased among the public, particularly through the popular media, universities have been adding aspects of forensic toxicology to their curricula at all levels (Stankiewicz et al., 2007). It has not only served to prepare students with the latest knowledge and skills, but also assisted in preparing a new breed of toxicologists better equipped to deal with new threats and challenges in forensic investigations. In addition, workshops and symposiums to acclimate students and practitioners with new techniques and technology are being organized. These courses play a critical role in bringing the workforce up to speed on developments, ultimately resulting in more accurate and authentic outcomes in toxicology findings in forensic pathology. The globalization of forensic toxicology education has enhanced information and best practice exchange between experts across nations (Stankiewicz et al., 2007). Forensic science, as a more globalized science, has witnessed international collaboration and conferences playing an important role in addressing such contemporary issues as new synthetic drugs and their often unforeseen toxicological profiles (Stankiewicz et al., 2007). Such gatherings not only allow for sharing of research and knowledge but also foster the sharing of common practices that can help enhance investigation outcomes worldwide. In times of crises, such as outbreaks of new psychoactive substances, a well-coordinated international response that incorporates advanced forensic toxicology can effectively manage public health risks. All this innovation and international cooperation ensure that forensic toxicologists not only possess adequate knowledge to analyze complex cases but are also active in updating themselves with the evolving situation of forensic pathology.

9.5.1. Emerging Technologies and Methodologies

With the development of pathology, the use of emerging technologies significantly enhances toxicological examination of human cases. High-resolution mass spectrometry, for instance, has radically changed the detection of drugs and toxins in biological materials. The technology is now more specific and sensitive than ever before, enabling forensic pathologists to detect more substances than before. Therefore, this can be used to move our knowledge of poisoning cases and cases of overdose, which are usually a mix of drugs, forward.

Additionally, new methods such as proteomics and metabolomics provide insight into biological responses to toxicants and open up a greater understanding of the way substances affect human physiology. With these innovations, science is not only expanding its analytical capability but also enhancing the integrity of toxicological proof in forensic proceedings. Another technology with major innovation in forensic toxicology is the application of artificial intelligence (AI) and machine learning. These technologies allow forensic scientists to work more efficiently with large sets of data, detecting patterns and correlations that may not immediately be visible to human analysts. Through the use of predictive algorithms and data mining, AI can help determine cause-and-effect relationships between exposures and outcomes of health, thereby enhancing the reliability of forensic evaluations. In addition, real-time data integration and analysis can help respond to new threats, including emerging psychoactive substances potentially spreading in illegal markets. The applications of AI in forensic toxicology, other than its speed and efficiency, lie also in its capacity to guide investigation approaches, thereby increasing case closure and justice delivery. The potential of marine biotechnology in forensic toxicology cannot be ignored. Recent studies indicate the investigation of marine-derived biocompatible materials, which can be utilized in environmental sampling to analyze for forensic purposes.

Marine biomarkers isolated from marine organisms have the potential to offer new pathways into knowing the effects of environmental pollutants on human health. Such inter-disciplinary work encourages industry-academic collaboration, and this opens up the field to new fundraising and research growth. As illustrated in educational interest stories in marine biotechnology, this paradigm represents a growing appreciation of the importance of holistic methods involving multiple scientific disciplines to reinforce forensic processes. Through fostering such convergence, the field of toxicology in forensic pathology can continue to evolve with the integration of cutting-edge technologies in order to conduct scrupulous investigations in the pursuit of justice (Figure 9.17).

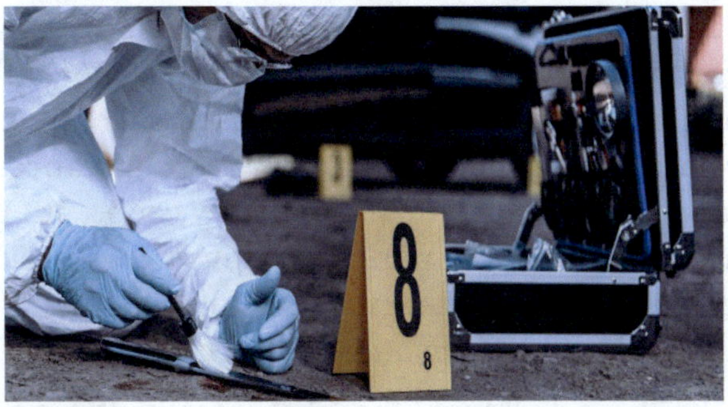

Figure 9.17. Mass spectrometry applications in forensic analysis.

Source: https://conquerscientific.com/wp-content/uploads/2023/10/Mass-Specs-Forensic-Analysis.jpg.

9.5.2. Integration of Toxicology with Other Forensic Disciplines

The incorporation of toxicology in the forensic sciences is a cornerstone in death investigation, particularly when death is suspected to result from poisoning or drug overdose. Toxicologists have a unique skill of analyzing biological fluids such as blood, urine, and tissue for the presence of toxic substances. This capability enhances the criminal investigation process because toxicological evidence may be the deciding factor in proving the cause of death or incapacitation of criminal activity. Furthermore, the interaction of forensic pathologists and toxicologists provides adequate knowledge of the physiological effects of toxins, which is important in the determination of accurate forensic conclusions.

By linking toxicological data to pathological analysis, the research can establish the mode of death and whether it is accidental, suicidal, or homicidal, thereby enriching the forensic examination with an essential element that feeds into legal judgments and public safety (Poalelungi et al., 2023). The inclusion of toxicology into other forensic disciplines enables a holistic approach that enhances the reliability and validity of forensic evidence. Inquirers usually collaborate with toxicologists, pharmacologists, and other specialists in examining complex relationships between numerous substances found in samples. Multidisciplinary cooperation achieves a more comprehensive insight into the influence of substances on human behavior, particularly in drug and alcohol cases.

As an instance, the pharmacokinetic and pharmacodynamic properties of substances can help trace events that led to a fatal outcome. This integration not only strengthens the foundation of evidence presented in court but also emphasizes the importance of interdisciplinary collaboration in forensic research. Each field advancing individual knowledge on toxic substances and their effect on the human body moves the field forward in its compilation of the body of forensic science (Morales et al., 2020). Moreover, technological advancements have significantly played a role in merging toxicology with forensic sciences and leading to increased detection techniques and analytical strategies. For example, the use of mass spectrometry and gas chromatography has enhanced toxicological tests by allowing one to detect minute traces of drugs and chemicals that may otherwise go unnoticed. These technological advances allow the identification of novel psychoactive substances and intricate drug mixes frequently encountered in forensic cases of interest. Forensic toxicologists and law enforcement must thus collaborate in their response to evolving trends in substance abuse and illegal drug use. Collaboration not only aids in solving cases but also educates public health programs and legal policy to address issues surrounding substances more effectively. Lastly, the synergy that results from toxicology's integration into other forensic sciences serves to enhance a better appreciation for the contribution of toxicity to forensic pathology (Poalelungi et al., 2023).

9.5.3. Future Directions and Research Opportunities

With increased interaction between forensic pathology and toxicology in the future, there are opportunities for more understanding and handling of toxic substances by the deceased. Among the key areas of research is continued exploration of new biomarkers, particularly the employment of Ethyl glucuronide (EtG) as a reliable marker of alcohol use. Even with the promising use of EtG in forensic circles due to the possibility of being detectable for numerous days after ethanol clearing, more studies must be done on the interference of EtG with other drugs. For instance, research could assess how common adulterants, such as Zinc Sulfate, influence EtG test results according to the evidence that has revealed such interference alters the interpretation of alcohol use in autopsies (Cawley et al., 2016). Examination of these complexities would render their evaluation in forensic analysis much more reliable and precise. With advancing analytical techniques, forensic toxicologists should perform research that involves the most sophisticated instruments of the trade, such as mass spectrometry and high-performance liquid chromatography. Not only do they give enhanced sensitivity and specificity, but they also provide enhanced overall insight into poly-drug toxicity that is increasingly prevalent in the modern world.

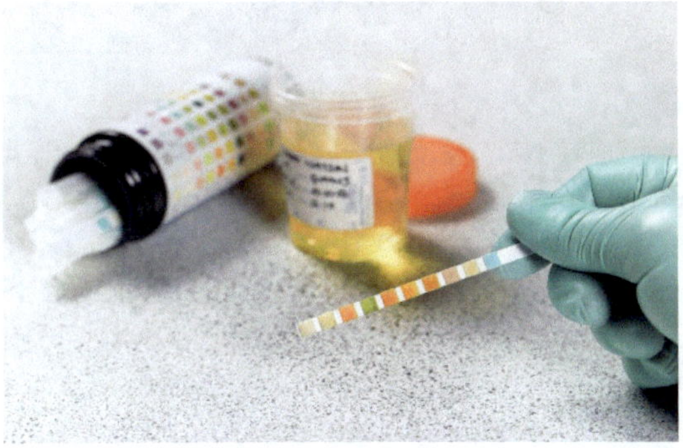

Figure 9.18. EtG test for confirming alcohol abstinence.

Source: https://www.verywellmind.com/thmb/AzjkNTl4pMVy-t8FMpFMJUyB35Q=/1500x0/filters:no_upscale():max_bytes(150000):strip_icc()/137357467-569fe6793df78cafda9efe59.jpg.

For instance, new studies can be addressed to the interactive effects of opioids, stimulants, and synthetic cannabinoids—a grim trend in samples encountered by forensic centers. This research will be essential since co-exposures can interfere with clinical presentation and toxicological interpretation. By creating detailed profiles of drug interactions and their forensic relevance, researchers may be able to help pathologists determine whether a death was due to accidental overdose or intentional poisoning, thereby reinforcing the overall integrity of forensic toxicology (Capiau et al., 2016).

Finally, interdisciplinary collaboration is a critical full-circle strategy for moving forward with the dynamic character of forensic toxicology. Facilitating collaboration between forensic pathologists, chemists, and data scientists can enable improved research models, particularly in population-specific drug responses. Collaboration can be further extended to developing databases tracking toxic substance trends over the long term and comparing them with demographic and geographic factors. These could possibly yield patterns that are transferable to public health and safety, particularly where new drug threats are concerned. Moreover, the application of technologies such as artificial intelligence has the potential to streamline data analysis, enabling easy differentiation and prediction of trends in toxicological findings. Interdisciplinary practice, acknowledging the complexity of the nature of forensic toxicology, is an untapped frontier with vast potential for rewarding research and practice in the field (Cawley et al., 2016) (Figure 9.18).

Test Your Knowledge

1. What are the emerging technologies?
2. What is the primary role of a forensic toxicologist?

SUMMARY

The intricacies of toxicology in forensic pathology are brought to the fore by the intricate association between substance abuse and mortality. Forensic experts are faced with a number of challenges while interpreting post-mortem concentrations of drugs, primarily in terms of when drugs were taken, post-mortem redistribution, and individual tolerance levels. Solving these issues requires not only a vast understanding of toxicological concepts but also the application of high-level methods such as Bayesian networks, which possess the ability to enhance predictive power in terms of the causative effect of drugs in death. Such enhancement reflects a shifting scene for forensic science, where case correlation and data analysis play a vital role in drawing accurate conclusions regarding drug deaths (Bolton et al., 2015). Through these techniques, forensic pathologists can make a real contribution to the validity and efficacy of death certifications, which ultimately enter public health statistics and mortality rates. Toxicology in forensic pathology is also tasked with examining the motives and behavior of criminal perpetrators, as in notorious cases such as Jeffrey Dahmer's. Autopsy findings and toxicology tests give valuable information regarding the psychological and emotional status of perpetrators and how drug interaction is involved in violent crime. On this basis, intelligence regarding the toxicology profile of an offender gives valuable background information to help understand the behavior, indicating the importance of the impact of drugs on criminal psychology. By integrating toxicological data with autopsy findings, forensic experts can construct a well-rounded picture of the interaction between drugs and existing psychological states and then guide court cases and enhance the overall picture of crime (Ho et al., 1994).Finally, the integration of forensic pathology and toxicology not only illuminates the dynamics of individual instances but also fosters the construction of public health programs. By the identification of drug-related mortality trends, forensic toxicology feeds into broader public debate concerning the misuse and use of drugs within society. Lastly, the findings from conclusions drawn using toxicological analysis have the potential to spur policy development, improve interventions for health, and inform educational programs for reducing substance abuse. It is therefore the exact methodology used in forensic toxicology that not only increases the integrity of individual cases but also contributes immensely to addressing public health crises resulting from drug abuse and addiction. As the field continues to evolve, the integration of new technologies and methodologies will continue to increase its contribution to forensic pathology and society in general.In forensic pathology, one must have a precise understanding of the importance of toxicology in determining the causes and modes of death. Toxicological analysis becomes the center of attention for examining a number of substances present in human tissues, such as drugs, alcohol, and poison. Toxicology reports have direct implications for legal decisions as forensic pathologists play a key role in correlating clinical presentations and autopsy results with toxicology reports. As highlighted in previous research, on-scene accuracy of evidence collection enhances the validity of autopsy results and aids public health programs. This calls for adequately trained personnel in first-time scene investigation since evidence contamination can render toxicological analysis invalid, thereby influencing the judicial process (Cecchi et al., 2023). Another core element in forensic toxicology is the knowledge of drug pharmacokinetics and pharmacodynamics. For instance, the interaction between ethanol and drugs is laced with some risk, particularly in vulnerable populations such as neonates and infants. Lack of knowledge regarding the safety levels of exposure to ethanol in these populations has created consequential interest among medical professionals and regulators as well (Kraft et al., 2014). Toxicological interpretation thus needs to take into account age-specific differences in metabolism by forensic pathologists. This complexity is further compounded by the potential for co-exposures, which calls for an integrated examination of all the substances in question when death is under investigation. These types of intricate analysis highlight the greater significance of toxicology in the legal and public health arenas, where accurate assessments can assist in avoiding such future fatalities. Interdisciplinary cooperation among forensic agencies is fundamental to delivering quality results in cases of toxicological analysis. An integrated approach encourages experience sharing, and thus proposals for enhanced protocols concerning medical and non-medical personnel at the crime scene. Interdisciplinary research is capable of enabling research-strong evidence collection, which is important in facilitating subsequent toxicological analysis. Also, the establishment of standard operating procedures, as suggested in research to develop improved forensic procedures, can simplify the investigation, thereby improving the general reliability of findings. The intersection of experience across disciplines not only increases the evidentiary value of forensic pathology but also confirms the pivotal position of toxicology in answering complex legal issues surrounding death and substance exposure (Cecchi et al., 2023).

KEY TERMS FROM THIS CHAPTER

- Automated systems
- Biological samples
- Chemical agents
- Chemistry
- Drugs
- Forensic traumatology
- Heavy metals
- High-performance liquid chromatography
- Pathology
- Pesticides
- Pharmaceuticals
- Pharmacology
- Poisons
- Thanatology

CRITICAL THINKING QUESTIONS

1. **What is the primary role of toxicology in forensic pathology?**
   a. Estimating time of death
   b. Determining whether poison or drugs contributed to or caused death
   c. Identifying blunt force trauma
   d. Detecting DNA at the crime scene
2. **Which of the following samples is most commonly used for postmortem toxicology testing?**
   a. Skin
   b. Hair follicles
   c. Blood and urine
   d. Bone fragments
3. **Which toxicological finding is most relevant in a suspected opioid overdose case?**
   a. High levels of lead
   b. Presence of ethanol
   c. Elevated morphine or fentanyl levels
   d. Low glucose concentration
4. **In forensic cases, the presence of which organ is especially valuable for drug concentration analysis postmortem?**
   a. Liver
   b. Lung
   c. Heart
   d. Kidney
5. **What is the significance of vitreous humor in toxicology?**
   a. It is resistant to decomposition and useful for measuring electrolytes and alcohol levels
   b. It provides information about carbon monoxide poisoning
   c. It is ideal for DNA extraction
   d. It detects gunshot residues

Short Answer Questions

1. What is toxicology?
2. List the various types of toxic substances.
3. What heavy metals are most commonly associated with contaminated groundwater and are known for their carcinogenic effects?
4. What are the methods of toxicological analysis?
5. What is death investigation toxicology?

Answer to Critical Thinking Questions

1. (b) 2. (c) 3. (c) 4. (a) 5. (a)

References

1. Achparaki, M., Chatzinikolaou, F., Mastrogianni, O., et al. (2012). Heavy metals toxicity. https://core.ac.uk/download/267932602.pdf (accessed on 12th July 2025).
2. Adley, M. (2017). DrugWatch information sheet: Fentanyls. https://core.ac.uk/download/89950633.pdf (accessed on 12th July 2025).
3. Almakrami, H. A. H., Saleh alsogoor, H. M., Alsulayyim, T. S. A., Alhokash, H. A. H., Jali, A. S. A., Lasloum, S. O. H., Al Sallum, D. O. H., et al. (2024). Forensic pathology and unnatural death investigations: A systematic review of case studies and procedures. *Journal of Ecohumanism*. https://www.semanticscholar.org/paper/3c6a8fa783c05b8e61537e0c070bef1592c784fb (accessed on 12th July 2025).
4. Alves, H., Botelho, C., Cardoso, M., et al. (2017). Parasites in forensic science: A historic perspective. https://core.ac.uk/download/154161377.pdf (accessed on 12th July 2025).
5. Anantharam, P., Burrough, E., Imerman, P. M., et al. (2016). Improved tissue-based analytical test methods for orellanine, a biomarker of *Cortinarius* mushroom intoxication. https://core.ac.uk/download/287623839.pdf (accessed on 12th July 2025).
6. Aromatario, M., Cappelletti, S., Piacentino, D., et al. (2015). Caffeine: Cognitive and physical performance enhancer or psychoactive drug? https://core.ac.uk/download/54528776.pdf (accessed on 12th July 2025).
7. Bagnall, R. D., Weintraub, R. G., Ingles, J., Duflou, J., Yeates, L., Lam, L., Davis, A. M., et al. (2016). A prospective study of sudden cardiac death among children and young adults. *New England Journal of Medicine, 374*, 2441–2452. https://doi.org/10.1056/nejmoa1510687 (accessed on 12th July 2025).
8. Barrett, R. H., Brown, R. N., Clifford, D. L., et al. (2015). Patterns of natural and human-caused mortality factors of a rare forest carnivore, the fisher (*Pekania pennanti*) in California. https://core.ac.uk/download/323081089.pdf (accessed on 12th July 2025).
9. Beer, L. J., Crichton, M. L., De Paoli, G., et al. (2018). Postmortem tissue distribution of morphine and its metabolites in a series of heroin-related deaths. https://core.ac.uk/download/228178478.pdf (accessed on 12th July 2025).
10. Blanckaert, P., Coopman, V., Cordonnier, J., et al. (2016). A case of acute intoxication due to combined use of fentanyl and 3,4-dichloro-N-[2-(dimethylamino)cyclohexyl]-N-methylbenzamide (U-47700). https://core.ac.uk/download/84044061.pdf (accessed on 12th July 2025).
11. Bolton, J., Carlin, M., Langford, A., et al. (2015). Post-mortem toxicology: A pilot study to evaluate the use of a Bayesian network to assess the likelihood of fatality. https://core.ac.uk/download/41072180.pdf (accessed on 12th July 2025).
12. Bottinelli, C., Bévalot, F., Cartiser, N., et al. (2016). State of the art in bile analysis in forensic toxicology. https://core.ac.uk/download/pdf/81153209.pdf (accessed on 12th July 2025).
13. Bottinelli, C., Cartiser, N., Bévalot, F., Fanton, L., & Guitton, J. (2020). Is insulin intoxication still the perfect crime? Analysis and interpretation of postmortem insulin: Review and perspectives in forensic toxicology. *Critical Reviews in Toxicology, 50*, 324–347. https://www.semanticscholar.org/paper/2a55facc953000a9b65c8c94766baaf1ed4b527b (accessed on 12th July 2025).

14. Brooke, H. L., Talbäck, M., Hörnblad, J., Johansson, L., Ludvigsson, J. F., Druid, H., Feychting, M., et al. (2017). The Swedish cause of death register. *European Journal of Epidemiology, 32*, 765–773. https://doi.org/10.1007/s10654-017-0316-1 (accessed on 12th July 2025).

15. Capiau, S., Stove, C., & Velghe, S. (2016). Opening the toolbox of alternative sampling strategies in clinical routine: A key-role for (LC-)MS/MS. https://core.ac.uk/download/84043363.pdf (accessed on 12th July 2025).

16. Cawley, S. M. (2016). The effects of zinc sulfate on ethyl glucuronide immunoassay urine testing. https://open.bu.edu/bitstream/2144/16768/1/Cawley_bu_0017N_11829.pdf (accessed on 12th July 2025).

17. Cecchi, R., Gherardi, M., Marchetti, C., et al. (2023). On-site inspection form in veterinary cases: The Parma veterinary form. https://core.ac.uk/download/590395582.pdf (accessed on 12th July 2025).

18. Corazza, O., Elgharably, Y., Martinotti, G., et al. (2017). Synthetic cannabinoids: Psychopharmacology, clinical aspects, and psychotic onset. https://core.ac.uk/download/148790765.pdf (accessed on 12th July 2025).

19. Fakiha, B. (2024). Forensic analysis of adult acute poisoning in Makkah region: A retrospective study. *African Journal of Biomedical Research*. https://www.semanticscholar.org/paper/49865aea748054669341c37084a3d4ebd4daca20 (accessed on 12th July 2025).

20. Fellmann, F., van El, C., Charron, P., Michaud, K., Howard, H., Boers, S. N., Clarke, A., et al. (2019). European recommendations integrating genetic testing into multidisciplinary management of sudden cardiac death. *European Journal of Human Genetics, 27*, 1763–1773. https://doi.org/10.1038/s41431-019-0445-y (accessed on 12th July 2025).

21. Genç, Ş., Zadeoğluları, Z., Fuss, S. H., & Genç, K. (2012). The adverse effects of air pollution on the nervous system. *Journal of Toxicology, 2012*, 1–23. https://doi.org/10.1155/2012/782462 (accessed on 12th July 2025).

22. Greer, B., Chevallier, O., Quinn, B., Botana, L. M., & Elliott, C. T. (2021). Redefining dilute and shoot: The evolution of the technique and its application in the analysis of foods and biological matrices by liquid chromatography mass spectrometry. *TrAC Trends in Analytical Chemistry, 141*, 116284. https://doi.org/10.1016/j.trac.2021.116284 (accessed on 12th July 2025).

23. Heo, M., Kwak, M., An, K. S., Kim, H. J., Ryu, H., Lee, S. M., Song, K., et al. (2020). Oral toxicity of titanium dioxide P25 at repeated dose 28-day and 90-day in rats. *Particle and Fiber Toxicology, 17*. https://www.semanticscholar.org/paper/b2758f59386a26ecbb6046d4b4cda96fe4a0a91a (accessed on 12th July 2025).

24. Hernández-Guerra, A. I., Moreno Tapia, J., Menéndez-Quintanal, L. M., & Lucena, J. (2019). Sudden cardiac death in anabolic androgenic steroids abuse: Case report and literature review. *Forensic Sciences Research, 4*, 267–273. https://doi.org/10.1080/20961790.2019.1595350 (accessed on 12th July 2025).

25. Ho, K. C., Jentzen, J., Johnson, L. T., et al. (1994). Destructive hostility: The Jeffrey Dahmer case: A psychiatric and forensic study of a serial killer. https://core.ac.uk/download/213059368.pdf (accessed on 12th July 2025).

26. Kraft, M. D., Walter, K., Marek, P. D., & Elizabeth. (2014). Ethanol pharmacokinetics in neonates and infants. https://core.ac.uk/download/46973454.pdf (accessed on 12th July 2025).

27. Morales, L., Gambhir, Y., Bennett, J., & Stedman, H. H. (2020). Broader implications of progressive liver dysfunction and lethal sepsis in two boys following systemic high-dose AAV. *Molecular Therapy*, *28*, 1753–1755. https://doi.org/10.1016/j.ymthe.2020.07.009 (accessed on 12th July 2025).

28. Mougenot Mores, C., Castro, M. B., & Barros de Melo, C. (2025). Forensic examinations in the investigations of crimes involving animals: A review. *Ciência Rural*. https://www.semanticscholar.org/paper/23398fee39fc9e3f3d3cfcb4f0252e741e3e3deb (accessed on 12th July 2025).

29. Nneoyi-Egbe, A. (2024). Assessment of heavy metal contamination in shrimp and water from the Great Kwa River: Implications for human health and aquatic ecosystems. *International Journal of Biochemistry Research & Review*. https://www.semanticscholar.org/paper/6cf157459984e3c08a24543a8f2d9c966fd5339c (accessed on 12th July 2025).

30. Poalelungi, D. G., Mușat, C. L., Fulga, A., Neagu, M., Neagu, A. I., Piraianu, A. I., & Fulga, I. (2023). Advancing patient care: How artificial intelligence is transforming healthcare. *Journal of Personalized Medicine*, *13*, 1214. https://doi.org/10.3390/jpm13081214 (accessed on 12th July 2025).

31. Sánchez-Sellero, I., Cabarcos-Fernández, P., Jaureguízar-Rodríguez, M. E., Álvarez-Freire, I., Tabernero-Duque, M., & Bermejo-Barrera, A. (2024). Development and validation of a sonication-assisted dispersive liquid–liquid microextraction procedure and an HPLC-PDA method for quantitative determination of zolpidem in human plasma and its application to forensic samples. *Molecules*, *29*. https://www.semanticscholar.org/paper/c412914269518e16188799d30bf0af9d3a6a4567 (accessed on 12th July 2025).

32. Seaman, W., & Whitehouse, J. H. (2001). Florida marine biotechnology: Research, development, and training capabilities to advance science and commerce. https://core.ac.uk/download/11016354.pdf (accessed on 12th July 2025).

33. Stankiewicz, H. (2007). Investigating the worldwide popularity of forensics. https://core.ac.uk/download/56509355.pdf (accessed on 12th July 2025).

34. Szeremeta, M., Janica, J., & Niemcunowicz-Janica, A. (2024). Artificial intelligence in forensic medicine and related sciences–selected issues. *Archiwum Medycyny Sądowej i Kryminologii*, *74*(1), 64–76. https://www.semanticscholar.org/paper/2bf24e85fc33ded30024feff789e796d61624106 (accessed on 12th July 2025).

35. Wezi, K., Mbawe, Z., Chisanga, A., Ellison, M., Frenshus, T., Zulu, H., Adutwum-Ofosu, K., et al. (2025). Forensic pathology research priorities for Zambia: Strengthening justice and public health through evidence-based practice. *International Journal of Research and Scientific Innovation*. https://www.semanticscholar.org/paper/9d98f1e748117ac7525cb8c3d1e4388a0af064a9 (accessed on 12th July 2025).

36. Woo, S., Lee, J. H., Lee, C., Lee, Y., Lee, H. J., & Kim, J. S. (2021). Single-dose and 4-week repeated dose toxicity of *Aconitum sinomontanum* Nakai pharmacopuncture: An experimental study. *Toxicology*, *38*, 47–59. https://www.semanticscholar.org/paper/6cfb88e20fdd94aa30e2c946bae47d01b8daffe0 (accessed on 12th July 2025).

THERMAL INJURIES

10

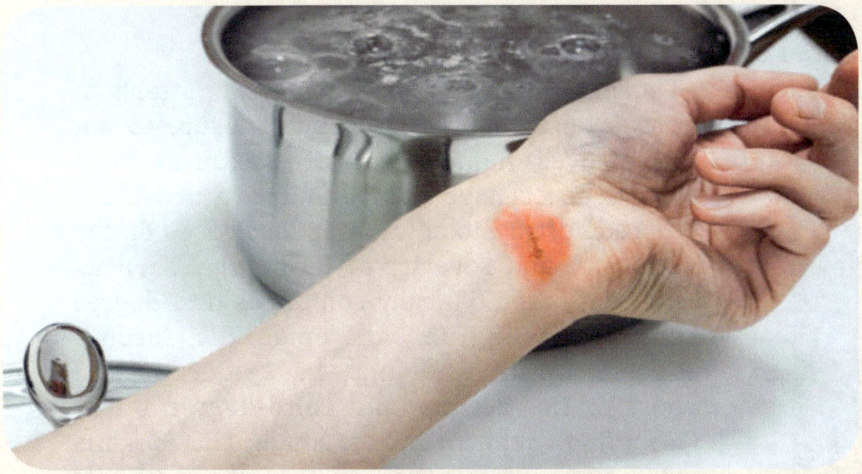

LEARNING OBJECTIVES

After studying this chapter, you will be able to:

1. Describe the types of thermal injuries;
2. Know the causes of thermal injuries;
3. Understand the mechanisms of injury associated with thermal trauma;
4. Classify the burns;
5. Describe the treatment and management of thermal injuries;
6. Know the psychological impact of thermal injuries.

Introduction

The study of heat injuries in man is an interdisciplinary investigation of the pathophysiologic mechanisms, manifestations, and implications of thermogenic disease. Heat injuries occur in a vast diversity of forms, like burns, scalds, and heat exhaustion, with heterogeneous etiologies like accidents to self-inflicted injuries. It is necessary to comprehend the pathophysiologic process of such injuries in order to plan effective management and prevention strategies. Research in the last few years has progressively emphasized the psychosocial factors in pain and outcome following thermal trauma, suggesting the need for an integrated approach to the management of thermal injuries. By exploring the synergy of the environment with human responses to thermal trauma, clinicians are better able to handle the complex requirements of thermally injured patients. Management. The care of thermal injuries has been revolutionized, led by developments in medical science and a greater understanding of pain mechanisms. Various treatment strategies, from surgery to drug therapies, to more recent modalities like tissue engineering and regenerative medicine, are employed to promote healing and restore function. Chronic pain management, which is a common sequelae of heat injury, plays a pivotal role in improving the patient's quality of life, as highlighted by recent findings on the role of stress and environmental factors in chronic pain syndromes. Specifically, current findings indicate that the environment plays a key role in pain experience and sensitivity, and thus the necessity of an integrative model of treatment for both physical and psychosocial healing (Reddy et al., 2016).

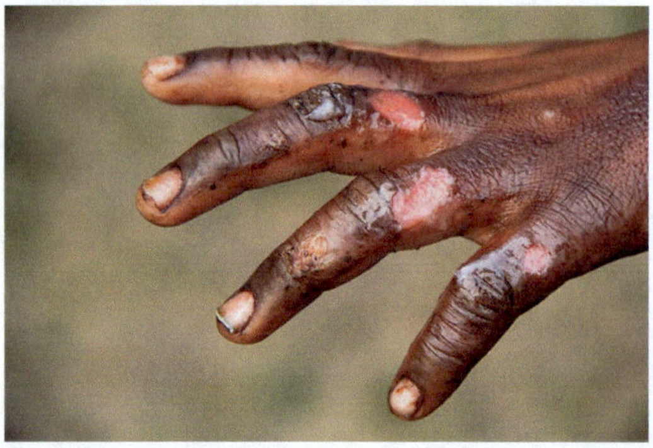

Figure 10.1. Thermal injuries.

Source: https://img.medscapestatic.com/pi/features/slideshow-slide/thermal-burns/updated/fig8.jpg?resize=645:439.

Furthermore, the global scope of thermal trauma extends beyond individual cases and includes issues of public health and policy intervention. Mass incidents, such as fire and factory accidents, underscore prevention strategies by emphasizing readiness and prevention in various industries. Education needs to focus on interventions for preventing heat hazard exposure and preventing injury, and common circumstances that are prone to cause thermal injuries, as well as recovery and rehabilitation factors, can be beneficial as leads for public education campaigns and developing emergency response plans. Sustainable solutions to decrease the prevalence of thermal injuries are crucial to the development of safer communities and general community health improvement (Nattiv et al., 2020). Through research and collaborative effort from various disciplines, it becomes feasible to increase our knowledge and control of thermal injuries, gradually improving outcomes for the victim and society at large (Figure 10.1).

Definition of Thermal Injuries

Thermal injuries are a complex pattern of tissue destruction caused by exposure to hot substances, flames, scalds, or extreme heat. The injuries have the potential to activate a cascade of physiological reactions based on the intensity and severity of the injury. Thermal injury grading typically comprises first-degree burns, affecting only the epidermis, second-degree burns, affecting the epidermis and part of the dermis, and third-degree burns affecting penetration through the dermis into more interior tissues. Severity is usually measured not just by depth, but also by the extent of the area of the total body surface area (TBSA) involved, which is very important in deciding the treatment plan as well as the complications of large-scale injury. Knowledge of the different classifications is vital for health care providers in managing treatment planning as well as estimating outcomes in individuals afflicted by these injuries. The pathophysiology of heat injury is characterized by the acute inflammatory response, which can trigger instantaneous systemic changes, affecting fluid balance, temperature regulation, and metabolic demand. Pro-inflammatory cytokines and other mediators are released at the time of injury, leading to local edema, changing permeability, and finally necrosis of the tissue if not treated in a timely manner. In severe burns, the patients acquire systemic manifestations that are indistinguishable from sepsis, that is, shock and multi-organ failure. Aside from physical damage, thermal trauma produces a number of psychological impacts, ranging from post-traumatic stress disorder (PTSD) to body image change, which complicate the recovery process. These multi-dimensional factors highlight, in turn, the importance of holistic therapy interventions in the acute care and rehabilitation stages of treatment for victims. Thermal injury management depends on the severity and complexity of the injury, requiring an interdisciplinary treatment regimen that can involve surgeons, nurses, and rehabilitation therapists.

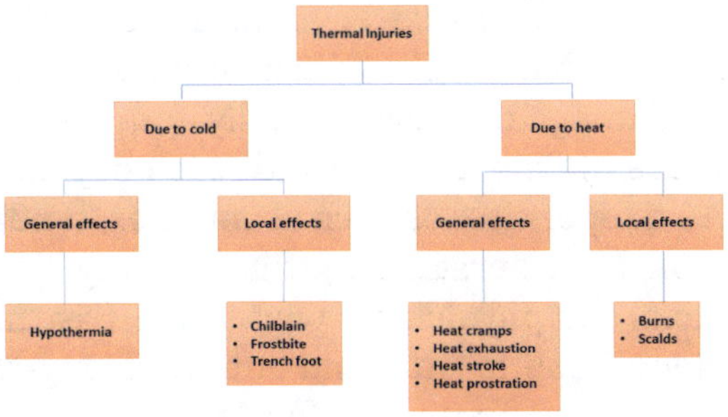

Figure 10.2. Classification of thermal injuries.

Source: https://blogger.googleusercontent.com/img/b/R29vZ2xl/AVvXsEjs04WEE86wlyKuLBHPwmzMwTW2v4DANz04G6KyekHUqIr2Z4GqcERXbTFLOeVQthLIwS1O9bWCemvjywkblOFtjIQRXkr7ExqeiVP6d7Qz-pD3kv1iQI-g4DMIHYwud0ehlChohl9-D2Sh1e6LPoXullMM-csNeTYLLdHylNAbAqSy8UUt-HQ1cTkc/s1280/Classification-of-thermal-injuries.png.

Acute care can focus on fluid resuscitation, pain management, and infection prophylaxis. Advanced therapeutic maneuvers, such as tissue engineering or skin grafting, can be used for more severe injuries to restore form and function. Rehabilitation is equally significant and may comprise physical therapy and counseling to ensure functional recovery as well as emotional adjustment. Moreover, community education regarding prevention of thermal injuries is necessary, particularly in areas with higher risk exposure, like industrial workplaces or households with vulnerable populations. Encouraging the utilization of protective measures can significantly reduce instances of such disabling injury, ultimately contributing to improved public health results for thermal trauma (Figure 10.2).

Importance of Studying Thermal Injuries

The study of thermal burns is vitally essential from a medical as well as preventive point of view as thermal burns range from minor burns to fatal conditions. The understanding of mechanisms of thermal damage gives the treating physician improved tools for investigating, classifying, and treating the victim with maximum effectiveness. This knowledge is necessary for designing interventions and improving rehabilitation protocols for the victim. Moreover, information gained from learning about thermal injury may be applied to inform public health interventions, particularly in high-risk environments such as workplaces and areas prone to wildfires. Through acknowledging the circumstances under which thermal injuries occur, effective safety practices may be implemented, which results in reduced occurrence rates and strengthened community resilience against thermal trauma (N/A). Secondly, understanding the physiological and psychological impacts of thermal burns enables a comprehensive understanding of the long-term outcomes suffered by survivors. Research reveals that patients experiencing severe burns can suffer not only from physical challenges but also from psychological issues, including post-traumatic stress disorder (PTSD) and disturbances of body image. A study investigating cutaneous skin blood flux through exercise illustrates the processes through which thermal regulation is influenced in older individuals, justifying the need for age-specific considerations within burn rehabilitation and treatment (Klonizakis et al., 2012). The applicability of the thermal injury study thus goes beyond immediate clinical application since it also encompasses the broader significance of recovery and adaptation processes that need to be undertaken by patients after injury. Also, advancements in technology to treat and rehabilitate burns come from continuous research in thermal injury. Technologies that involve skin grafting techniques, advanced wound care items, and computerized therapy aids that help relieve pain have emerged as a direct consequence of knowledge gained from cautious research in such a field. A forward-thinking understanding of thermal injuries focuses not only on urgent treatment but also on building strong healthcare systems ready for sudden events. As the world experiences increased extreme temperatures and climate change, the study of thermal injuries has grown increasingly necessary to justify the need to equip both doctors and patients with the intelligence necessary to understand this complex world (Klonizakis et al., 2012).

10.1. Types of Thermal Injuries

Learning Outcome

1. Describe the burns and scalds.
2. Understand the frostbite.

Thermal burns can be categorized into a number of different types depending on the origin of heat exposure. The most universal categories are burns, scalds, and thermal contact burns. Burns usually result from exposure to fire flames, hot surfaces, or chemicals that lead to instant destruction of skin and deeper tissues. From medical literature, superficial burns affect only the outer layer of skin and are red and painful but do not form blisters, while deep partial and full-thickness burns affect deeper layers, and they have greater adverse effects like loss of tissue and potential complications like infection. Scalds are especially caused by hot liquid or steam, which can inflict severe and rapid damage, particularly in susceptible areas such as children and the elderly. These groups highlight the various mechanisms and manifestations of thermal burns, and with a plea for different treatment and prevention strategies in different settings. Another significant division of thermal burns is on the basis of severity. This ranges from first-degree through fourth-degree burns, each of which represents a progressively more severe degree of tissue damage. First-degree burns are very mild, producing pain and redness, but with the skin's integrity still intact. On the other hand, second-degree burns are deeper in nature, causing blisters and severe pain, while third-degree burns cover all layers of skin and are usually charred or whitish with no sensation due to damage to nerves. Finally, fourth-degree burns are the most severe and reach beyond the skin to deeper tissues such as muscles, tendons, and bones. Understanding this grading system is crucial for physicians, who guide treatment regimens, hospital stay, and potential long-term rehabilitation protocols for the healing and recuperation process of the affected individuals. Aside from these divisions, it is important to consider the effect of thermal damage on the physiological operation of the body. When the skin is compromised by scalds and burns, the barrier of the body is disrupted, leading to fluid loss, an infection that is predisposed, and a systemic inflammatory response. This may manifest as shock, tachycardias, and alterations in blood pressure, drastically complicating the clinical management of burn patients. Evidence confirms the utility of early intervention, such as fluid resuscitation and wound care, in preventing these systemic effects and improving patient outcomes. Moreover, the psychological effects of thermal injury, such as potential post-traumatic stress disorder and anxiety from disfigurement, validate the utility of treatment regimens that incorporate physical and psychological requirements. It is thus essential that a coordinated management of heat injuries is done to ensure optimum recovery and quality of life for the victims (Figure 10.3).

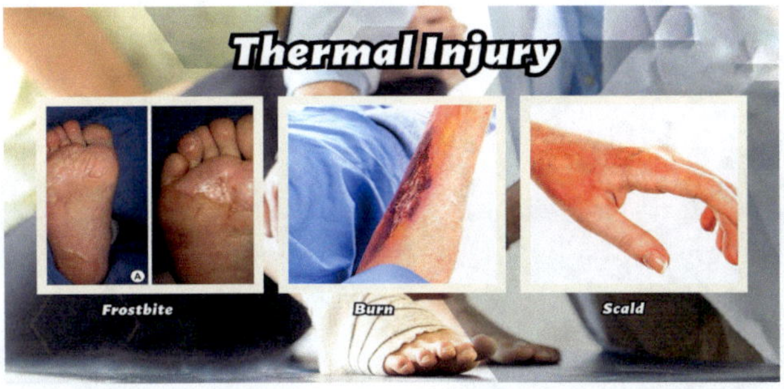

Figure 10.3. Types of thermal injuries.

Source: https://blogger.googleusercontent.com/img/b/R29vZ2xl/AVvXsEgEsIN1dNby4Tx8UjFcKkLGBm02IHGlmyK3lSpOTRmU8lMNdZOUHrn__YR8L3prVT5FlbBAg8tDZPInUV4m Kgrughg dtwepPGD4DEq7XTvQRZlag0TO449HwOgedBfsMQ6 bEr7ekbIqWAt akan3fw49oLkHk91DaXLFIM6nH1Zni36Xy9yNePqPznzCaA/s2240/2.jpeg.

10.1.1. Burns

The prevalence of burns as a serious medical issue renders it necessary that their classification and importance are completely understood. Burns can be classified in terms of several degrees of severity and depth of tissue damage, ranging from superficial burns where only the epidermis is damaged to full-thickness burns with involvement of deeper skin structures and underlying tissues. Classification is fundamental to treatment planning and to the expectation of recovery outcome. Moreover, the significance of good and timely care should not be overestimated; inappropriate treatment will cause complications such as infection, scarring, and prolonged rehabilitation time. In addition, factors outside the body, such as availability to medical facilities and public education against burns, also play a crucial role in reducing the impact of this heat injury. It is thus important that health practitioners working in critical care and rehabilitation settings possess adequate knowledge regarding burns. Over the past few decades, the research on burn management has experienced significant developments in managing not only the short-term stabilization but also the long-term recovery processes. Prevention of infection and maximization of functional recovery are specialists' top priorities, and this has resulted in enhanced patient outcomes. New advancements in the field of wound care, like the incorporation of biologics and sophisticated dressings, play a major role in the healing process. New technologies, including telemedicine, introduce new means of monitoring the health of patients with burns and continuous care. Research emphasizes the need for individualized treatment programs that consider the particular scenario of every patient, especially in high-risk populations, such as children and the elderly. As more information about burns is gained, further studies in the future will continue to advance techniques for recovery and prevention of thermal injury overload in the patient as well as in the healthcare system (Matthew et al., 2015). Along with advancing therapy techniques, causes of burn injury from the environment are also worthy of serious consideration. The increasing use of plastics in consumer goods and packaging puts the hazard of thermal burns involving these materials into focus. Because plastics are produced in greater quantities, flammability issues also emerge; the majority of modern furnishings and materials contain plastic components that can increase fire hazards. In addition to physical risks, chemicals emitted when plastics are burned cause serious health hazards, such as toxic inhalation and long-term exposure effects. Therefore, integral waste management and safety protocols on plastics are needed to ensure environmental contamination prevention and human health preservation. It is necessary to realize the intersection of material science and thermal trauma to facilitate a safe society and the necessity of preventive measures, as well as the development of treatment modalities of burns (John et al., 2017) (Figure 10.4).

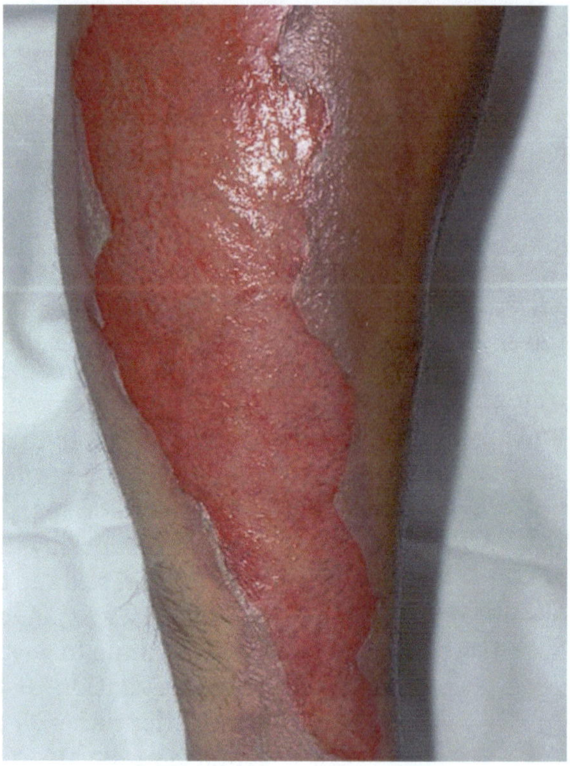

Figure 10.4. Burns.

Source: https://www.mayoclinic.org/-/media/kcms/gbs/patient-consumer/images/2013/08/26/10/08/ds01176_im04387_mcdc7_second_degree_burnthu_jpg.jpg.

10.1.2. Scalds

Scalds, being frequent thermal injuries, can most often be attributed to exposure to steam or hot liquids, leading to tissue damage based on temperature, duration, and body area affected. Scalds most often happen among vulnerable populations, particularly young children, whose exploratory patterns expose them to hazards in domestic environments. It has been shown that the etiology of these injuries can be attributed mostly to factors that can be modified, including insufficient supervision, absence of protective devices, and inadequate parental education regarding safe home habits. Children's centers play an important part in the dissemination of injury prevention strategies, with an emphasis on increasing parental awareness and increasing home safety measures for preventing scalds. By backing initiatives limiting children's exposure to hot substances and campaigning for safer temperatures in water, these centers can decrease the frequency of scalds and strengthen overall childhood safety protocols, as seen in recent studies (Ablewhite et al., 2017). The public health importance of scald injury is very great, as they not only inflict immediate physical damage but also result in long-term health costs. Scalds can lead to extended medical treatment, from first acute intervention to rehabilitation care, thus placing a burden on healthcare systems. Accidental burns, which include scalds, continue to be a major cause of morbidity and mortality in various populations, and consequently, enhance health inequalities among the victims, according to recent research. Positively, intervention programs effective in educating caregivers with safe prevention strategies have been demonstrated to be effective. Enhanced understanding of safety measures, such as reducing water heater temperatures and the use of protective shields to prevent access by hot liquids, has been shown to minimize the occurrence of such injuries in children (Weyhing et al., 2020). Implementation of evidence-based interventions can thus minimize the medical load for thermal burns and ensure safer living environments. In conclusion, addressing the issue of scalds is a matter of balanced understanding of their risk factors and joint action by various stakeholders.

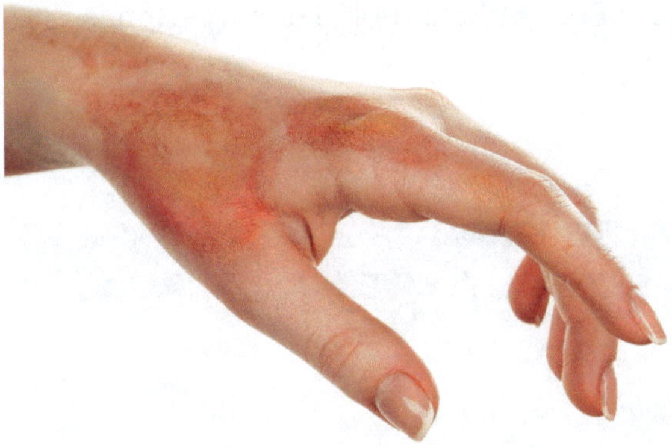

Figure 10.5. Scalds.

Source: https://urgentcaresouthaven.com/wp-content/uploads/2020/09/burn-care.jpeg.

Public health initiatives need to give high priority to evidence-based programs involving education, community action, and policy change to be in a position to reduce the incidence of such injuries substantially. All measures that empower parents with information and means to protect their children are particularly important in preventing injury. In addition, collaboration among healthcare workers and social organizations will be important in creating awareness and enforcing safety measures that lead to radical declines in scald injuries. Research and evaluation of the interventions will be essential in simplifying methods and guaranteeing effectiveness, not only in preventing scalds, but also in improving the overall safety and well-being of communities (Ablewhite et al., 2017; Weyhing et al., 2020) (Figure 10.5).

10.1.3. Frostbite

Frostbite is a severe problem among thermal injuries, particularly for those subjects subjected to very cold temperatures. Frostbite occurs when tissues and skin become frozen, leading to cellular damage due to the crystallization of ice inside cells. The most susceptible areas are areas with poor circulation of blood, such as fingers, toes, ears, and the nose. Early signs are typically manifested as cold, numb skin that may develop into a tingling sensation. As the condition advances, the injured skin turns white or blue, indicating reduced blood supply. Understanding the pathophysiology of frostbite is significant in proper prevention and treatment protocols because the outcome may lead to severe complications like necrosis and even amputation in extreme cases. The management of frostbite is grounded on an evidence-based knowledge of its pathophysiology and the application of best practice guidelines. The Wilderness Medical Society brought together a panel of experts to develop a comprehensive system of recommendations for the prevention and management of frostbite. The guidelines target the principal interventions, such as ensuring proper dressing and looking out for initial signs, for the prevention of injury progression. In established frostbite, management can be through slow rewarming of the affected tissue, which must not be done suddenly to avoid injury to the tissue when it thaws. The treatment applied to frostbite must blend individual patient assessments with generalized rules and emphasize that effective treatment protocols significantly enhance recovery outcomes (McIntosh et al., 2019). Long-term effects and preventive measures are still of prime concern in the debate of frostbite and heat injury. Evidence shows that individuals who experienced frostbite may develop long-term pain and persistent cold sensitivity in the affected areas. As such, public health education about cold-induced injury is necessary for risk prevention. Along with it, research on the treatment of frostbite, such as updated guidelines from professional panels, empowers practitioners with tools for maximizing patient care and minimizing the development of complications. In light of continued developments in knowledge within the discipline, it is necessary to embrace up-to-date practices that transcend standard knowledge, thereby supporting the safety and well-being of individuals at risk of thermal injury like frostbite (Liu et al., 2020) (Figure 10.6).

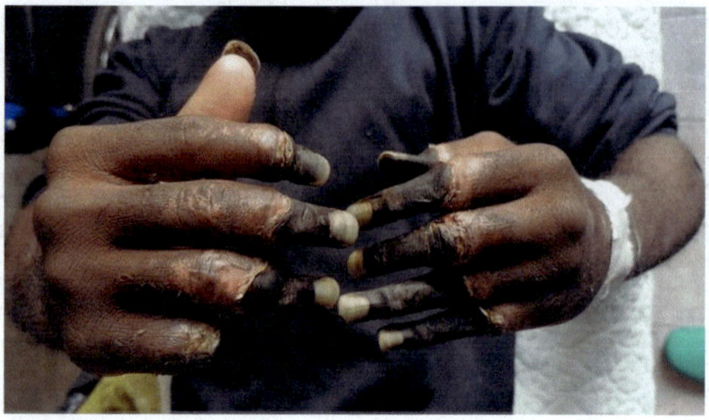

Figure 10.6. Frostbite.

Source: https://assets.cureus.com/uploads/figure/file/451695/article_river_1e972d70307e11ed8e28492cf24f4471-Figure-1.png.

Test Your Knowledge

1. Which type of burn affects only the epidermis?
2. What role do children's centers play in scald prevention?

10.2. Causes of Thermal Injuries

Learning Outcome

1. Describe the environmental factors of thermal injuries.
2. Learn about occupational hazards.
3. Examine household accidents.

The broad range of thermal injury is due to multiple causes, largely falling under the headings of burns, scalds, and contact injury. Burns are caused by heat from fire, hot objects, or toxic substances, causing tissue destruction. Scalds, frequently due to coming into contact with hot liquids, are especially common among children and may follow accidental spillage or improper cooking. Contact burns typically involve direct contact with hot surfaces, such as metal components in appliances or vehicles. The severity of thermal injury varies with exposure time and heat. Demographic characteristics like age and health status may also affect susceptibility. For instance, the elderly and infants have thinner skin and are more likely to suffer serious thermal injuries. The identification of these causes is important in developing effective prevention methods and public safety measures aimed at lowering cases of such injuries. Environmental factors also play a significant role in the cause of thermal injuries, particularly where natural catastrophes are prevalent. Higher frequency and severity of fires have been found in recent research to lead to a surge of thermal injuries, as evidenced in California, where humans and animals were badly burned by exposure to wildfires. Complications after a burn, such as respiratory distress due to smoke inhalation, have a tendency to aggravate the effect of thermal injuries. The impact of wildfires on human health is considerable, with many suffering both physical and psychological trauma associated with destructive fire events. In veterinary medicine, similar burn events have been found to have cardiovascular implications; recovery requires widespread monitoring and management.

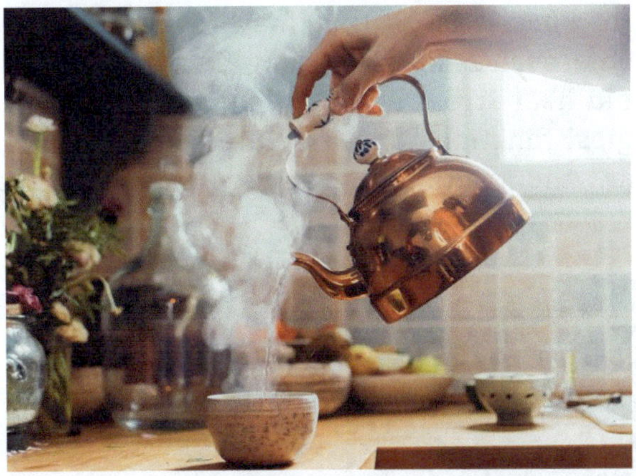

Figure 10.7. Causes of thermal burns.

Source: https://media.post.rvohealth.io/wp-content/uploads/2022/06/hot_water_pour_steam-732x549-thumbnail.jpg.

This cross-animal perspective identifies the more general effects of heat injury and the need for wide-ranging examination in human and veterinary medicine (Epstein et al., 2020). Additionally, systemic and organizational reasons lead to thermic injuries, particularly in institutional and industrial settings. In Brazil, large-scale studies assessed the welfare of broiler chickens, revealing suboptimal thermic comfort and its implications for injuries. These welfare tests emphasized that unacceptable thermal comfort ratings can lead to tremendous distress and mortality in animals, with an analogy drawn towards potential effects on human populations exposed to harsh working conditions or inefficient safety measures. The findings reveal that neglect of adequate standards of safety can lead to the onset of thermal injury, which is a threatening intersection of animal and human well-being. By identifying the organizational deficits that caused the thermal injuries, stakeholders are able to enhance safety procedures and regulations to better protect both humans and animals under their care (Federici et al., 2016) (Figure 10.7).

10.2.1. Environmental Factors

The setting is also important in the determination of the degree and severity of thermal burns in humans. Climatic factors like temperature and humidity provide a setting within which thermal burns may occur. Increased temperatures may amplify the possibilities of heat-related conditions, especially in substandard living conditions or overcrowded settings where there is inefficient air movement. For example, work conditions devoid of adequate shade or cool respite will predispose individuals to heat exhaustion or heat stroke. These conditions are common in factories or working outdoors under hot conditions, where workers may be unaware of their rising body temperatures due to working activities. Consequently, design and regulation of the work environment play a key role in reducing risk from thermal injuries. The interaction between environmental factors and individual physiological adjustments is critical within the context of heat injury. The capacity for acclimatization to heat of each individual will vary with age, fitness level, and hydration status. Young athletes, for instance, may tolerate heat better than older individuals but are generally more likely to push their physical limits under competitive conditions. Moreover, dehydration, especially under hot conditions, reduces the ability of the body to thermoregulate, increasing vulnerability to thermal damage. From sporting performance research, there is a showing that climate stressors affect both physical and psychological well-being of persons exposed to inordinate heat, ultimately affecting their heat-stress outcomes (Van der Merwe et al., 2018). Secondly, the role of urbanization and infrastructure development cannot be overlooked in the case of thermal burns. When urban land grows and natural land shrinks, urban heat islands are bound to form, resulting in elevated ambient temperatures. This trend enhances thermal stress among urban residents, especially among vulnerable populations who have no access to water, cooling centers, and other means to manage during peak heat. Along with that, housing conditions, such as low insulation and a lack of ventilation, can trap heat, increasing the risk of thermal injuries. Thus, modification of those environmental factors by urban planning and policy can create a healthier environment, hence decreasing the rate of thermal injuries and public health resilience overall (Federici et al., 2016).

10.2.2. Occupational Risks

In other workplaces, workers are usually exposed to special risks that may result in severe thermal burns. Unhealthy high-temperature environments, such as metalworking, construction, and firefighting, necessitate meticulous precautions to avoid heat stress and burn injuries. Prolonged exposure to high temperatures can weaken physiological functions and, in extreme cases, result in heat exhaustion or heat stroke. It is essential to know the health risks of heat exposure so that effective prevention programs can be adopted.

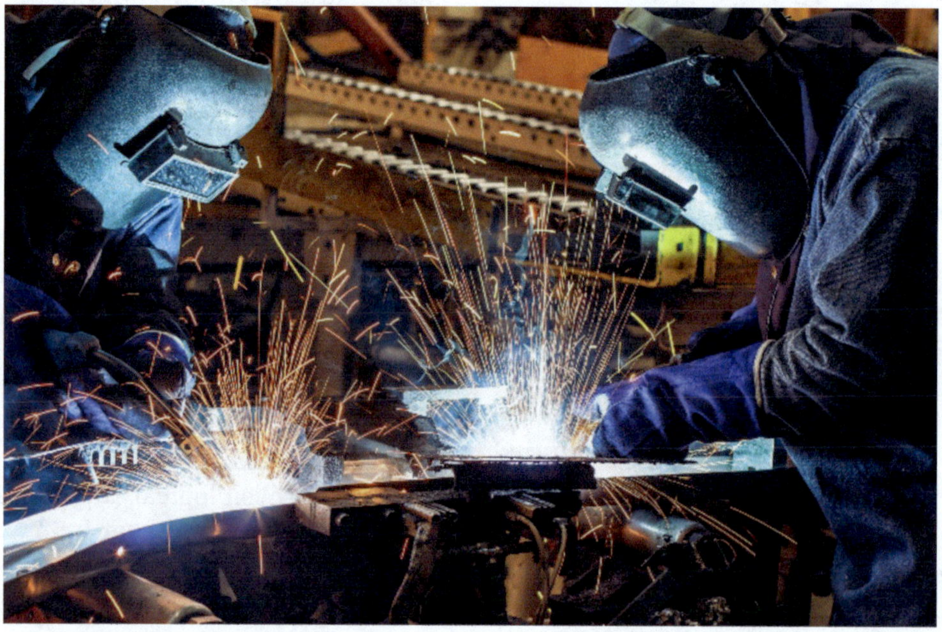

Figure 10.8. Occupational hazards.

Source: https://industrialmachinerydigest.com/wp-content/uploads/2022/11/iStock-488539284-scaled.jpeg.

Through a study of contrasts among various systems of energy, there is a critical imperative for assessing health and safety implications of severe heat within these systems, quantifying severity and uncertainty as a function of occupational hazard (Brown et al., 1980). This progressive program not only protects employees but also optimizes overall system efficiency and productivity in the workplace. Workstation design plays an important role in the incidence of thermal injury, excluding heat illness. Occupational ergonomics investigates the mechanisms by which poorly designed workplaces can result in increased risk of injury, particularly due to excessive heat exposure. For instance, inadequate ventilation, inappropriate protective gear, and poorly maintained equipment can raise thermal stress. A solid ergonomics program addresses problems such as worker placement, tool reach, and environmental factors, which have a direct influence on both thermal exposure and the rate of injury.

Through the use of proper ergonomic designs, organizations can successfully minimize the risk of thermal injury as well as the overall category of occupational hazards that influence the health of workers (Stramler et al., 2025). This indicates the link between workspace design and employee safety, underscoring the need for an integrated approach to occupational health. Finally, psychosocial considerations need to be incorporated into the evaluation of occupational hazards from thermal injuries. Employees working in hot environmental conditions could be more stressed and anxious, and hence less capable of effectively coping with thermal loads. Social isolation and communication deficits in isolated work settings, such as those endured by employees working remotely or in space, may also exacerbate thermal problems (Stramler et al., 2025). Encouraging a healthy work setting in terms of mental well-being, as well as physical security, is something that businesses can do to better equip their laborers to handle thermal stresses. Knowledge of such psychosocial dynamics is vital to designing full-spectrum safety measures that include both the physical and the psychological well-being of the employees. By doing so, the general resilience of the workforce against heat injuries and associated occupational threats could be improved (Figure 10.8).

10.2.3. Household Accidents

While researching home accidents, one must appreciate that they encompass a wide range of accidents that include falls, cuts, and, most particularly, thermal injuries. Thermal injuries in the guise of burns typically arise from common household activities that involve cooking, the use of heating appliances, or accidental exposure to hot materials. In addition to causing massive physical harm, these injuries inflict a high psychological burden on the victims and their families. Identification of the most frequent reasons behind such incidents is required to devise effective prevention plans. Domestic cooking spaces, which involve hot temperatures and sharp knives coming together, form a highly unsafe platform for thermal burns. Awareness drives educating individuals on healthy cooking techniques, along with the healthy usage of domestic appliances, can serve to reduce such accident frequencies significantly. Adding to the issue of accidents at home are the unique dangers that confront some groups of people, such as children and the elderly. Research indicates that children are also at higher risk of thermal burns because they are unaware of the dangers presented by hot liquids or surfaces. Meanwhile, adults who are elderly have trouble moving around with ease and have slower reflexes, putting them at higher risk for falls and accidental burns. The consequences of thermal injury in such groups can be considerable, often leading to long-term health consequences or death. Addressing the special requirements of such vulnerable groups is paramount while formulating prevention programs.

Caregivers and families must be made aware of the distinct risks involved in thermal injuries in the domestic environment in order to lower the risks to children and the elderly. Prevention of home thermal injuries also includes the use of safety gadgets and proper education. Smoke detectors, fire extinguishers, and skid mats can considerably reduce the hazard of injury from falling or fire. Moreover, community-based public health programs for information dissemination on safe kitchen and home management practices can be a primary preventive factor. For instance, encouraging the use of oven mitts and other protective gear while cooking can guard against direct contact burns. Psychological effects occurring as a result of accidents must also be taken into account because the victims and their families are exposed to trauma or anxiety when they encounter such accidents. Thus, promoting awareness through carrying out outreach and education campaigns is essential in reducing accidents in homes and developing secure homes for all in the community (Figure 10.9).

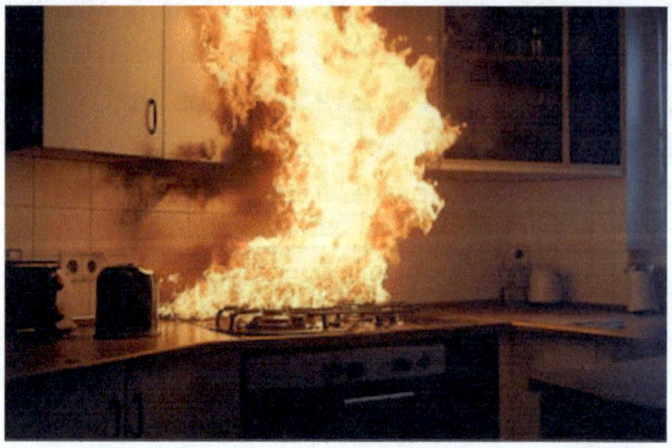

Figure 10.9. Kitchen fire hazards are a serious domestic accident in a home environment during the day.

Source: https://img.freepik.com/premium-photo/kitchen-fire-hazards-serious-domestic-accident-home-environment-day_447653-36088.jpg?w=360.

Test Your Knowledge

1. What are the environmental factors of thermal injuries?
2. What is meant by occupational hazard?

10.3. Mechanisms of Injury

Learning Outcome

1. Describe the process of heat transfer.
2. Describe the cellular response to thermal damage.
3. Know the systemic effects of thermal injuries.

The mechanisms of injury produced with thermal trauma are complex and multifaceted, with both the immediate effect of heat exposure and the subsequent biological response of the body. When the body is subjected to extreme heat, proteins within cells begin to denature, leading to the malfunction of the cell and eventually necrosis. This serves to initiate a cascade of inflammatory responses that act to further damage tissues. In addition, compromise of the skin integrity compromises the body's capacity for maintenance of temperature regulation and resistance against pathogens, thereby further increasing susceptibility towards infection and systemic complications. The most important effect of thermal trauma is the increase in inflammatory markers, which are crucial in the coordination of healing but, if poorly regulated, lead to secondary damage. Understanding of these mechanisms will be crucial in the development of effective treatment regimens for victims of thermal trauma. In muscle damage caused by thermal trauma, literature indicates that various thermal treatments will impact the outcome in recovery. To be precise, evidence has shown that heat therapy will predispose muscle regeneration after injury by promoting increased blood flow as well as pain reduction. In comparison among different thermal modalities, hot water immersion has been reported to exert beneficial effects in decreasing indices of muscle damage, such as circulating creatine kinase and myoglobin levels, simultaneously alleviating perceived muscle soreness. Notably, cold water immersion has been unable to exert a significant effect, highlighting the importance of temperature in therapeutic use. The differential impact of heat treatments reveals the mechanisms underlying tissue repair and the need for personalized approaches in rehabilitation regimens after thermal burns (Dablainville et al., 2025). Furthermore, the intersection of thermal wounds with cardiovascular reactions brings an additional layer to the understanding of injury mechanisms. Studies on animals with wildfire-induced thermal burns reveal that large burns induce hypercoagulability and thrombosis due to altered platelet activation and response. Hypercoagulability is characterized by the disappearance of platelet-derived macrovesicles, which are likely to play a central role in the triggering of thrombus development within injured tissues. The recognition of this response underlines the necessity for an integrated strategy toward thermal trauma, where not only the local effects of heat are treated but also the systemic effects, such as increased susceptibility to thrombosis or myocardial dysfunction. The exploration of such interrelated mechanisms underscores the necessity for further research with a view toward enhancing the current understanding of the pathophysiology of thermal trauma in humans (Avalene et al., 2022).

10.3.1. Heat Transfer Processes

Heat transfer mechanisms are central to the comprehension of thermal injuries among humans, since these processes determine how energy transfers from and to bodies and their surroundings. Conduction, convection, and radiation are the main mechanisms by which heat transfer is brought about. Heat in such a process is conducted by immediate contact between materials, which is retained especially well in the context of burn injuries because of direct contact with hot surfaces that leads to rising temperatures of tissue and cellular death in a short span of time. Convection, on the other hand, is heat transfer through fluids like water or air, where hot particles rise and cold particles descend. This process can have the effect of exacerbating heat injuries under warm conditions to cause heat stroke. Understanding these mechanisms can be used to develop prevention methods and treatment approaches, and hence the application of thermal management in guaranteeing protection of human health. A core element of processes of heat transfer is the role of thermoregulation in maintaining core body temperature, especially under the stress of atypical environmental conditions. The human body employs various physiological mechanisms in maintaining body temperature, including sweating and vasodilation, that make possible heat loss through evaporation and augmented blood circulation to the skin. Failure to dissipate heat can cause injury from heat, with excessively high inside temperatures leading to organ failure and systemic complications. These thermoregulatory responses are efficient, as they depend on extrinsic factors like wind speed and humidity, pointing out the intricate interaction between the conditions of the environment and thermoregulatory processes. Researchers have investigated innovative therapeutic practices, therapeutic ultrasound specifically, to enhance healing in patients who have been traumatized thermally, offering opportunities for improved procedures for recovery (Bloyer et al., 1999). Besides, advanced imaging modalities such as thermographic imaging are growing more valuable in the research of heat transfer and its implications in clinical applications. The non-invasive method provides precise temperature mapping of temperature gradients on body surfaces, which allows clinicians to detect abnormalities that may indicate underlying thermal trauma or conditions that must be treated. Studies on dogs as subjects have confirmed the application of thermographic imaging to establish surface temperatures, deeming it potential for use in human medicine (Vainionpää et al., 2014). By using these variations of thermal patterns, doctors can diagnose and treat heat injuries more precisely. Therefore, combining a deep knowledge of heat transfer mechanisms with cutting-edge imaging technologies not only optimizes our diagnostic resources but also ultimately enhances the management and outcomes of thermal burns in man (Figure 10.10).

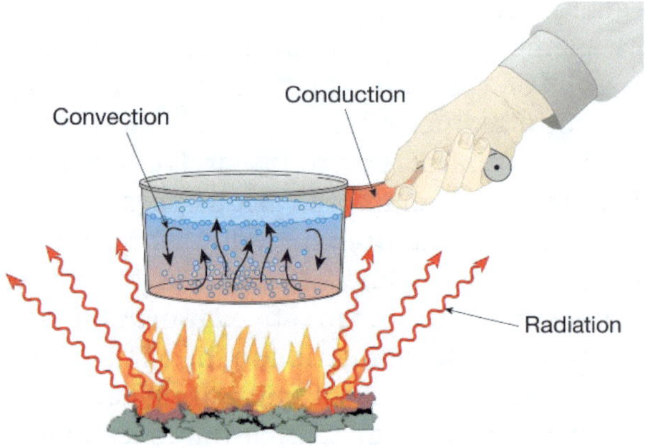

Figure 10.10. Heat transfer methods.

Source: https://www.simscale.com/wp-content/uploads/2020/04/heat-transfer-methods-1.jpg.

10.3.2. Cellular Response to Thermal Damage

Cellular response to heat injury is a multifaceted and significant aspect of human physiology that highlights the delicate mechanisms of resistance to extreme thermal stress. When exposed to elevated temperatures, cells trigger a variety of defense responses in an attempt to avoid injury. Among the critical responses is the induction of heat shock proteins (HSPs), which function as molecular chaperones. These proteins facilitate the proper folding of other proteins that have already been heat-denatured and are thus protecting cellular integrity. Activation of HSPs may also trigger cascading signals that lead to enhanced cell survival and repair mechanisms. These answers are interpreted, and they not only clarify the cellular adaptive response of thermal injury but also determine the therapeutic interventions to enhance cell recovery in a clinical scenario. Moreover, thermal damage induces a cellular response involving gene expression modification. Following thermal injury, thermal stress-responsive genes are upregulated, which contribute to the development of a protective cellular environment. For instance, induction of essential transcription factors such as NF-kB and AP-1 leads to the transcription of inflammation and survival genes. This suggests that the acute response to heat involves an inflammatory process that has the potential to enhance healing of tissues or increase damage depending on the degree and duration of thermal exposure. As such, the control of protective and deleterious effects of such inflammatory responses becomes crucial in order to understand how cells deal with thermal injuries, as failure to exert this control has deleterious consequences, like apoptosis. The cellular responses to thermal injury have not only immediate physiological outcomes but also subsequent ecological consequences. With global warming still on the rise and ambient temperatures increasing, cells in various organisms, including bacteria, exhibit altered mechanisms of survival against heat stress. Research has shown that increasing temperatures can influence mechanisms of antibiotic resistance in microbial populations, with a shocking overlap between thermal exposure and microbial survival. As highlighted in recent studies, the reversible physiological changes induced by heat stress not only elicit cellular defense mechanisms but also compel the development and survival of antibiotic-resistant isolates (Cruz-Loya et al., 2020). This dynamic growth highlights the necessity for comprehensive insight into thermal responses at cellular and ecosystem levels, forecasting the implications of thermal injuries in humans will have far-reaching effects on public health and environmental sustainability (Dereeper et al., 2012) (Figure 10.11).

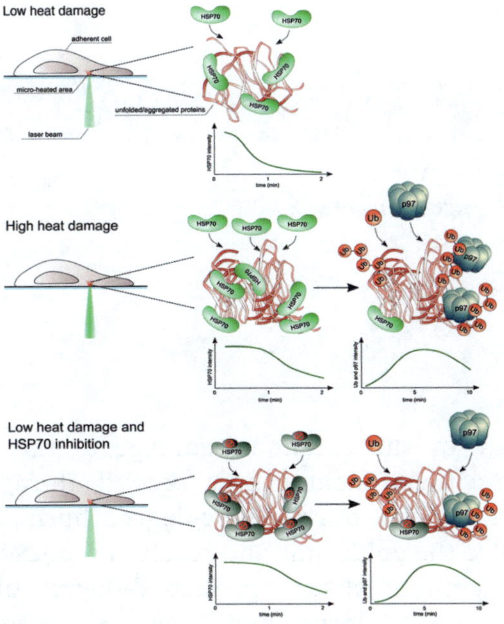

Figure 10.11. Schematic representation of the cellular two-wave response to micro-heat damage.

Source: https://www.researchgate.net/publication/348885591/figure/fig6/AS:985911781236736@1612071094026/Schematic-representation-of-the-cellular-two-wave-response-to-micro-heat-damage-The.png.

10.3.3. Systemic Effects of Thermal Injuries

The systemic effects of heat injuries go far beyond the initial insult to the skin and underlying tissue, and evoke a cascade of physiological responses that can have a profound effect on a patient's healing process. Burn injury evokes a period of hypermetabolism, with an increased expenditure of energy and alterations in immune function that make healing more problematic. The metabolic response is characterized by increased heart rate, increased oxygen consumption, and increased protein catabolism. These types of alterations have a significant effect on the overall physical status of burned patients, which can lead to complications such as infections, secondary organ dysfunction, and prolonged hospitalization. Proper knowledge of these system reactions is a must in order to develop appropriate treatment plans that not only treat the local aspect of burn damage but also address the overall effect on health and healing. Research has found that cardiovascular complications are often encountered as a primary concern in severely injured patients following burns. Cutaneous and visceral tissue damage will result in systemic inflammatory response syndrome, which is associated with changes in cardiac function. For example, data have established that cardiac injury after burns is common and may serve as a predictor of mortality in burned patients. Echocardiographic evaluations have revealed alarming results, such as myocardial thickening and signs of thrombi development, calling for strict cardiovascular monitoring among patients who are burned (Epstein et al., 2020). The synergistic risk of myocardial damage combined with systemic inflammatory responses poses a challenge that necessitates clinicians seeking out new ways of cardiac testing and treatment in the critical phases of burn injury recovery. The effect of thermal injury is realized in multiple organ systems and therefore needs to be managed integrally by the patient. The respiratory system, for instance, may be injured through inhalational injuries that introduce extra systemic complications. These injuries may lead to pulmonary edema, reduced lung compliance, and susceptibility to respiratory infection, further contributing to the patients risk (Van der Merwe et al., 2018). Furthermore, homeostatic breakdown resulting from the loss of large volumes of fluid may cause renal impairment, which is expressed as acute kidney injury. Physicians thus must maintain a high degree of suspicion for potential renal complications alongside the management of the primary thermal injuries. These correlated effects validate the necessity of an interdisciplinary treatment plan of thermal injury with emphasis on immediate and late consequences in order to optimize prognosis in seriously burned patients (Figure 10.12).

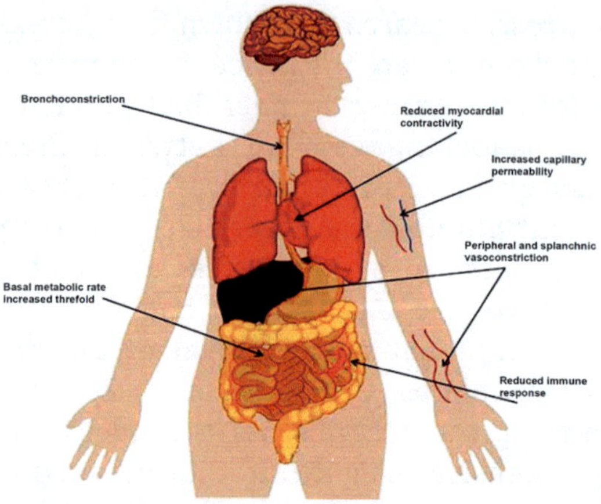

Figure 10.12. Systemic changes that occur after a burn injury.

Source: https://cdnintech.com/media/chapter/57336/1512345123/media/F1.png.

Test Your Knowledge

1. Which heat transfer processes involve direct contact between materials?
2. Which physiological mechanism helps in heat loss by increasing blood flow to the skin?

10.4. Classification of Burns

Learning Outcome

1. Understand the first-degree burns.
2. the second-degree burns.
3. Learn about third-degree burns.

Categorization of burns is a significant consideration in the understanding of thermal trauma among human subjects because it dictates treatment modalities and prognosis. Burns are traditionally categorized based on depth, or the extent of damage to the skin layers; these include first, second, third, and fourth-degree burns. First-degree burns only involve the epidermis and result in redness and pain without blistering. Second-degree burns penetrate the dermis and develop swelling and tender blisters. Third-degree burns penetrate the epidermis and dermis and potentially affect deeper tissue, and are often white, charred, or leathery in appearance. Finally, fourth-degree burns penetrate the skin into fat, muscle, or bone underneath and generally result in widespread damage requiring special medical attention. An understanding of the above categories is crucial in deciding proper medical intervention and predicting recuperation. Other than the extent of injury, the cause of burns predominantly influences their category and therapy. Thermal burns, being the most common, are due to exposure to scalding water, hot objects, or flames. One of the specific issues in recent years has been an increase in cases related to wildfires, with significant implications for both human and veterinary health. For example, a study of veterinary patients harmed by wildfires recently highlighted the way that thermal burns from wildfires exacerbate cardiac disease, leading to complications and high mortality. This linkage of burn classification with subsequent health risks highlights the necessity of individualizing treatment modalities in terms of causation and the nature of burn injury.

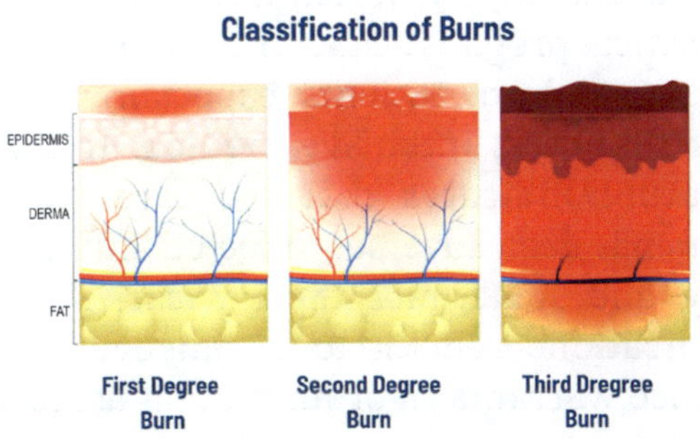

Figure 10.13. Classification of burns.

Source: https://cdn.prod.website-files.com/635940de6d286505c38236fe/66e2d38455efd6e098cf4a16_66e2d2d54e25097b67ce49e8_Classification%2520of%2520Burns.webp.

A clear comprehension of burn classification, hence, enables a greater recognition by medical professionals not only of the immediate physical injury but also the eventual resulting health outcomes. Moreover, the psychological impact of burn trauma also needs consideration, as grading of burns goes beyond physical recovery. The trauma of severe burns, particularly third or fourth-degree burns, may cause intense psychological trauma in the form of anxiety, depression, and PTSD. Severe burn survivors are likely to require extensive rehabilitative measures addressing emotional and physical needs. It has been discovered through studies that integrating psychological care into the treatment of burn patients can significantly improve patient outcomes. Because burns are so complex, health practitioners must approach burn patient treatment holistically, addressing physical and emotional aspects of their lives. Thus, classification not only is a procedure for medical treatment but also is a basis for overall care approaches that include the patients' healing process (Figure 10.13).

10.4.1. First-Degree Burns

First-degree burns or superficial burns primarily affect the outermost skin layer, or epidermis. These burns result from direct exposure to the heat sources, such as sunburn, hot water, or fire. The presenting complaint and signs and symptoms are redness, swelling, and pain over the burnt area. Unlike more severe burns, first-degree burns don't cause blistering or injury to the inner skin layers and can thus heal relatively quickly. The patients will typically have some pain for a few days to a week, and then the skin will peel as it heals. First-degree burns are not rare and typically can be treated at home with cold water, aloe vera, or over-the-counter painkillers to ease pain and heal. While first-degree burns are otherwise trivial wounds, they also deserve appropriate care to prevent complications. Management for these burns is aimed at pain reduction and maintaining skin integrity. Cooling the burn with running water for 10 to 15 minutes reduces pain and swelling in a notable way. Topical medications in the form of aloe vera gel or anti-inflammatory creams can also facilitate healing and soothe the affected skin. It is also necessary to monitor the burn area for evidence of infection, especially in cases where the wound might cover extensive portions of the body. Sticking to proper wound care procedures not only promotes healing but also prevents secondary infection, which would complicate what appeared to be a superficial thermal burn initially. Although less serious than second- and third-degree burns, first-degree burns can also cause psychosocial distress and quality-of-life issues, particularly if in conspicuous areas such as the face or hands. Anxiety about scarring or a change in appearance is one issue that patients might experience and, subsequently, affect their ability to function psychologically and emotionally. Also, recurrent sunburns, a common form of first-degree burns, may potentially increase the risk for skin cancer in the future, and prevention measures such as the application of sunscreen and protective equipment are paramount. Sounding the alarm about the potential outcomes of first-degree burns and the importance of treatment is essential to fostering a better understanding of thermal injuries in humans and minimizing their overall health impact in society (Figure 10.14).

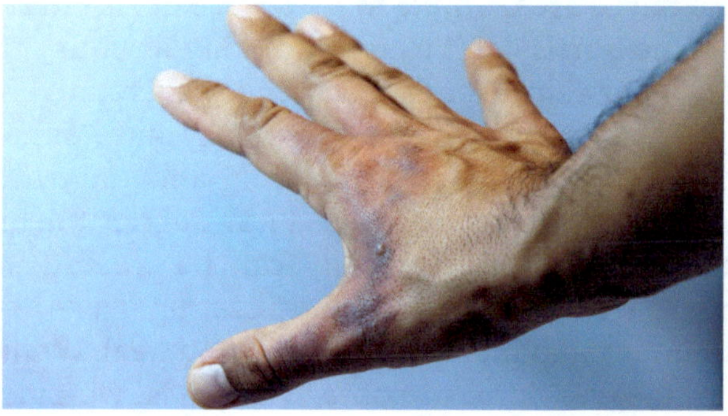

Figure 10.14. First-degree burns are superficial burns affecting only the outer layer of skin.

Source: https://post.medicalnewstoday.com/wp-content/uploads/sites/3/2022/01/first-degree-burn_iStock171265966_slide-1024x575.jpg.

10.4.2. Second-Degree Burns

Second-degree, or partial-thickness burns, are characterized by damage that extends past the epidermis and into the dermis, the skin structure made up of connective tissue, hair follicles, and sweat glands. The injury produces more clinical presentation than first-degree burns, which is usually blistering, edema, and significant pain. The activation of the dermis provides for exposure to nerves, which is responsible for the heightened sensitivity of the involved tissues. Varying with the nature of the specific burn, that is, duration of exposure and intensity of the thermal agent, second-degree burns can be of variable intensity, necessitating varying methods for management and treatment. The healing process of second-degree burns typically involves re-epithelialization and granulation tissue formation, both of which are fundamental to achieving skin integrity. However, this process is not complication-free. An example is post-burn cardiac injury, which has been identified as a critical prognostic factor for morbidity and mortality in burn patients, especially in severe cases requiring intensive medical treatment. Literature indicates that the cardiovascular system has been adversely affected after thermal injury, and sometimes the intricacies of such complications remain to be uncovered. This evidence warrants rigorous patient assessment after burns and encompasses monitoring of the cardiovascular status after the injury, as evidenced in recent burn patient literature, including information gained from animal models (Episcopal et al., 2020). In addition to cardiovascular conditions, the role of endothelial progenitor cells (EPCs) in repairing wounds has been an area of interest in learning about second-degree burns. EPCs have a significant role in neovascularization, which is required to bring nutrients and oxygen to the healing tissue. Mobilization of EPCs after burn injury can be employed as a biomarker when assessing the extent of the burn and healing potential. Though existing literature reveals inconclusive evidence of the relationship between EPC mobilization and the severity of burns, it is well-documented that EPCs play an important role in the regeneration processes following thermal burns. Advances in the knowledge about EPCs can pave the way for novel treatment strategies focused on enhanced recovery among second-degree burn victims, expanding research potential within the field (Adnani et al., 2016) (Figure 10.15).

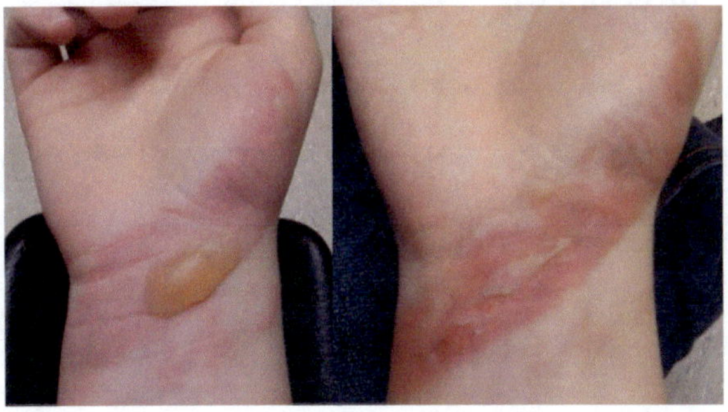

Figure 10.15. Second-degree burns are painful. Blisters and moderate skin peeling are present.

Source: https://post.medicalnewstoday.com/wp-content/uploads/sites/3/2022/01/VerbrennungGrad2a_slide-1024x575.jpg.

10.4.3. Third-Degree Burns

Third-degree or full-thickness burns are the most severe form of thermal burn, extending down through the dermis and epidermis to involve deeper tissue, such as subcutaneous fat and muscle. Full-thickness burns are characterized by loss of skin integrity with a leathery, dry appearance that is usually white, charred, or waxy. Unlike partial-thickness and superficial burns, where certain skin function and sensation are preserved, third-degree burns can be painless due to nerve-ending loss. Such painlessness can lead to underestimation of the severity of the injury and delayed medical intervention. Third-degree burns intricacy in the healing process necessitates comprehensive treatment protocols including surgery and skin graft to regain function and aesthetics of the burned tissue, signifying the urgent need for effective management protocols in thermal injury. Healing after a third-degree burn is significantly prolonged and plagued by the risk of complications. Secondary infections are common due to the weakened protective barrier that intact skin otherwise provides, and scarring can be correlated with long-term psychosocial impairment for patients if the burns traverse highly visible locations. Contractures can also be correlated with functional impairment in patients, restricting movement to a great extent, depending on the location of the burn.

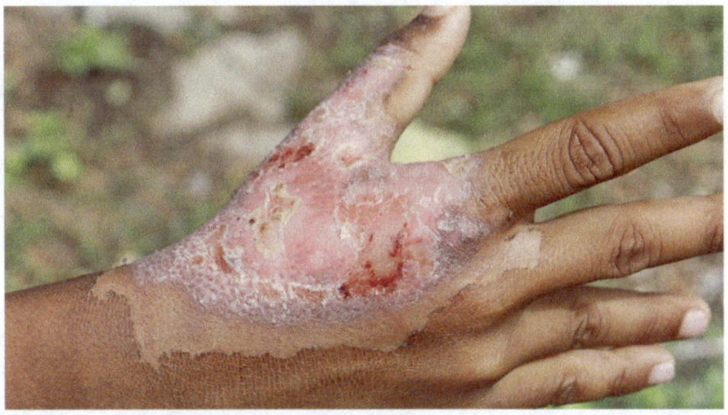

Figure 10.16. Third-degree burns.

Source: https://post.medicalnewstoday.com/wp-content/uploads/sites/3/2021/02/TDB3.jpg.

Managing these complications needs a multidisciplinary strategy, including not just surgical and medical interventions but also psychological care and rehabilitation services to facilitate recovery. As the prevalence of third-degree burns keeps increasing in different settings, including wildfire-related and industrial accident-related (Epstein et al., 2020), it becomes critical to understand the overall implications of third-degree burns to enhance patient outcomes for victims. There is evidence to indicate that well-designed treatment protocols for third-degree burns are important in minimizing their long-term impacts. For example, advances in dressings and skin substitutes have been shown to promote wound healing and protect against infection. Early intervention with surgical debridement to remove dead tissue and properly manage the wound is now emphasized by most medical practitioners. Interestingly, more recent studies also point to the cardiovascular distress that is related to serious burn trauma, and they emphasize vigilant monitoring of the affected patients for timely identification of complications (Adcock et al., 2018). Such newer information regarding the pathophysiology of third-degree burn again emphasizes the necessity for ongoing study and improved clinical methods for the sake of optimizing care for thermal burn patients. By considering both short-term and long-term therapeutic goals, the recovery pathways in healthcare systems can be enhanced and a better quality of life ensured among survivors of burns (Figure 10.16).

Test Your Knowledge

1. First-degree burns primarily affect which layer of the skin?
2. What is a second-degree burn called?

10.5. Treatment and Management

Learning Outcome

1. Learn about immediate first aid measures.
2. Describe the medical interventions for thermal injuries.
3. Understand the rehabilitation and recovery process.

Effective treatment and care for heat injuries are essential to minimize complications and enhance recovery rates among sufferers. First response, also called first aid, involves the evacuation of the individual from the source of heat and the cooling of the injured areas through the application of running water for a duration of not less than 20 minutes. This is a quick response that minimizes heat damage and discomfort. Following the cooling process, assessment of burn severity is important because it will direct treatment subsequently. Burns are classified on the basis of their severity and depth, with first-degree burns being the least severe and third-degree burns highly risky for complications in the form of infection and systemic response. Distinguishing this categorization allows health care providers to implement the corresponding interventions from simple wound management for minimal burns to complex surgical treatment for major burns. In major thermal injury, multidisciplinary treatment is often warranted. Special treatment teams like burn surgeons, dermatologists, and rehabilitation experts deliver complete treatment, including physical and psychological rehabilitation. More advanced treatments, such as grafting, debridement, and the use of bioengineered skin substitutes, are used for wound care and healing of deep burns. Along with this, the psychological impact of the thermal injury must be managed because most patients are indeed affected by PTSD and trauma-related anxiety. Incorporation of mental health interventions in treatment can go a long way in improvement. The use of sophisticated research and technologies, such as skin substitutes, mirrors the dynamic nature of burn management, illustrating the need for continuous improvement in this field to maximize patient outcomes. As well, due to the effect thermal trauma has on general health, long-term care is a component of care. Patients may need to continue physical rehabilitation to restore movement, especially in the instance of extensive skin grafting or surgery. Complications monitoring, for instance, infections or airway compromise for inhalation injuries, is important in ensuring patient safety. Further, scar management education and lifestyle modifications can direct the healing of patients more effectively. Empirical evidence also indicates that patients suffering from severe burns are prone to cardiovascular complications, as evidenced by veterinary population studies evaluating comparable injuries (Epstein et al., 2020). With an understanding of these interrelated health issues, health professionals can take a holistic stance, thereby maximizing the quality of life of patients recovering from thermal injuries (Figure 10.17).

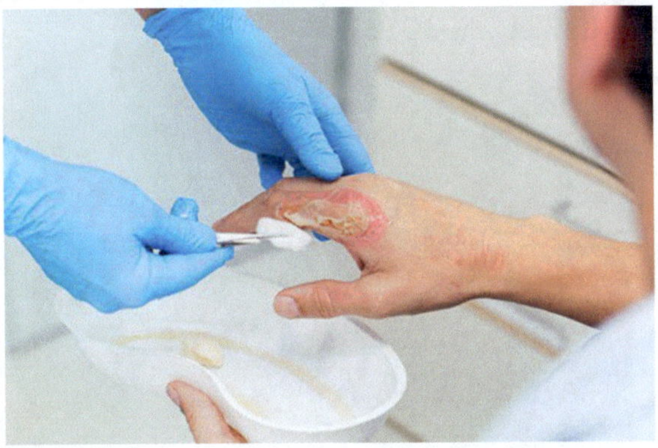

Figure 10.17. Thermal injury treatment.

Source: https://www.medicoexperts.com/wp-content/uploads/2021/10/symptoms-of-burn-injuries.jpg.

10.5.1. Immediate First Aid Measures

Thermal burns treatment involves early and systematic intervention, particularly during the very immediate post-trauma period. The use of immediate first aid is critical to avoid or limit the impact of heat, which can be an acute complication if not immediately addressed. Cooling the affected area is the primary objective in early treatment, which can dramatically prevent tissue damage and pain. It can be cooled by lukewarm (not cold) water streamed lightly over the burned area for a minimum of 10 to 20 minutes. This not only releases the heat but also calms burning and prevents further damage to the skin. Besides this, the dressing of the burn with a sterile non-stick dressing can also protect the area from infection and further damage, making these initial steps important to burn healing and treatment. In addition to cooling and dressing the burn, assessing the extent of the thermal trauma is important in guiding further treatment. The assessment relies on whether the trauma is superficial, partial-thickness, or full-thickness and informs medical-related decisions. For instance, those injuries that were graded as third-degree burns, involving all structures in the skin and potentially disintegrating supporting tissue, typically require specialist medical care. Aside from the administration of burn treatment, it is also important to evaluate the victim for shock to have developed, which can be caused by severe pain or dehydration due to more severe burns. The presentation of pale, clammy skin, a racing heart, or confusion demands immediate attention by a qualified medical operator. Awareness of the severity of the injury allows responders to elevate care accordingly and guarantees that the victim is provided with prompt and adequate assistance. Last but not least, it is crucial that a patient and comforting environment is created while providing first aid. Psycho-emotional support has the potential to significantly impact the psychological consequences for burn victims at this vulnerable phase. Comforting the affected individual serves to minimize panic and anxiety, which are automatic responses to traumatic injuries like burns. Where appropriate, having the victim recline and raising the injured part above the heart level could also assist in minimizing swelling and pain. Furthermore, providing accurate information on steps being taken helps to build confidence in the treatment being provided. Having provided initial first aid, a professional medical evaluation is required to further assess and treat the injury, particularly if the burn is severe or shows signs of infection. These early interventions not only help in physical recovery but also facilitate a better healing experience for patients with thermal injuries (Figure 10.18).

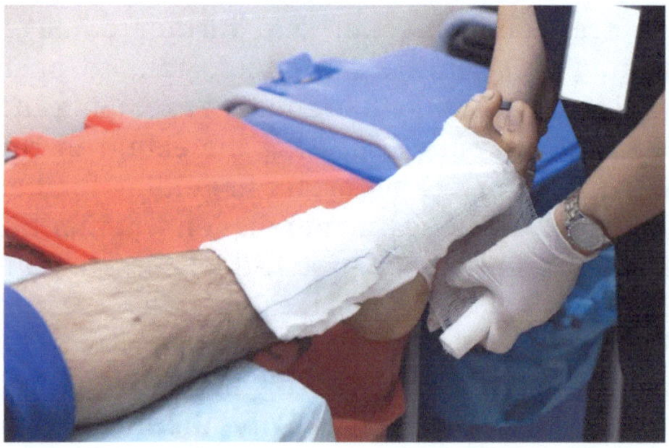

Figure 10.18. First aid treatment for thermal burns.

Source: https://www.mhg.sg/wp-content/uploads/2021/02/cover-burn-with-blanket-1024x683.jpg.

10.5.2. Medical Interventions

Thermal trauma medical treatment is significant in enhancing the patient outcome and diminishing complications. The first treatment is often to assess the severity of the burn, which is categorized into first, second, or third-degree burns. Each category dictates a varying medical strategy. For instance, first-degree burns may be treated with local creams and painkillers, while more serious second-degree burns may require expert wound treatment to prevent infection and aid faster healing of the burns. In third-degree burns, where the dermal layers are completely destroyed, surgery in the form of skin grafting may be necessitated to facilitate regeneration and restore the integrity of the skin (Van der Merwe et al., 2018). Furthermore, management of systemic complications such as fluid loss and hypothermia is essential as part of the overall management, necessitating advanced medical care to be able to control the vital signs along with intravenous hydration. Pain relief is another essential component of the medical management of thermal injuries. Victims of severe burns experience acute as well as chronic pain, which needs both pharmacological and non-pharmacological interventions for relief. Analgesics may include opioids and nonsteroidal anti-inflammatory drugs, while adjunctive therapy, such as cognitive-behavioral therapies, can aid in psychological support. Psychosocial implications of burn injuries are also significant to manage because they considerably impact emotional well-being and overall quality of life. Incorporating multidisciplinary teams, including pain specialists and mental health professionals, is the foundation for designing interdisciplinary care plans based on individual patient needs (Maulder et al., 2018).

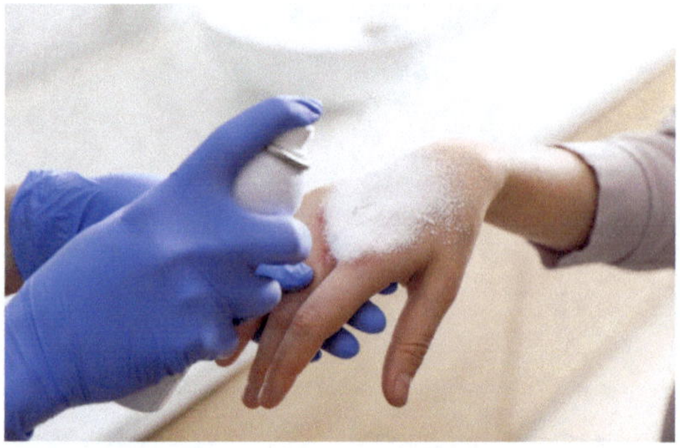

Figure 10.19. Thermal trauma medical treatment.

Source: https://drzaydon.com/wp-content/uploads/2022/07/burns-specialist-miami.png.

Such teamwork ensures that the focus also extends beyond the healing of the body to encompass emotional and psychological healing as well. Lastly, rehabilitation plays a very important role in the medical management of heat burns. Once the initial danger of pain and infection has been treated, patients typically require extensive rehabilitation to restore function and mobility to affected areas. Physical therapy can be necessary to regain strength, flexibility, and coordination in affected areas. This can include certain exercises, occupational therapy, and the use of specially designed splints to prevent contractures, which, if untreated, can lead to permanent disability. Additionally, the psychological impact of thermal injury disfigurement should not be underestimated; counseling and group therapy can facilitate adaptation, making the patient able to deal with his or her new situation following injury. Thus, an integrated treatment plan consisting of physical rehabilitation, psycho-support, and continuous medical evaluation is vital to the overall success of thermal injury care (Van der Merwe et al., 2018) (Figure 10.19).

10.5.3. Rehabilitation and Recovery

The rehabilitation and recovery process following heat injuries requires a multidimensional methodology, directly applicable to the patient's individualized requirements. Maximal recovery depends on the integration of physical recovery with psychiatric care, especially given the intense and often traumatic nature of such injury. Rehabilitation guidelines target physical restoration to function and movement, and address the emotional and psychological needs of the victim subsequent to injury. This two-way approach is crucial, as many have issues with their mind and body when they've incurred extensive burns or other heat trauma. The treatment of these psychological issues is as important as the physical recovery that occurs, providing a milieu for healing and reintroduction to daily living. One of the facilitative aspects of the treatment for thermal injury patients is the application of on-scene rehabilitation (OSR). Literature shows that OSR is capable of curbing the physiological stress that is expressed through acts that are commonly performed by firefighters, such as working in emergencies under conditions of hot weather. Literature has shown that firefighters undergo increased cardiovascular and thermal stress, which can lead to serious health conditions, including mortality, when not kept under control. A report stated the necessity of researching efficient recovery protocols, including a comparative study of improved and control OSR interventions. Highlighting these findings may be helpful in imparting informative knowledge for improving recovery protocols, thereby reducing health hazards from excessive physical activity, which is precisely the need for thermal injury recovery. The application of technology to formulate procedures in rehabilitation cannot be overlooked, particularly with the utilization of devices such as GPS to monitor recovery phases and physical activities during training and rehabilitation. While predominantly applied in sports medicine, these technologies have promising applications for any rehabilitation facility, including thermal injury setups. For instance, monitoring activity levels and metabolic responses will allow tailored rehabilitation programs to adapt to the exact challenges faced by each patient in the rehabilitation process. Identifying specific recovery milestones allows practitioners to administer an effective and targeted rehabilitation process that maximizes recovery. Through the integration of new techniques, such as constant monitoring and personalized fitness programs, there is an important step forward in enhancing the rehabilitation of patients recovering from the debilitating effects of heat injury.

Test Your Knowledge

1. What is the primary goal of immediate first aid in thermal injuries?
2. What medication is used for thermal burns?

10.6. Psychological Impact

Learning Outcome

1. Describe the emotional trauma from thermal injuries.
2. Know the long-term psychological effects of thermal injuries.
3. Describe the support systems and counseling.

Thermal trauma, particularly that which is suffered in extreme conditions, can cause significant psychological distress among the survivors. The psychological impact may be caused by injury severity, recovery duration, and potential long-term changes in body function or body image. Victims experience a myriad of emotions such as depression, fear, and anxiety, in addition to the pain caused by their injuries. The stress of undergoing invasive treatment, coupled with the hope of rehabilitation, can profoundly affect mental health. A complex interrelationship between psychological and physical recovery emerges, which necessitates an integrative approach to healing that addresses emotional as well as physical issues. In therapists treating thermal injury, a sense of the psychological ramifications is essential. Effective interventions can be initiated to establish both physical and psychological resilience. This can include providing counseling with a coping skills and emotional support emphasis. Research documents that early psychological interventions can diminish long-term effects such as post-traumatic stress disorder (PTSD) and long-term depression. In particular, efforts to establish systems of social support may be most important because isolated victims may find it particularly challenging during the recovery process. Therefore, the psychological impact of burn injuries needs to be acknowledged while establishing care procedures. Mental health professionals also play a vital part in rehabilitation. They can give essential support in dealing with trauma complications arising after injury. Following the research related to physical effort in dangerous professions, such as firefighting, it is evident that mental health problems need to be included in discussions about physical training and recovery methods. The utilization of prolonged on-scene rehabilitation procedures, as exemplified in the study of the health of firefighters, reflects the value of psychological evaluation following thermal trauma. Through the integration of mental health treatment within rehabilitation practices, the potential to enhance recovery rates significantly is present, creating a more holistic and informed approach based on a broader understanding of the human experience of trauma (Fahey et al., 2010; Van der Merwe et al., 2018) (Figure 10.20).

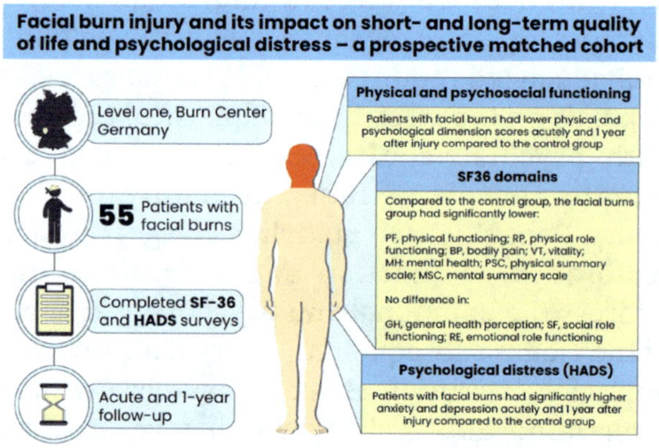

Figure 10.20. The impact of facial burns on short- and long-term quality of life and psychological distress.

Source: https://pub.mdpi-res.com/jcm/jcm-12-05057/article_deploy/html/images/jcm-12-05057-ag.png?1690861714.

10.6.1. Emotional Trauma from Thermal Injuries

The implications of thermal injuries extend well beyond the burns, which permanently brand the victim's body. Thermal injuries also have a deep psychological impact on the victim. Victims of burns are likely to experience emotional trauma, which may be in varying forms like depression, anxiety, and post-traumatic stress disorder (PTSD). Emotional disturbance is usually compounded by the social stigma of injuries in public, since it leads to social withdrawal and low self-esteem. The psychological effect is of particular concern in children, who may struggle to comprehend their injuries and responses from others. Furthermore, the recovery process can be emotionally stressful, with victims facing significant lifestyle adjustments, long-term medical treatment, and, in some cases, tolerated pain, all of which yield heightened stress levels and emotional disorientation. Psychological interventions have a critical role to play in the management of the emotional trauma associated with thermal injuries. Effective interventions may help develop coping skills and resilience in victims of burns. Cognitive behavior therapy (CBT) has proved useful in treating anxiety and depression caused by traumatic events, enabling patients to challenge maladaptive thinking and adopt more adaptive perspectives. Group therapy, and often peer support, can assist patients in the sharing of experiences and alleviation of feelings of isolation. Such interventions are essential for the improvement of mental health and reintegration into society, particularly in children. Treatment of the emotional impacts of thermal injuries is as crucial as treatment of the physical wounds; neglect of this element can lead to long-term psychological disturbances that are setbacks to recovery. New research underscores the significance of integrated care, considering both the physical and emotional health of survivors of burns. A new veterinary study involving patients exposed to heat burns from wildfires delineated the effect of trauma to cause grave consequences, such as cardiac injury, as an analogy for human cases (Epstein et al., 2020). According to this medical research, it goes without saying that interdisciplinary approaches would have a big return on human burn patients. Having mental health professionals as part of burn teams can ensure that patients receive a holistic treatment plan that caters to the nuances of emotional injury, as well as nurturing physical healing. This multifaceted treatment is required, since emotional trauma knowledge and healing may enable healing in general, which will allow victims to regain their lives after the widespread impacts of thermal injuries.

10.6.2. Long-Term Psychological Effects

The psychological implications of thermal trauma extend much beyond the direct physical effects, typically having profound long-term effects on those affected. The sufferers of major burns or other thermal trauma often develop long-term symptoms of post-traumatic stress disorder (PTSD), depression, and anxiety. The psychological scarring done by such injuries can also be added to by the lengthy rehabilitation process, which may include several surgeries, lengthy hospital stays, and radical lifestyle modifications.

Patients are likely to suffer from body image issues and problems of social readjustment. Not only are the psychological impacts individual, but they are also family and social relationship related, creating a domino effect that complicates the rehabilitation and recovery process. The study of such long-term psychological effects necessitates a complete understanding of the traumatizing nature of thermal injury and the ongoing struggle to maintain emotional strength. Moreover, the interaction between physical pain and emotional suffering can produce psychological illnesses that will persist long after the wound heals physically. Burn survivors and veterans often need to deal with embracing a new physical identity while struggling with shame and loneliness. The resultant social isolation of the stigma of observable scarring results in social withdrawal and inability to form new relationships, with a secondary layer of loneliness and despair. Psychological intervention with therapeutic interventions, support groups, and community programs, facilitating participation and acceptance, is necessary to treat such psychological problems. The understanding that such psychological problems are the norm serves to break down the stigma and get patients into treatment.

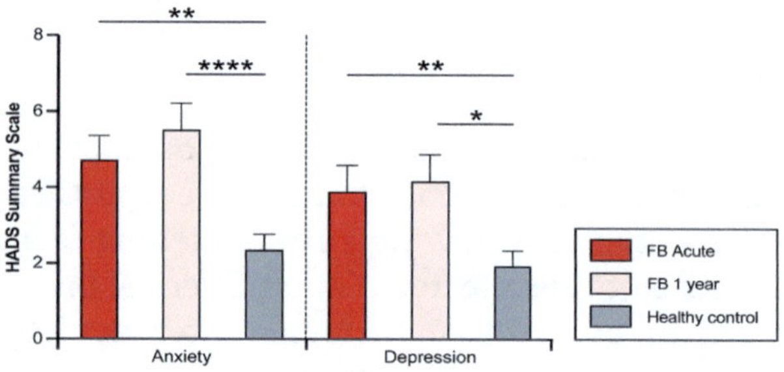

Figure 10.21. Short (acute) and long-term (one year) assessment of hospital anxiety and depression scale (HADS) scores after facial burn. Visualization of the scores in facial burn (FB) patients versus the healthy cohort.

Source: https://www.mdpi.com/jcm/jcm-12-05057/article_deploy/html/images/jcm-12-05057-g003.png.

Through such schemes, the long-term care of the elderly caused by the psychological effect of thermal injury can be substantially improved. Finally, in understanding the long-term psychological effects of thermal injury, there is a need to consider the part played by comprehensive treatment protocols that integrate mental health care with rehabilitation. Evidence suggests that patients receiving psychological attention throughout recovery have better outcomes in terms of emotional well-being and quality of life. For instance, interventions toward cognitive behavioral therapy and trauma-informed care are a long way in addressing some of the burdens of PTSD and anxiety disorders. In addition, designing spaces for mutual aid and shared experience can allow individuals to walk the path to healing together. As is suggested through research, effective treatment methods not only address the psychological dimensions of recovery but also develop resilience and restore a sense of agency in individuals who are healing from thermal trauma (Maulder et al., 2018; Van der Merwe et al., 2018) (Figure 10.21).

10.6.3. Support Systems and Counseling

Thermal trauma from industrial accidents, natural disasters, or personal mishaps may extend beyond the actual physical trauma, creating psychological effects that demand extensive support systems and counseling. Patients experiencing deep burns or heat trauma often have trouble with emotional challenges such as anxiety, depression, and post-traumatic stress disorder (PTSD). Support systems help facilitate psychological recovery after trauma. This also involves the addition of mental health professionals who are able to treat the emotional and psychological consequences of thermal injuries and provide coping and resilience techniques. Developing a system of organized support, which encompasses peer support groups, counseling services, and educational material, ensures that the survivors not only receive medical treatments for their bodily wounds but also receive proper assistance for their emotional wounds, which is typically overlooked in traditional medical practices. Counseling services, targeted at those who endure thermal injuries, must be responsive to a multidisciplinary treatment acknowledging the individual issues of such patients. Healthcare providers should collaborate with mental health care providers to develop integrated treatment plans that incorporate physical healing and mental treatment. Cognitive-behavioral therapy (CBT) and trauma-informed care are therapeutic interventions that have the potential to assist survivors in redefining their identity and establishing a sense of normalcy. Above all, in the scenario of disasters like Hurricane Katrina, where society experienced large-scale trauma, institutions must be oriented toward implementing effective psychological support systems (Edwards et al., 2009). By establishing resilience through counseling and peer bonding, survivors are able to cultivate a support system that is instrumental in empowering them towards recovery after being injured. Moreover, the participation of society in support systems is instrumental in coping with the far-reaching impact of thermal injuries on social systems. Involving community leaders and local organizations in the creation of support networks can encourage outreach and provide victims with a sense of belonging. Education for awareness that raises their knowledge of the psychological impact of thermal injuries can also foster sympathy from society, working to diminish stigma towards seeking treatment. Efficacious support systems need to both respond at the individual survivor level and be coordinated at the community level to create elaborate recovery and resilience plans. By integrating counseling as part of community programs directly, it is possible to consolidate emotional pillars of societies that have been traumatized by thermal trauma, with the outcome being healthier societies that can deal more effectively with impending disasters (Edwards et al., 2009).

Test Your Knowledge

1. What is the emotional trauma from thermal injuries?
2. What are the long-term psychological effects of thermal injuries?

SUMMARY

In simplifying the intricacies of thermal injuries in humans, it is clear that these injuries are highly challenging across various settings, ranging from routine environmental exposures to extreme instances arising from chemical burns or scalds. The physiological, psychological, and socio-economic effects of such injuries can be far-reaching, affecting not only the victim but also healthcare systems and societal norms. Effective preventive measures, including tolerance to temperature and risk factor awareness, play a central role in thermal injury prevention. These need to be included in public health campaigns so that the population is equipped with information concerning the risks involved in unfavorable temperatures and protective methods. Additionally, the therapy of thermal injuries relies on both immediate first aid and subsequent medical treatment. Literature emphasizes the necessity of individualized treatment protocols that match the patient's specific level of injury, from superficial burn to increased tissue injury. Evidence from research indicates that individually tailored rehabilitation interventions, such as the application of novel topical solutions and psychological management, can effectively maximize recovery patterns and quality of life among impacted patients. Of interest, blending new technologies potentially can maximize clinical outcomes, emphasizing the need for further research on new modalities of treatment for burn victims. Finally, as demonstrated in discussions regarding the performance of athletes, discussions regarding physiological adaptation and psychological resilience on the part of the patient are of main concern with regard to recovery and rehabilitation from thermal trauma. Methods involving both mental and physical conditioning, like those in sports science, have the potential to greatly assist victims who are recovering from thermal trauma. More studies need to be conducted in these related fields, not only to advance treatment models but also to have a complete picture of how individuals are managing recuperation. As quoted in a study examining exercise and performance, leveraging multidisciplinary approaches may give vast insights into thermal injury patients' rehabilitation systems and improve outcomes through integrated care procedures (Van der Merwe et al., 2018; Maulder et al., 2018).

The large prevalence of heat injuries among human beings, particularly in perilous occupations such as firefighting, calls for caution in the prevention and recovery processes. Around 100 firefighters lose their lives every year in the course of duty, while numerous others suffer from injuries that are caused by the physical demands of their occupation, in addition to the heat. Almost 45% of firefighter fatalities are linked with heart attacks, which take place mostly after intense firefighting activities. Studies have indicated that the main cause of injury while battling fires is related to overexertion and strain, indicating that awareness of the physiological effects of heat exposure is critical in designing protective steps in fire brigades (Fahey et al., 2010). These findings support the importance of ongoing research on recovery treatments that can act against the cardiovascular and thermal strain endured by firefighters while working. Moreover, advances in technology, such as infrared thermography (IRT), have also been useful in supplementing our understanding of thermal injuries. In a clinical environment, the application of IRT allows us to measure skin temperature in real-time, which is a key factor in evaluating thermal exposure. This technology has gained popularity in the field of sports and exercise medicine, where data collection guidelines still do not exist. From a Delphi study involving experts from different fields, a very comprehensive checklist for the proper application of IRT was formulated. This questionnaire, the Thermographic Imaging in Sports and Exercise Medicine (TISEM), was intended to standardize data collection and allow clinicians to evaluate thermal reactions in numerous varied scenarios, such as thermal injury to human beings (Adamczyk et al., 2017). The setting of these standards highlights the significance of having a procedure system for thermographic assessment. Finally, thermal injuries need a multi-dimensional strategy with preventive and post-exposure treatment protocols. For firefighting, on-scene rehabilitation (OSR) has been suggested to minimize the stresses of hard work, but the effectiveness of various OSR interventions remains to be examined systematically. New research tries to explain the acute physiological reactions to firefighting and the recovery process, providing crucial data on cardiovascular reactions and heat stress. By comparing different strategies for rehabilitation, researchers are contributing to the knowledge base on best practices in promoting recovery and reducing the incidence of severe thermal injuries. As a result, continued study of these strategies is essential to optimizing safety and performance in high-risk environments, ultimately protecting human health (Fahey et al., 2010).

KEY TERMS FROM THIS CHAPTER

- Burns
- Flames
- Heat exhaustion
- Physical therapy
- Rehabilitation
- Scalds
- Thermal injuries
- Chronic pain
- Frostbite
- Heat-related afflictions
- Psychological support
- Scalding liquids
- Skin grafts
- Thermal trauma

CRITICAL THINKING QUESTIONS

1. **Which of the following is classified as a first-degree burn?**
   a. Burn involving epidermis and dermis with blistering
   b. Burn involving only the epidermis with redness and pain
   c. Burn involving muscle and bone
   d. Burn with complete charring of skin
2. **What is the primary cause of death in cases of extensive thermal burns?**
   a. Sepsis
   b. Hemorrhage
   c. Hypoglycemia
   d. Anaphylaxis
3. **Which of the following is a hallmark of antemortem burns?**
   a. Cherry red discoloration
   b. Absence of inflammation
   c. Vital reaction such as blister formation
   d. Fixed lividity
4. **Which type of burn is most commonly associated with electrical injuries?**
   a. Flash burns
   b. Deep tissue burns with small entry and exit wounds
   c. Superficial scalds
   d. First-degree burns only
5. **In forensic pathology, "pugilistic posture" is indicative of:**
   a. Antemortem struggle
   b. Electrical burns
   c. Postmortem drying
   d. Heat stiffening due to high temperature

Short Answer Questions

1. What is the definition of a thermal injury?
2. List the types of thermal injuries.
3. What is the cause of a thermal injury?
4. What is the mechanism of thermal injury?
5. What is the classification of a burn?

Answer to Critical Thinking Questions

1. (b) 2. (a) 3. (c) 4. (b) 5. (d)

REFERENCES

1. Ablewhite, J., Achana, F., Benford, P., et al. (2017). Keeping children safe: A multicenter programmed of research to increase the evidence base for preventing unintentional injuries in the home in the under-fives. https://core.ac.uk/download/84637006.pdf (accessed on 12th July 2025).
2. Adamczyk, J. G., Ammer, K., Bach, A. J. E., et al. (2017). Thermographic imaging in sports and exercise medicine: A Delphi study and consensus statement on the measurement of human skin temperature. https://core.ac.uk/download/288395288.pdf (accessed on 12th July 2025).
3. Adcock, S., Rajapaksha, E., Tucker, C., et al. (2018). Branding practices on four dairies in Kantale, Sri Lanka. https://core.ac.uk/download/323070107.pdf (accessed on 12th July 2025).
4. Adnani, B. O., Araniego, C. A., Banyard, D. A., et al. (2016). Endothelial progenitor cells and burn injury–exploring the relationship. https://core.ac.uk/download/323075412.pdf (accessed on 12th July 2025).
5. Bloyer, M. H. (1999). The effects of therapeutic ultrasound on open wounds. https://core.ac.uk/download/46950553.pdf (accessed on 12th July 2025).
6. Brown, C., Gasper, J. R., & Habegger, L. J. (1980). Health and safety: Preliminary comparative assessment of the Satellite Power System (SPS) and other energy alternatives. https://core.ac.uk/download/pdf/42860725.pdf (accessed on 12th July 2025).
7. Burak, I. I., & Cherkasova, O. A. (2013). Labor safety. https://core.ac.uk/download/53873565.pdf (accessed on 12th July 2025).
8. Caggiano, G., DE GIGLIO, O., Montagna, M. T., et al. (2016). Knowledge, attitudes, and behavior concerning dental trauma among parents of children attending primary school. https://core.ac.uk/download/84928145.pdf (accessed on 12th July 2025).
9. Cruz-Loya, M., Lozano-Huntelman, N., Rodríguez-Verdugo, A., et al. (2020). Compounding effects of climate warming and antibiotic resistance. https://core.ac.uk/download/323082801.pdf (accessed on 12th July 2025).
10. Dablainville, V., Mornas, A., Normand-Gravier, T., Al-Mulla, M., Papakostas, E. T., Olory, B., Marín Fermín, T., et al. (2025). Muscle regeneration is improved by hot water immersion but unchanged by cold following a simulated musculoskeletal injury in humans. *The Journal of Physiology*. https://www.semanticscholar.org/paper/cf71a68b6c8902379c1341445bfd73444c64d232 (accessed on 12th July 2025).
11. Dereeper, A., Hartl, A., Hubel, A., Shonhai, A., Walther, A., Yamamoto, A., Sanchez, A. A., et al. (2012). Small but crucial: The novel small heat shock protein Hsp21 mediates stress adaptation and virulence in *Candida albicans*. https://core.ac.uk/download/11303948.pdf (accessed on 12th July 2025).
12. Edwards, F., & Goodrich, D. C. (2009). The role of transportation in campus emergency planning, MTI Report 08-06. https://core.ac.uk/download/70413477.pdf (accessed on 12th July 2025).
13. Epstein, S. E., Gunther-Harrington, C. T., Li, R. H. L., et al. (2020). Cats with thermal burn injuries from California wildfires show echocardiographic evidence of myocardial thickening and intracardiac thrombi. https://core.ac.uk/download/323070249.pdf (accessed on 12th July 2025).

14. Fahey, G. C., Fernhall, B., Horn, G. P., Illinois Fire Service Institute, et al. (2010). The effects of firefighting and on-scene rehabilitation on hemostasis. https://core.ac.uk/download/4837716.pdf (accessed on 12th July 2025).

15. Federici, J. F., Molento, C. F. M., Sans, E. C. O., et al. (2016). Assessment of broiler chicken welfare in Southern Brazil. https://core.ac.uk/download/55742528.pdf (accessed on 12th July 2025).

16. Freeman, C. (2019). The effects of pre and post-exercise low-level laser therapy on biochemical markers of skeletal muscle fatigue in equines. https://core.ac.uk/download/215464245.pdf (accessed on 12th July 2025).

17. Gurjar, B. R., & Mohan, M. (2002). Environmental risk analysis: Problems and perspectives in different countries. https://core.ac.uk/download/72056551.pdf (accessed on 12th July 2025).

18. Hahladakis, J. N., Velis, C. A., Weber, R., Iacovidou, E., & Purnell, P. (2017). An overview of chemical additives presents in plastics: Migration, release, fate, and environmental impact during their use, disposal, and recycling. *Journal of Hazardous Materials*, *344*, 179–199. https://doi.org/10.1016/j.jhazmat.2017.10.014 (accessed on 12th July 2025).

19. Horta, R., Almeida, A., Horta, P., & Oliveira, H. (2020). No rib cartilage, no prosthesis: Partial ear reconstruction using a composite chondrocutaneous peninsular flap associated with a retro auricular flap. *Microsurgery*, *40*. https://www.semanticscholar.org/paper/05575c3ae45a6442530babf7bc5de3b990b91db6 (accessed on 12th July 2025).

20. Hyde, R. (2019). Conversations in architectural science. *Architectural Science Review*, *62*, 193–194. https://www.semanticscholar.org/paper/bc021a66841d738a80cf5678d67caadd8077807b (accessed on 12th July 2025).

21. Klonizakis, M. (2012). Studying the cutaneous microcirculatory response during upper-limb exercise in healthy, older, sedentary people. https://core.ac.uk/download/1645737.pdf (accessed on 12th July 2025).

22. Liu, S., Song, J., Mao, H., Zhao, J., & Song, Q. (2020). Expert consensus on the diagnosis and treatment of heat stroke in China. *Military Medical Research*, *7*. https://doi.org/10.1186/s40779-019-0229-2 (accessed on 12th July 2025).

23. Maulder, P. S., & McDonald, K. (2018). The effects of morning preconditioning protocols on testosterone, cortisol, and afternoon sprint cycling performance [conference presentation]. https://core.ac.uk/download/187724674.pdf (accessed on 12th July 2025).

24. McIntosh, S., Freer, L., Grissom, C. K., Auerbach, P. S., Rodway, G. W., Cochran, A., Giesbrecht, G. G., et al. (2019). Wilderness Medical Society clinical practice guidelines for the prevention and treatment of frostbite: 2019 update. *Wilderness and Environmental Medicine*, *30*, S19–S32. https://doi.org/10.1016/j.wem.2019.05.002 (accessed on 12th July 2025).

25. N/A. (2025). Aerospace medicine and biology: A continuing bibliography with indexes (supplement 331). https://core.ac.uk/download/pdf/42824791.pdf (accessed on 12th July 2025).

26. Nattiv, A., Philp, A., Loucks, A. B., Loucks, A. B., Jeukendrup, A. E., Jeukendrup, A. E., Jeukendrup, A. E., et al. (2020). Nutrition strategies for triathlon. https://core.ac.uk/download/249364290.pdf (accessed on 12th July 2025).

27. Reddy, A. (2016). The effect of environment on post-surgical overall well-being and pain sensitivity in an animal model. https://open.bu.edu/bitstream/2144/14941/1/Reddy_bu_0017N_10538.pdf (accessed on 12th July 2025).

28. Rowan, M. P., Cancio, L. C., Elster, E. A., Burmeister, D. M., Rose, L. F., Natesan, S., Chan, R. K., et al. (2015). Burn wound healing and treatment: Review and advancements. *Critical Care, 19.* https://doi.org/10.1186/s13054-015-0961-2 (accessed on 12th July 2025).

29. Stramler, J. (2025). Occupational ergonomics in space. https://core.ac.uk/download/pdf/42810341.pdf (accessed on 12th July 2025).

30. Tan, A. W. K., Li, R. H. L., Ueda, Y., Stern, J., Hussain, M., Haginoya, S., Sharpe, A. N., et al. (2022). Platelet priming and activation in naturally occurring thermal burn injuries and wildfire smoke exposure is associated with intracardiac thrombosis and spontaneous echocardiographic contrast in feline survivors. *Frontiers in Veterinary Science*, *9*. https://www.semanticscholar.org/paper/c4094ee726f1367aa83d67ce2ce6cebb7713b33d (accessed on 12th July 2025).

31. Vainionpää, M. (2014). Thermographic imaging in cats and dogs: Usability as a clinical method. https://core.ac.uk/download/20441286.pdf (accessed on 12th July 2025).

32. Van der Merwe, F. H. (2018). GPS analysis of a team competing at a national Under 18 field hockey tournaments. https://core.ac.uk/download/187724717.pdf (accessed on 12th July 2025).

33. Weyhing, W. (2020). Care after burn trauma: A burn toolkit for providers. https://core.ac.uk/download/368317133.pdf (accessed on 12th July 2025).

SUDDEN DEATHS

11

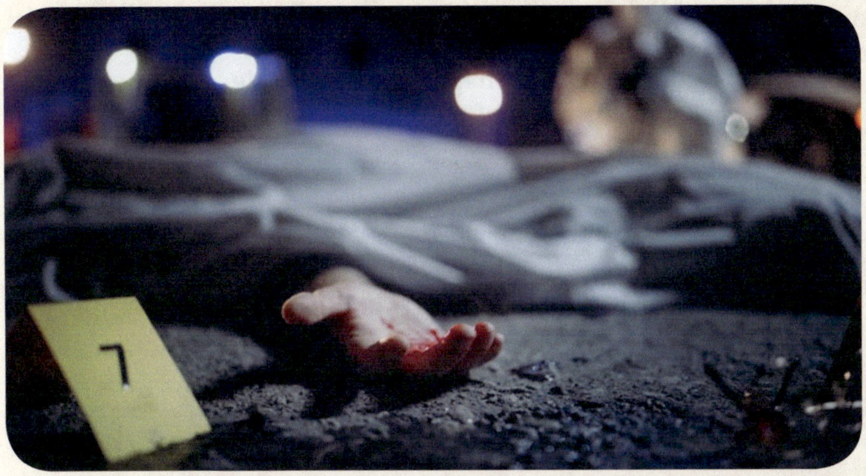

LEARNING OBJECTIVES

After studying this chapter, you will be able to:

1. Know the causes of sudden death;
2. Describe the demographics of sudden death
3. Know the psychological impact of sudden death;
4. Describe the preventive measures in addressing the issue of sudden deaths;
5. Understand the role of technology in understanding sudden death.

Introduction

The syndrome of sudden death in man encompasses a range of medical conditions and situations that can lead to sudden death without any warning. One of the chief causative factors in this phenomenon is the role of inherited conditions, one of the most prevalent hereditary cardiomyopathies, and a foremost cause of sudden cardiac death, being hypertrophic cardiomyopathy (HCM). The complexity of HCM lies in its variable presentation among patients, which is influenced by genetic heterogeneity and environmental factors. Despite advancements in cardiology therapeutics for managing this disease, current treatments are inadequate to cover the full spectrum of HCM conditions. Therefore, a systems biology approach is required to dissect the signaling pathways of cardiomyocyte hypertrophy to discover individualized treatment options that can mitigate the immediate risk associated with this disease (Luanpaisanon et al., 2024). Beyond genetics, natural disasters are a huge contributor to influencing human mortality rates, particularly concerning cardiovascular health. Earthquakes, for instance, respond with acute physiological and psychological symptoms, which have been found to trigger adverse cardiovascular events like myocardial infarction and cardiac mortality. According to science, even victims who do not suffer physical injuries under these traumatic experiences are at risk of developing stress reactions that affect their cardiovascular systems negatively. Stress triggers all the body's systems, leading to higher chances of cardiac complications. Increased research into how environmental stressors interact with traumatic cardiovascular conditions is needed, given that a lot of the evidence yields conflicting results regarding their impact. Public health policy and readiness improvement in traumatic events depend on evaluating short- and long-term effects of such exposure (Özge Turgay Yıldırım et al., 2024).

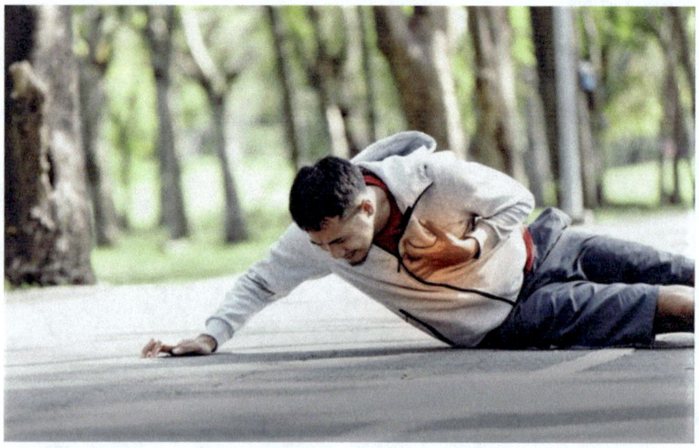

Figure 11.1. Sudden deaths.

Source: https://neu.edu.tr/wp-content/uploads/2022/06/13/ani-kalp-olum-1.jpg?ver=8435da3ac4849c59bfe1eecc5626ae4f.

Merging both genetic risk factors and environmental stressors might produce a more detailed explanation of the multifactorial etiology of sudden death in humans. Synergy between researchers from various disciplines, including genetics, cardiology, and disaster management, is crucial in developing effective interventions and prevention programs. With continued clarification of cardiac signaling network complexity via systems biology, identification of potential therapeutic targets presents novel paradigms for precision medicine in individuals with HCM and other related cardiovascular diseases. In addition, an enhanced understanding of the cardiovascular effects of environmental stressors, including those generated by earthquakes, may result in better public health programs aimed at reducing the ill effects of such occurrences. Finally, resolution of the interplay between genetic components and environmental factors is important in preventing sudden deaths in humans and thus improving overall health outcomes in society (Figure 11.1).

Definition of Sudden Death

Sudden death describes a chain of unanticipated fatalities occurring instantaneously and without prior warning, challenging the boundaries of medical understanding and emergency responses. Sudden death can result from a variety of underlying conditions, including cardiac arrest, neurological disorders, and other external factors like trauma. Distinguishing sudden death due to recognizable medical conditions from those occurring unexpectedly among apparently healthy patients is crucial. Such unpredictability necessitates exhaustive examination of risk factors such as genetic predispositions, lifestyle behaviors, and environmental hazards. Such an understanding of the intricacies will facilitate maximizing preventive strategies and optimizing early detection in an attempt to minimize the incidence of sudden death in high-risk populations. The most feared cases of sudden death are those occurring in individuals with epilepsy, known as sudden unexpected death in epilepsy (SUDEP). This condition is a significant public health issue that highlights the need for additional research into the pathophysiological processes of this disorder. Research has shown that some of the structural brain alterations can predispose patients with epilepsy to SUDEP, and they consist of areas such as the amygdala and hippocampus in their etiology. These neurologic substrates have been noted to impact autonomic regulation and cardiac rhythm, rendering the patients particularly susceptible to lethal arrhythmias. SUDEP has been correlated with larger amounts of grey matter in certain regions of the brain, underscoring the complex connection between neurological health and sudden death (Balestrini et al., 2015). This overlap between brain and cardiovascular health underscores the need for interdisciplinary treatment and research approaches. Aside from neurological factors, cardiovascular disease remains the leading cause of sudden death among racially, ethnically, and socioeconomically diverse populations.

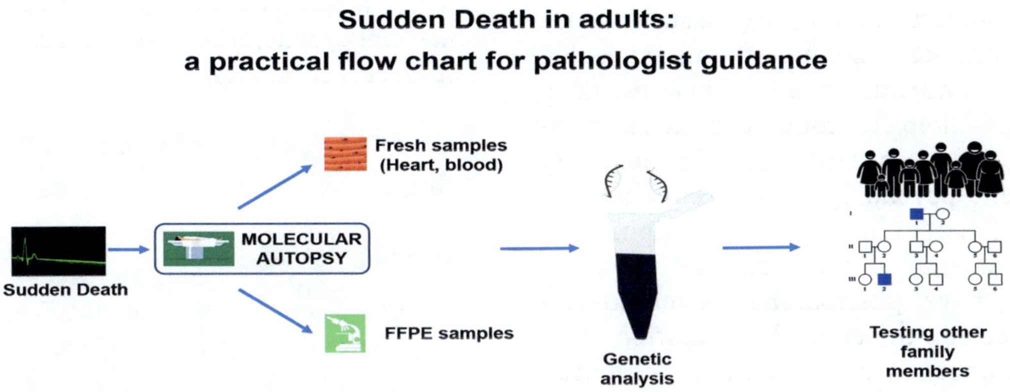

Figure 11.2. Sudden death in adults: A practical flow chart for pathologist guidance.

Source: https://pub.mdpi-res.com/healthcare/healthcare-09-00870/article_deploy/html/images/healthcare-09-00870-ag.png?1625832768.

Examples of these are arrhythmias and myocardial infarctions, which are often not diagnosed until they are seen acutely. Arrhythmias, in particular, are a consequence of many disease processes, including cardiac remodeling and inflammatory diseases, which are dangerous even in the absence of obvious heart disease. New research shows the dialogue between insular and temporal lobe neurogenic signals and their arrhythmogenic effects, suggesting that changes in autonomic control are a major contributor to cardiac function (Loh et al., 2014). This complex dialogue suggests that sudden death cannot just be a result of electrical dysfunction of the heart but a convergence of neurocardiac communication systems. It is critical to understand these complex relationships in order to form successful preventive approaches and enhance patient outcomes in individuals at risk for sudden death (Figure 11.2).

Importance of Studying Sudden Deaths

It is significant to investigate sudden human death because sudden deaths have countless health, social, and economic impacts. Sudden death comes from the occurrence of many unforeseen events, such as heart attacks, accidents, or natural catastrophes that surprise individuals and destroy families and communities. Understanding the epidemiology of sudden death episodes informs investigators and public health experts about patterns and risk factors, which ultimately enable preventive interventions. For instance, the knowledge of the occurrence of sudden cardiac events can be used to enhance screening protocols and lifestyle interventions for at-risk populations. By carrying out in-depth research on sudden deaths, the professionals can attempt to design appropriate public health interventions that would reduce the occurrence of such incidents, thereby enhancing overall community resilience and health. The necessity of carrying out research on sudden deaths extends to the mental health effects on the bereaved and those who are involved directly or indirectly in such events. Sudden deaths leave behind an unmanageable sense of loss and trauma, which may result in long-term psychological conditions such as post-traumatic stress disorder (PTSD). The necessity to document psychological consequences in instances of sudden deaths is also emphasized by research that some disasters, such as landslides, have phenomenal psychological consequences on the affected population, with resultant increased rates of PTSD compared to other disasters (Kennedy et al., 2015). By comprehending such psychological effects of trauma, intervention strategies can be developed to support individuals dealing with their loss and trauma, thus emphasizing the need to examine sudden human death from multiple angles. Additionally, findings from sudden death research lie at the heart of developing disaster readiness and response initiatives. Governments and healthcare agencies must anticipate the potential for sudden death scenarios in cases of natural disasters or pandemics. It is such anticipation that drives policy decisions, as seen from the massive hoarding of medication during cases like the H1N1 flu pandemic (Roemer-Mahler et al., 2014). Understanding reasons for and outcomes of acute death can inform policymakers to introduce sweeping emergency measures. Lastly, this research not only seeks to enhance near-term reactions to unanticipated death event incidents, but it also seeks to strive towards a broader theme of public health and safety preparedness to make communities better prepared to respond to unanticipated tragedies (Figure 11.3).

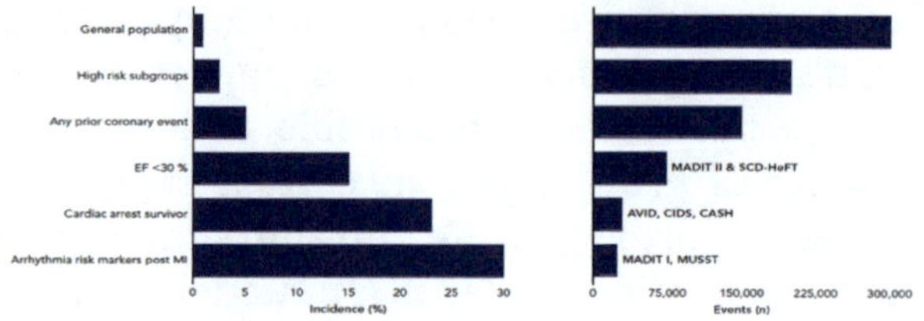

Figure 11.3. Incidence and occurrence of sudden cardiac death over 1 year.

Source: https://assets.radcliffecardiology.com/s3fs-public/article/2020-12/figure1-incidence-and-occurrence.png.

11.1. Causes of Sudden Death

Learning Outcome

1. Learn about cardiovascular events.
2. Describe the accidents and trauma.
3. Describe the medical conditions and diseases.

There are a variety of causes for sudden death, with cardiovascular events accounting for the majority of cases. Myocardial infarction as well as arrhythmias often arise without warning and kill people who appear healthy. Genetic predisposition and lifestyle factors, and even environmental stressors add to the sudden nature of these cardiovascular events. For the majority, routine medical exams may overlook underlying heart issues until it is too late. As such, a grasp of the pathophysiological processes through which these cardiovascular conditions operate is pertinent to the formulation of prevention. Higher knowledge and education concerning heart health can subsequently eradicate the risks that are associated with sudden cardiac events and thereby reduce overall mortality rates associated with these unexpected events. Another important but often overlooked cause of sudden death is the action of substances, particularly stimulants like caffeine. While caffeine is a widely used and accepted substance in moderation, instances of overdose can result in a fatal response, particularly in individuals with pre-existing medical conditions. Events reported in the medical literature illustrate that death due to caffeine is possible, although rare, and has been linked to its cardiac stimulant effect, which leads to fatal arrhythmias or an increase in heart rate. (Corkery et al., 2012) emphasizes monitoring of death due to caffeine, particularly with its growing use in the forms of energy drinks to nutrient supplements.

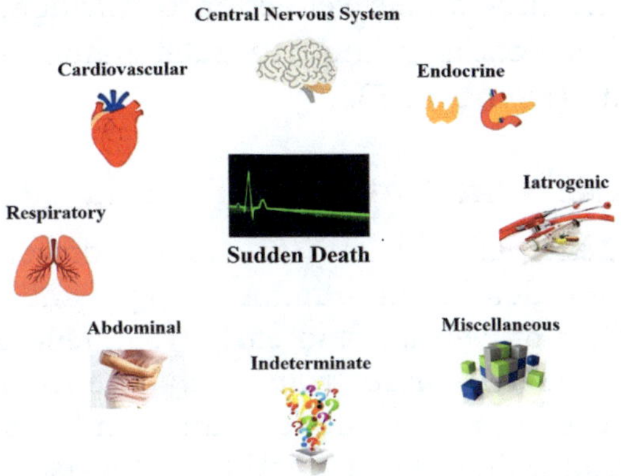

Figure 11.4. A classification of the possible causes of death in cases of SD.

Source: https://www.mdpi.com/healthcare/healthcare-09-00870/article_deploy/html/images/healthcare-09-00870-g001.png.

Continued research and documentation of such incidents are necessary to enhance public health responses to stimulant use and provide more precise directives for safe consumption amounts to prevent sudden death from caffeine. In addition to extrinsic factors such as drug abuse, intrinsic factors based on aging contribute significantly to the rate of sudden death. The aging process naturally increases an individual's susceptibility to a spectrum of illnesses, from cardiovascular disease to neurodegenerative illness. With aging, physiologic systems grow weak in a manner that can make them susceptible to precipitous deterioration when illness does strike. (Harry et al., 2003) condemns the aging regulation as a primary cause of death, yet demands a wider understanding of the manner in which aging is entwined with mechanisms of disease in older individuals. Acceptance of the multifaceted function that aging plays in unexpected deaths fosters a broader perspective of healthcare, with a focus on evidence-driven interventions and particular attention to the specific needs of elderly people, ultimately for improved health outcomes in this vulnerable population (Figure 11.4).

11.1.1. Cardiovascular Events

The occurrence of cardiac events as indicators of sudden mortality in human beings cannot be overstressed, particularly among young athletes and otherwise healthy individuals. Postmortem studies reveal that undiagnosed cardiac illnesses are most of the time responsible for such tragedies, thereby emphasizing learning about the intricacy behind the diagnosis and treatment of such subjects. On the incidence of sudden death, especially among youth, coroners are likely to request autopsies to establish the cause of death, with cardiac pathology often being at the center. As explained in recent research, consultant histopathologists bear a pivotal role in dissecting causes of sudden cardiac death, such as coronary artery disease and cardiomyopathy, among sports individuals engaging in vigorous physical exercise (Sheppard et al., 2012). Thus, a deep understanding of cardiovascular events and associated pathophysiologic processes is required for prevention as well as the detection of threats to life at an early stage. The relationship between cardiovascular events and sudden death is not limited to anatomical defects but encompasses disturbances in function, for example, arrhythmias. Arrhythmias, that is, electrical abnormalities in the activation of the heart, can result in fatal outcomes, especially when stress is high, for example, during exercise. This relationship highlights the difficulty of diagnosing asymptomatic conditions that culminate in sudden death. There is increasing evidence for the involvement of neurogenic pathways in arrhythmogenesis, with areas of the brain involved in autonomic regulation affecting the heart. Central autonomic regulation would appear to be a key issue in such an instance, suggesting that understanding the neurophysiological substrate of arrhythmias would be more beneficial to the prevention of events in susceptible groups (Loh et al., 2014). Hence, the recognition of arrhythmias as a leading cause of cardiovascular events necessitates multidisciplinary input in terms of reconsideration of athletic participation standards.

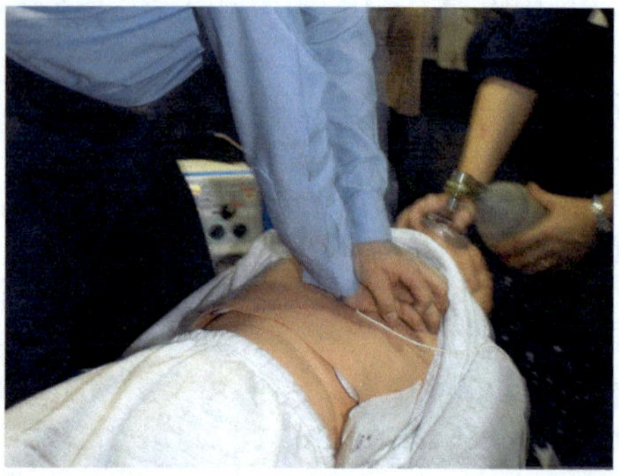

Figure 11.5. Cardiac arrest.

Source: https://upload.wikimedia.org/wikipedia/commons/2/20/US_Navy_040421-N-8090G-001_Hospital_Corpsman_3rd_Class_Flowers_administers_chest_compressions_to_a_simulated_cardiac_arrest_victim.jpg.

Furthermore, cardiovascular events also have a secondary impact that extends beyond individual risk and is a serious public health issue. Sudden and unexpected deaths due to cardiovascular complications have severe consequences for preventing such events in the population. As trends show rising involvement in high-intensity sports in all age groups, preventive measures in terms of pre-participation cardiovascular screenings need to be rendered standardized to prevent risks. Identification of individuals at risk for cardiovascular episodes can be encouraged by the interaction between clinical assessment and advanced diagnostic techniques, and in the process save lives (Sheppard et al., 2012). Moreover, heightened awareness of signs and symptoms of cardiovascular distress, particularly among young athletes, will allow individuals to seek critical medical attention before the event of disaster. Ultimately, a proactive stance in addressing cardiovascular health will contribute significantly to the reduction of incidents of sudden deaths related to such pathological events (Figure 11.5).

11.1.2. Accidents and Trauma

Accidents and trauma are major drivers of sudden deaths in human beings, and this calls for prevention and early treatment. Such incidents can arise from many events, such as automobile accidents, falls, and violent confrontations. Most notable is the fact that the deleterious health impact of such events extends beyond the primary physical trauma. Other factors, such as environmental agents, may exacerbate trauma severity; so, knowledge of the underlying principles of physiological response can help in creating effective treatment protocols. Considering the energy systems such as nuclear and coal, it is apparent that the health consequences of accidents can be closely related to systemic issues beyond, affecting how the accidents are viewed and handled in clinical and public health realms (Afifi et al., 1978). This multifaceted definition of trauma reveals the sheer intricacy of deaths by accident and necessitates global measures to reduce their impact. Among the vast types of trauma, head injuries are an extremely complex element in the discussion of accidents and unanticipated deaths. Most of these injuries are directly linked to accidents among children and adults, especially in settings like sports, falls, and road traffic accidents. Of importance is that head trauma symptoms and outcome do change considerably among different age groups, making the early diagnosis and intervention overly challenging. For instance, in children, the impact of what may seem a trivial event can result in dangerous complications, while adults are likely to experience more severe and life-threatening forms of injury. Subtlety of head trauma establishes the importance of prompt and individualized medical management, which can significantly influence prognosis. Greater understanding regarding closed and penetrating wounds is also of utmost importance, as prompt diagnosis and management are crucial in improving survival rates for traumatic brain injury (Chang et al., 2013).

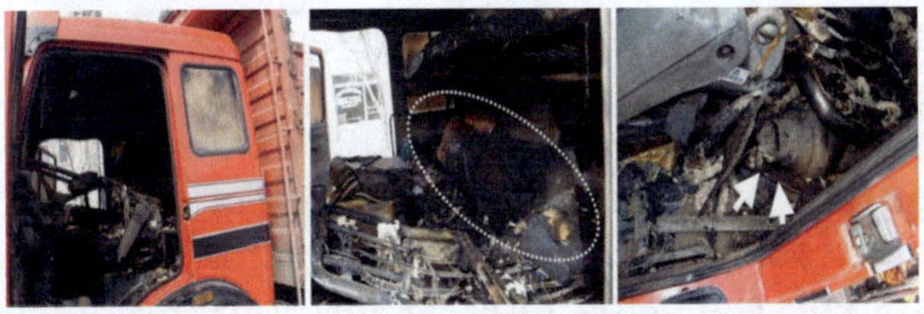

Figure 11.6. A 48-year-old male truck driver (ellipse) was found dead due to a fire in a truck parked in an open area of the truck garage. Scene investigation revealed that the cause of the fire was a broken supplementary heater (arrows) in the truck.

Source: https://cdnintech.com/media/chapter/19160/1512345123/media/image26.jpeg.

Moreover, the impact of accidents and related traumas extends far beyond instantaneous fatalities, affecting the survivors' long-term health and healthcare systems. Seriously injured survivors of major disasters often have long-term complicating health problems from their traumas and need ongoing treatment and rehabilitation. The combination of trauma and healthcare discourse highlights the requirement for comprehensive data collection and analysis to inform prevention interventions as well as management guidelines. Having an awareness of how environmental concerns can pose additional challenges to injury response enables healthcare professionals to develop plans that address not only the injuries but also the systemic concerns that exacerbate them. As public health interventions evolve to address these complexities, it is apparent that a comprehensive response to trauma and accidents is intrinsic in reducing the rate of sudden deaths and thus improving overall community health outcomes (Afifi et al., 1978) (Figure 11.6).

11.1.3. Medical Conditions and Diseases

The abrupt death of people, especially with pre-existing medical conditions, highlights the significance of knowing a variety of diseases and illnesses. Cardiovascular illnesses, for instance, arrhythmias and myocardial infarction, have a reputation for causing death instantly. These have no advance symptoms, so prevention is not easy to have. Data have indicated that there are specific groups, for instance, individuals with known risk factors like hypertension or diabetes, who are most vulnerable to these sudden deaths. Early diagnosis and the management of these risk factors can be a matter of life and death, but many of the reports identify gaps in patient education and accessibility of healthcare. This gap in awareness highlights the need for continuous public health interventions aimed at improving cardiovascular health to prevent sudden deaths due to such conditions, thereby fostering a healthier society as a whole. Other than cardiovascular disease, infection has been a major underlying cause of sudden death among vulnerable populations. Vaccination has been instrumental in maintaining control over diseases like measles and tuberculosis. It has been implicated by a study conducted by Kristensen et al. that the measles and BCG vaccines may have mortality protection independent of their specific effects on the target diseases, although evidence is not yet sufficient (Boyce et al., 2003). The implications of such findings cannot be overstated, especially since public health policies move towards prioritizing vaccinations not only for their immediate protective functions but as a preventive measure of general mortality risk.

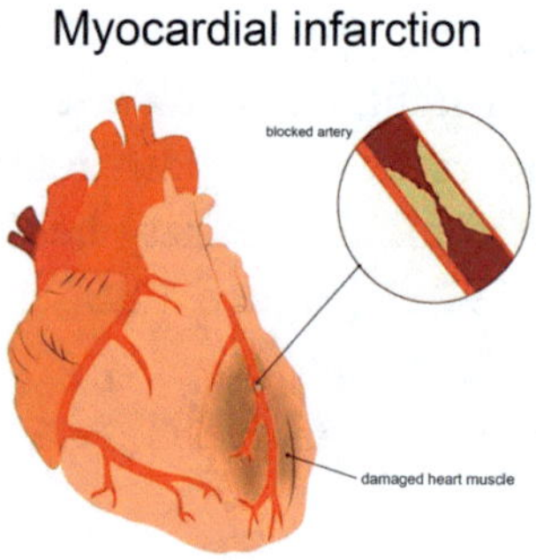

Figure 11.7. Over time, the buildup of fatty cholesterol deposits in the coronary arteries occludes blood flow to the heart muscles and deprives them of oxygen and nutrients.

Source: https://www.australiawidefirstaid.com.au/media-library/acute-myocardial-infarction-923w.webp.

ublic awareness and education on the importance of vaccinations are crucial factors in averting the incidents of unexplained fatalities related to infectious preventable diseases, thereby ensuring better health outcomes among communities. Finally, maternal and neonatal health needs to be examined closely in the sudden death discourse, specifically with regard to stillbirth, which is frequently not included in international health accounts. The evidence indicates that stillbirth contributes a significant proportion of perinatal deaths but forms an invisible account of public health discourse (Abdel-Aleem et al., 2009). Gathering accurate data on the incidence, conditions, and etiology of stillbirth can be extremely enlightening in relation to maternal and infant health. Improved registration systems, harmonized definitions, and comprehensive data sets are necessary to establish why such disasters are taking place and how they can be avoided. By putting priority on the improvement in quality of care and understanding the nature of stillbirths, health systems can better forecast and prevent sudden deaths and hence healthier generations ahead (Figure 11.7).

Test Your Knowledge

1. What type of examination is typically performed to determine the cause of sudden death in young individuals?
2. Which specialists play a key role in analyzing causes of sudden cardiac death during autopsies?

11.2. Demographics of Sudden Death

Learning Outcome

1. Understand age-related statistics.
2. Understand gender differences in sudden death rates.
3. Describe the role of geographic variations in understanding the phenomenon of sudden deaths.

The factor of sudden death among human beings poses a great concern about how demographics matter with regard to incidence and prevalence. Significantly, older persons remain the most vulnerable demographic population, accounting for a whopping percentage of sudden death resulting from numerous health conditions. Studies indicate that the bulk of these accidents happen to people aged 65 years and above, frequently as a result of having underlying diseases that make them susceptible to sudden occurrences. Moreover, the reluctance of this age group to adopt preventive health interventions, such as vaccinations, exacerbates the situation. According to research on the vaccination decisions of an elderly group, it was found that individual factors, such as age, sex, and comorbidity, determine the status of health, especially during health crises like flu epidemics (MK et al., 2008). All these factors combined highlight the importance of certain public health interventions to reduce sudden deaths among high-risk groups. In addition to age, the influence of sex as a determinant of the incidence of sudden deaths is also observed. Recurrent epidemiological surveys consistently point out that males are at higher risk than females for sudden deaths. Increased mortality among men may be due to either biological or behavioral factors, like higher levels of risk behavior and lifestyle that expose them to those diseases leading to acute death, like cardiovascular disease and substance abuse. Moreover, the stressors and health problems that go with male roles in society may be the cause of this group's higher risk. These results align with host mortality studies of parasitic etiology, wherein populations such as males, juveniles, and the elderly were found to be significantly at risk (Hayward et al., 2017). Demographic details such as these emphasize the several aspects of sudden death and the multidisciplinary scope of study and prevention initiatives. Socioeconomic status is also a major determinant of predicting the demographics of sudden death. Individuals from lower socioeconomic status have disparities in health access and quality, resulting in poor health outcomes and higher risks of sudden death events.

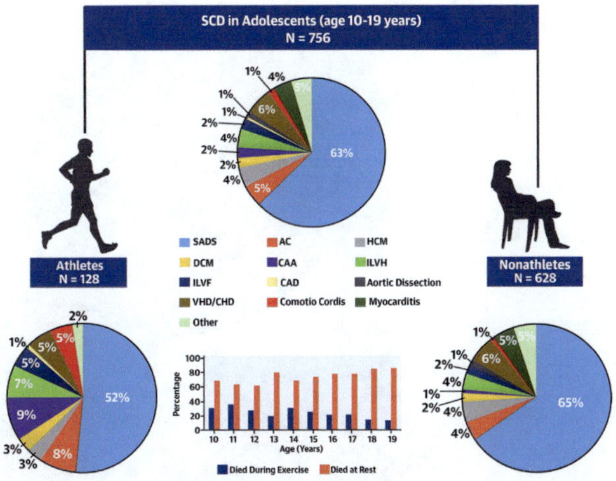

Figure 11.8. Sudden cardiac death among adolescents in the United Kingdom.

Source: https://ars.els-cdn.com/content/image/1-s2.0-S0735109723003315-fx1_lrg.jpg.

Such individuals have more comorbidities, which complicate their health states and increase the likelihood of sudden mortality. The disparities in health literacy and access to preventive treatments among different socioeconomic strata further contribute to existing inequalities in sudden death events. Addressing these disparities requires not only systemic policy shifts in healthcare but also targeted educational programs aimed at increasing awareness and knowledge about health risks associated with sudden death. A deeper comprehension of the manner demographics intersect with health vulnerabilities can inform the development of more effective public health interventions aimed at containing the instances of sudden death across the population (Figure 11.8).

11.2.1. Age-Related Statistics

It is essential to comprehend age-related statistics when analyzing abrupt mortality in humans because they reveal the demographic patterns that drive death rates. For example, young groups could be more likely to be impacted by certain causes of sudden death, for example, lethal accidents or violence, whereas older groups are more exposed to certain risks posed by chronic diseases like cardiovascular disease or stroke. According to emerging analyses, a significant percentage of unexpected death among youth, particularly children and adolescents, is due to causes related to maltreatment.

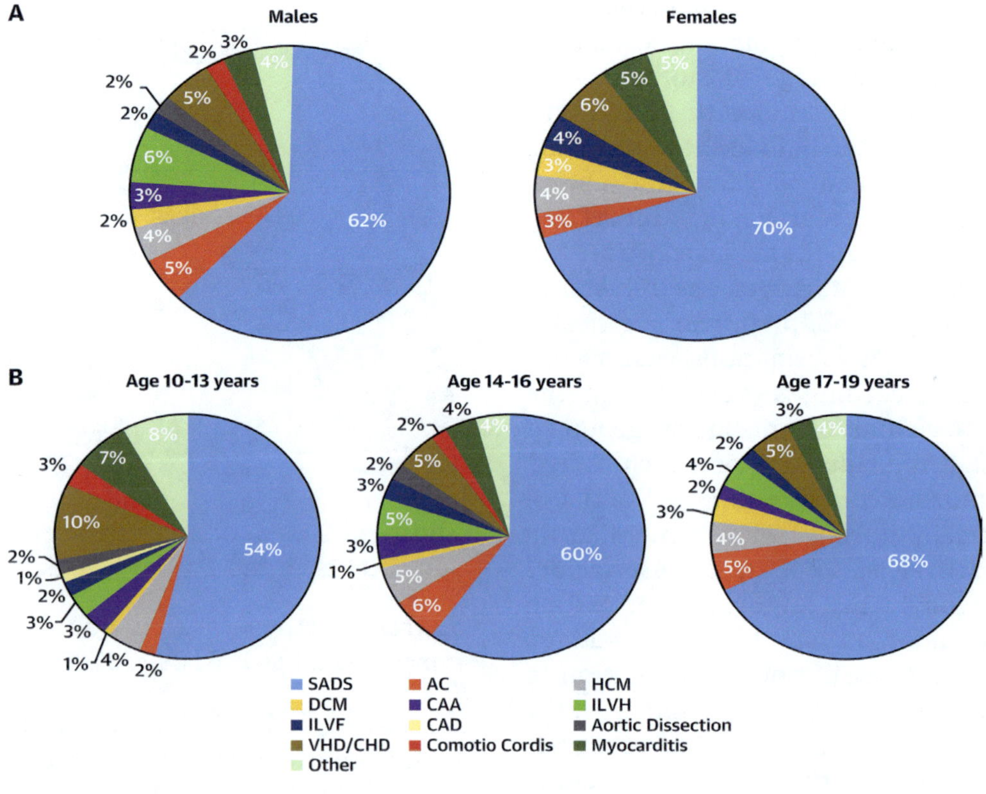

Figure 11.9. Causes of sudden cardiac death according to sex (A) and age (B) are shown.

Source: https://ars.els-cdn.com/content/image/1-s2.0-S0735109723003315-gr1_lrg.jpg.

The description of the tragic incidents in terms of the underlying cause suggests that extreme physical violence is the leading cause of lethal child maltreatment and points to an essential target for public health intervention and prevention efforts (Belsky et al., 2011). Thus, by respecting these figures, it not only underscores the importance of age as a determinant of mortality but also demands measures tailored for a particular age group. In examining sudden deaths, one has to respect the diversity of causes that are correlated with disparate age groups. For instance, causes of sudden deaths differ significantly between infancy and late old age. In young populations, sudden deaths are usually accounted for in terms of preventable causes, that is, accidents or neglect, while the elderly are explained away due to health-related issues that are often lifestyle and genetic in origin. The results of various studies indicate that, though obvious homicide and concealed acts of violence feature frightening figures among children, deaths due to natural causes rise exponentially with age. In fact, no less than 40% of cases examined showed some indication of neglect, even where neglect was not the direct cause of death, corroborating that interventions of a multifaceted nature are necessary to address the various aspects of issues of mortality among different age groups (Belsky et al., 2011). Furthermore, age-related statistics of reasons for sudden death underscore the necessity of multidisciplinary approaches to prevention and intervention. There are other determinants, such as social setting, access to medical care, and social resources, which are all important influences on mortality rates in specific age groups. For example, although deaths due to the use of substances like caffeine combined with other drugs will be found in different forms among various age groups, campaigns and education specifically targeting a particular age group are necessary to ensure effective prevention. Although healthcare systems will strive to address evident etiologies, there is an increasing recognition of the subtle but influential contributions of causes like fatalities due to caffeine intake, where fatalities go unobserved and unreported. By comprehending the context within which these numbers are presented, stakeholders can create comprehensive efforts to reduce sudden death, ultimately promoting longevity and optimal health among various populations (Figure 11.9).

11.2.2. Gender Differences in Sudden Death Rates

It is essential to comprehend gender disparities in rates of sudden death in order to design preventive strategies and interventions. Evidence points towards higher rates of sudden cardiac events and death in males relative to females, especially under conditions such as sudden cardiac arrest. These factors may include biological variation in cardiovascular wellness, lifestyle factors, and stress responses. For example, men are more likely to indulge in risky lifestyles and have higher incidences of conditions such as hypertension and prior myocardial infarction. Thus, the combination of such factors significantly contributes to the rise in male sudden death, finally putting the onus on specifically targeting health awareness campaigns and medical attention towards such populations to effectively manage their risks. Aside from cardiovascular disease, gender inequality also occurs in instances of sudden unexpected death in epilepsy (SUDEP), a fatal comorbidity of epilepsy. Research based on Kcna1 knockout mice, an SUDEP model, has determined significant results about disparity between sexes in such incidences. Outcomes indicate that the female Kcna1-/- mice live longer than the male mice, suggesting a decreased probability of SUDEP events in females, even if there are no contrasts between seizure occurrence and length. Oddly enough, females also experienced a greater frequency of bradycardia during seizures and were resistant to certain arrhythmias, again suggesting an essential difference in brain-heart interactions. These biological determinants would account for the varying rates of sudden unexpected deaths in individuals with epilepsy, and their clinical determination has been called for in order to advance gender-sensitive identification and intervention methods for SUDEP susceptibility (Paulhus et al., 2025). Provision of preventive interventions against sudden death also indicates significant gender variation, particularly in cardiovascular care. A retrospective analysis conducted on patients who were eligible for an implantable cardiac defibrillator (ICD) implantation reported that 33% of female eligibles and 47% of males were treated with the device, showing a significant difference in the treatment of women. This is indicative of the broader health disparities issue in which gender not only influences rates of prevalence but also access to potentially life-saving treatment. Other factors like age, ethnicity, and socioeconomic status only make these inequalities more complex, and healthcare delivery requires sophisticated solutions. In addressing all the above factors comprehensively, it is possible for healthcare professionals to further customize prevention measures to lower rates of sudden death in both genders, hence enhancing improved health outcomes in vulnerable groups (Elsaygh et al., 2025) (Figure 11.10).

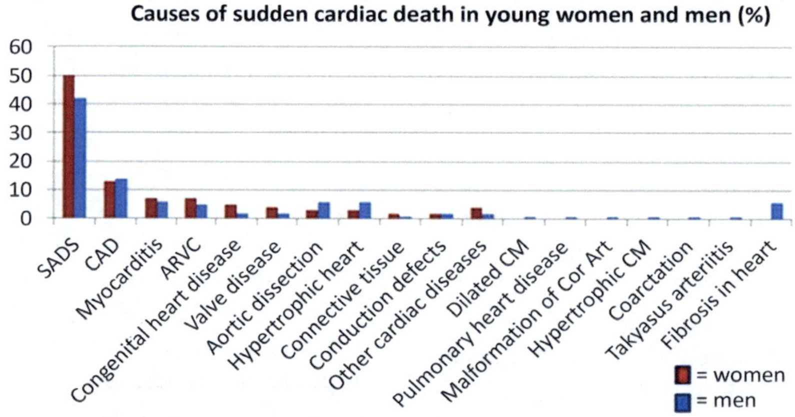

Figure 11.10. Causes of SCD in young women and men (aged 1–35 years) in percent of total SCD in the same gender in 2000–2009 in Denmark.

Source: https://media.springernature.com/full/springer-static/image/art%3A10.1186%2Fs12872-016-0446-5/MediaObjects/12872_2016_446_Fig2_HTML.gif?as=webp.

11.2.3. Geographic Variations

Geographical variations play a vital role in the research of sudden deaths in human beings because they reveal the manner in which some areas experience different mortality patterns and rates. Environmental factors, socio-economic status, and access to healthcare could be responsible for the existence and causes of sudden deaths. For instance, rural areas may suffer more from sudden cardiac events due to the inaccessibility of emergency services, whereas urban dwellers may suffer from pollution and lifestyle hazards. Furthermore, health and wellness cultural activities vary extensively on a regional basis, generating yet another reason for such variations. Assessment of these geographic differences is critical to public health policy, making it possible to have effective interventions that can reduce the incidence of sudden death in different populations and settings. These interactions also extend to the effects of climate and the local ecological setting. High ultraviolet radiation areas, for instance, may observe increased incidences of skin-related sudden death, particularly among individuals with fair skin. Geographic location influences the balance between beneficial exposure to sunlight and lethal UV radiation risks, as indicated by the varying public health recommendations for various populations. In addition, the disparate availability of resources at the local scale, such as healthcare services and preventive treatment policies, can enhance these risks. A critical assessment of such geographic differences can reveal inherent patterns that ultimately guide health programs intended to combat sudden deaths due to region-specific factors. With a grasp of these subtle differences, public health systems can create more effective and targeted response systems. Geographical differences also bleed over into the sociocultural realm, where dietary habits, diet, and regional customs generally determine health outcomes. For example, countries that eat high levels of omega-3 fatty acids have lower rates of sudden cardiac deaths than those relying on fast foods. The intersection of indigenous knowledges and practices with modern health systems can reveal new protective factors against sudden death. In addition, differential exposures to stressors such as economic hardship or environmental poison exposures are manifested differently across geographies, necessitating geographically targeted mental well-being and mental health interventions. As a reaction to sudden death, the understanding of these social and emotional determinants by geography is essential. A comprehensive approach considering both biological and sociocultural determinants can significantly enhance public health practice and outcomes with respect to sudden death events (Figure 11.11).

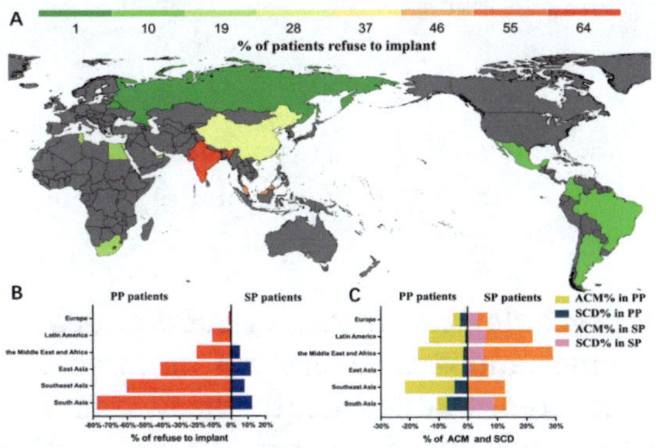

Figure 11.11. Graphical display of implantation by region. a World map showing the percentage of patients without implantable cardioverter-defibrillators/cardiac resynchronization therapy-defibrillators (ICDs/CRT-Ds). b Percentage of PP and SP patients without ICDs/CRT-Ds. c Percentage of primary prevention (PP) and secondary prevention (SP) patients with all-cause mortality (ACM) and sudden cardiac death (SCD).

Source: https://media.springernature.com/full/springer-static/image/art%3A10.1186%2Fs12916-024-03310-5/MediaObjects/12916_2024_3310_Fig1_HTML.png?as=webp.

Test Your Knowledge

1. What is a common cause of sudden death among children and adolescents.
2. What gender is reported to have a higher prevalence of sudden cardiac death?

11.3. Psychological Impact of Sudden Death

Learning Outcome

1. Understand the effects of sudden death on family and friends.
2. Know the grief and coping mechanisms.
3. Describe the long-term psychological consequences.

The psychological impact of sudden death on surviving family members can be intense and multifaceted. Sudden death throws survivors into a disorganized emotional state of shock, bewilderment, and grief. The nature of this grief can vary greatly based on the relationship to the deceased, the circumstances of death, and the social support systems available to the widowed. Such abrupt loss has the ability to perturb the whole emotional life of the survivors and evoke responses such as depression, anxiety, and even post-traumatic stress disorder (PTSD). Research is eager to indicate that the intensity of such psychological reactions is typically in response to the abrupt nature of the loss, indicating a paramount necessity for appropriate support and coping mechanisms for individuals who experience sudden deaths (N/A, 2007). Moreover, information regarding these emotional challenges is critical for mental health professionals who will be carrying out personalized interventions for bereaved individuals. When it comes to sudden death, the phenomenon of complicated grief must be grasped, in which people experience exacerbation and prolonged grief reactions that interfere with their functioning. Complicated grief is commonly manifested in dwelling on the loss, emptiness, or feeling stuck in life. Evidence indicates that unless individuals are given proper psychological interventions following a sudden loss, they may be more vulnerable to mental disorders like anxiety disorders and depressive episodes (Kennedy et al., 2015). The absence of interventions to reverse the psychological trauma of sudden death merits a proactive approach to mental healthcare. Promoting peer support groups and community mental health services can facilitate a collective grief process, in which survivors have an opportunity to express their emotions and experiences within a supportive and safe environment.

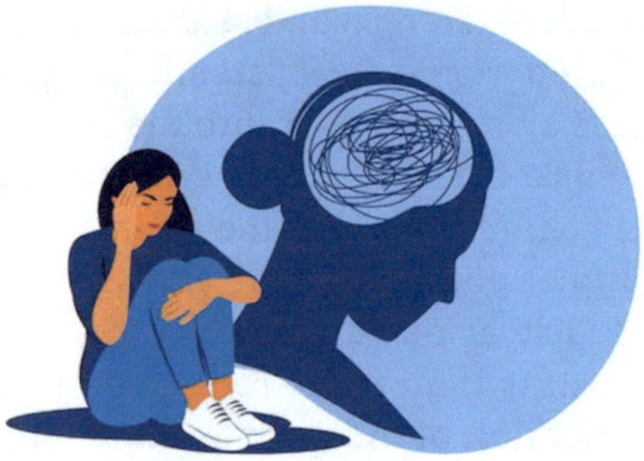

Figure 11.12. Impact of sudden death on mental health.

Source: https://www.emoneeds.com/wp-content/uploads/2023/12/3-large.jpg.

11.3.1. Effects on Family and Friends

Coping with an unexpected loss of a loved one impacts members of a family and friends, who are typically pushed into emotional turmoil. Individuals mourning may face a multi-faceted combination of different emotions like shock, denial, and immense grief, which can have severe implications for their everyday living. Such emotional distress frequently derails family relationships, as family members cannot manage their grief within themselves and attempt to console one another. Family dynamics can shift through the process of grieving, precipitating fights or struggles that can further challenge the toughness of relationships and leave those going through it isolated. The ripple effect of sudden loss illustrates the manner in which personal loss can alter family dynamics to highlight the importance of free communication and support during such a trying endeavor. The psychological implications of sudden death extend beyond immediate emotional trauma; they can also manifest as prolonged mental illness among mourning family members and friends. Research has demonstrated that untreated bereavement might even lead to more severe mental health issues, including depression, anxiety, and sometimes even complicated grief disorder. Inadequate coping skills could even aggravate these issues, thus forming a cycle of mental illness and bereavement. Relatives and friends tend to become helpless when they also face their own bereavement as well as others' suffering. In the long run, this may lead to scattered social networks, in which individuals withdraw from others due to their overwhelming feelings or fear of bringing about more sorrow. This withdrawal facilitates magnified overall experienced loss and thus complicates healing processes. With abrupt fatalities, especially, societal expectations for bereavement can affect the process of how family members and friends cope with their loss as well. Social customs usually dictate how and for how long one should grieve, and not conforming to these social expectations can bring on guilt or feelings of inadequacy. The need to be strong and stoic can also bring on emotional weight, for victims of loss will struggle with being truthful about how they feel. Within other communities, cultural stigmatization of mental health excludes sincere discussions of mourning, and as a result, there is a generalized silence that suppresses the recovery process. It takes empathy for the meaning of sudden death for family and friends to take those cultural environments into account, as well as the need for supportive environments that allow individuals to mourn sincerely and with impunity and hence build resilience and recovery against disaster (Figure 11.13).

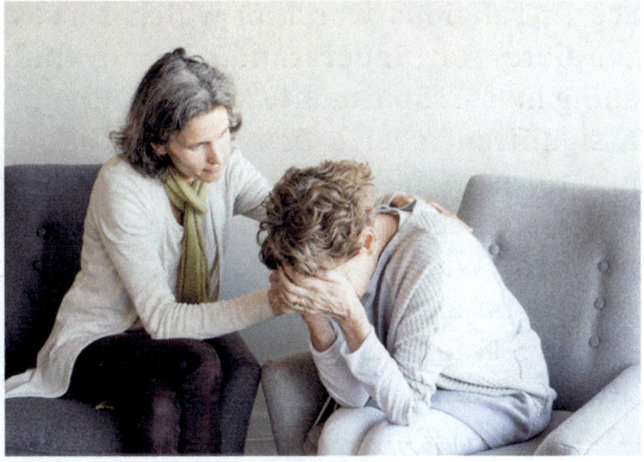

Figure 11.13. Effects of sudden death on family and friends.

Source: https://domf5oio6qrcr.cloudfront.net/medialibrary/1982/w0709b16207232845769.png .

11.3.2. Grief and Coping Mechanisms

The mourning process following an unexpected death is highly complex, as it involves a group of emotional responses that have much to do with the mental health of an individual. Sudden deaths usually leave the surviving people in shock and denial, hence making the mourning process challenging. The traditional theories of grief concentrate on stages such as denial, anger, bargaining, depression, and acceptance, but these are not necessarily processed in sequence. Instead, they can have reliving emotions or at the same time experience more than one emotion, which causes them coping problems (N/A, 2021). Sudden death is generally unpredictable in origin, and the consequent feeling of powerlessness leads the survivors to resort to means of finding things to make themselves powerful once again in their lives. It is critical to comprehend this dynamic interaction of emotions for achieving effective coping mechanisms that cater to the unique issues the sudden loss poses. Coping mechanisms employed by individuals who undergo sudden death can vary extensively, based on diverse individual and cultural beliefs. Some will find solace in religious worship, which serves as a template for understanding and finding meaning in loss. Spirituality has been identified as a significant source of resilience, allowing people to make meaning of their experiences and feel connected to an entity greater than themselves (Wiggins et al., 2025). Conversely, spiritual bypassing, or using spirituality to avoid distressing emotions, can prove unhealthy to long-term resilience, underlining the intricacy of grieving (Wiggins et al., 2025).

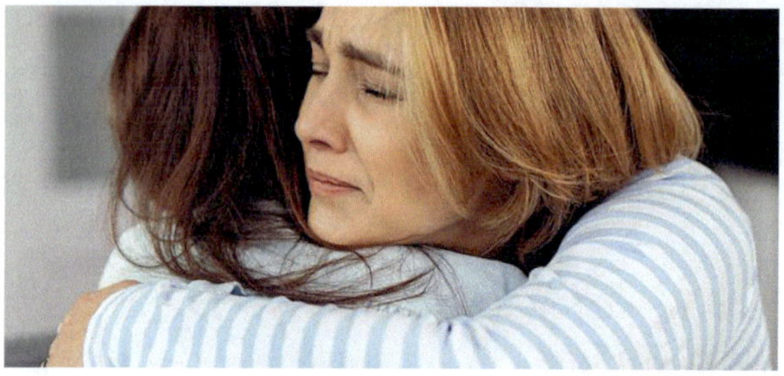

Figure 11.14. Coping with a sudden death.

Source: https://images.ctfassets.net/iqbixcpmwym2/2rEw4piBBxYhdUhEF9OFix/694c0fd531994b6cc4c04efc98f35c08/MicrosoftTeams-image__20_.png?fm=jpg&q=60&w=740&h=347&fit=fill&fl=progressive.

Attending community-based support groups can also be a constructive strategy to cope with the trauma, as people can vent their emotions and bond with other survivors of loss. Such interactions provide empathy and validation, which are vital in overcoming feelings of isolation that commonly occur with sudden deaths. In addition, coping strategies in real life, such as the establishment of a routine or exercise, can also become a part of healing. Incorporation of self-care interventions into daily life may bring a sense of stability in the midst of the chaos that follows sudden death. Journal writing or creative writing can also assist individuals who undergo loss because these methods give a place for emotional release and processing. In addition, professional assistance from therapists or grief work-trained counselors can be an important resource of guidance in this difficult period. This consultation with mental health experts allows one to analyze their grief in a safe and supportive environment and ultimately enhance their coping skills (N/A, 2021). With the examination of these varied coping strategies, one realizes that an interdisciplinary approach must be employed to address the complex world of grief pertaining to sudden deaths (Figure 11.14).

11.3.3. Long-Term Psychological Consequences

Sudden loss of a loved one or a prominent figure can result in severe psychological effects on the survivors. Bereavement in this situation could be transformed from acute mourning to prolonged mental illness, including anxiety, depression, and complex grief, which could last for a period of several years. Such reactions to sudden loss necessitate a closer look at the psychological consequences since the survivors are still grappling with their untimely absence. Ironically, survivors will be prone to fluctuate among anger, guilt, and denial in attempting to comprehend the senseless nature of unexpected death. This delicate emotional ground justifies having appropriate support structures to prevent long-term psychological distress. Research has proven that traumatic events, such as sudden deaths, tend to result in differential magnitudes of Post-Traumatic Stress Disorder (PTSD) among survivors. PTSD prevalence will always be much higher in instances of sudden loss because the affected persons will feel they are bogged down by the traumatic memory of the loss. While most of the literature presents physical health consequences after traumatic events, such as landslides, the fact remains that the psychological consequences can equally be debilitating. Natural disaster research highlights that the psychological consequences, in particular PTSD, may be exacerbated after such a sudden loss of life as opposed to other disaster environments, with reference to a significant literature gap regarding sudden fatalities and long-term psychological consequences (Kennedy et al., 2015). Furthermore, the long-term psychological consequences of sudden fatalities also reach beyond the immediate family environment to broader social networks and communities. The psychological strain has a reach that extends to the interpersonal relationships, creating tensions that are caused by feelings of powerlessness and the need for support among loss survivors. Evidence documents that long-term bereavement impacts not only individual functioning but can also be quantified as broader social and community disorganization. The demand for greater mental health care and support from the community after a sudden death cannot be overstated, as such care plays an important role in facilitating coping mechanisms and enhancing resilience. This ongoing need for psychological interventions mirrors the fact that the effects of sudden deaths persist way beyond the very instant of bereavement, affecting mental health in perhaps unexpected ways (Corkery et al., 2012) (Figure 11.15).

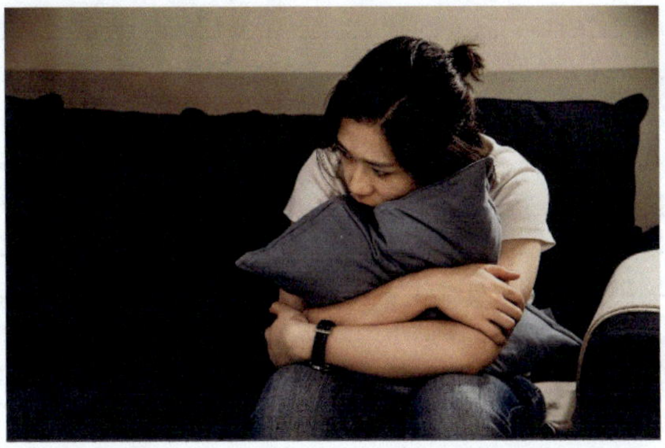

Figure 11.15. Long-term psychological consequences.

Source: https://www.verywellmind.com/thmb/Tsz_71Pb5qGpfcMPcY4-GhZL2j4=/2121x0/filters:no_upscale():max_bytes(150000):strip_icc()/GettyImages-1265371206-70fd954269b34baf946b4ceb6c95caa6.jpg.

Test Your Knowledge

1. What are the effects of sudden death on family and friends?
2. What emotional reaction is most commonly associated with the immediate aftermath of sudden death?

11.4. Preventive Measures

Learning Outcome

1. Describe the health screenings and awareness.
2. Understand the emergency response training.
3. Describe the lifestyle changes and risk reduction.

In addressing the issue of sudden human deaths, preventive policies have a critical role to play when it comes to risk reduction. Effective prevention is founded on careful information collection on death causes, particularly in categories such as stillbirths. Collecting good-quality data allows public health officials to identify patterns and root cause determinants behind such tragic outcomes. For instance, systematic investigation of stillbirths can augment obstetric care and maternal health interventions and reduce even the most difficult-to-predict loss occurrences. (Abdel-Aleem et al., 2009) emphasizes the requirement for accurate registration and investigation, with evidence that awareness of the timing and circumstances of such deaths can inform better healthcare practice and policies to enhance the quality of care offered for pregnant women. In addition, newly emerging infectious diseases like Ebola emphasize the necessity of preventive measures beyond the traditional healthcare paradigms. The rapid spread of Ebola in 2014 indicated the necessity for countries to implement effective preparedness measures. Proposals ranged from improving the treatment of patients, formulating adequate isolation centers, and training health workers in responding to emergencies. The combined effort by organizations such as the WHO to enhance the availability of resources has been instrumental in preventing the spread of outbreaks and saving lives. (Pace et al., 2014) explains the way the availability of personal protective equipment is improved and effective reporting systems are established to prevent the spread of infectious diseases that lead to sudden deaths. These preventive measures are not only required within endemic regions but globally because the global risk of transmission is a continued threat. Education and community involvement are also the most important features of the prevention system for sudden death. It is imperative that individuals get educated about lifestyle practices that contribute to avoidable illness like heart disease, drug use, and psychiatric illness to reduce the rate of death. Community programs providing information and support can enable individuals to make well-informed health choices, leading to fewer sudden deaths from preventable conditions. Educating communities and families on a regular basis about threats to health and prevention fosters an environment in which individuals are more likely to take advantage of prompt medical treatment. An integrated approach with education, effective healthcare systems, and well-organized emergency response policies can significantly improve the public health impact and ultimately reduce the prevalence of sudden deaths in human beings (Figure 11.16).

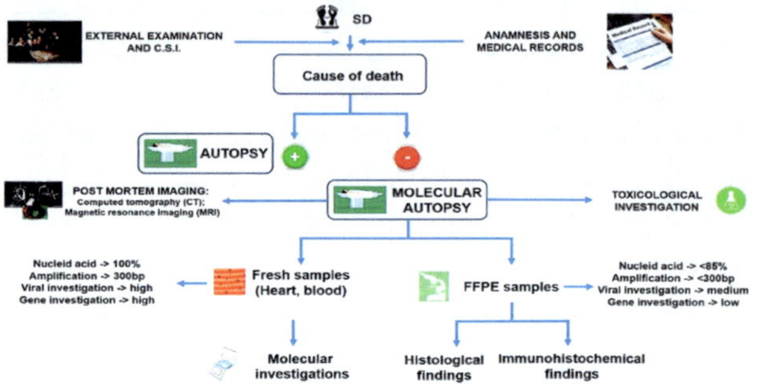

Figure 11.16. A practical flowchart that should be applied in all cases of SD.

Source: https://www.mdpi.com/healthcare/healthcare-09-00870/article_deploy/html/images/healthcare-09-00870-g002.png.

11.4.1. Health Screenings and Awareness

Health screenings form a critical component in the prevention of hazards of sudden death in human beings, as they allow for the diagnosis of predisposed underlying conditions prior to asymptomaticity. Cardiovascular programs are particularly crucial given that heart issues are a leading cause of sudden death both in athletes and non-athletes. Studies have shown that applications of cardiac screenings, especially among adolescent athletes, are effective in identifying irregularities that would expose young individuals to life-threatening events during periods of strenuous physical activities. The findings of a study on coaches and athletic trainers support routine cardiac examination prior to partaking in sports, acknowledging that such preventive intervention can significantly enhance overall health outcomes and reduce cases of sudden cardiac death among adolescents (Smith et al., 2021). Health screening awareness is not confined to cardiovascular disorders alone; it also involves early detection of other illnesses like colorectal cancer, which is a considerable public health issue. Increased incidence of colorectal cancer among African Americans underscores the need for intervention to increase awareness and utilize screening services among high-risk populations. Despite the availability of efficient screening tests, many individuals remain under-screened due to perceived low risk and socio-cultural reasons. Results of qualitative studies on family experiences of colorectal cancer highlight the importance of education and awareness in the community in order to mobilize individuals to combat cancer through increased awareness and preventive healthcare practices (Loggins et al., 2018).

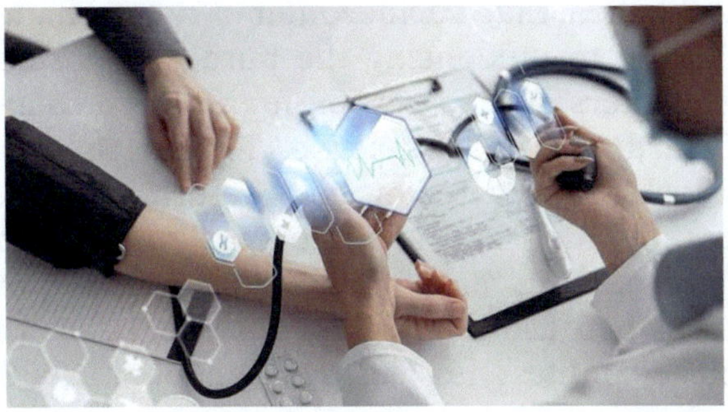

Figure 11.17. Health screenings.

Source: https://ghost-cms.s3.ap-south-1.amazonaws.com/2023/06/Health-Screening_corporate-wellness-program_Truworth-wellness-1.jpg.

Here, health screening emerges as a vital tool for not only individual health maintenance but also for enhanced insights into disease prevention at the population level. Above all, increased uptake of health screening is the solution to reducing sudden deaths from conditions that are preventable or treatable. Efforts to increase awareness need to correct demographic disparities and construct outreach efforts aimed at meeting diverse community needs. Open dialogue with health providers on the importance of screenings can develop the culture of prevention and allow individuals to act on controlling their health. Campaigns that promote education on the importance of frequent check-ups and screenings, and the use of valid data in demonstrating their effectiveness in saving lives, will have a critical role in shaping public sentiment. Through these multi-faceted approaches, reducing sudden deaths can be more effectively achieved through an environment where preventive health practices are recognized and put into action as integral components to individual and community well-being (Figure 11.17).

11.4.2. Emergency Response Training

Emergency response training plays a critical role in averting the consequences of sudden deaths in humans, particularly where rapid medical help can make a significant difference. Such training is also pertinent in most environments, including schools and workplaces, where there is potential for heightened sudden cardiac events. For instance, an efficient emergency response system encompasses communication and coordination of actions during crises. Trained personnel and instructors, such as CPR and the use of automated external defibrillators (AEDs), are important in guaranteeing survival for those who undergo cardiac arrest. Research indicates that school nurses, for instance, reported that even in instances where resources are available, they felt unprepared, hence the need for joint training sessions that equip employees with skills and competency to act suitably in the event of an emergency (Dahlen et al., 2014). Besides that, it is also essential to continually evaluate and streamline emergency response training so that it remains effective. The dynamic evolution of medical science and practice necessitates frequent updates in training curricula so that responders can utilize the latest evidence-based practices. The emergence of unexpected complications during emergency events underscores the need for flexibility and responsiveness in training programs. Therefore, organizations must have a structured process to assess the adequacy of existing training practices, which may lead to the de-implementation of ineffective, outdated practices that lack today's health requirements. This examination and realignment are crucial since noneffective or unnecessary interventions can subtract from more effective interventions, thus compromising the quality of emergency response plans (Brownson et al., 2018). Adding scenario-based training exercises enhances the preparedness of individuals exposed to sudden death emergencies. Through the simulation of real emergency situations, trainees develop their technical skills and pressure management skills, which are essential in high-risk environments. The simulations may also enhance team and communication among rescuers, which is essential during actual emergencies when timely coordination could be a matter of life and death. The level of confidence gained from such thorough training sessions can prove more effective in real life, emphasizing the point that preparedness is an ongoing process requiring constant practice and evaluation. In efforts to reduce fatalities due to sudden medical conditions, providing emergency response training with priority and ongoing enhancement remains vital to achieving effective intervention and ultimately saving lives (Figure 11.18).

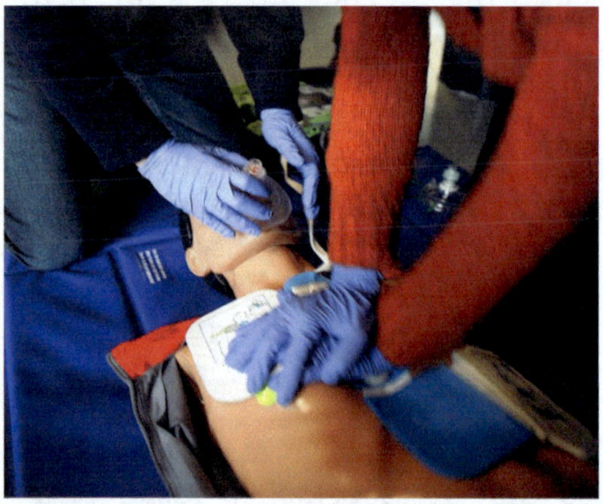

Figure 11.18. CPR training.

Source: https://upload.wikimedia.org/wikipedia/commons/5/58/CPR_training-04.jpg.

11.4.3. Lifestyle Changes and Risk Reduction

The intricate relationship between lifestyle adjustments and risk mitigation in human instances of sudden death underscores the importance of preventive health interventions. Lifestyle adjustments, such as a change to a healthy diet pattern, higher rates of physical exercise, and the cessation of tobacco use, are important in reversing the risk factors for cardiovascular diseases and other instances of sudden health events. Research has established that socioeconomic determinants are vital to influencing the burden of disease risk factors and have been found to be causes of cardiovascular disease. Pinpointing the underlying socioeconomic determinants of such health risks is important to adopting effective interventions for reducing sudden deaths because their removal can enhance the efficacy of lifestyle changes (Vogli et al., 2008). Moreover, the pharmacological intervention versus lifestyle modification comparison sets the stage for the promise of holistic approaches to risk reduction. Statins have been proven effective in lowering lipid levels and in the prevention of cardiovascular events; yet lifestyle modification presents a strong rival that is powerful and generates no side effects. Research has demonstrated that good lifestyle practices, including avoiding smoking, a body mass index (BMI) of under 25, exercising regularly, and an adequate diet, are associated with dramatic reductions in cardiac risk. Unlike statins, whose impact on total mortality may be restricted and whose limitations relate to long-term treatment, these lifestyle changes are cheap and can be made for a lifetime, which translates to enhanced overall health (Chagas et al., 2011).

Implementing these lifestyle changes requires a collective effort that transcends an individual's vow. Behavioral change is often coupled with difficulties, requiring a multifaceted intervention based on medical, nutritional, and psychological interventions. Successful interventions must involve more than one sector of society, like schools, government departments, and health institutions. Involvement of the community at more than one level generates a facilitating environment for healthy lifestyles to be taken up and maintained. Lastly, cessation of the epidemic of sudden death from lifestyle diseases involves individual behavior change in addition to systemic intervention for encouragement of widespread availability of resources conducive to healthy living and thus significantly reduced risks of cardiovascular events and other life-threatening conditions (Figure 11.19).

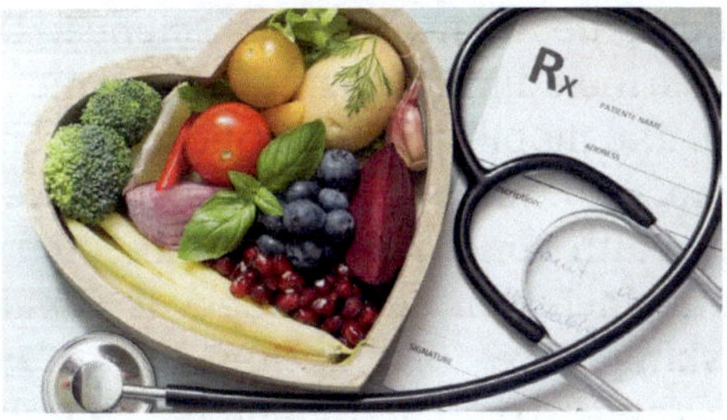

Figure 11.19. Heart-smart eating: diet tips to lower risk of sudden cardiac arrest.

Source: https://bsmedia.business-standard.com/_media/bs/img/article/2025-06/18/full/1750242920-9157.jpeg?im=Resize,width=826,height=465,aspect=ignore.

Test Your Knowledge

1. What do you mean by health screening?
2. What is the emergency response training?

11.5. Role of Technology in Understanding Sudden Death

Learning Outcome

1. Describe the advances in medical imaging.
2. Understand the data collection and analysis.
3. Describe the wearable health technology.

Improvements in technology have significantly altered the character of sudden death in human beings, with new technologies for diagnosis and analysis. Medical technology, specifically imaging technologies such as MRI and CT scans, has the ability to conduct extensive analyses of sudden deaths. These technologies are able to reveal underlying health conditions that could have been contributing factors in a sudden death, such as undiagnosed cardiac diseases or neurological conditions. Apart from this, machine learning and data analysis also contribute significantly to processing large amounts of health data and identifying patterns and risk factors that may not be immediately identifiable. This synergy between technology and medicine not only enhances the accuracy of post-mortem analysis but also informs healthcare professionals about preventive actions, which they can use to combat life-threatening conditions before they worsen. Thus, technology emerges as an important contributor in understanding the sophisticated factors that lead to sudden death, ultimately contributing to health outcomes among populations. Technology is a prominent contributor in understanding the factors of sudden death in forensic science. Digital forensics, including analysis of electronic health records and mobile health applications, enables examiners to establish an entire perception of the health condition of an individual prior to death. Inclusion of such data is capable of unmasking core information about patient comportment, treatment guideline compliance, or exposure to environmental hazards, thus creating a link between technology and public health and safety. Moreover, genomic sequencing and bioinformatics technologies facilitate the identification of genetic predisposition to sudden death that may otherwise remain unobserved. By utilizing these technological resources, researchers can create more complex accounts of how biological and environmental determinants interact to affect rates of mortality and feed into a broader narrative of health within society. This engagement between forensic science and technology demonstrates the importance of interdisciplinarity in accounting for sudden deaths. Technology is also central to responding to the rising rates of environmental explanations for sudden deaths. As observed, the increasing incidences of environmental catastrophes pose a great challenge to public health in terms of the demand for a better understanding of potential implications. Environmental observation technologies, such as satellite images and remote sensing, provide useful information on hazards associated with natural disasters and their consequences on human health. Through the evaluation of historical environmental events in combination with ongoing health data, scientists are establishing connections between environmental stressors and health, paving the way for the development of focused interventions. This intersection of geosciences and health technologies is important because it bridges the distance between what was once known and what is currently faced and ultimately feeds into public policy and readiness efforts. Besides, with the world having difficulties in understanding the reality of sudden deaths brought about by environmental circumstances, the contribution of technology also increases in order to empower a society to be resilient and informed, designed for countering future uncertainties (Figure 11.20).

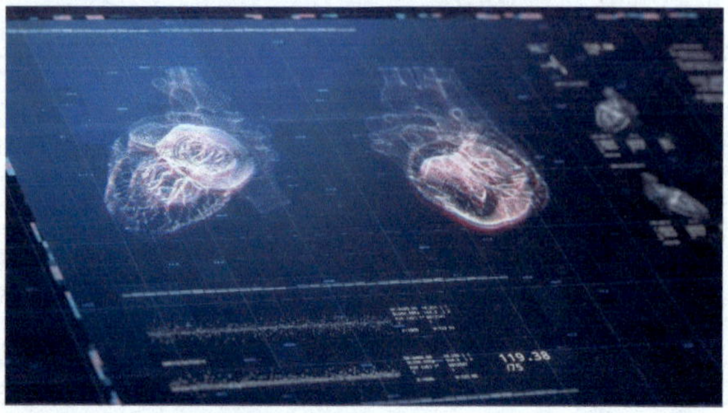

Figure 11.20. Arrhythmic sudden death survival prediction using deep learning analysis of scarring in the heart.

Source: https://www.news-medical.net/image-handler/ts/20220524125449/ri/950/src/images/news/ImageForNews_714632_16533680880418469.jpg.

11.5.1. Advances in Medical Imaging

Technological strides in medical imaging have transformed the realm of diagnosing cardiovascular defects, a significant causative agent for sudden human deaths. Sophisticated techniques such as magnetic resonance imaging (MRI), computed tomography (CT), and echocardiography have enabled physicians to visualize structures of the heart with excellent clarity and precision. These modalities not only enhance the detection of congenital heart defects (CHDs) but also permit the grading of their severity and functional effects. As CHDs account for a high proportion of sudden deaths in youth, augmenting diagnostic accuracy with newer imaging is a high priority. Furthermore, marrying imaging data with artificial intelligence algorithms can potentially enhance risk stratification to enable timely intervention that can prevent potentially fatal complications from the underlying cardiac pathology resulting from CHDs (Reemtsen et al., 2017). The role of high-resolution imaging in the identification and definition of genetic differences that cause cardiovascular disease cannot be overstated. As technology advances in next-generation sequencing, medical imaging has emerged as an adjunct strategy in understanding the interrelationship between phenotypic expressions and silent genetic derangements. Enhanced imaging technology allows for better knowledge of how specific gene-environment interactions can lead to conditions that predispose individuals to sudden cardiac death. For context, physicians are better positioned to characterize CHDs' range of phenotypes, which includes being most important in the case of creating tailored therapy to offset threats posed by defects. Thus, the intersection of advanced imaging methods and genetic testing presents avenues for enhanced diagnostics along these lines, as well as tailored treatment strategies, which ultimately save lives (N/A, 2012). Secondly, the creation of biobanks with high-quality biological samples of properly characterized patient populations is a crucial step towards precision medicine in cardiovascular medicine. In combination with sophisticated imaging methods, these biobanks enable massive research to elucidate the molecular basis of various cardiac diseases. The construction of an integrated CHD BioCore involving imaging, genetic sequencing, and clinical data is an infrastructural move required to facilitate innovation in diagnosis and treatment. Through systematic examination of the correlations between phenotypes identified in imaging studies and genotypes revealed by sequencing, investigators can discern key molecular networks involved in the pathogenesis of CHDs. With this procedure, the medical community is that much closer to developing targeted therapy that not only enhances survival rates but also the quality of life of those afflicted with cardiovascular disease (Reemtsen et al., 2017) (Figure 11.21).

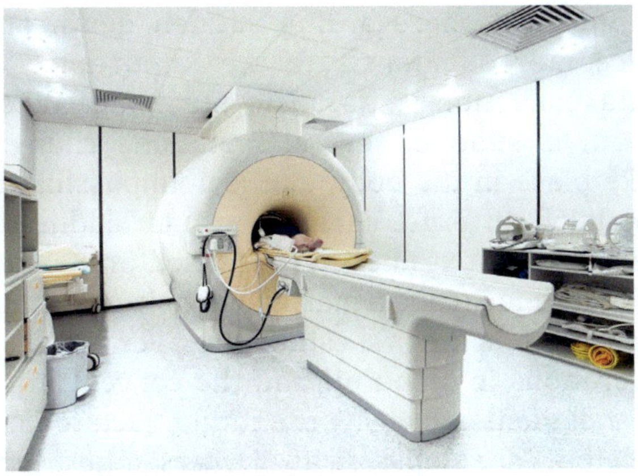

Figure 11.21. Cardiac MRI.

Source: https://www.verywellhealth.com/thmb/cEz7DpaR3TrkH_u7afZ2TQh38j4=/1500x0/filters:no_upscale():max_bytes(150000):strip_icc()/GettyImages-1053413820-9cd44f0634b3485fab8a18d4b7ad3728.jpg.

11.5.2. Data Collection and Analysis

The pathogenesis of sudden death in man demands careful data collection and processing in an attempt to identify causal factors. Coroners play a major role in this process, particularly in the instance of young patients whose sudden deaths prompt investigation. The coroners' choice to conduct an autopsy, led by consultant pathologists, represents a seminal action in establishing the cause of death. Such an analysis makes it possible to gather vast amounts of data in relation to various potential diseases that could have caused the death. Based on tissue samples examined and specific pathological changes identified, experts can uncover underlying diseases, in this instance primarily the cardiovascular ones, which frequently dictate sudden mortality among young people. The findings of such autopsies contribute to the improved understanding of the epidemiology of sudden death and inform future prevention strategies, hence the even greater significance of conducting thorough data analysis in such a field (Sheppard et al., 2012). Post-mortem biochemical alterations offer another source of information regarding sudden death and once more demonstrate the importance of data collection in forensic medicine. When death is sudden, several metabolic changes take place in the body, and it is impossible to establish an exact chain of events leading to death. Recent studies have focused on looking at these biochemical markers to help maximize post-mortem interval estimations. For instance, alterations in blood pH and the concentration of metabolites like hypoxanthine, lactate, and ammonia are employed as markers of how long ago the person died. Such data are not just helpful in the understanding of sudden death mechanisms but also aid in the differentiation between natural and potential foul play. This novel approach to data gathering emphasizes the demand for sophisticated analytical techniques in forensic science (Donaldson et al., 2013). Sophisticated data analysis techniques also enhance the ability to ascertain and rectify the causes of sudden death. With multi-disciplinary analytic approaches, researchers are able to compile data acquired from autopsy results, biochemical examinations, and medical histories. Such a multi-disciplinary approach facilitates closer examination of the common causes like coronary artery disease, cardiomyopathies, and other electrical conduction abnormalities that are generally implicated in such disastrous events. In addition, the findings assist in educating healthcare practitioners as well as policy-makers in terms of risk factors among high-risk populations, most importantly, athletes and young people. Thus, efficient data collection and analysis not only provide for prompt response to sudden deaths but also aid long-term population health interventions aimed at reducing incidence rates and enhancing preventive services (Sheppard et al., 2012; Donaldson et al., 2013).

11.5.3. Wearable Health Technology

Wearable health technology has revolutionized the way individuals monitor their physiological condition to the point of impacting disease preventive measures. Smartwatches and fitness trackers can be used to monitor vital signs in real time, thereby enabling real-time data analysis. This continuous monitoring is crucial because it enables real-time feedback regarding health parameters that can serve as early warning signs for potentially fatal diseases. For instance, integrating these technologies into daily life allows one to monitor one's oxygen levels, heart rate, and even the electrical activity of the heart, which can be extremely helpful in identifying risks for sudden cardiac events. As described, the implementation of WBAN is an advancement on such capabilities through the application of a sensor network that can transmit vital health information promptly and effectively, making it possible for early detection of anomalies not only to be a possibility but a reality (Blondia et al., 2012). Also, wearables have a key role in predictive healthcare by applying complicated algorithms to process data gathered. These devices have the capability to identify abnormal heart rhythms, which may be a sign of potentially life-threatening arrhythmias. The integration of machine learning techniques with wearable data can lead to highly accurate predictive models. Heart rate variability analysis and real-time ECG monitoring are central features in this context. As can be observed, current research emphasizes the importance of such analysis towards forecasting of negative health events before they escalate into adverse states, ultimately serving the purposes of timely intervention strategies (Walinjkar et al., 2017). The predictive capability inherent in these technologies serves to shift the paradigm from reactive care to proactive care, where the users are provided with warnings for deteriorating health states, which have the potential to reduce the incidence of sudden death. Implementation of wearable health technology into traditional healthcare is not problem-free, particularly with regards to data quality, privacy, and reliability of the devices. While there has been rapid advancement in significantly increasing the capacity of wearable devices to monitor key health indicators, variability of data accuracy can affect predictive outcomes. It is important that the devices be in compliance with rigorous regulatory standards and yield high-quality data to facilitate widespread adoption. Also, ethical considerations of data privacy raise the very serious questions regarding how health data are transmitted and stored. With the health tech community continuing to expand, solving these problems effectively will be essential for realizing the maximum potential of wearable health technology. Ultimately, these innovations have enormous potential not only in understanding the dynamics of human health but also in implementing steps that could possibly reduce the risks involved with sudden deaths in human beings (Figure 11.22).

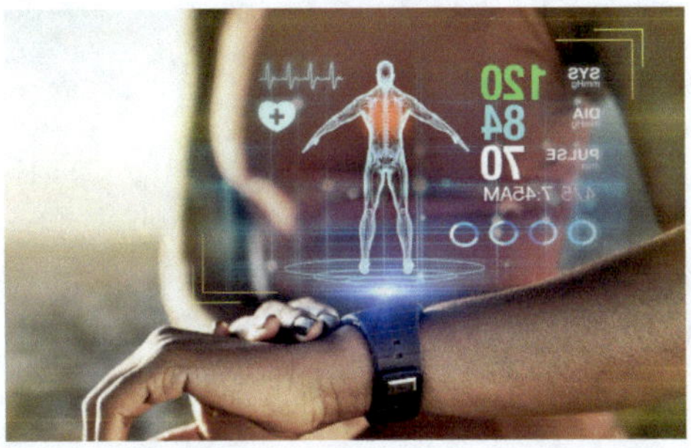

Figure 11.22. Wearable health technology.

Source: https://media.licdn.com/dms/image/v2/D5612AQHXUUifUqkAHA/article-cover_image-shrink_720_1280/article-cover_image-shrink_720_1280/0/1713831871929?e=2147483647&v=beta&t=7h-HVtmt-8F9PqIh1yGlnZa6zYzQozG8BE62VJLCFyk.

Test Your Knowledge

1. Which imaging techniques provides detailed visualization of heart structures?
2. Which sudden health condition can wearable tech potentially help prevent?

SUMMARY

In encapsulating the research of sudden death in man, particularly with reference to cardiac risk, it is apparent that a method of multidisciplinary character is indispensable for the unraveling and prevention of these fatal deaths. The evidence indicates that patients who carry implantable cardioverter-defibrillators (ICDs) provide valuable predictors of appropriate and inappropriate device therapy interventions, respectively, and both are causally linked to occurrences of sudden cardiac death (SCD). Specifically, data in Lebedeva et al. (2024) demonstrate that nearly half of the observation patients revealed frequent ventricular tachyarrhythmias, highlighting attentive observation and therapy of high-risk patients. The high rate of inappropriate shocks reflects the necessity for immediate enhanced diagnostic precision and treatment protocols because these malfunctioning devices not only provide insufficient protection but may even increase psychological distress in patients. Evidence in other areas derives from global observations that illustrate heterogeneity of SCD risk profiles by regions of the world. For instance, Zhao et al. (2024) assert that primary prevention by implantation of ICD reduces all-cause mortality and SCD risks significantly, particularly in developing nations. The revelations regarding the differential efficacy of such interventions by region highlight the importance of regionalized healthcare policy that considers local risk factors, including socioeconomic and environmental. Understanding the geographic variation in SCD incidence and the impact of ICD use will enable improved resource allocation and better patient outcomes by healthcare systems. This implies an appeal for an urgent response to comprehensive public health initiatives to enhance awareness and access to preventive care. Lastly, the implication of this assessment is the need for continuous research and development in reducing sudden deaths. Identification of risk factors and implementation of effective prevention strategies, such as targeted ICD placement and lifestyle modifications, can effectively lower the incidence of sudden cardiac deaths. The data shows that patients and the medical workforce equally have to be more proactive in identifying solutions appropriate to certain health challenges, thus establishing a responsive healthcare system. By encouraging interdisciplinary collaboration among scientists, public health specialists, and cardiologists, the problem of sudden deaths can be addressed more effectively, ultimately enhancing survival rates and quality of life for susceptible populations.

Unexplained human deaths are a multifaceted event with a variety of conditions and contexts, often carrying immense medical and social burdens. The cause of such occurrences calls for an exhaustive examination of causative factors, which may consist of natural health status, lifestyle, and exogenous environmental causes. For instance, cardiac arrest or cerebrovascular accident may suddenly happen in otherwise healthy individuals, emphasizing the need for widespread education and prevention. This information not only educates public health policy but also directs health workers in developing successful interventions for controlling the prevalence of these sudden deaths. In addition, the utilization of concepts in reliability theory, particularly relating to transitions in mortality rates, can provide an in-depth description of how sudden deaths may occur in different populations and ages, such as in the Transient Shock conjecture predictions regarding diverse organisms, including the human (Berrut et al., 2016). Besides clinical conditions, environmental factors are important causes of sudden death. For example, widespread diseases, such as Ebola, have rung alarm bells globally and forced an international response and preparedness system. This view on Ebola hemorrhagic fever encapsulates the importance of establishing robust health systems with emphasis on early detection and intervention, which can avoid the risk of sudden deaths from the disease propagating over geographical distances. With re-evaluation of the historical context and scientific studies of Ebola, it is clear that proactive measures such as having trained health workers at strategic locations like airports and seaports will be essential in stemming outbreaks. These measures not only save lives but also save countries from the brunt of sudden health crises (Adu-Gyamfi et al., 2019). Moreover, the broader implications of sudden deaths reach into society, touching communities and medical systems far and wide. The fabric of families themselves can be irrevocably shaken by a member's death, exposing them to emotional trauma and economic strain. The importance of immediate healthcare response following sudden deaths is great, because rapid medical intervention can prevent, at times, escalation from acute to chronic health crises. In addition, studies of demographic disparities in sudden death rates have the potential to shed light on dimensions of unequal access to healthcare and socioeconomic status. Ultimately, addressing the vagaries of sudden deaths is a group effort involving public health organizations, healthcare workers, and society at large to develop evidence-based interventions and policies that can cut these tragedies off at the pass. This minute-by-minute analysis not only confirms the necessity of addressing sudden deaths but also underscores the necessity of ongoing vigilance and preparedness in the wake of unexpected health events.

KEY TERMS FROM THIS CHAPTER

- Arrhythmias
- Cardiology
- Cardiovascular stability
- Epidemiology
- Hypertrophic cardiomyopathy
- Mental health
- Natural disasters
- Brain health
- Cardiomyocytes
- Disaster management
- Genetics
- Hypertrophy
- Myocardial infarctions
- Pandemics

CRITICAL THINKING QUESTIONS

1. **Which of the following is the most common cause of sudden natural death in adults?**
   a. Pulmonary embolism
   b. Acute myocardial infarction
   c. Subarachnoid hemorrhage
   d. Epilepsy
2. **Which of the following is least likely to cause sudden death?**
   a. Ruptured aortic aneurysm
   b. Myocardial infarction
   c. Pancreatic cancer
   d. Pulmonary embolism
3. **Which of the following is a major risk factor for sudden cardiac death?**
   a. Anemia
   b. Asthma
   c. Ventricular fibrillation
   d. Type 2 diabetes
4. **In forensic practice, sudden death is defined as death occurring:**
   a. Within 24 hours of symptom onset
   b. Within 12 hours of hospitalization
   c. Instantly, with no known disease
   d. Within 1 hour of the onset of acute symptoms
5. **SUDEP stands for:**
   a. Sudden Unidentified Death in Elderly Patients
   b. Sudden Unexpected Death in Epilepsy
   c. Sudden Unconsciousness Due to Electrolyte Problems
   d. Sudden Unprovoked Death in Emergency Patients

Short Answer Questions

1. Define sudden death.
2. Why is studying the epidemiology of sudden deaths important?
3. What is the most common cause of a sudden death?
4. What is the psychological impact of sudden death?
5. What is the role of technology in understanding sudden death?

Answer to Critical Thinking Questions

1. (b) 2. (c) 3. (c) 4. (d) 5. (b)

REFERENCES

1. Abdel-Aleem, H., Bergsjø, P., Betran, A., Duke, et al. (2009). Making stillbirths count, making numbers talk: Issues in data collection for stillbirths. https://core.ac.uk/download/13117512.pdf (accessed on 12th July 2025).
2. Adu-Gyamfi, S. (Samuel). (2019). Ebola hemorrhagic fever in Africa: A necessary highlight. https://core.ac.uk/download/480549437.pdf (accessed on 12th July 2025).
3. Afifi, A. A., & Sagan, L. A. (1978). The biological basis for standard setting for environmental pollutants: A critique. https://core.ac.uk/download/33892324.pdf (accessed on 12th July 2025).
4. Andrew, M. K., Cornford, C. S., Department of Health, Goldrick, B., Gross, P. A., Morgan, R., Plotkin, S. L., et al. (2008). A review of the factors involved in older people's decision making with regard to influenza vaccination: A literature review. https://core.ac.uk/download/82906958.pdf (accessed on 12th July 2025).
5. Balestrini, S., Diehl, B., Duncan, J. S., et al. (2015). Structural imaging biomarkers of sudden unexpected death in epilepsy. https://core.ac.uk/download/323077527.pdf (accessed on 12th July 2025).
6. Belsky, B., Berkowitz, B., Blair, B., Bourget, B., Bourget, B., et al. (2011). Fatal child maltreatment in England, 2005-9. https://core.ac.uk/download/44459.pdf (accessed on 12th July 2025).
7. Berrut, S., Pouillard, V., Richmond, P., et al. (2016). Deciphering infant mortality. Part 1: Empirical evidence. http://arxiv.org/abs/1603.04007 (accessed on 12th July 2025).
8. Blondia, C., Braem, B., Higgins, H., et al. (2012). A comprehensive survey of wireless body area networks on PHY, MAC, and network layers solutions. https://core.ac.uk/download/55705205.pdf (accessed on 12th July 2025).
9. Boyce, G. T., Cooper, O. W., Griffin, R. M., et al. (2003). Do childhood vaccines have non-specific effects on mortality? https://core.ac.uk/download/pdf/11307006.pdf (accessed on 12th July 2025).
10. Brownson, R. C., McKay, V. R., Morshed, A. B., et al. (2018). Letting go: Conceptualizing intervention de-implementation in public health and social service settings. https://core.ac.uk/download/287888057.pdf (accessed on 12th July 2025).
11. Chagas, A. C. P., Da Luz, P. L., & Nishiyama, M. (2011). Drugs and lifestyle for the treatment and prevention of coronary artery disease: Comparative analysis of the scientific basis. https://core.ac.uk/download/pdf/37452566.pdf (accessed on 12th July 2025).
12. Chang, C. F., Chen, S. J., Fan, H. C., et al. (2013). Current approaches to the treatment of head injury in children. https://core.ac.uk/download/pdf/81144539.pdf (accessed on 12th July 2025).
13. Collier, N. (2010). What's unusual in online disease outbreak news? https://core.ac.uk/download/pdf/8425577.pdf (accessed on 12th July 2025).
14. Corkery, J. (2012). UK fatalities associated with caffeine: Annex 3. https://core.ac.uk/download/1643837.pdf (accessed on 12th July 2025).
15. Dahlen, P. (2014). School district assessment for sudden cardiac arrest preparation. https://core.ac.uk/download/162576263.pdf (accessed on 12th July 2025).

16. De Vogli, R., & Marmot, M. (2008). Should socioeconomic factors be considered as traditional risk factors for cardiovascular disease, as confounders, or as risk modifiers? https://core.ac.uk/download/1678308.pdf (accessed on 12th July 2025).

17. Donaldson, A. (2013). Biochemistry changes that occur after death: Potential markers for determining post-mortem interval. https://core.ac.uk/download/322841937.pdf (accessed on 12th July 2025).

18. Elsaygh, J., Bradel, L., Pink, K., Chen, L., Arnedo, J., Reddy, B. M., Wong, B. C., et al. (2025). Do gender differences persist in ICD implantation in patients with acute on chronic heart failure? *Future cardiology*. https://www.semanticscholar.org/paper/c72d42f46ec17b32d3dc917e95de172e7c04fceb (accessed on 12th July 2025).

19. Feelisch, M., Kolb-Bachofen, V., Liu, D., et al. (2010). Is sunlight good for our heart? https://core.ac.uk/download/46361.pdf (accessed on 12th July 2025).

20. Hayward, A. D., Lummaa, V., Lynsdale, C. L., et al. (2017). Parasite-associated mortality in a long-lived mammal: Variation with host age, sex, and reproduction. https://core.ac.uk/download/156827839.pdf (accessed on 12th July 2025).

21. Kennedy, I., Murray, V., Petley, D. N., et al. (2015). A systematic review of the health impacts of mass earth movements (landslides). https://core.ac.uk/download/41989325.pdf (accessed on 12th July 2025).

22. Koreyba, K. A., Minabutdinov, A. R., & Gatina, L. N. (2024). Modern synthetic bioplastic materials with functional properties in the surgery of ulcerative defects of diabetic foot syndrome. https://doi.org/10.34660/inf.2023.99.96.160 (accessed on 12th July 2025).

23. Lebedeva, V. K., & Levinova, O. E. (2024). Analysis of electrotherapy in patients with implantable cardioverter-defibrillator for primary prevention of sudden cardiac death according to remote monitoring data. *The Siberian Journal of Clinical and Experimental Medicine*. https://www.semanticscholar.org/paper/fae21f70b2370a8a78632bcc1e2121a322d23b3e (accessed on 12th July 2025).

24. Leroy, S. A. G. (2006). From natural hazard to environmental catastrophe: Past and present. https://core.ac.uk/download/336621.pdf (accessed on 12th July 2025).

25. Loggins, C. (2018). The meaning of a family history of colorectal cancer in Black families in the United States. https://core.ac.uk/download/217323274.pdf (accessed on 12th July 2025).

26. Loh, D., & Pullicino, P. (2014). Neurogenic disturbances of cardiac rhythm. https://core.ac.uk/download/46602507.pdf (accessed on 12th July 2025).

27. Luanpaisanon, P., Wolf, M., & Saucerman, J. (2024). Abstract We133: *In silico* model of cardiomyopathy caused by a MYBPC3-induced HCM mutation. *Circulation Research*. https://www.semanticscholar.org/paper/fe6bf0b942821e428dccf2e4c2489ce9e812b05a (accessed on 12th July 2025).

28. Maximova, M. N., & Akhmerova, V. M. (2024). Analysis of factors affecting the effective work of a civil servant in the Ministry of Labor, Employment and Social Protection of the Republic of Tatarstan and the Ministry of Digital Development of the State Administration of Information Technologies and Communications of the Republic of Tatarstan. https://doi.org/10.34660/inf.2023.79.19.147 (accessed on 12th July 2025).

29. Moody, H. R., & Hayflick, L. (2003). Has anyone ever died of old age? https://core.ac.uk/download/71356368.pdf (accessed on 12th July 2025).

30. N/A. (2007). Pandemic influenza: Warning, children at-risk. https://core.ac.uk/download/71353662.pdf (accessed on 12th July 2025).

31. N/A. (2012). Outlook magazine, autumn 2012. https://core.ac.uk/download/70380678.pdf (accessed on 12th July 2025).

32. N/A. (2021). Exploring nurses' experiences and perspectives with patient death due to drug overdose: Implications for future practice. https://core.ac.uk/download/395449644.pdf (accessed on 12th July 2025).

33. Pace, D., & Torpiano, P. (2014). Ebola: Too far or so close? https://core.ac.uk/download/46602506.pdf (accessed on 12th July 2025).

34. Paulhus, K., Kumar, P., Kneale, K., Hutson, T., Gautier-Hall, N. M., Shiau, D., Watts, M., et al. (2025). Sex-specific differences in mortality and neurocardiac interactions in the Kv1.1 knockout mouse model of sudden unexpected death in epilepsy (SUDEP). *The Journal of Physiology*. https://www.semanticscholar.org/paper/b32db9c26cc845a6916d91c364d8dd609d379e09 (accessed on 12th July 2025).

35. Reemtsen, B., Finn, J. P., Alejos, J., Touma, M., Touma, M., Halnon, N., Nelson, S. F., et al. (2017). A path to implement precision child health cardiovascular medicine. https://core.ac.uk/download/323077346.pdf (accessed on 12th July 2025).

36. Roemer-Mahler, A., Long, C., Clarke, A., Cooper, M., Elbe, S., Elbe, S., Elbe, S., et al. (2014). Securing circulation pharmaceutically: Antiviral stockpiling and pandemic preparedness in the European Union. https://core.ac.uk/download/30608191.pdf (accessed on 12th July 2025).

37. Sheppard, M. N. (2012). Etiology of sudden cardiac death in sport: A histopathologist's perspective. https://core.ac.uk/download/29469414.pdf (accessed on 12th July 2025).

38. Smith, V. C. (2021). Perceptions of cardiac screening of high school athletes among athletic trainers and high school coaches. https://core.ac.uk/download/425542239.pdf (accessed on 12th July 2025).

39. Walinjkar, A., & Woods, J. C. (2017). ECG classification and prognostic approach towards personalized healthcare. https://core.ac.uk/download/96933809.pdf (accessed on 12th July 2025).

40. Wiggins, K. A. (2025). Analysis of the relationship of spirituality and spiritual bypass on the resilience of survivors of homicide in the U.S. https://core.ac.uk/download/657262515.pdf (accessed on 12th July 2025).

41. Yıldırım, Ö. T., Tunay, D. L., & Turgay, A. (2024). The impacts of the earthquake on the cardiovascular system. *Çukurova Anestezi ve Cerrahi Bilimler Dergisi*. https://www.semanticscholar.org/paper/f0230d2716f5bd396d0a1ee599c427f87d878b62 (accessed on 12th July 2025).

42. Zhao, S., Ching, C. K., Huang, D., Liu, Y. B., Rodriguez-Guerrero, D. A., Hussin, A., Kim, Y. H., et al. (2024). Regional disparities and risk factors of mortality among patients at high risk of sudden cardiac death in emerging countries: A nonrandomized controlled trial. *BMC Medicine, 22*. https://www.semanticscholar.org/paper/abf41ff16e882b7e129a4db750c23e22c7b14867 (accessed on 12th July 2025).

PEDIATRIC FORENSIC PATHOLOGY

12

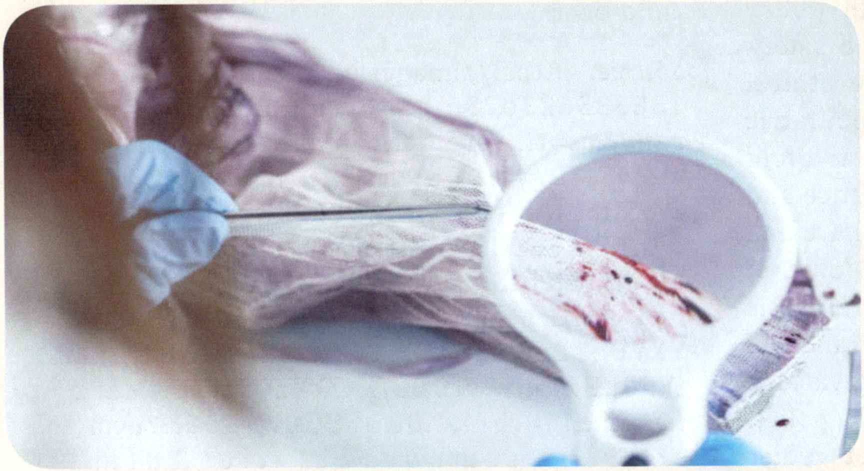

LEARNING OBJECTIVES

After studying this chapter, you will be able to:

1. Describe the role of pediatric forensic pathologists;
2. the common causes of death in pediatric cases;
3. Describe the techniques and methodologies in pediatric forensic pathology;
4. Understand the current trends and challenges in pediatric forensic pathology.

Introduction

The pediatric forensic pathologist is also responsible for rigorous investigation of child death, which often happens in suspicious circumstances or due to trauma. The specialty of pediatric forensic pathology is a significant intersection of the law and medicine with precise knowledge of child health, injury patterns, and medico-legal responsibility. The subtlety of this area is exacerbated by the need to differentiate between natural fatalities and abuse- or neglect-induced fatalities. As argued, the clear-cut definition is far off in the field, thus making it problematic to analyze child-related deaths (Argo et al., 2019). This challenge emphasizes the need to develop uniform criteria to analyze pediatric deaths and to enhance the education and training of professionals working with such sensitive cases. As the incidence of violence and trauma increases in contemporary society, pediatric forensic pathology has never been more necessary. Equally important is an urgent response to the legal and ethical issues of pediatric forensic pathology. Such a sensitive aspect of the investigative process in the case of minors demands a strong ethical framework through which to navigate the potentiality of bias, misinterpretation, and family psychological impact. As professionals encounter more high-tech situations, maintaining the integrity of the forensic investigation and avoiding premature conclusions that could adversely affect judicial decisions is essential.

Moreover, pathological findings may have implications extending beyond immediate legal ramifications to affect public health policy and community attitudes toward child safety. Understanding the subtlety of these ethical dilemmas is most important as pediatric forensic pathologists balance their twofold obligations: to serve the interest of justice and to advocate for the interests of the welfare and well-being of the concerned children (Sage et al., 2018). The evolution of pediatric forensic pathology also highlights the importance of interprofessional collaboration among various experts. Pathologists, medical examiners, police, and child protective services must work together to untangle the intricate issues that arise in each case. One such example is the interplay between physical evidence and psychological assessment of child witnesses, whose interplay can greatly impact investigations. Furthermore, recent developments in pediatric neurotrauma, including Chronic Traumatic Encephalopathy (CTE), have generated debate regarding long-term consequences of those injuries incurred in youth, particularly within the context of sports (Sage et al., 2018). Therefore, an integrative approach that addresses advances in medical science, changing societal views of child protection, and stronger legal provisions is needed for further advancement of the discipline. Lastly, pediatric forensic pathology serves not only to explain the causes of death but also as a necessary mechanism in advocacy for safer lives for children (Figure 12.1).

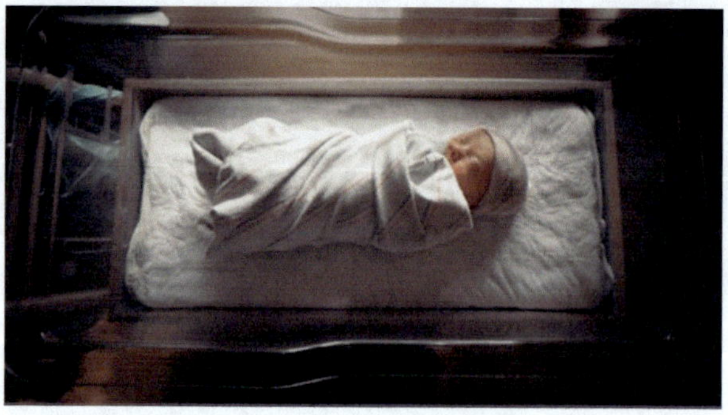

Figure 12.1. Forensic pathology of infant and child death.

Source: https://images.unsplash.com/photo-1583356230736-b5b9ecb85605?crop=entropy&cs=tinysrgb&fit=max&fm=jpg&ixid=M3w3MDgyMDR8MHwxfHNlYXJjaHwxfHxmb3JlbnNpYyUyMHBhdGhvbG9neSUyQyUyMGluZmFudCUyMGRlYXRoJTIwaW52ZXN0aWdhdGlvbiUyQyUyMGNoa WxkJTIwZGVhdGglMjBpbnZlc3RpZ2F0aW9uJTJDJTIwYXV0b3BzeSUyMGluJTIwY2hpbGQlMjBkZWF0aHxlbnwwfDB8fHwxNzQ5OTEwMzczfDA&ixlib=rb-4.1.0&q=80&w=500&?utm_source=numberanalytics&utm_medium=referral.

12.1. Role of Pediatric Forensic Pathologists

Learning Outcome

1. Understand the responsibilities of pediatric forensic pathologists in death investigations.
2. Collaborate with law enforcement and legal entities.
3. Understand the importance of expert testimony in court.

Pediatric forensic pathologists are at the forefront of examining unexplained child and infant deaths. They provide crucial expertise to determine the circumstances surrounding a child's death, especially when the cause is doubtful or suspicious. With meticulous autopsies and state-of-the-art forensic examination, these specialists can diagnose underlying medical conditions, trauma, or toxicological conditions that may have resulted in a fatal outcome. Such inquiries are essential, since misclassifications or misdiagnoses mean grieving families may never receive closure and can also interfere with public health measures designed to stop such disasters from recurring. Though Sudden Infant Death Syndrome (SIDS) has remained a serious cause of infant death for a long time, the recent discussion at the 3rd International Congress on Unexplained Deaths in Infants and Children has put the focus on enhancing classifications and definitions, so that proper recording of such catastrophic events can be ensured (Richard et al., 2019). Moreover, pediatric forensic pathologists play an important role in addressing the consequences of sudden cardiac death (SCD) in children. As research has demonstrated that SCD is a substantial cause of death in children, and its relation to genetic elements, the aforementioned specialists must be involved in postmortem genetic testing as well. Postmortem genetic testing can provide valuable information about hereditary cardiac disease not evident during life. Institutionalizing rigorous autopsy practices is to establish a more specific etiology of death that can have implications for not only the medical treatment of surviving family members but also inform public health policy. Expert advice demands more recognition of the value of postmortem genetic testing, which necessitates focus on multidisciplinary and coordination among healthcare professionals to ensure that families are provided with applicable information and attention throughout the process (Fellmann et al., 2019). Pediatric forensic pathologists are not only essential contributors to examinations but also vitally significant teachers and community supporters. They are responsible for disseminating information on pediatric forensic issues, including the importance of recognizing signs of abuse or neglect, which can lead to devastating consequences. Moreover, through partnerships with law enforcement and protective agencies, these professionals can assist in constructing procedures that enhance safety and prevention factors within the community. Awareness campaigns can aid both the public and professionals, significantly impacting children's health outcomes by emphasizing the importance of early intervention and precise diagnostic methods. As pediatric forensic pathology continues to evolve, its professionals play a central role not just in investigating individual cases but in ensuring society's devotion to the child's health and preventing disasters (Figure 12.2).

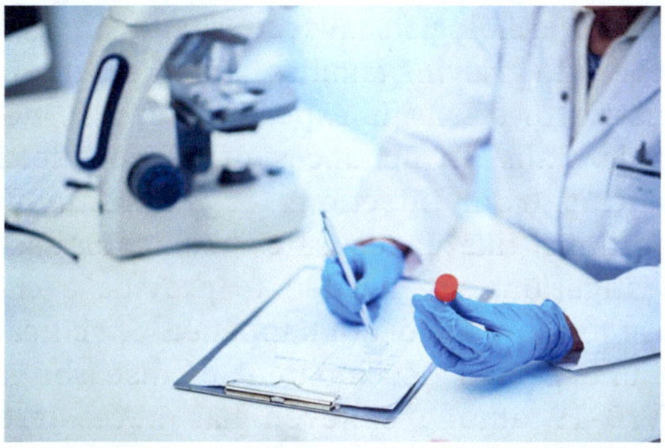

Figure 12.2. Role of pediatric forensic pathologists.

Source: https://medical.rossu.edu/sites/g/files/krcnkv261/files/styles/atge_3_2_crop_md/public/2022-04/Forensic-Pathology.jpg?h=a6da41a2&itok=CXEF2voV.

12.1.1. Responsibilities in Death Investigations

In pediatric forensic pathology, the role in death investigations is complex and requires a great understanding of the medical as well as legal procedures. Forensic pathologists are responsible for identifying the cause and manner of death through performing detailed autopsies involving gross and microscopic examinations of the dead body. Autopsy offers a way of identifying underlying reasons that could have contributed but not been detected prior to death, such as those in the case of SIDS or other unexplained outcomes. The use of toxicological analysis and laboratory testing is further significant in ascertaining contributory reasons that may influence the causation determination. To this end, accurate reporting of histopathological findings is essential, as it aids in correlating clinical observations with autopsy reports, finally contributing to effective public health measures and prevention strategies (Rai et al., 2024). The challenges of pediatric death examinations also necessitate acknowledgment of social and psychological concerns that affect families and investigators. Forensic pathologists must cope with emotional issues with grieving families, and this is not just a matter of scientific expertise but also good people skills. In instances of sudden deaths resulting from infections or environmental conditions, like exposure to toxins, extensive investigations are needed to provide a clear cause for how the death happened. Specifically, the unexpected development of diseases like COVID-19 among children has necessitated improvement in investigative processes, including neuroimaging, to identify subtle brain lesions that may not be apparent during autopsy (Michelle et al., 2022). Hence, forensic experts have a function that goes beyond technical assessment; there is also a responsibility to report results empathetically to affected families and cautiously address social implications. Lastly, the complete responsibilities in pediatric forensic death investigations emphasize the necessary bridge between medical expertise and moral principles. While death investigations expose significant information regarding sudden deaths, they can also propel additional research that may advance the knowledge on diseases of children and their prevention. The role of forensic pathology not only informs legal cases and public health policy but also the broader medical community's collective knowledge base, ultimately enhancing child health. By being attuned to the subtleties of pediatric cases and the inherent frailties of this population, forensic pathologists can promote policies that ensure children are protected from preventable disease. This integrative strategy for investigations into death, therefore, becomes a critical aspect of developing pediatric forensic pathology in humans and reflects the continued devotion to child welfare across all levels of society (Figure 12.3).

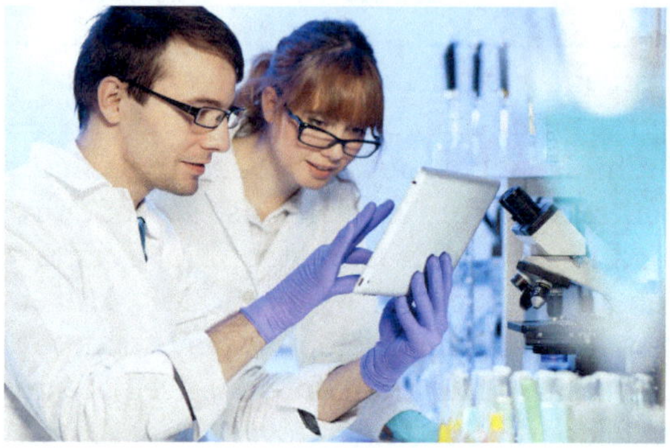

Figure 12.3. Responsibilities of forensic pathologists in death investigations.

Source: https://theforensicdoc.com/wp-content/uploads/2019/06/Male-and-Female-Researchers-Examining-Tablet-in-Lab-scaled.jpg.

12.1.2. Collaboration with Law Enforcement and Legal Entities

Collaboration between law enforcement and pediatric forensic pathologists is crucial to facilitate quality investigation of child deaths. In cases where suspicion arises of suspicious circumstances, early action by forensic experts facilitates law enforcement in gathering vital evidence and identifying the cause of death. Pediatric forensic pathologists provide valuable information regarding the unique anatomical and physiological characteristics of children, which are quite distinct from those of adults. This information enables police to act on cases of child death in the care and precision required, improving investigations as a whole. Also, mutual support in the form of sharing findings with police forces enables everyone concerned to know and react accordingly to ensure justice, enabling a better response in cases where there can be criminal involvement. Legal agencies like legal representation and protective services for children are also key in the collaborative framework of pediatric forensic pathology. Support in providing liaison among these agencies and forensic pathologists is vital in providing effective case management. Upon the incidence of a child's death, which calls for a legal inquiry, the involvement of forensic experts may sustain the explanation of medical data that can influence legal verdicts. Pediatric forensic pathologists serve a supporting role by providing expert testimony in court so that legal professionals are able to better comprehend the complexities of pediatric death and trauma. Additionally, their specialist can contribute to ensuring such vulnerable populations are provided with necessary safeguards and interventions, thus harmonizing clinical findings and legal requirements. Such an association not only enriches the investigative process but also reinforces the protection of the rights of children in legal proceedings. Effective collaboration is not just between police and medical practitioners but also with community partners and advocacy groups. These organizations are typically engaged in sensitization concerning the welfare and protection of the child, identifying families who are susceptible to neglect and abuse of the child, and advocating for child abuse and neglect prevention policy. Pediatric forensic pathologists can collaborate with these teams to spread awareness regarding the indicators of abuse and the need for early medical intervention. Multi-disciplinary team responses, which could include social workers and mental health counselors, can also better bolster the concerted action against child fatalities. By bringing together lenses of diverse types and experience, collaborative work has the potential to design more comprehensive solutions, ultimately leading to improved results for families and children in diverse communities (Dogonova, 2024).

12.1.3. Importance of Expert Evidence to Court

The role of expert opinion in the legal process cannot be overstated, particularly within the domain of pediatric forensic pathology. Expert opinion serves as a vehicle for communicating challenging medical facts to the legal understanding, allowing judges and jurors to make knowledgeable determinations based on specialized knowledge. In cases of child abuse or suspicious trauma, specialty witnesses such as child abuse pediatricians offer data based on medical exams and research that can throw light on the nuances of child injuries. Expertise is essential in establishing the credibility of evidence, thus influencing the persuasiveness of court decisions. But issues arise when prejudice and vagueness enter the expert testimony, potentially warping the system of justice. Thus, it is important for the experts to adhere to strict standards of objectivity in an effort to maintain the integrity of their findings as well as the overall legal process, thus signaling the importance of expert evidence in such sensitive cases. There are extremely serious concerns regarding bias in expert evidence in pediatric forensic pathology cases, including child abuse claims. The presence of biases such as adversarial bias and confirmation bias has the ability to undermine the objective nature of medical opinions, leading to skewed interpretations and findings that may be used in support of a prosecutor's case rather than presenting unbiased evidence. As has been found in recent literature, the aforementioned biases have the potential to exchange objectivity for advocacy; the professionals must be careful against such influences so that the reliability of their testimonies is maintained. In cases that involve contentious issues like Shaken Baby Syndrome (SBS), the identification of specific symptoms is extremely critical relative to the making of broader legal conclusions. Differentiating from this would result in expert witnesses unintentionally corroborating myths, emphasizing the absolute significance of having a transparent, unbiased method of testing forensic evidence (Skellern et al., 2015). Shaken Baby Syndrome, or Abusive Head Trauma, controversies show the complexity and challenge that pediatric forensic pathologists face in their testimony. As legal outcomes often rest on the recommendations of medical professionals, definitions and interpretations provided by these specialists have a direct impact on judicial processes of child abuse cases. There are fears that some pediatricians may be making absolute findings of abuse on a limited, contentious medical evidence base and quite possibly blurring medical opinion with legal findings. Blending the medical opinion with legal action highlights the importance of clear guidelines that delineate the boundaries of expert evidence. Legal professionals and medical experts must join in an effort to guarantee that evidence-based testimony remains based on corroborative medical facts and does not resort to hyperbolic claims or advocacy positions. This collaboration is vital to establish a judicial environment within which expert witness testimony can guide and uphold the principles of justice (Barnes et al., 2020) (Figure 12.4).

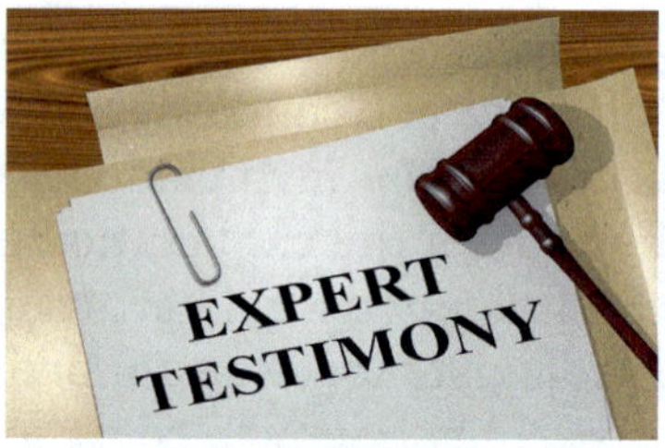

Figure 12.4. Expert testimony in court.

Source: https://www.simmonsandfletcher.com/wp-content/uploads/2018/03/expert-testimony.png.

Test Your Knowledge

1. What is a primary responsibility of forensic pathologists in pediatric death investigations?
2. Why is collaboration between pediatric forensic pathologists and law enforcement important in child fatality investigations?

12.2. Common Causes of Death in Pediatric Cases

Learning Outcome

1. Know the natural causes of death and their forensic implications.
2. Investigate accidental deaths in children.
3. Describe the role of forensic pathologists in homicide cases.

It is important in the establishment of pediatric forensic pathology to have knowledge of the common causes of death in children. Natural causes, that is, congenital disorders and infectious diseases, account for a large percentage of mortality in children. Infant deaths caused by natural death are often caused by congenital disorders, with congenital heart diseases and neural tube defects ranking top. Moreover, illnesses such as pneumonia and sepsis remain prominent contributors to the deaths of children, particularly those aged under five years. Because these natural processes have a tendency to resemble features of trauma or child abuse, forensic pathologists must be equipped with training in order to make discriminations between the two in order to facilitate correct diagnoses and court proceedings. Accidental deaths are also another critical element in studies on child deaths, primarily resulting from preventable injuries. Statistics indicate that child accidents, which include a range of incidents like drowning, motor vehicle crashes, and falls, constitute a majority of childhood fatalities, primarily among children aged one to four years. The unfortunate reality is that the majority of such accidents occur within the home or in known surroundings, prompting one to speculate that environmental safety measures can play a critical role in preventing such fatalities. By treating certain behaviors like the supervision of children playing and the institution of proper safety measures, including protocols, within the home setting, pediatric forensic pathologists can determine public health awareness strategies to combat these accidents. Perhaps the most grim statistic related to pediatric homicide is the reality of its frequency, which usually appears as abuse or neglect. Breathtaking percentages of the deaths of children reported as homicides have had causes such as blunt force trauma and asphyxia, and huge percentages have had shaken baby syndrome as the cause. There has been some new research mentioning a shocking coincidence between the age of the victim—an infant, in many cases—where the possible violent crime has been perpetrated by family members. Identification of such patterns is not only essential to forensic investigation but also throws light upon the necessity of interdisciplinary strategies toward child protection. Comprehensive techniques based on the combination of medical knowledge and legal terminology are required both in response to the evolving forms of child homicide and in the successful enforcement of preventative measures (Collins et al., 1999; Patterson et al., 1814) (Figure 12.5).

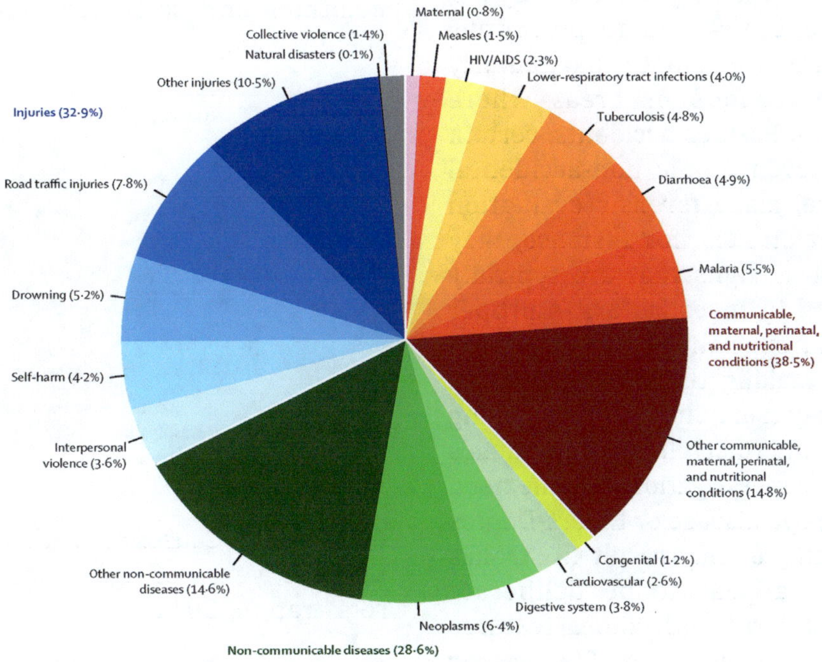

Figure 12.5. Global causes of death in 5–19-year-olds in 2019.

Source: https://www.thelancet.com/cms/10.1016/S2214-109X(21)00566-0/asset/8f5e4ba0-f8de-449d-a7a9-02b674c85679/main.assets/gr1_lrg.jpg.

12.2.1. Natural Causes and Their Forensic Implications

Unexpected natural causes of death, especially pediatric fatalities, present special forensic pathology challenges. Unlike adult fatalities, where chronic illness or a longstanding condition provides more definition to the cause of death, children may suddenly die from unanticipated natural phenomena. Such events include accidents due to tree failure, which lead to instant death in children at play outside. A two-decade-long study of cases in South Australia where trees or branches falling caused accidental fatalities emphasized variables within environmental conditions and tree species, showing the possibility of such tragic incidents occurring without extreme weather (Byard, 2024). Forensic investigation in such cases mainly shows blunt force trauma, further emphasizing the need to learn about natural incidents in the context of pediatrics (Byard, 2024). This awareness can guide preventive measures in community safety, particularly in children's playgrounds or areas where children congregate. Besides accidents, certain medical illnesses even mimic non-accidental trauma and, hence, make forensic evaluation challenging. Infant strokes, for instance, may be misinterpreted as signs that are typically anticipated of NAHI by investigators. A proper history taking and specialized investigations are important in making the right diagnosis. Genetic diseases may cause such life-threatening strokes, and hence interdisciplinary approaches in pediatric forensic investigations are the need of the hour. Moyamoya disease or Ehlers-Danlos syndrome, for example, may result in strokes that may initially appear to be deliberate injuries. Hence, familiarity with clinical features of such disorders becomes a must for forensic pathologists to differentiate between natural and homicidal (Treves et al., 2024). Through the integration of genetic assessments into forensic practice, pathologists are more effectively able to examine difficult pediatric cases. The results of natural causes of childhood death have multiple uses beyond forensic medicine; they can be used to inform the public regarding matters of health and influence public policy. Understanding how specific natural events or conditions lead to lethal outcomes can help guide preventive measures aimed at lessening risk to the pediatric population. For example, epidemiological reports on tree-related deaths can guide town planning and landscaping activities, making living spaces safer for children. Likewise, identifying genetic susceptibility to pediatric strokes can result in better screening programs, allowing for timely intervention and management of those who are at risk. Therefore, the role of forensic pathology in these natural causation cases is critical not just from a legal standpoint but also for general child health outcomes and community safety initiatives. By making these natural causes more manageable, the field can be an incredible asset in creating healthier and safer communities in general (Figure 12.6).

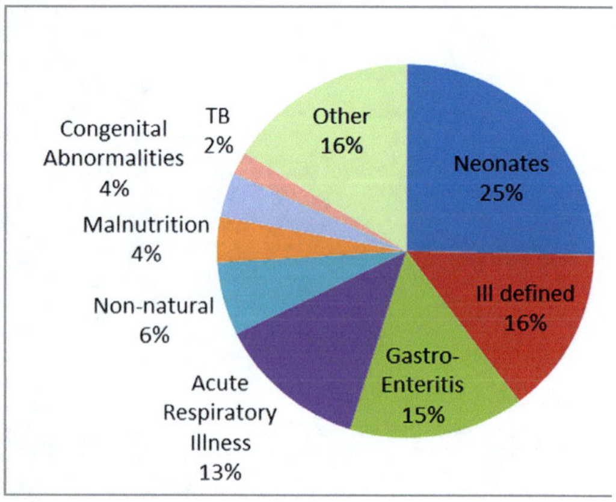

Figure 12.6. Causes of death of death in children under 5 years of age reported through vital registration, 2011.

Source: https://www.researchgate.net/profile/Mphelekedzeni-Mulaudzi/publication/333673728/figure/fig3/AS:768175000023046@1560158600953/Cause-of-death-of-deaths-in-children-under-5-years-of-age-reported-through-Vital.ppm.

12.2.2. Accidental Deaths and Their Investigation

Sudden infant death is a difficult case for forensic pathologists because of its multi-causal nature and complex nature of inquiry. The accidents typically occur in ordinary circumstances, where children are engaged in their routine activities, which unexpectedly lead to death. Forensic scientists have to differentiate between natural, accidental, and unnatural causes of death through careful examination and analysis. The role of the forensic pathologist is particularly important when it comes to determining the manner of death, which not only informs the medical community but also aids legal authorities in resolving disputes regarding parental responsibility or medical negligence. To that end, the detailed categorization of causes and manner of death is required for the sake of establishing an appropriate narrative around the death, thus obtaining preventive measures for future instances. The increase in inadvertent child fatalities has put focus on the need for extensive examinations using modern diagnostic methods. The diagnostic methods enable one to understand the root cause, especially where the cause of death cannot be identified. Recent research indicates the application of sophisticated imaging procedures, such as MRI, in analyzing child fatalities. Integrating imaging is able to reveal details that are overlooked by autopsy and thus enables improved investigation into possible causes of death. These modalities are especially useful to distinguish between accidental fatalities and other underlying disease conditions that are not visually apparent. Despite the apparent advantages, their ethical implications are yet another imposing obstacle, in constant need of debate to establish a model for their application in the use of pediatric forensic investigation (Beck et al., 2014). Accidental deaths necessitate a serious response, particularly on the ethical side of forensic analysis. With children, the impact extends beyond the individual loss to affected families and communities as well. Researchers have to thread the tightrope around the sensitive circumstances surrounding cases of child deaths so that their data informs constructively the public health and safety efforts. Recent research has highlighted the role of medical practitioners in enhancing perioperative environments towards minimizing risks that come with death resulting from accidental injury through a medical procedure. As highlighted by the understanding of anesthesia and perioperative mortality, it is important that medical practice embraces quality control measures for enhancing patient safety (Argo et al., 2019). Through identification of the multifactorial causation of lethal accidents and adherence to evidence-based preventive steps, forensic pathologists can play a crucial role in preventing future cases while ensuring accountability and empathy in pediatric medical practice (Figure 12.7).

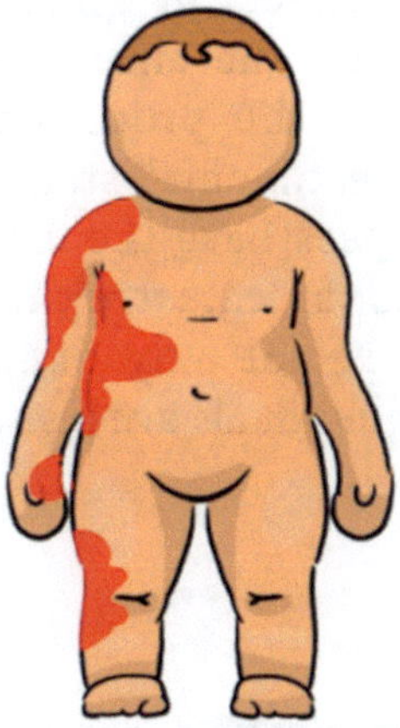

Figure 12.7. Accidental burns.

Source: https://cdnintech.com/media/chapter/19165/1512345123/media/image7.jpeg.

12.2.3. Homicides and the Role of Forensic Pathology

In pediatric forensic pathology, the role of forensic pathologists in homicide cases involving children is multifaceted and essential.

As significant players in the criminal justice system, forensic pathologists examine the conditions under which a child's death occurred to determine the cause and manner of death. These experts conduct more than physical examination autopsies; they must consider medical history, developmental stage, and environmental elements that may have caused the death of a child. By careful analysis of such cases, forensic pathologists help to uncover potential homicides or neglects, data that is precious and can be utilized to aid law enforcers and legal practitioners in administering justice to criminals, hence bolstering the value of their contribution towards pediatric forensic pathology. But the link between forensic pathology and wrongful conviction is a critical subject of concern in the field of child homicide investigation. A study of wrongful convictions indicates that the majority of forensic mistakes are not identification or categorization errors, but are the products of systemic flaws that have an effect on the entire criminal justice system, such as the processing of forensic evidence and testimonial standards (Morgan, 2023). Such lapses have the capability to lead to accusations of catastrophic proportions where justice is not only denied to victims, but innocent individuals are also involved in the legal system. In children, these miscalculations may result in premature conclusions about the cause of death and further complicate the process of justice for vulnerable persons, like children, who are often unable to speak for themselves. New research also illustrates the role of environmental forces in influencing the health, indeed possibly the lives, of children. In urban areas, exposure to nanoparticles and other pollutants has been linked to profound neurological damage and disease that could present as homicides if overlooked (Calder et al., 2022). When forensic pathologists are investigating child fatalities, they must watch out for such environmental contaminant exposures that might not have been accounted for in typical homicide cases. Understanding the interplay between environmental exposures and child health outcomes is essential; not only does it allow for accurate death determination, but also for more general public health interventions aimed at reducing risk factors in a community-based setting. Thus, the forensic pathology contribution to cases of child homicide extends beyond individual autopsy and the investigation process; it includes a holistic approach emphasizing environmental and systemic considerations necessary for reliable judgments and child welfare advocacy.

Test Your Knowledge

1. What are the natural causes of death?
2. What is the role of forensic pathologists in homicide cases?

12.3. Techniques and Methodologies

Learning Outcome

1. Know the autopsy procedures specific to pediatric cases.
2. Describe the use of imaging and toxicology in investigations.
3. Understand the importance of documentation and evidence collection.

In pediatric forensic pathology, the application of advanced techniques and methodologies plays a crucial role in determining the cause and manner of death in children. Incorporation of digital imaging technology in enhancing the visualization of body trauma or pathological changes that are minute or difficult to visualize with the regular methods is a significant approach. Imaging techniques such as computed tomography (CT) and magnetic resonance imaging (MRI) have been central in providing a non-invasive window of insight during post-mortems. These methods enable a thorough examination of internal structures, and hence, forensic pathologists can identify injuries or abnormalities that may indicate foul play or internal diseases. This multi-disciplinary imaging strategy underlines the importance of technology within contemporary forensic practice, as it allows for closer examination of observations that might otherwise go unnoticed during routine autopsies. Molecular techniques have also increasingly emerged in pediatric forensic pathology, significantly enhancing the ability to diagnose and identify genetic disease potentially lying behind a death in a child. For instance, the use of the polymerase chain reaction (PCR) and next-generation sequencing (NGS) allows forensic pathologists to analyze intricate DNA and identify mutations that underlie various diseases. Such molecular methodologies prove invaluable when analyzing cases of sudden unexpected death in infancy (SUDI) since they offer clues towards potential hereditary factors involved in the risk of mortality. Furthermore, a combination of these approaches gives a clear comprehension of the toxicological tests routinely conducted in forensic autopsies. By introducing molecular analysis in conjunction with advanced imaging techniques, the investigations are interdisciplinary and provide an avenue for establishing sound cause-of-death conclusions.

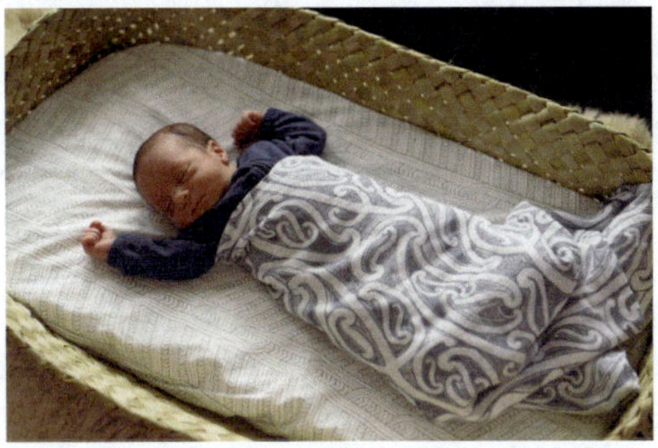

Figure 12.8. Sudden unexpected death in infancy (SUDI).

Source: https://www.plunket.org.nz/assets/General-images/DSC_2125__ResizedImageWzYwMCw0MDFd.jpg.

Besides technological advancements, interdisciplinary approaches have played an imperative role in the utilization of pediatric forensic pathology. The cooperative effort between forensic pathologists, pediatricians, child psychologists, and law enforcement personnel constitutes a holistic model for conducting case investigations. By combining the knowledge base of various professions, the team is in a better position to place findings from autopsy and clinic in an appropriate perspective. The combined effort facilitates exhaustive probing into family histories, habits, and environment pertinent to the death of a child. As underscored in current literature, the use of artificial intelligence and machine learning for examining large databases of children's deaths presents promising avenues for future studies.

The evolving face of pediatric forensic pathology demonstrates the necessity to adopt diverse methodologies in order to ensure a holistic and empathetic exploration of each case with the ultimate goal of upholding justice and clarity for the involved families (Figure 12.8).

12.3.1. Autopsy Procedures Specific to Pediatric Cases

The autopsy protocols unique to child cases call for a customized method to support the unique differences in child physiology and development relative to adults. In forensic pathology, an intimate appreciation of the medical history and the circumstances of a child's death is critical. Forensic pathologists must conduct a diligent external inspection, taking into account age-related anatomical features such as organ weight and size, and the position of growth plates. This is particularly important because developmental phases may influence the interpretation of findings. Sampling methods for histopathological analysis must also be adjusted in a way that involves specimens that are representative based on the age and developmental stage of the child in order to enhance diagnostic accuracy. Such systematic reviews are not only crucial to establish the cause of death but also in handling the potential legal consequences in the event of suspected child abuse or neglect. Deaths among children are typically multifactorial; hence, an exercise of both natural and unnatural causes of death is necessary. Forensic pathologists must scrutinize possibilities such as infections, congenital malformations, and traumatic injury closely. Where there is a suspicious circumstance, for example, in shaken baby syndrome cases, the autopsy is even more significant. For example, finding specific pathological changes such as subdural hemorrhage and retinal hemorrhages can direct the forensic inquiry towards suspected cases of child abuse. All these findings must be understood in the context of the developmental stage, as pediatric trauma varies from that occurring in adults. The application of advanced imaging devices and complementary laboratory studies allows pathologists to deliver expert opinions while avoiding misdiagnosis and guaranteeing justice for vulnerable victims (Apostol et al., 2017). Besides, some challenges in pediatric autopsies are posed by ethical issues and the emotional burden of cutting open a child's body. Forensic pathologists have to handle families with empathy, along with proper communication throughout the process. Mental as well as emotional stability of professionals handling pediatric autopsies is equally critical because these cases carry a very profound effect on grief and trauma. For this purpose, there needs to be training schemes in psychological resilience and support systems for pathologists working in this field. On top of this, the autopsy reports in child cases, for example, those concerning death due to natural disease or accidents, are not necessarily solely for legal purposes but are also an integral component of public health efforts in general. Experience gained from such autopsies can assist in the development of preventive measures against diseases of children and can direct ongoing medical education programs toward improving pediatric patient care (Argo et al., 2019) (Figure 12.9).

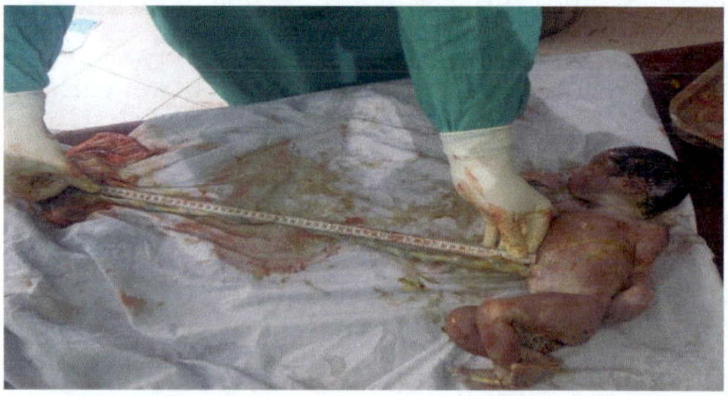

Figure 12.9. Measuring the length of the umbilical cord.

Source: https://cdnintech.com/media/chapter/72362/1512345123/media/F1.png.

12.3.2. Use of Imaging and Toxicology in Investigations

Advanced imaging modalities are significant in pediatric forensic pathology when the examination of child mortality takes place. The autopsies using routine procedures, while incredibly insightful, can be augmented using modalities such as computed tomography (CT) and magnetic resonance imaging (MRI). Advanced imaging modalities allow experts to visualize structures from the inside out without using invasive methods, which is an important factor in cases involving minors since it is a sensitive process. For instance, post-mortem imaging can identify small fractures, soft tissue injuries, and other anatomical abnormalities that might be difficult to detect by routine autopsy practice. Such a non-invasive technique not only preserves the integrity of the body but also enables accurate documentation of injury, thus enhancing the quality of evidence presented during legal proceedings (Fragkou et al., 2025). Therefore, the imaging has a crucial role in ensuring that child homicide cases involve thorough knowledge of potential trauma or abuse. Toxicology also plays a critical role in pediatric forensic pathology, especially in determining causes of death in children who may have come into contact with harmful substances. By toxicological analysis, forensic pathologists can detect the presence of drugs, poisons, or other toxic agents that can lead to a child's death or signs of foul play. Toxicology is also instrumental in suspected child abuse or neglect cases, where it can uncover hidden patterns of drug use or poisoning not otherwise readily visible. This process is often a case of specialized age-specific metabolic response to toxin expertise and the probability of accidental versus criminal exposure (Mores et al., 2025). By describing how toxic agents impact children, forensic experts are able to better distinguish natural causes from criminality and meet the complexities of child fatalities. Moreover, the merging of imaging and toxicology enhances the potential for multidisciplinary dialogue among forensic scientists, law enforcement agents, and legal professionals. Such collegial interaction promotes a comprehensive investigation that integrates traditional forensic fields with the use of modern technology. Through ongoing improvement in pediatric forensic pathology, the integration of these specialized techniques guarantees greater insight into the circumstances under which children perish. By increasing the diagnostic capacity of forensic examiners, both imaging and toxicology are significantly involved in contributing to the level of certainty and reliability of the evidence presented in child homicide cases. The multidisciplinary system not only ensures bringing justice to the victim but also establishes preventative measures for future abuse or neglect, critical towards the protection of generations to come (Fragkou et al., 2025) (Figure 12.10).

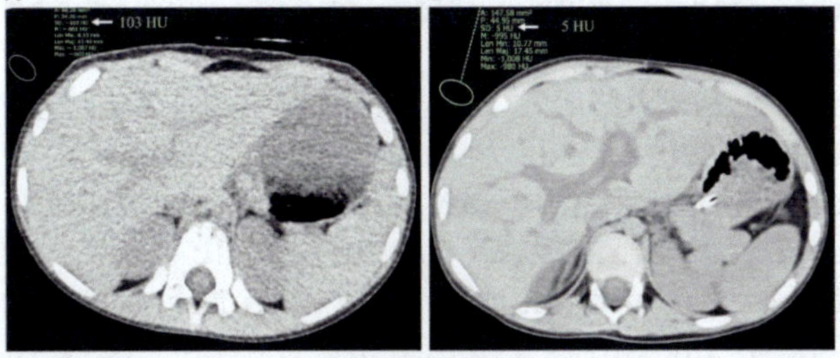

Figure 12.10. Pediatric forensic postmortem computed tomography.

Source: https://media.springernature.com/lw1200/springer-static/image/art%3A10.1007%2Fs00247-024-06014-3/MediaObjects/247_2024_6014_Fig9_HTML.png.

12.3.3. Importance of Documentation and Evidence Collection

In pediatric forensic pathology, the need for careful documentation and evidence collection cannot be emphasized sufficiently. There must be proper procedures to ensure that forensic evidence is correctly identified, preserved, and made available for legal analysis. Pediatric cases are prone to pose special challenges due to the vulnerability of child victims and the sensitivity involved in handling families. Through a lack of proper documentation, critical information is never recorded, thus inhibiting investigations and, in effect, denying victims justice. For instance, institutions lacking trained forensic experts can process evidence poorly, and cases of important ballistic evidence not being taken or stored properly, for instance, are reported on "orphans" of bullets that had not been handed over to law enforcement agencies. This failure not only incapacitates the judicial process but also brings about critical emotional damage to the affected families who depend on justice for closure (Derek et al., 2024). Moreover, evidence collection procedures have to be standardized to preserve the integrity of forensic examination. Formulation of complete guidelines ensures equal treatment of evidence in various cases and that handling procedures and documentation procedures are always followed. In Australia, for example, the establishment of forensic testing standards entailed consultation with stakeholders like law enforcement officials and consumers to build public trust in forensic information and interpretations. These measures underscore the necessity of serially documenting each step of the evidence collection and processing steps, which can serve as an audit trail during court cases. The better organized and accountable the evidence-gathering process, the more solid and justifiable its results will be in court, thus safeguarding the rights of victims and enhancing the quest for justice (Michael, 2016). Proper evidence gathering and documentation also serve as the foundation for building expert testimony in court. The credibility of forensic pathologists relies not only on experience but also on the accuracy and integrity of the evidence collected. Where children are involved, with the emotional complexities being many, the ability to provide well-documented findings adds strength to the credibility of the case. This applies most where forensic evidence, such as ballistic analysis, is directly based on the circumstances in which a child has been injured or murdered. If forensic processes are adhered to in a religious manner, the risk of misinterpretation or conflict significantly declines. Eventually, compliance with proper documentation and evidence collection enhances the overall efficiency of pediatric forensic pathology so that justice is delivered while also serving as a learning opportunity for both physicians and lawyers involved in such sensitive matters (Derek et al., 2024) (Figure 12.11).

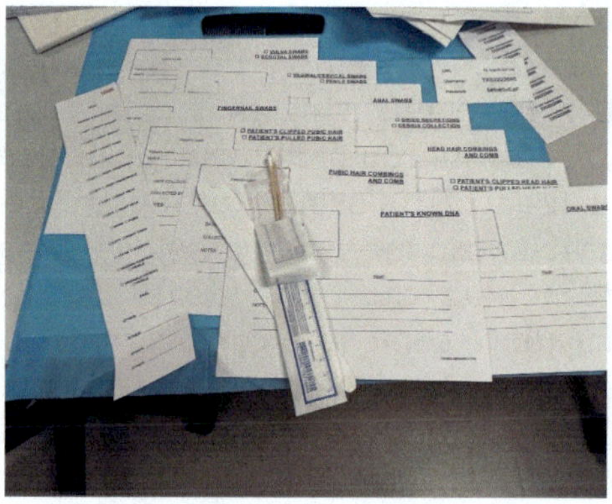

Figure 12.11. Medical forensic assessment documentation.

Source: https://tecp.forensic-nursing.tamu.edu/wp-content/uploads/2023/06/kit-nine.jpg.

Test Your Knowledge

1. What is the use of imaging and toxicology in investigations?
2. What is the importance of documentation and evidence collection?

12.4. Current Trends and Challenges

Learning Outcome

1. Know the advances in technology and their impact.
2. Describe the training and education for forensic pathologists.
3. Address the shortage of pediatric forensic specialists.

The progressive pediatric forensic pathology landscape is dominated by high-priority trends that converge around the evolution of technologies and enhanced knowledge regarding multidisciplinary approaches. Most notable among these is the integration of artificial intelligence (AI) in redesigned pathology services. AI technologies offer promising applications in diagnostic processes via platforms such as digital pathology and whole slide imaging (WSI) that facilitate high-resolution image analysis. This innovation not only enhances the efficiency of child forensic examinations but also addresses the growing workforce shortage in the field. The blend of AI, however, continues to be plagued by issues in the form of the need for robust regulatory systems as well as the quality assurance of evidence. With improvements in technology, pediatric forensic pathology will greatly benefit from improvements if the business can effectively address such challenges in a manner to realize the maximum potential of the technology (Wezi et al., 2025). Besides technological improvements, the current challenges in pediatric forensic pathology also illustrate broader systemic issues that impact the delivery of forensic services. Resource constraints, coupled with manpower deficits, hinder the capacity for thorough investigations and accurate autopsies. Among the primary problems is the scarcity of qualified forensic pathologists, whose demand is highest in low-resource settings. Utilization of established protocols is crucial to the effective investigation of child deaths, but standardization is not present across various regions. Recent research has identified these issues as a priority, highlighting the need for urgent investment in forensic pathology facilities and training initiatives. By addressing these systemic problems, stakeholders can better position the field to address the complexities of pediatric forensic examinations and reinforce its potential for public health and justice (Wezi et al., 2025). Furthermore, the impact of infectious diseases, such as COVID-19, introduces an added layer of complexity to pediatric forensic pathology. Not only have health systems been inundated by the pandemic, but forensic services, too, have been derailed, leading to backlog cases and delayed investigations. The problem raises serious questions about the efficacy of existing protocols against emerging health crises. Forensic pathologists are tasked with weathering these new challenges while safeguarding the integrity and validity of their findings. As a result, there is more emphasis on developing adaptive measures that can respond to public health emergencies. By applying new studies and institutions' collaboration, the field can better prepare itself for future challenges, finally leading to improved quality and integrity of pediatric forensic pathology (Sebire et al., 2024).

12.4.1. Advances in Technology and Their Impact

The revolution in technology has advanced pediatric forensic pathology significantly through enhanced knowledge and investigation of child deaths. Improved imaging technologies, such as high-definition CT scans and MRIs, have maximized the diagnostic capability to detect minor injuries that cannot be seen using conventional autopsy scans. The modalities enable the use of non-invasive testing, particularly vital in children's cases, where an autopsy can be traumatic to families. Furthermore, the employment of digital tools allows forensic pathologists to access and examine large databases, leading to more accurate conclusions regarding the cause of death. In turn, technology not only aids in the detection of trauma but also enhances the overall accuracy and efficiency of forensic investigation in cases of children, ensuring justice and responsibility in highly tragic incidents. The field of genetics also plays a pivotal role in enhancing pediatric forensic pathology. Emerging genetic technologies, such as whole-exome sequencing and next-generation sequencing, provide forensic scientists with the means to identify genetic abnormalities that may be causing some injuries or conditions among child victims. These technologies are also very important in the study of hereditary illnesses, which can be crucial in determining whether the cause of the death of a child was natural or otherwise. Furthermore, genetic testing in forensic science offers a window for resolving cold cases through linking the genetic material obtained at crime scenes to possible perpetrators or victims' relatives. Such a union of genetic data strengthens the worth of forensic evidence, making it more potent in the courts and ultimately contributing towards a proper estimation of the circumstances surrounding pediatric deaths, as described in the literature (Avena et al., 2018). In addition to the enhancement of genetics, machine learning, and the application of artificial intelligence (AI) are presently revolutionizing the pediatric forensic pathology scene. These technologies enable the assessment of enormous quantities of information, making it simple to recognize trends and patterns in child mortality that would otherwise not have been noticed through hand inquiries. For instance, AI programs can predict likely causes of death using medical histories, environmental data, and presenting injuries and assist pathologists in rendering better diagnoses. Besides, AI technologies can aid forensic education and training for experts with simulated case studies applied to laboratory exercises. Through the application of such technological advancement, the career is poised to not only improve outcomes from forensic analyses but also enhance interdisciplinary practice by bringing pathologists, geneticists, and data scientists to collaborate toward better comprehending pediatric death, such as in existing research (University NS, 2014) (Figure 12.12).

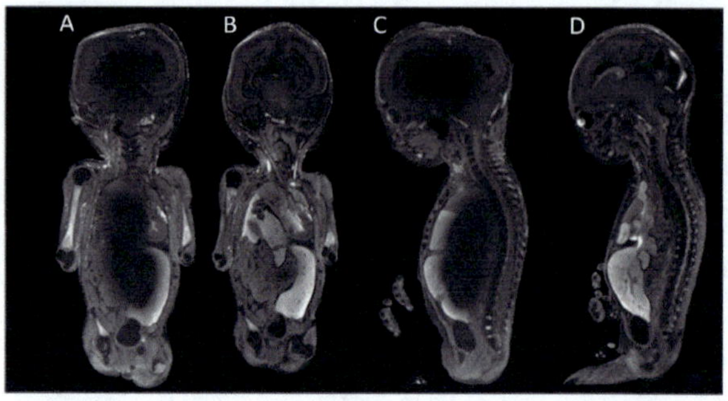

Figure 12.12. Advanced imaging techniques.

Source: https://media.springernature.com/lw685/springer-static/image/chp%3A10.1007%2F978-3-031-69694-7_6/MediaObjects/523952_1_En_6_Fig6_HTML.jpg.

12.4.2. Training and Education for Forensic Pathologists

Forensic pathologists' education and training are essential to developing such professionals who can properly analyze and interpret complex medical evidence in the context of law. Typically, entry into such a professional career begins with a degree in medicine, completed by residency training in anatomical pathology. Such initial training is necessary, for it provides prospective forensic pathologists with the minimal competence in autopsies, tissue analysis, and overall diagnostics necessary to evaluate trauma and disease processes. Further education programs focusing on pediatric forensic pathology specifically also prioritize more discussion of the special concerns of child victims, such as topic areas like intentional versus accidental injury, which are much different from those of adults. Consequently, the education system must also change to include child-focused modules that equip future pathologists with the knowledge to manage the intricate intricacies of fatal child abuse. In addition, pediatric forensic pathology practice depends on ongoing learning, which demands ongoing education even after initial training. This is particularly important due to the dynamic nature of forensic science, which keeps developing new techniques and technologies. Forensic pathologists must be committed to ongoing learning by means of conferences, workshops, and certification courses that enhance their expertise. Implications of miscommunication or inattentiveness in forensic testimony make stringent quality control in practice and training indispensable. In line with previous research, the majority of wrongful convictions result from improper forensic practice and inadequate forensic professional training (Morgan 2023). Therefore, legal requirements and ethical mandates should also be included in ongoing training so that pathologists can effectively present their findings in court. Lastly, the growing disparity in the population of workers in the United States in comparison with other nations, including Canada, directs us toward increased recruitment and retention strategies for pathologists, particularly pediatric (Metter et al., 2019). With increasing demand for forensic pathology services, as reflected by increased diagnostic workloads, schools should assign training programs to fill these gaps. The decrease in active pathologists per capita is a major hazard in the timely and correct analysis of child victim cases. Educational programs that focus on interdisciplinary collaboration would enhance the workforce by pairing forensic pathology training with other professions, such as law enforcement and child advocacy. By doing this, we not only enhance the forensic pathologist's expertise but also ensure that they will be prepared to address the complexities that come with pediatric forensic cases (Figure 12.13).

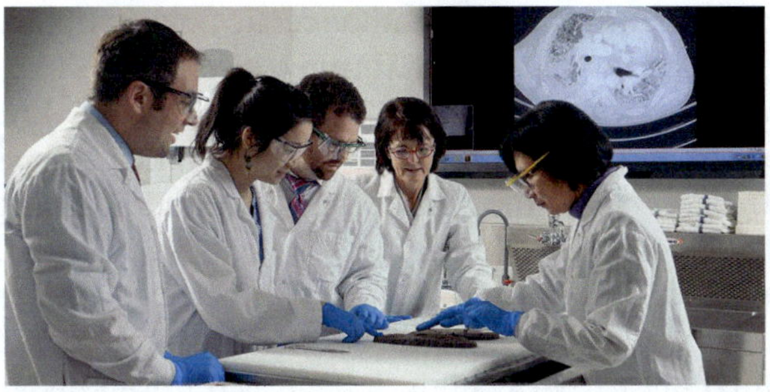

Figure 12.13. Training and education for forensic pathologists.

Source: https://pxl-mayoedu.terminalfour.net/fit-in/1024x2000/filters:quality(75)/prod01/channel_2/media/mccms/content-assets/academics/explore-health-care-careers/pathologist-assistant-career-3336846-0040-hero-tablet.jpg.

12.4.3. Addressing the Shortage of Pediatric Forensic Specialists

The shortage of pediatric forensic specialists is an essential problem for the field of pediatric forensic pathology, as it affects the ability to adequately serve cases of child abuse, neglect, and sudden death. In addition to impacting the quality of investigations, this shortage compromises the justice system that relies on accurate and rigorous forensic analysis to protect vulnerable populations. Schools and medical training institutions have not yet taken adequate steps to bridge this gap, in light of the fact that new forensic pathologists working on pediatric cases lack specific training and infrastructure. The seriousness of the issue warrants stakeholders to give top priority to the establishment of sound education programs to bring forth a fresh generation of specialists proficient in this important area of forensic medicine. Increased awareness and investment in pediatric forensic pathology are required to counter the shortage of experienced professionals. Organizational and governmental activism can lead to increased investment in pediatric forensic training facilities and equipment, which will enhance the infrastructure required for successful training. Interdisciplinary partnerships involving medical schools, law enforcement, and child protection agencies need to be formed to create well-rounded training strategies. These partnerships have the potential to foster best practices in pediatric forensics and provide assurance that those who come into contact with children have a comprehensive understanding of the complexities of such delicate examinations. Embedding state-of-the-art technology and methodology into training curricula could also be a key consideration to inspire interest and improve competency levels among trainees, addressing existing gaps in the discipline. Finally, pediatric forensic pathology fellowship and mentorship opportunities may close the aforementioned gap. With the assistance of experienced practitioners and young professionals, the field cannot just impart lessons but also shape a new batch of pathologists. Hands-on training by way of these mentorship opportunities may expose trainees to real cases, thereby enhancing their actual skills and their confidence in handling delicate forensic cases involving children. The integration of pediatric forensic pathology into wider debates on public health can likewise drive it to higher prominence, thus sparking greater understanding of its importance by future physicians. The synergy of these efforts has the potential to reinvigorate the field so that it is well able to address rising demands for protection and welfare of children, marking the enormous need for advanced training and expertise in pediatric forensic practice.

Test Your Knowledge

1. Why are non-invasive imaging techniques especially important in pediatric cases?
2. How does the shortage of pediatric forensic specialists impact investigations involving children?

SUMMARY

In summarizing pediatric forensic pathology in human beings, it is important to accept that there exists a complicated interface between child health concerns and forensic science. In working on pediatric cases, there has to be a balanced understanding of the biological and environmental factors of human health outcomes. This applies particularly to the situation of advanced decomposition, in which the resistance of human teeth as a DNA source is integral in the identification of remains. Research highlights that the maintenance of DNA in teeth is greatly affected by various intrinsic and extrinsic conditions, such as dental pathology and conditions of burial, which directly correlate to the methods applied in forensic investigations (Mar Aía Salazar et al., 2025). Understanding such dynamics is essential for forensic scientists to devise more effective methods for detecting child victims and obtaining accurate case resolutions, thereby paving the way towards seeking justice. Secondly, moral concerns are of utmost relevance in pediatric forensic pathology. Forensic practice should be based on codes that respect the well-being and rights of children. In pediatric victim situations, the potential psychological impact on surviving siblings and family members makes careful handling of forensic evidence and findings paramount. This perspective is supported by arguments in analogous fields, where maximization of performance via pharmacological improvement comes at the cost of maintenance of individual health and thus creates an ethical concern (Burguete et al., 2025). With growth in the field, it is necessary to have an ethical framework in place that is aware of the specific vulnerabilities of children so that any forensic examination puts their dignity on an equal pedestal with the pursuit of truth. Ultimately, the challenges and complexities inherent to pediatric forensic pathology necessitate a multidisciplinary approach that brings together legal, medical, and ethical issues. Forensic pathologists must be proficient not only in science but also learn to become advocates for the children they serve. The future pediatric forensic examination will most likely be regulated by advances in technology and interdisciplinary collaboration towards refining identification and resolution methods. In addition, further research is needed to develop predictive models that account for the multifaceted impacts on DNA recovery rates and other forensic findings (Mar Aía Salazar et al., 2025). Through a continued commitment to ethical practice and concern for the specialized nature of pediatric cases, the profession can enhance its role in delivering justice and enabling healing in affected families.

Pediatric forensic pathology is a specific field that addresses the peculiar challenge involved in ascertaining the cause of death in children. The core discussions identified anatomical and physiological differences between the adult and the child, necessitating specially modified techniques in forensic analysis. Notably, the development stages significantly influence the pathology of injury and conditions underlying in pediatric cases, necessitating a professional understanding of child development and signs of health. Not only is it necessary to be proficient in routine autopsy techniques, but also sensitive to potential social and psychological matters involving children. Pediatric forensic pathologists, thus, play a pivotal role in providing detailed examinations that can be utilized to guide legal systems and guide public health interventions, their expertise being priceless in the pursuit of justice for vulnerable individuals. In addition to knowledge relevant to children's anatomy, controversy has brought into focus interdisciplinary collaboration. Pedontology cases routinely intersect with other fields like law enforcement, social work, and medical personnel. Effective collaboration is essential to gathering the whole evidence and background, especially in neglect or abuse cases involving children. For instance, medical professionals can identify signs of trauma or abuse that, when communicated to forensic pathologists, can be employed to inform protective action and legal proceedings. Besides this, the inclusion of newer technologies such as artificial intelligence in analysis and diagnostics is under research since these support further enhancement of the capacity to assess trauma and produce valid pathological reports. Such multidisciplinary convergence significantly impacts child welfare and legal outcomes, further emphasizing the need for forensic examination collaboration. Finally, continuous education and conformity to evolving methodologies are also significant issues discussed in pediatric forensic pathology. The lessons of existing research dictate that forensic pathologists must keep up to date with the latest advances in medical imaging and diagnostic practices, as well as child health trends. For example, increasing use of online resources for training in dental anatomy has been found to be effective in improving education models for forensic practice to ensure that practitioners gain the expertise needed in correct analysis (Lind et al., 2024). Additionally, the use of artificial intelligence in trauma diagnosis will also enhance the accuracy of diagnoses in clinical practices, particularly in pediatric trauma patients (Tuan et al., 2024). As such, a culture that supports continuous professional development not only enhances individual competence but also practice standards as a whole in pediatric forensic pathology.

KEY TERMS FROM THIS CHAPTER

- Asphyxia
- Child abuse
- Chronic traumatic encephalopathy
- Congenital heart defects
- Injury patterns
- Pediatric neurotrauma
- Sepsis
- Blunt force trauma
- Child welfare
- Congenital disorders
- Infectious diseases
- Medical research
- Pneumonia
- Trauma

CRITICAL THINKING QUESTIONS

1. **Which of the following is the most common cause of sudden unexpected death in infants?**
   a. Neonatal sepsis
   b. Pneumonia
   c. Sudden Infant Death Syndrome (SIDS)
   d. Aspiration
2. **In forensic pathology, the "triad" of subdural hematoma, retinal hemorrhage, and encephalopathy is classically associated with:**
   a. SIDS
   b. Congenital heart disease
   c. Shaken Baby Syndrome
   d. Meningitis
3. **Which fracture type is most suggestive of child abuse?**
   a. Greenstick fracture of the radius
   b. Spiral fracture of the femur in a non-ambulatory infant
   c. Transverse fracture of the clavicle during delivery
   d. Colles' fracture of the distal radius
4. **What is the most critical step in investigating a suspected case of pediatric neglect or abuse death?**
   a. Immediate burial of the body
   b. Toxicology testing only
   c. Complete autopsy, including skeletal survey and scene investigation
   d. Verbal confirmation from caregiver
5. **Lucid intervals are most commonly seen in which pediatric intracranial condition?**
   a. Subarachnoid hemorrhage
   b. Subdural hematoma
   c. Epidural hematoma
   d. Hydrocephalus

Short Answer Questions

1. What is the primary responsibility of pediatric forensic pathologists?
2. Why is an ethical framework crucial in pediatric forensic pathology?
3. What is the most common cause of death in a pediatric patient?
4. Which age group is particularly vulnerable to accidental deaths such as drowning or falls?
5. What is a key setting where most pediatric accidents occur?

Answer to Critical Thinking Questions

1. (c) 2. (c) 3. (b) 4. (c) 5. (c)

REFERENCES

1. Apostol, I., Belis, V., Calota, R. G., et al. (2017). Forensic and clinical diagnosis in shaken baby syndrome, between child abuse and iatrogenic abuse. https://core.ac.uk/download/144553178.pdf (accessed on 12th July 2025).
2. Argo, A., Buscemi, R., Karch, S. B., Lanzarone, A., Roccuzzo, R., & Zerbo, S. (2019). Perioperative and anesthetic deaths: Toxicological and medico-legal aspects. https://core.ac.uk/download/224993621.pdf (accessed on 12th July 2025).
3. Avena, B., Barbero, B., Borrajo, B., Borrajo, B., Botto, B., et al. (2018). Genetics and genomic medicine in Argentina. https://core.ac.uk/download/287881679.pdf (accessed on 12th July 2025).
4. Barnes, P. D., Bohan, T. L., Findley, K. A., Mack, et al. (2020). Feigned consensus: Usurping the law in shaken baby syndrome/abusive head trauma prosecutions. https://core.ac.uk/download/289231245.pdf (accessed on 12th July 2025).
5. Beck, B., Blickman, J., Brogdon, B., Burton, L., Busuttil, R., Carty, J., Cohen, et al. (2014). Can cross-sectional imaging contribute to the investigation of unexplained child deaths? A literature review. https://core.ac.uk/download/20024692.pdf (accessed on 12th July 2025).
6. Burguete, E., Peydro, L., & Ventura, I. (2025). Bioethical evaluation of methylphenidate and atomoxetine for pediatric ADHD and cognitive enhancement. *Philosophy, Ethics, and Humanities in Medicine: PEHM, 20*. https://www.semanticscholar.org/paper/65bf16b697a4bffff823c156961926f283d0b58c (accessed on 12th July 2025).
7. Byard, R. (2024). Tree failure – A natural phenomenon with forensic implications. *Forensic Science, Medicine, and Pathology*. https://www.semanticscholar.org/paper/6c15538e535df26f52ce49ece5e28acae266e7c6 (accessed on 12th July 2025).
8. Calderón-Garcidueñas, L., González-Maciel, A., Reynoso-Robles, R., Silva-Pereyra, H. G., Torres-Jardón, R., Brito-Aguilar, R., Ayala, A., et al. (2022). Environmentally toxic solid nanoparticles in noradrenergic and dopaminergic nuclei and cerebellum of metropolitan Mexico City children and young adults with neural quadruple misfolded protein pathologies and high exposures to nano particulate matter. *Toxics, 10*, 164–164. https://doi.org/10.3390/toxics10040164 (accessed on 12th July 2025).
9. Collins, K. A., & Nichols, C. A. (1999). A decade of pediatric homicide: A retrospective study at the Medical University of South Carolina. *The American Journal of Forensic Medicine and Pathology, 20(2)*, 169–172. https://www.semanticscholar.org/paper/1a0f01deeb4ebb9f0cc634763f1424edde3799ea (accessed on 12th July 2025).
10. Dogonova, N. A. (2024). Digital rights and freedoms. https://doi.org/10.34660/inf.2024.16.49.334 (accessed on 12th July 2025).
11. Fellmann, F., van El, C., Charron, P., Michaud, K., Howard, H., Boers, S. N., Clarke, A., et al. (2019). European recommendations integrating genetic testing into multidisciplinary management of sudden cardiac death. *European Journal of Human Genetics, 27*, 1763–1773. https://doi.org/10.1038/s41431-019-0445-y (accessed on 12th July 2025).
12. Fragkou, K., Ketsekioulafis, I., Tousia, A., Piagkou, M., Bacopoulou, F., Ferentinos, P., Peyron, P., et al. (2025). From fragile lives to forensic truth: Multimodal forensic approaches to pediatric homicide and suspect death. *Diagnostics, 15*. https://www.semanticscholar.org/paper/63ebac527a63fda5f14ded21b3d1bd0f0e6cc6b9 (accessed on 12th July 2025).

13. Giannakopoulos, K., Kavadella, A., Salim, A. A., Stamatopoulos, V., & Kaklamanos, E. G. (2023). Evaluation of the performance of generative AI large language models ChatGPT, Google Bard, and Microsoft Bing Chat in supporting evidence-based dentistry: Comparative mixed methods study. *Journal of Medical Internet Research*, *25*, e51580–e51580. https://doi.org/10.2196/51580 (accessed on 12th July 2025).

14. Goldstein, R. D., Blair, P. S., Sens, M. A., Shapiro-Mendoza, C. K., Krous, H. F., Rognum, T. O., & Moon, R. Y. (2019). Inconsistent classification of unexplained sudden deaths in infants and children hinders surveillance, prevention, and research: Recommendations from The 3rd International Congress on Sudden Infant and Child Death. *Forensic Science Medicine and Pathology*, *15*, 622–628. https://doi.org/10.1007/s12024-019-00156-9 (accessed on 12th July 2025).

15. Lindén Overskott, H., Markholm, C. E., Sehic, A., & Khan, Q. (2024). Different methods of teaching and learning dental morphology. *Dentistry Journal*, *12*, 114–114. https://doi.org/10.3390/dj12040114 (accessed on 12th July 2025).

16. Marlor, D. R., Crandall, M., Elman, M., Stewart, S., Cruz-Centeno, N., Kim, D., Ginger-Wiley, M., et al. (2024). Misplaced evidence, missed opportunities: Protocols for handling ballistic evidence in pediatric patients. *Journal of Trauma Nursing*, *31*, 40–48. https://www.semanticscholar.org/paper/8a5502b8e2ef2422ea2cd468535e8418c88961b9 (accessed on 12th July 2025).

17. Metter, D., Colgan, T. J., Leung, S. T., Timmons, C. F., & Park, J. Y. (2019). Trends in the US and Canadian pathologist workforces from 2007 to 2017. *JAMA Network Open*, *2*, e194337–e194337. https://doi.org/10.1001/jamanetworkopen.2019.4337 (accessed on 12th July 2025).

18. Michael, K. (2016). Can good standards propel unethical technologies? [Editorial]. *IEEE Technol. Soc. Mag.*, *35*, 6–9. https://www.semanticscholar.org/paper/6009a197faffd2ce86da2c25a5e464e53996f61c (accessed on 12th July 2025).

19. Morgan, J. (2023). Wrongful convictions and claims of false or misleading forensic evidence. *Journal of Forensic Sciences*, *68*, 908–961. https://doi.org/10.1111/1556-4029.15233 (accessed on 12th July 2025).

20. Mougenot Mores, C., Castro, M. B., & Barros de Melo, C. (2025). Forensic examinations in the investigations of crimes involving animals: A review. *Ciência Rural*. https://www.semanticscholar.org/paper/23398fee39fc9e3f3d3cfcb4f0252e741e3e3deb (accessed on 12th July 2025).

21. N/A. (1999). Jefferson alumni bulletin–Volume XLIX, Number 1, December 1999. https://core.ac.uk/download/46972857.pdf (accessed on 12th July 2025).

22. N/A. (2003). Jefferson alumni bulletin–Volume 52, Number 3, June 2003. https://core.ac.uk/download/46972845.pdf (accessed on 12th July 2025).

23. Nova Southeastern University. (2014). Academic impressions, 2014. https://core.ac.uk/download/51073269.pdf (accessed on 12th July 2025).

24. Patterson, K., & Silverman, R. (1814). Book reviews. *The Medical and Physical Journal*, *31*, 55–79. https://www.semanticscholar.org/paper/97e63a1ebccb2a048e36181026d2f302e2bca7b9 (accessed on 12th July 2025).

25. Pham, T. D., Holmes, S., & Coulthard, P. (2024). A review on artificial intelligence for the diagnosis of fractures in facial trauma imaging. *Frontiers in Artificial Intelligence*, *6*. https://doi.org/10.3389/frai.2023.1278529 (accessed on 12th July 2025).

26. Rai, R., Dawani, A., Sukheja, C., Panchonia, A., Mittal, M., & Yerawar, M. (2024). Case series of pediatric special cases on autopsy. *Indian Journal of Forensic Medicine and Pathology*. https://www.semanticscholar.org/paper/09de3f4828b83d1a8c4007a092c54dd2ff21a998 (accessed on 12th July 2025).
27. Sage, M. (2018). Neurocognitive findings in adults who played youth football. https://open.bu.edu/bitstream/2144/33032/5/Sage_bu_0017N_14075.pdf (accessed on 12th July 2025).
28. Salazar, A. M., Huerta, P. A., Coliboro-Dannich, V., Castro, A. F., & Barbaro, A. (2025). Evaluation of DNA in human teeth—Ante-mortem and post-mortem factors affecting degradation and preservation: A literature review. *Genes, 16*. https://www.semanticscholar.org/paper/c341088ff6fecf92d92ca25dc16425bdcb076911 (accessed on 12th July 2025).
29. Sebire, N. J., & Hutchinson, C. (2024). Whole slide imaging, artificial intelligence, and machine learning in pediatric and perinatal pathology: Current status and future directions. *Pediatric and Developmental Pathology*, *28*, 91–98. https://www.semanticscholar.org/paper/f95b67e6df8d2cbdaa1c4d3f109bf34bca290ccc (accessed on 12th July 2025).
30. Skellern, C. (2015). Minimizing bias in the forensic evaluation of suspicious pediatric injury. https://core.ac.uk/download/43374514.pdf (accessed on 12th July 2025).
31. Stram, M. N., Seifert, A., Cortes, E. P., Akyatan, A., Woodoff-Leith, E., Borukhov, V., Tetlow, A. M., et al. (2022). Neuropathology of pediatric SARS-CoV-2 infection in the forensic setting: Novel application of *ex vivo* imaging in analysis of brain microvasculature. *Frontiers in Neurology, 13*. https://www.semanticscholar.org/paper/2cf46a297f07c934dbf30bed6372986fa1e1e7b2 (accessed on 12th July 2025).
32. Thurzo, A., Urbanová, W., Novák, B., Czakó, L., Siebert, T., Stano, P., Mareková, S., et al. (2022). Where is the artificial intelligence applied in dentistry? Systematic review and literature analysis. *Healthcare*, *10*, 1269–1269. https://doi.org/10.3390/healthcare10071269 (accessed on 12th July 2025).
33. Treves, B., Sonnini, E., La Russa, R., Del Duca, F., Ghamlouch, A., De Matteis, A., Trignano, C., et al. (2024). Can hemorrhagic stroke genetics help forensic diagnosis in pediatric age (<5 years old)? *Genes, 15*. https://www.semanticscholar.org/paper/8ca272f5e11445f979c9f49d57358de3f01b8248 (accessed on 12th July 2025).
34. Wezi, K., Mbawe, Z., Chisanga, A., Ellison, M., Frenshus, T., Zulu, H., Adutwum-Ofosu, K., et al. (2025). Forensic pathology research priorities for Zambia: Strengthening justice and public health through evidence-based practice. *International Journal of Research and Scientific Innovation*. https://www.semanticscholar.org/paper/9d98f1e748117ac7525cb8c3d1e4388a0af064a9 (accessed on 12th July 2025).

IDENTIFICATION OF HUMAN REMAINS

13

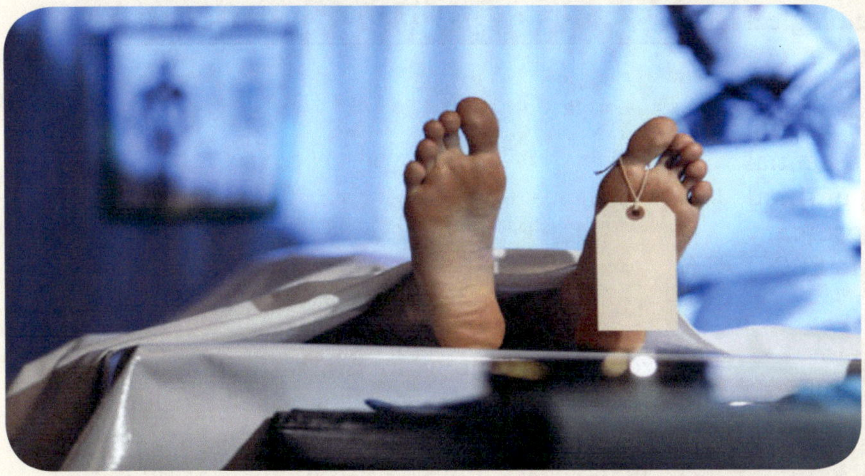

LEARNING OBJECTIVES

After studying this chapter, you will be able to:

1. Describe the methods of identifying human remains;
2. Understand the role of forensic pathologists in identifying human remains;
3. Describe the challenges in identification of human remains;
4. Understand the technological advances in identification of human remains.

Introduction

Forensic pathology plays a central function in the identification of human remains, particularly in instances of unidentified deceased and mass fatalities. With society now demanding accountability and closure in case of unexplained death, technological developments in forensic science have redefined the methods employed in this sphere. Human remains identification is based on a multidisciplinary method that combines old methods like anthropometry and odontology with advanced technologies such as DNA profiling and computerized imaging. The merger maximizes the accuracy and validity of the identifications, which in turn are aimed at serving both legal and humanitarian objectives. By an examination of the complexities of forensic pathology, it is hoped that this chapter will clarify the dynamics of human remains identification, emphasizing its role in law, ethics, and social justice. In addition, medical device use, particularly hip and knee prostheses, has also played a pivotal role in aiding human remains identification. Recent studies highlight the potential for the implants to create identification, especially when combined with other physical information. A systematic documentation of these devices, their manufacturers, and implant numbers will significantly reduce the likelihood of identification. Growing use of Joint Replacement Registries implies that this technique will soon become a standard in forensic analysis, and with potential for more efficient identifications during and after the post-mortem examination. As presented in current literature, the pursuit of properties of these implants and radiological findings propels the field forward with an eye toward integrating technological innovation into traditional methodology (Bryson et al., 2015). Forensic science incorporation is also essential in addressing legal aspects of unidentified remains, for example, in the Extraordinary Chambers in the Courts of Cambodia (ECCC) case.

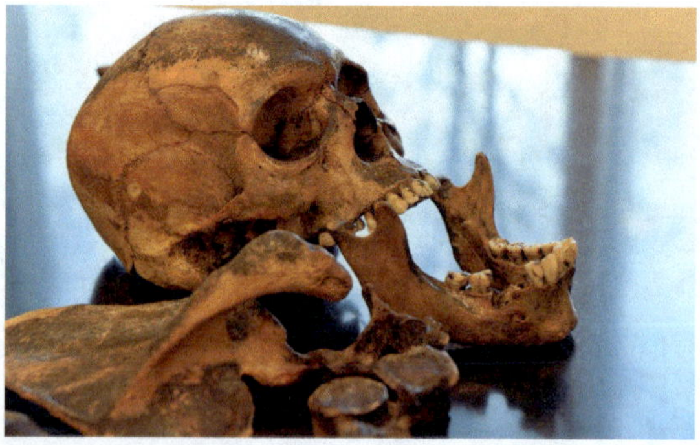

Figure 13.1. Human remains.

Source: https://www.towson.edu/fcsm/images/human-remains-m.jpg.

The historical significance of mass graves from the Khmer Rouge era justifies a critical examination through forensic evidence, which can assist in pursuing justice for thousands of victims. The use of forensic methods in this legal framework not only serves to identify the victims but also attempts to provide closure to victims' families and communities that have been affected by such atrocities. The intersection of forensic science and the law, researched in present studies, determines the profound meaning for humanitarian intervention and the value of forensic evidence to aid legal accountability (Klinkner et al., 2008). Through such investigations, the chapter will seek to highlight the imperative role played by forensic pathology in the identification of human remains and its broader implications for society (Figure 13.1).

13.1. Methods of Identification

Learning Outcome

1. Understand the visual identification.
2. Describe the application of DNA analysis in forensic pathology.
3. Compare the dental records.

Forensic pathology identification of human remains employs a wide array of techniques that rely on biological, morphological, and technological studies. The traditional techniques, on which most reliance is placed with regard to dental records and fingerprints, remain the foundation for establishing identity but are typically limited by the condition of the remains or the availability of historic documentation. Subsequent developments, such as the study of palatal rugae patterns, provide an emerging potential for identification that can be particularly useful in circumstances when typical markers are not available. Research in this area illustrates the individualizing characteristics of palatal rugae, validating their value in forensic application, but acknowledges the absence of widespread popularity in the discipline currently. By establishing a new system of classification based on the unique parameters of palatal rugae, forensic experts can enhance the set of methods for identifying remains, enhancing the precision and dependability of the identification process (Filipe et al., 2021). Complementing these techniques, forensic anthropology contributes by creating biological profiles from the skeletal remains. By analyzing variables such as sex, age-at-death, ancestry, stature, and trauma, forensic anthropologists can produce powerful evidence that narrows potential identities of unidentified remains. The skeletal analysis is typically focused on morphoscopic characteristics, the cranium and pelvis being particularly important because they have distinctive characteristics. Various limb measurements are also important in determining a biological profile correctly. This methodology not only aids in direct identification but also helps in the confirmation of other identification procedures, yielding a multi-aspect approach to tackling the issues raised in forensic cases. These in-depth analyses are illustrative of the need for multiple approaches in identification techniques in order to enhance our ability to identify human identity correctly, particularly in complex scenarios (Ramey et al., 2018). Aside from physical attribute-based biological profiling and palatal rugae, DNA technology has revolutionized the techniques of human identification in forensic science.

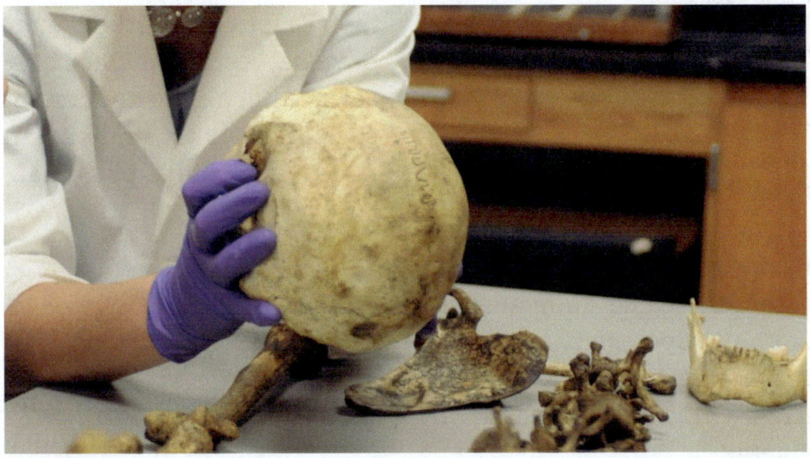

Figure 13.2. Forensic anthropologists work to identify human skeletal remains and uncover the stories of the unknown dead.

Source: https://news.clemson.edu/wp-content/uploads/2020/08/16x9-Katherine-Weisensee-Bone-1536x864.jpg.

The ability to retrieve, amplify, and compare DNA from bones or soft tissue has brought DNA profiling to the forefront of the list of modes of establishing identity, particularly for degraded samples. Due to the genetic marker heterogeneity, DNA testing can yield very specific results that corroborate or even supersede morphological evidence. Furthermore, DNA technology offers the potential of genealogical inquiry through which tracing of relationships with living relatives is made possible, thereby offering additional identification avenues. With further expansion of forensic science, the use of strong DNA methods with traditional and emerging identification techniques will enhance our overall ability to solve cases, bringing justice to the deceased and their families (Figure 13.2).

13.1.1. Visual Identification

Visual recognition is a significant component of human remains identification within forensic pathology, particularly during the early phases of an investigation. It involves the identification and scrutiny of physical features that can potentially aid in confirming the identity of remains.

Visual identification is frequently employed by forensic experts to establish preliminary connections between unidentified remains and missing persons. However, this method is subjective in itself and relies heavily on the experience and ability of the individuals involved in making the identification. In forensic cases, precision is totally critical since misidentification can lead to erroneous conclusions and decide the fate of judicial processes.

Visual identification also calls on other methods, such as DNA profiling or dental identification, to develop an integrated approach toward human remains identification. While, as with all means of visual recognition, subjective, tremendous reliability has been achieved due to technological advancement. Existing techniques, such as the mesh-to-mesh value comparison (MVC), allow forensic anthropologists to match the digital images of skeletal material with high sensitivity and specificity in a pair-matching of commingled components.

In the MVC method, the geometric parameters of the bones are also analyzed digitally to derive a similarity value as a measure of likely matches. All such developments significantly minimize human error and augment the process of visual identification to make it a more potent tool for forensic pathologists. With the manual MVC being 100% accurate, the automatic version also promises a lot, albeit with specificity improvements that are to be performed. All these developments highlight the evolving dynamics of visual identification as a crucial element of forensic investigations towards obtaining improved results. Other than forensic application, visual identification has ancillary significance in bioarcheological studies when researchers can establish family relationships and health information from ancient remains. A case in point is a study in the Tomb of the Shroud in which visual identification could be used to examine skeletal remains in conjunction with genetic screening. This inter-disciplinary study revealed mitochondrial haplotypes that indicated shared ancestry among the people who were interred in the tomb. Identification of specific pathogens, including *Mycobacterium tuberculosis* and *Mycobacterium leprae*, further demonstrates how visual analysis can reveal significant information about ancient populations.

These observations underpin the relevance of visual recognition not only in today's forensic science but also to understand human behaviors, social structures, and past diseases, thus filling in our knowledge of human history.

13.1.2. DNA Analysis

Employment of DNA analysis in forensic pathology has transformed the science of identification of human remains to a great extent. The molecular technique enables forensic specialists to define genetic relationships between subjects, providing them with valuable information about family relationships.

A sentimental example is found in the archeological research of the Jerusalem Shroud Tomb, in which mitochondrial DNA was applied to examine the genetic heritage of remains found inside a family tomb. The presence of three shared mitochondrial haplotypes amongst a group of individuals signified a family relationship, underscoring the importance of DNA analysis to reconstruct genealogical relations between human remains. Moreover, genetic data indicated the presence of causative pathogens of tuberculosis and leprosy diseases, highlighting forensic analysis's interdisciplinary emphasis as well as DNA's key role in enhancing historical understanding as well as contemporary medical information (Donoghue et al., 2009).

Last, beyond history, DNA analysis plays its most dramatic role in contemporary forensic use, specifically in the case of disaster victim identification. Following catastrophic occurrences, normal procedures of identifying remains can be faulty or marred by extraneous environmental factors. In such a situation, DNA analysis has become a mandatory method, which facilitates the identification of victims with an accuracy never previously envisioned.

The evidence in high-profile cases, such as those following the September 11th attacks and the Asian Tsunami in 2004, speaks to the significant impact of DNA technology in handling tragedies. As its application has become widespread, there is more pressure from the public and the media that DNA analysis be employed as the first identification technique and lead forensic pathology operations (Bourdieu et al., 2014).

Despite the advantages of DNA analysis, its application in all cases is not free from challenges. In certain environments, particularly in those that have rigidly defined socio-political conventions and cultural ordering, the imposition of DNA testing could actually work counter to local customs and belief systems unintentionally. To suppose that the use of DNA technology is feasible everywhere ignores the complexity presented by diverse cultural contexts. For instance, in nations like Cambodia and Iraq, the application of DNA analysis in identification procedures has raised debates on whether it is appropriate and why it is being used. They are of the opinion that the bias towards this prestigious technology is more a result of a political and social need for approval rather than a benevolent interest, and the critical evaluation of the circumstances under which DNA analysis is applied is merited (Bourdieu et al., 2014) (Figure 13.3).

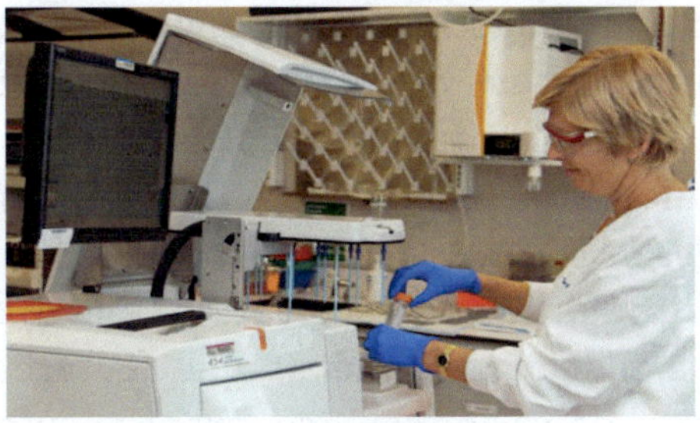

Figure 13.3. DNA Analysis: The backbone of modern forensic pathology.

Source: https://images.unsplash.com/photo-1583912372112-e2908da68383?crop=entropy&cs=tinysrgb&fit=max&fm=jpg&ixid=M3w3MDgyMDR8MHwxfHNlYXJjaHwxfHxETkElMjBhbmFseXNpcyUyQyUyMGZvcmVuc2ljJTIwcGF0aG9sb2d5JTJDJTIwbmV4dC1nZW5lcmF0aW9uJTIwc2VxdWVuY2luZyUyQyUyMEROQSUyMHBoZW5vdHlwaW5nfGVufDB8MHx8fDE3NDk5MDk5ODd8MA&ixlib=rb-4.1.0&q=80&w=500&-?utm_source=numberanalytics&utm_medium=referral.

13.1.3. Dental Records Comparison

Dental record comparison is a key role in human remains identification in forensic pathology. The distinctiveness of each individual's dental anatomy makes dental evidence a possible method of identification. The rest of the body remains can degenerate from the environment, but not teeth. Thus, they are a lasting source of identifying information even after total decomposition. As noted by forensic books, the coincidence between antemortem and postmortem dental records allows forensic odontologists to establish a strong identification profile. Thus, the success of the process is based on the presence and accuracy of certain dental records for comparison with incident site or crime scene remains, making proper dental records kept in clinical practice very important. While traditional methods have laid the foundation for comparison of dental records, recent advances have also contributed to the field's capability.

The introduction of 3D digital technology has created new opportunities for capturing and examining dental records, which offer a detailed source of information beyond the confines of 2D imaging. These new technologies enable practitioners to create detailed digital records that record the unique features of a patient's dentition, which are important in forensic analysis. Nevertheless, even after their production, a concerning lacuna is present within practitioners' knowledge of their implications in forensic uses. As noted in contemporary studies, most dental practitioners lack adequate information regarding how to utilize these records for forensic examination, ultimately hindering the advantages that can be achieved from such advanced technology in the identification of human remains (Perkins et al., 2024). Reasonable procedures for retaining dental records are also critical to guarantee that comparative analysis can be conducted when required. There is wide variation among dental practices in the handling and keeping of antemortem and postmortem records. This inconsistency will hinder the forensic process of identification because incomplete or missing records can lead to the remains being matched to an incorrect person. With the growing need for accurate identification, particularly following disasters or homicides, there has been a need to enhance the handling of dental records. Thus, awareness and education on the forensic application of dental records among dentists is a necessity since this knowledge can efficiently move the identification process forward and improve overall forensic outcomes in human remains cases (Ahmed, 2024) (Figure 13.4).

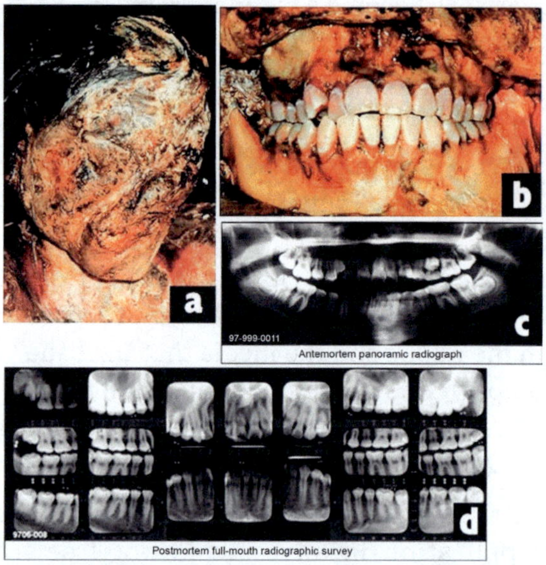

Figure 13.4. Example of a comparative dental identification case.

Source: https://media.springernature.com/full/springer-static/image/art%3A10.1038%2Fsj.bdj.4800972/MediaObjects/41415_2001_Article_BF4800972_Fig3_HTML.jpg?as=webp.

Test Your Knowledge

1. What is commonly used to supplement visual identification?
2. What is the application of DNA analysis in forensic pathology?

13.2. Role of Forensic Pathologists

Learning Outcome

1. Describe the responsibilities of forensic professionals in the identification process.
2. Collaborate with law enforcement.
3. Understand the role of expert testimony in court proceedings.

Forensic pathologists' participation in the identification of human remains is critical, given that these specialists are bridges between the law and medicine. Forensic pathologists do thorough autopsies that offer significant information regarding the cause of death, post-mortem interval, and victim identity. This is particularly important in decomposed or fragmented remains cases when older techniques such as fingerprints or dental records are not viable. Forensic pathologists apply a variety of methods, ranging from radiography and histological studies, to clarify the circumstances surrounding death. Their conclusions often are pivotal bits of testimony in court, therefore enhancing knowledge of legal and forensic sophistication involved in criminal investigations, as in instances brought at the International Criminal Tribunal for the former Yugoslavia (Klinkner et al., 2008). The implications of forensic pathology extend beyond simple acknowledgment; they contribute to establishing a forensic reality that is consistent with the legal versions presented in court. Forensic pathologists take meticulous collection and analysis of evidence so that it is consistent with scientific standards and rigor. The role is particularly important in extremely high-profile cases, such as the analysis of serial killers. In the case of serial killer Jeffrey Dahmer, for example, forensic scientists conducted autopsies that showed important information about the motivating factors behind the foundation of his criminal behavior. These analyses not only aid in the identification of remains but also assist in obtaining a deeper understanding of the psychopathology of perpetrators, which affects the pursuit of justice (Ho et al., 1994). Second, the interdisciplinary collaboration among forensic pathologists, law enforcement, and legal professionals is instrumental to enable that human remains are identified and interpreted in the social context of crime. This collaboration is crucial when dealing with mass casualty incidents or events that are very difficult, such as natural disasters or terrorist attacks. Forensic pathologists generally work alongside anthropologists and geneticists, who contribute additional methods for the identification of remains by skeletal analysis and DNA testing. These robust procedures are reflective of a heightened respect for the sophistication of human identification in forensic pathology, where the crossing of multiple scientific disciplines enhances the entire investigative process. This convergence not only aids in the resolution of individual cases but also facilitates greater societal insight and justice for victims' families as well (Figure 13.5).

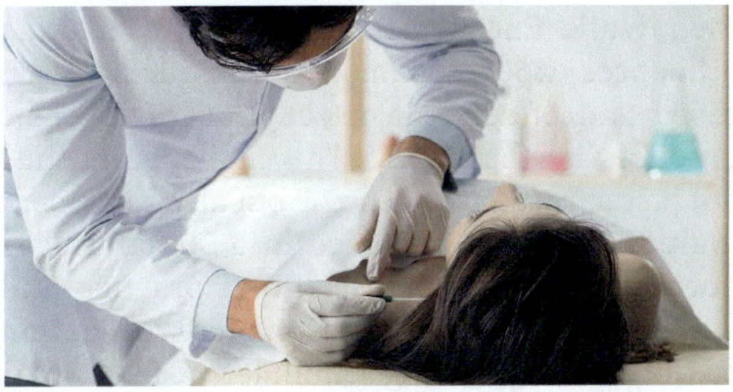

Figure 13.5. Role of forensic pathologists.

Source: https://mallory.com.au/cm/wp-content/uploads/forensic-pathology-body-examination.jpg.

13.2.1. Responsibilities in the Identification Process

In forensic pathology, the function of identification is of profound and intricate significance. At the top of the responsibilities is the one borne by the forensic experts to ensure the scientifically sound and ethically justified methods employed in the identification procedure of human remains. The forensic pathologists must employ a combination of techniques, including anthropological tests, DNA analysis, and comparative pathology, each applied conscientiously. This degree of precision not only aims to provide a distinct identification but also serves to uphold the credibility of the judicial process. Ultimately, any failure or lapse in this responsibility can lead to misidentification, which has grave consequences for both the parties involved and the general system of justice. Secondly, the responsibilities of forensic professionals are not simply that of identification; they must also critically consider the implications of their findings. It involves constructing so-called 'forensic truth,' which is a job that has a close association with legal and ethical demands. For example, as outlined in the latest studies, the intersection of forensic evidence and legal limits underscores the need for specialists who are aware of the legal environment for their work. Engagement with such a meeting influences expert testimony given during court cases and affects the perception of forensic practices by the public. The challenge is thus not just to recognize remains but also to present multidimensional evidence in a shape that is both compatible with scientific practice and with legal requirements, a complete realization of the forensic setting (Klinkner et al., 2008). Additionally, the ethical implications inherent in the identification process cannot be exaggerated. As can be seen in other comprehensive works, for example, the ALRC Report 96, the moral concerns related to genetic and forensic data include a wide array of implications for society (Opeskin et al., 2025). Forensic pathologists must walk the narrow, tightrope between ensuring criminal justice while maintaining the dignity and rights of the deceased and their families. Thus, the identification process must involve consideration of personal histories and cultural contexts, so that every case is examined sensitively and with awareness. In doing this, forensic practitioners offer families closure and enhance public confidence in the forensic system. This holistic approach to responsibility in the identity process demands the fusion of scientific professionalism, legal astuteness, and ethical awareness, thereby reaffirming the foundational ethic of forensic practice (Figure 13.6).

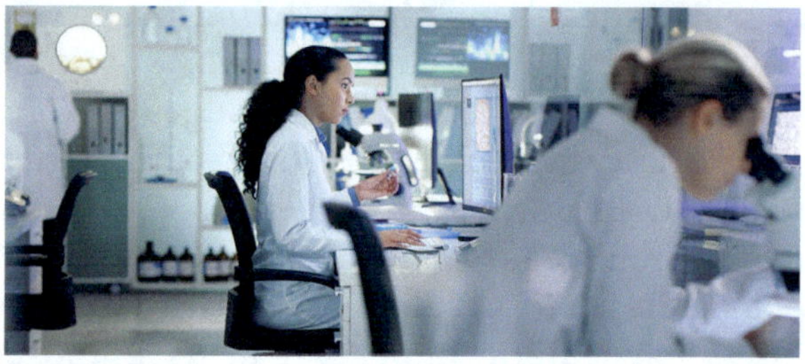

Figure 13.6. Responsibilities of forensic pathologists.

Source: https://www.sgu.edu/wp-content/uploads/what-does-forensic-pathologist-do-3.jpg.

13.2.2. Collaboration with Law Enforcement

Collaboration among law enforcement officials and forensic experts is essential in forensic pathology's identification of human bodies. The integration of forensic experts with law enforcers not only enhances the investigative process but also maximizes the use of available resources and skills. When police encounter unidentified human remains, the initial support of forensic pathologists offers an appropriate analysis of the physical evidence, identification of foul play, if any, and the establishment of timelines on the remains. Such integration is likely to enhance forensic unit and police department communication so that there can be a collaborative effort in crime solving and the recovery of the missing remains. Such partnerships turn out to be crucial in the delivery of justice through the provision of effective and credible identification processes. Procedural protocols in forensic investigations cannot be downplayed, as they ensure the credibility of evidence collected in the identification of human remains. The combination of forensic pathologists and law enforcement officers establishes the deployment of standardized procedures that should be adhered to throughout the process. These developed procedures not only allow for precise recording of evidence but also provide a foundation for quality control in forensic investigations. By adhering to these procedures, forensic teams are able to accurately analyze and interpret data obtained from the remains, something that is essential in presenting evidence in court. Be it through advanced biochemical instruments or dental records, proven to remain operational even after decompositions have begun, this cooperative effort makes forensic evidence more valid and potent while reducing room for misinterpretation or wrongful conclusion during legal trials (Auerkari et al., 2008). Furthermore, forensic and technological innovation provides a new roadmap for forensic pathology and law enforcement to cooperate. The expanding accessibility of DNA testing, for instance, has changed the way human remains are identified, with increasingly accurate results even in cases where conventional identifiers such as dental records are lacking (Auerkari et al., 2008). Such ongoing collaboration facilitates the development of forensic techniques to fit the particular needs of each case, as evidenced in the emergent necessity of diverse identification tools. Where there may be some resources lacking in areas, law enforcement can tap into the expertise of specialized forensic units, and thus be able to create a better-informed reaction to human remains cases. Last but not least, success in human remains identification relies significantly on the interactive nature of such disciplines to provide more comprehensive and better-informed investigations that can prove beneficial to the pursuit of justice.

13.2.3. Testifying in Court

The expert witness in judicial procedures has a critical function, especially that of identifying human remains in forensic pathology. Forensic experts, such as pathologists and anthropologists, provide knowledge that facilitates the legal process through verifying evidence derived from crime scenes. Their findings are often supported by stringent scientific processes and enhance the credibility of the submitted evidence. It is important to understand how forensic science interacts with legal systems in a way that ensures justice is served. This interaction is most apparent in international environments, such as the Extraordinary Chambers in the Courts of Cambodia (ECCC), where forensic science can make invaluable contributions to legal accountability for past atrocities, as seen in Klinkner et al. (2008). Thus, the synergy of legal procedures and forensic knowledge is a key component to provide a foundation of truth in the legal arena. Presenting forensic evidence in a court of law requires careful articulation to bridge the gap between sophisticated legal data and requirements. Expert witnesses must travel this difficult ground, ensuring that their testimony is understood by juries and judges untrained in specialties. They have to provide technical facts and procedures and thus establish what is termed forensic truth. This is not only a scientific familiarity but also the capacity to communicate and convince. The exhumations done in proceedings related to the former Yugoslavia International Criminal Tribunal are good examples of challenges faced by experts to communicate their evidence effectively. The interface of legal needs and forensic science eventually directs the perception of courts towards evidence, as explained in the synopsis of Klinkner et al. (2008). Moreover, the credibility of forensic evidence usually comes under questioning by opposing counsel in pursuit of justice. Legal advisors must critically review the process and conclusions presented by forensic experts to ensure that evidence satisfies codified legal standards. In high-stakes cases involving human remains, the stakes of introducing faulty forensic evidence are large, impacting not only individual convictions but also public perception of justice more broadly. As in recent attempts to correct historical injustices in Cambodia, the ability of forensic science to deliver a verdict in legal proceedings can generate significant humanitarian implications. The arguments regarding the role of forensic science in legal cases reflect on the requirement for scrupulous scientific practice and its implementation in court, upholding the fundamental principles of justice witnessed in Klinkner et al. (2008) (Figure 13.7).

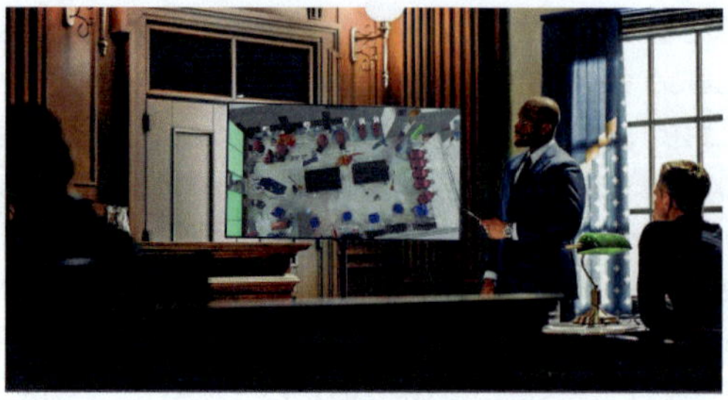

Figure 13.7. Expert testimony in court.

Source: https://media.faro.com/-/media/Project/FARO/FARO/FARO/Resources/Article/2022/2958_Article_Daubert-Challenge_Main_1400x760.jpg?rev=d2c0cdb60866456ca74ff2923b872215.

Test Your Knowledge

1. What is the primary responsibility of forensic pathologists in the identification process?
2. Why is expert testimony important in forensic cases involving human remains?

13.3. Challenges in Identification

Learning Outcome

1. Describe the decomposition and environmental factors.
2. Address the challenges posed by the lack of available records.
3. Understand the cultural and ethical considerations in the identification of human remains.

Identification of human remains in forensic pathology is riddled with numerous pitfalls that can significantly hamstring the pursuit of justice. Perhaps one of the biggest challenges is the condition and disarticulation of the remains themselves, aided by environmental factors and the passage of time. Decomposition procedures may conceal identifying features, such as characteristic dental records or bone structure, making it virtually impossible to identify the dead using standard means. This issue is even more pronounced in the case of mass graves, where multiple individuals' remains are intertwined, which renders identification challenging. As defined in the Cambodian setting, the existence of mass graves under the Khmer Rouge government points towards the applicability and need of forensic science in such a scenario, where legal justice remains intertwined with scientific interpretation of human remains (Klinkner et al., 2008). The correlation of legal frameworks and forensic science is another theme of challenge in the identification process. Forensic experts need to operate in complex legal scenarios without compromising the integrity of their evidence. How forensic evidence interacts with mechanisms for admitting it as court evidence can become confusing. In past cases, for instance, mechanisms by which forensic truths are produced and interpreted tend to change once within the judicial system (Klinkner et al., 2008). This provokes questions over the legitimacy of forensic evidence, as procedural differences between legal expectations and forensic techniques can lead to challenges of securing a conviction or closure for victims' families. Ultimately, this convergence underscores that there needs to be a standardized procedure and improved communication among forensic scientists and legal officials. Ethical and cultural considerations also complicate the identification of human remains in forensic pathology, particularly when dealing with sensitive issues such as war crimes or genocide.

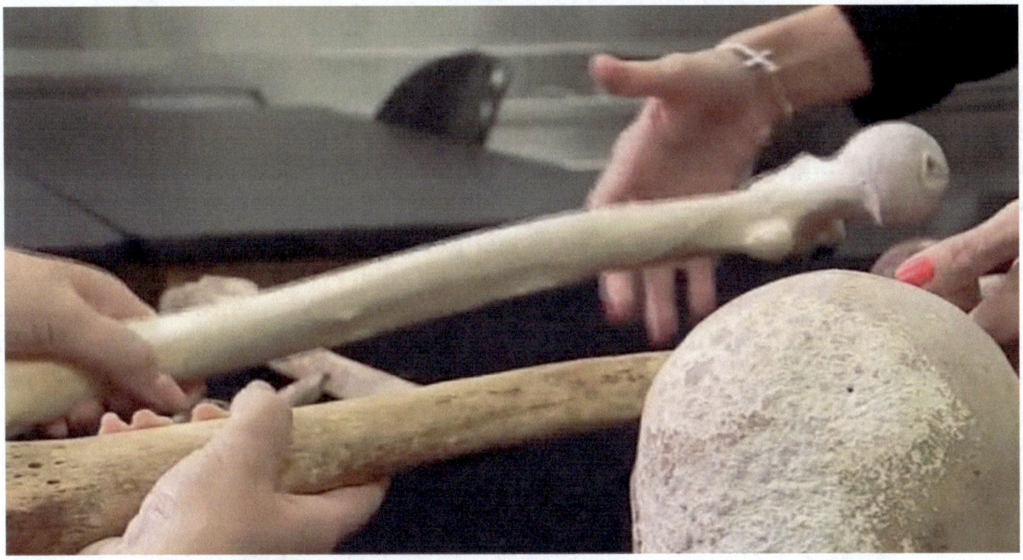

Figure 13.8. Process of identifying human remains.

Source: https://cdn.abcotvs.com/dip/images/1279889_040616-ktrk-human-remains-img.jpg.

The responsibility to treat remains in a respectful and dignified manner, which can be at odds with the demands of scientific investigation. This is particularly pertinent when dealing with mass grave scenarios, in which the victim's human rights are pitted against the need for forensic investigation. The Cambodian experience illustrates the potential for forensic science to play a transformative role in addressing historical injustices and facilitating reconciliation, but it also raises ethical dilemmas about the exploitation of remains in legal discourse (Klinkner et al., 2008). Hence, the challenge of identification extends beyond scientific methods to encompass a broader ethical framework that prioritizes humanity alongside scientific inquiry. It is important to address these multifaceted problems in order to enhance the efficacy of forensic identification in circumstances calling for both justice and compassion (Figure 13.8).

13.3.1. Decomposition and Environmental Factors

Decomposition is significantly influenced by a variety of factors in the environment, which also come into play when identifying human remains in forensic pathology. These include temperature, humidity, soil composition, and insects, all of which can hasten or retard the process of decomposition. Favorable temperatures, for example, can enhance microbial activity and hasten decay, whereas cold climates can slow down the integrity of the remains. In addition, high-humidity environments promote insects and fungi, which also contribute to the decompositional rate. It is paramount that forensic analysts are aware of these influences and how they combine so that they can properly interpret phases of decomposition when determining time since death and other key facts for the case. The urban setting complicates decomposition and recovery as well. Certain anthropogenic sources, such as pollution and construction disturbances, may alter the natural decomposition process. Even man-made materials, such as clothing or plastic, found in the remains can inhibit the decomposition of organic tissues. New methods, such as geophysical surveys, are being employed for the detection of buried remains, as demonstrated in a study using a mock grave to identify what works best. As the research revealed, decomposition and urban landscapes need a holistic strategy that combines traditional forensic practice and advanced technologies like ground-penetrating radar and electrical resistivity tomography for the enhanced capacity to recover remains in challenging environments (Cassella et al., 2008). Additionally, interdisciplinary tactics such as the analysis of biochemical markers during the process of decomposition offer promising developments in forensic science. Research has indicated that the chemical makeup of human remains changes profoundly over time, demonstrating possible biochemical signatures that could be identified even during the later stages of decay. This focus on postmortem biomarkers is aligned with novel forensic techniques such as iris recognition, which are focused on accurate identification in a postmortem context. Despite the uncertainty of their viability, preliminary results suggest possible integration into standard forensic protocol. The union of environmental examination and advanced identification techniques will certainly enhance the accuracy in the detection of human remains, attesting to the importance of decomposition knowledge and its environmental variables in forensic pathology (Sansola et al., 2015) (Figure 13.9).

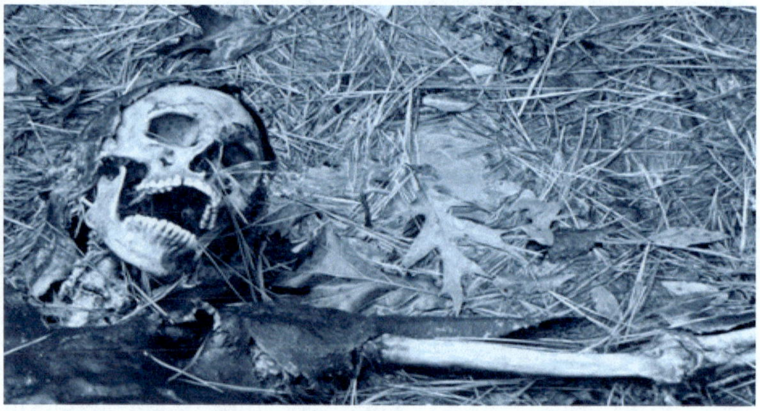

Figure 13.9. Life after death: the science of human decomposition.

Source: https://i.guim.co.uk/img/static/sys-images/Guardian/Pix/pictures/2015/5/5/1430830181724/6f5c83cb-d792-45ba-9d49-9aedc2a37b51-620x372.png?width=465&dpr=1&s=none&crop=none.

13.3.2. Lack of Available Records

One of the major challenges in human remains identification in forensic pathology is the lack of records. In cases where a patient's medical history is missing or unavailable, forensic investigators face a serious challenge regarding linking remains to identified patients. It is more challenging in cases where victims are from marginalized or war-torn areas, where records may have been ignored or deliberately destroyed. With proper medical records, the reliability of identifying unique features such as implants, scars, or dental records is diminished tremendously. As more researchers acknowledge the importance of such identifiers, the diversity in procedures for keeping records is a major obstacle to carrying out correct identifications, stressing the imperative for systematic documentation in medical as well as legal contexts. Also, the impact of inadequate records reaches far beyond singular cases and has implications for legal frameworks and overall justice. As an illustration, in war or genocide-ravaged regions, inadequate documentation can inhibit criminal cases aimed at prosecuting perpetrators. In Cambodia, inadequate forensic evidence in mass graves has precluded pursuing justice for Khmer Rouge era atrocities. The unique chambers for such cases demonstrate the possible role of forensic science in uncovering the truth regarding a specific history, yet without proper records, the main links between remains and events in history are tenuous. This scenario identifies the need to bring forensic methodologies into convergence with legal procedures, moving toward enhanced documentation as a means of solidifying justice results both at home and abroad, as noted in a number of scholarly controversies surrounding the topic (Klinkner et al., 2008). In overcoming the challenge posed by the lack of records, methodological and technological advances hold out the promise of enhancing identification methodologies. Techniques such as DNA testing, imaging, and database matching can, at times, bypass missing records, allowing forensic analysts to make connections that could not have been made otherwise. Merging of Joint Replacement Registries, for instance, improves the possibility of tracing people through surgical implants, as surmised in ongoing studies. But even with technology as advanced as that, the root issue of record insufficiency persists, indicating that technology can by itself not correct the problem. Relentless promotion for vast documentation of medical and forensic procedures is in place, so that the identification processes are not only effective but also morally ethical, filling the gap between technology and historical responsibility (Bryson et al., 2015).

13.3.3. Cultural and Ethical Considerations

Identification in forensic pathology is significantly linked with cultural and ethical issues. What one believes about death and how funerals are done will influence how the remains are treated and identified. In most cultures, for instance, death is held sacred, and hence there's a fear of opening graves. This wariness can make forensic inquiries difficult, especially where legal or investigative imperatives are at odds with cultural respect for the deceased. Ethical considerations also mean that forensic professionals must engage respectfully with culture, so that the process of identification respects the traditions significant to the deceased's community and does not breach or take advantage of them. This emphasis promotes the importance of respect and inclusivity so that it can work with local communities and maintain justice without breaching cultural expectations. Furthermore, ethical concerns are prevalent in consent as well as in utilizing human remains for forensic examination. In the majority of cases, remains can be identified through scientific methods such as DNA testing or comparative anatomy, and these have limitations on whether or not they are applicable in approaching the situation. Issues on informed consent then tend to emerge, particularly when dealing with exhumed remains from archaeological sites or mass graves, where descendants may not be aware that their ancestors' remains exist. Meeting these needs requires that the forensic practitioners employ sensitivity and openness to engage families and communities in dialogue about the identification processes. The ethical implications of such do not end at the case level but instead point toward an open debate on the moral obligations of the forensic professionals to the societies they are working within, especially those involving vulnerable individuals who are victims of violence or past injustice. Additionally, the capability of traversing cultural and ethical issues proficiently can advance forensic investigations to be more successful. Forensic pathologists are now recognizing the value of interdisciplinary consultation, inviting advice from anthropologists, historians, and pertinent cultural representatives. This multidisciplinary approach allows for better comprehension of the remains, promoting practices that respect the deceased's culture while meeting legal expectations. Additionally, as forensic technologies improve, priority must be given to creating methodologies that are sensitive to both cultural and ethical considerations. As each new tool becomes available, incorporating the voices of communities into forensic practice can make identification efforts more legitimate while fostering healing and closure for impacted communities and families. Ultimately, an emphasis on cultural and moral considerations in forensic pathology not only enriches the process of investigation but also ensures that the dignity of the deceased is preserved (Figure 13.10).

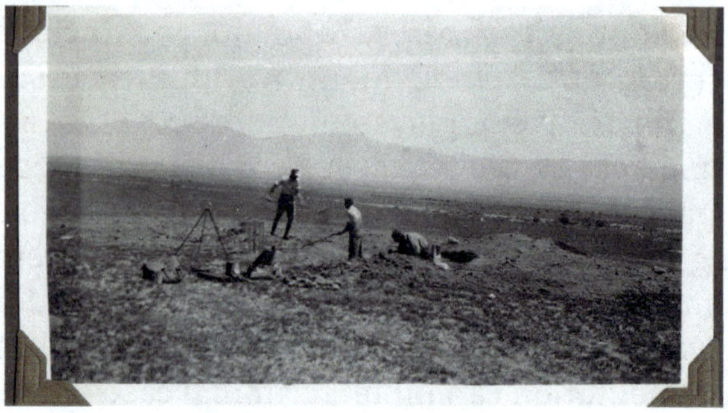

Figure 13.10. Ethical considerations for human remains.

Source: https://d26toa8f6ahusa.cloudfront.net/wp-content/uploads/2023/05/12102928/Anthropological_work_1931_05_HEADER.jpg.

Test Your Knowledge

1. Which environmental factors most directly influence the rate of human decomposition?
2. What modern advancement is helping to overcome the absence of traditional records?

13.4. Technological Advances

Learning Outcome

1. Understand the use of imaging techniques.
2. Know the innovations in DNA technology.
3. Describe the use of software for facial reconstruction.

Technological innovation is the primary dynamic force of evolution in human remains identification in forensic pathology. Some of the most discernible developments in the recent past include upgrading DNA analysis techniques. This has become more overt since being successfully utilized in high-profile cases, such as the post-9/11 and the Asian Tsunami of 2004. DNA analysis not just gives a high level of accuracy in victim identification of disasters, but also is now the public's accepted standard for such procedures. But the application of DNA technology has raised questions regarding its appropriateness in various contexts, as socio-political dynamics and cultural forces can dictate the success of its usage. Critics argue that, despite being a highly effective tool, the DNA analysis application is usually triggered by social and political legitimation needs instead of intrinsic humanitarian motivations, and point to the need for more advanced techniques in forensic identification (Bourdieu et al., 2014). In addition to DNA analysis, the use of craniofacial superimposition techniques is another technological advancement relevant to forensic pathology. This method proves most beneficial when the conventional identification methods, such as DNA profiling or dental matching, are not practical or impossible due to certain circumstances. Recent research indicates the efficacy of manual and computer-assisted craniofacial superimposition techniques, providing useful tools for disaster victim identification. The comparison with photographs in different orientations and skeletal collections' skulls has highlighted the significance of three-quarter and profile views for proper identification. Nevertheless, the research also identified the demerits of identification by frontal photos from databases, like the MPUB Interpol database, that are not detailed enough for safe identification. Thus, the findings encourage theoretical advocacy for the integration of diverse ante-mortem images to enhance identification procedures in diverse contexts (Lofthouse et al., 2025). Taken together, these technological advancements unveil the multifaceted aspects of human identification methods in forensic pathology. Interplays between DNA profiling and craniofacial superimposition not only exhibit the range of available technologies but also complement the urgencies of philosophical discourses surrounding their theoretical uses. As forensic scientists progress, they have to be mindful of the ethical issues, socio-political context, and cultural awareness that inform their practice. The challenge lies in reaching a balance between seeking proper identification and being critically mindful of how these technologies are woven into the existence of victims and their families. Granting a proper and respectful use of these technologies can lead to both effective and sensitive resolutions in forensic matters, finally maximizing the field's commitment to justice and regard for the departed (Figure 13.11).

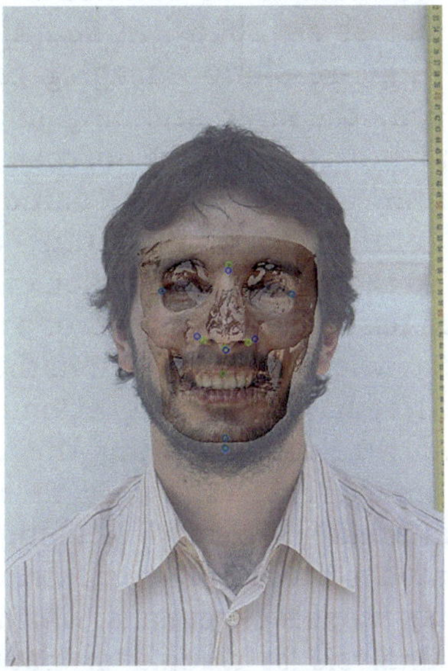

Figure 13.11. Identification of human remains using craniofacial superimposition.

Source: https://scx2.b-cdn.net/gfx/news/hires/2024/researchers-propose-an.jpg.

13.4.1. Use of Imaging Techniques

The role of imaging techniques in forensic pathology, particularly in the identification of human remains, cannot be overstated. The techniques have, in a huge way, revolutionized the process by enabling forensic science experts to capture tiny details of skeletal remains that are typically determinative for positive identification. Techniques like digital three-dimensional (3D) modeling have become an anthropologist's godsend, particularly when dealing with commingled remains. One of the new techniques is mesh-to-mesh value comparison (MVC), a numerical technique of comparing the geometric similarity between bones. The technique makes it possible to accurately identify bones and thereby enhance forensic analysis quality. The precision of manual and computer-aided MVC methods in pair-matching humeri has been demonstrated, recognizing their capacity to assist forensic anthropologists in determining individual identity in skeletally complex assemblages, as outlined in previous work (Frelat et al., 2016). In addition to 3D modeling, high-resolution imaging modalities such as confocal laser scanning microscopy (CLSM) have broadened the forensic arsenal. CLSM not only provides high-resolution images but also optical sectioning, thus allowing scientists to explore the distribution of cells and proteins in tissues. This ability is of paramount significance where inflammation in the vicinity of skeletal remains is being examined, and this could result in knowing the cause of death or injury. The technology incorporates both traditional microscopy techniques and sophisticated software to reconstruct three-dimensional models of remains, which provide accurate analysis of trauma or pathological changes. Moreover, these imaging techniques provide forensic examiners with adequate detail to assess the biological profiles of unidentified remains, and thereby improve the overall quality of forensic pathology investigations (Cantatore et al., 2015). But still another critical aspect of imaging techniques is their integration with other techniques, such as Western blotting, to augment forensic analysis of human tissues. With these ancillary techniques, researchers not only identify but also visualize the topographical distribution of proteins that are unique to different physiological or pathological conditions. Identification of these markers can offer a clearer understanding of trauma or disease at the moment of death, which is important in forensic situations. Furthermore, the combination of imaging modalities allows for a semi-quantitative evaluation of injury and inflammation-related proteins, ultimately leading to the identification of the sequence of events causing an individual to die. This integrated approach not only improves forensic pathology but also stabilizes the whole investigative process because it ensures that all the available data is utilized to identify human remains more correctly and reliably (Cantatore et al., 2015) (Figure 13.12).

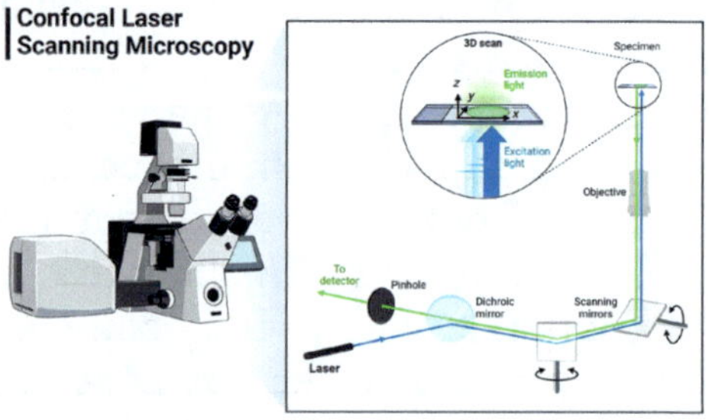

Figure 13.12. Confocal laser scanning microscopy.

Source: https://microbenotes.com/wp-content/uploads/2024/04/Laser-Scanning-Confocal-Microscopy.jpeg.

13.4.2. Innovations in DNA Technology

The advances in DNA technology have contributed immensely to forensic pathology, especially to the identification of human remains. High-throughput sequencing and polymerase chain reaction technologies have immensely increased the capacity to recover and analyze degradative and complex biological materials. The technology allows forensic specialists to generate genetic profiles from very small quantities of DNA, and that is making it possible to identify victims from mass disasters or where they have decomposed extremely. These methods also enhance the accuracy of biological sample matches to potential relatives, which is crucial for providing closure to families. With more forensic agencies embracing these advances, we see increased reliance on DNA evidence in courtrooms, underscoring its vital role in establishing identity and supporting criminal investigations. Moreover, integration of artificial intelligence (AI) in DNA analysis underscores the shifting landscape of forensic science. AI algorithms assist in the interpretation of complex genetic data so that forensic pathologists can notice patterns and abnormalities that can be easily overlooked by regular examinations. With the computerization of the processing of enormous data sets, AI enhances the speed and accuracy of forensic identification processes. Such a technological shift is particularly critical in cases of large-scale investigations, where identification speed is generally of paramount importance. Additionally, AI-driven systems can help estimate postmortem interval and contribute to virtual autopsy procedures, which align with the trend towards non-invasive techniques in forensic medicine. The implications of these technologies extend beyond the immediate solving of cases, with speculation moving towards other potential criminal justice uses with tasks like reconstruction of crime scenes (Piraianu et al., 2023). Despite the promising advancements, the union of DNA technology and forensic pathology is not without problems. Variability in forensic information, often attributable to outdated techniques or analyst errors, can lead to false convictions and compromise the justice system (Morgan, 2023). Excessive reliance on DNA as an infallible source of data is increasingly under scrutiny, with greater emphasis placed on procedure standardization and strict training for forensic specialists. Continuous monitoring of forensic processes, along with technological advancements, is crucial in reducing the risk of miscommunication or misinterpretation of DNA information. As forensic science develops, ethical issues surrounding data security and the use of AI in forensic applications will be central in ensuring that DNA technology advances fulfill their potential without compromising the integrity of forensic investigation.

13.4.3. Software for Facial Reconstruction

The application of software in facial reconstruction has become an important area of technological development within forensic pathology, especially when it comes to the identification of human remains. This type of software allows for the crucial process of craniofacial superimposition, in which facial structures are reconstructed using skeletal materials. While the manual process is subject to limitations, computerized applications provide increased precision and speed, enabling forensic experts to create 3D representations of an individual's face from cranial geometry. As defined in a comparative study of manual and computerized approaches, the efficacy of such systems depends on ante-mortem image quality and the specific algorithms used in reconstruction. For victim identification disasters where there are huge numbers of remains that must be quickly screened, the ability to efficiently utilize software helps to accelerate the investigative process and achieve successful victim identification through visual recognition with current photographic records (Lofthouse et al., 2025).

Aside from its technical application, the facial reconstruction software also addresses issues of ethics in forensic investigation. The work of getting the face of deceased individuals accurately is delicate, particularly in cases of extreme decomposition or trauma. Programs used have to walk the moral tightrope on how faces can be represented post-mortem, something that has evolved through the years in terms of social perception about images of this sort. Foreseeing possible misidentification by families, the reconstructions must be balanced against the psychological impact that such images could have on the families of the victims. Integration of software into such sensitive processes, therefore, requires a prudent approach so that reconstructions are used for identification purposes without introducing any indignity upon the deceased (Achenbach et al., 2014). With the advancement of forensic technology, software's role in facial reconstruction will only increase, requiring sustained research and development. With the integration of artificial intelligence and machine learning, future software can take the accuracy of facial reconstructions further to allow for even more nuanced interpretations of cranial features. Secondly, the employment of multiform sets of data with varied expressions and orientations of the human face will add even more accuracy to such reconstructive techniques. As cross-sectional research illustrates, the varying viewpoint angles of ante-mortem images, in fact, have a significant impact on influence identification rates, proving the need for global methods considering the varied factors impacting facial recognition. With the development of forensic science, the application of advanced computer programs will surely be a great factor not only in optimizing identification rates but also in dictating ethical levels in forensic pathology (Achenbach et al., 2014) (Figure 13.13).

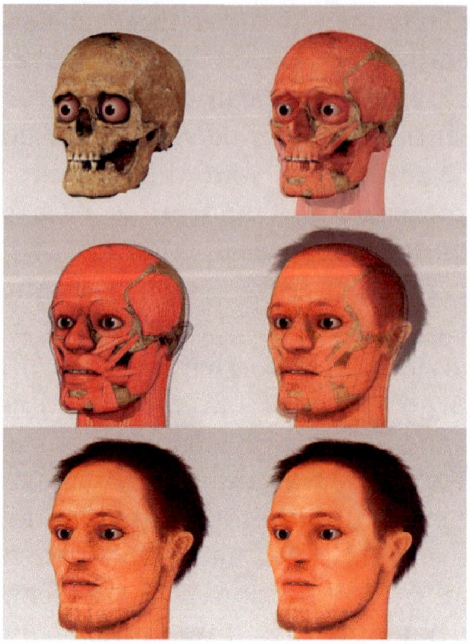

Figure 13.13. Forensic facial reconstruction of Alberto di Trento by Arc-Team and the 3D artist Cicero Moraes.

Source: https://upload.wikimedia.org/wikipedia/commons/d/d6/Forensic_facial_reconstruction_of_Alberto_di_Trento.jpg.

Test Your Knowledge

1. What is the use of imaging techniques?
2. What is the use of software for facial reconstruction?

SUMMARY

In summarizing forensic pathology analysis of human remains, one realizes that the use of several scientific methods significantly enhances the effectiveness of human identification. Various methods, such as radiographic imaging, provide critical details on pathological conditions that can be used to identify demographic profiles of individuals. For instance, the diagnosis of individual diseases, like Paget's disease, from skeletal analysis not only narrows down the list of possible identities but also leaves an indelible mark capable of withstanding forensic examination. This is a demonstration of how radiographic evidence can be the clincher in cases where other, more conventional methods of identification are unavailable or limited, which exemplifies the significance of a multi-prognostic methodology in forensic examination (Duffy et al., 2023). Moreover, breakthroughs in genetic analysis techniques have recently added to the identification procedure by divulging familial association and the presence of specific pathogens within human remains. The Tomb of the Shroud is a good instance of how mitochondrial DNA analysis, besides confirming familial association between remains, also reveals information on the health of ancient people. The simultaneous identification of pathogens such as *Mycobacterium tuberculosis* and *Mycobacterium leprae* acts to further reinforce the use of such forensic techniques in placing the mundane existence of the individuals buried within the tomb (Donoghue et al., 2009). Aside from providing multifaceted data to further assist in identifying the subject, it enhances our database for understanding historical health trends, thereby placing the study of human remains within broader socio-historical frameworks. The relevance of these findings resonates strongly within the field of forensic pathology to indicate that the cross-pollination of various scientific fields has the potential to reveal authoritative information regarding the identification and past of human remains. Through the means of developing forensic techniques, its professionals need to be attentive to the potential for bringing together radiographic, anthropological, and genetic techniques so as to provide more dynamic identity accounts. The process of reaching appropriate identification is not merely a quest for legal validity but one of finding a voice for lost lives and breathing life into history as it really transpired. Thus, an integrated application of contemporary techniques is required so that one can tackle the intricate problems in the field of forensic pathology, ultimately enabling a full comprehension of the dead as well as the social environments in which they existed.

The investigation of human remains is a forensically highly significant branch of forensic pathology with serious humanitarian and legal consequences. Central to this science is the understanding of how forensic experts operate at varying stages of investigation, especially in complex international cases. Notably, the environment in which such inquiries are conducted involves evidence gathering and interpretation towards the ultimate aim of creating a forensic narrative that can be useful within a court of law. This twofold stress on scientific effectiveness and legal reason effectively points to the intricate symbiotic association between forensic science and the judicial system and demonstrates the challenges of pursuing forensic truth in adversarial situations, as also emphasized during the events following the atrocities of Srebrenica in 1995 (Klinkner et al., 2008). Exhumations by forensic scientists are a poignant reminder of the way that evidence is rebuilt in an attempt to be credible in judicial situations. Expert witness testimony expertise is particularly important in international criminal trials, as findings from mass graves increasingly inform human rights abuses decisions. The coming together of forensic science and judicial judgment is a convoluted challenge for forensic pathologists: taking detailed scientific data and converting it into forms understandable and persuasive under legal structures. The nuances of this interaction are more striking in the mixed legal systems that exist within international tribunals, where preconceived notions of the law are confronted with the realities of forensic evidence recovery and analysis (Klinkner et al., 2009). In addition to methodologies employed in the recovery and analysis of human remains, the admissibility discussion of forensic evidence is also applicable. Cross-examination protocols within courtroom environments enter the picture to deal with methodological issues, especially in instances where expert opinions will have a high probability of dispute. Shortcomings in extensive advice on expert testimony necessitate an approach that is so practical that normative ideals are used to test the validity of forensic procedures. Acknowledging these dynamics helps not only in the identification of human remains but also is a sign of more universal measures of justice and accountability in contexts plagued by violence and conflict. This serves to underscore the significance of forensic pathology in both unveiling the past and shaping the future of legal proceedings (Klinkner et al., 2009).

KEY TERMS FROM THIS CHAPTER

- Anthropometry
- DNA analysis
- DNA technology
- Medical devices
- Mycobacterium tuberculosis
- Palatal rugae
- Terrorism
- Digital imaging
- DNA profiling
- Fingerprints
- Mycobacterium leprae
- Odontology
- Skeletal analysis
- Visual identification

CRITICAL THINKING QUESTIONS

1. **Which of the following is considered the most reliable method of positive identification in forensic cases?**
   a. Facial recognition
   b. Tattoo examination
   c. DNA profiling
   d. Clothing analysis
2. **Which of the following skeletal parts is most useful in determining biological sex?**
   a. Femur
   b. Skull
   c. Rib
   d. Sternum
3. **Dental records are especially useful in human identification because:**
   a. Teeth do not decay after death
   b. Dental restorations are unique and durable
   c. All individuals have the same dental pattern
   d. Teeth are immune to fire and trauma
4. **Which of the following is used to estimate the age of skeletal remains in children?**
   a. Skull suture closure
   b. Tooth eruption patterns
   c. Pelvic angle
   d. Cranial index
5. **The "superimposition technique" in forensic anthropology is used for:**
   a. Identifying species of origin
   b. Matching a skull to a photograph
   c. Estimating time since death
   d. Determining race

Short Answer Questions

1. What is the primary role of forensic pathology in the context of unidentified human remains?
2. What legal institution was mentioned in relation to the use of forensic evidence in historical mass fatality cases?
3. What are the methods of human remains identification?
4. What type of biological profile can forensic anthropologists typically construct from skeletal remains?
5. What is the role of forensic pathologists in identifying human remains?

Answer to Critical Thinking Questions

1. (c) 2. (b) 3. (b) 4. (b) 5. (b)

REFERENCES

1. Achenbach, A., Aitken, A., Algemeen, et al. (2014). A review of the changing culture and social context relating to forensic facial depiction of the dead. https://core.ac.uk/download/42477688.pdf (accessed on 12th July 2025).
2. Auerkari, E. (Elza). (2008). Recent trends in dental forensics. https://media.neliti.com/media/publications/282217-recent-trends-in-dental-forensics-522dfd43.pdf (accessed on 12th July 2025).
3. Bourdieu, P., Carey, N., Caruth, C., Cohen, A., Interpol, Lessig, R., Marshall, R. D., et al. (2014). Who knows who we are? Questioning DNA analysis in disaster victim identification. https://core.ac.uk/download/30704511.pdf (accessed on 12th July 2025).
4. Bryson, D. (2015). Towards a working methodology for using total hip and knee joint replacements to support identification. https://core.ac.uk/download/46170993.pdf (accessed on 12th July 2025).
5. Cameron, F. (2021). Investigation of palatal rugoscopy for forensic human identification. https://core.ac.uk/download/482116221.pdf (accessed on 12th July 2025).
6. Cantatore, S., De Carlo, D., Fineschi, V., et al. (2015). Confocal laser scanning microscope, raman microscopy, and western blotting to evaluate inflammatory response after myocardial infarction. https://core.ac.uk/download/54248088.pdf (accessed on 12th July 2025).
7. Cassella, J. P., Cassidy, N. J., Jervis, J., et al. (2008). Time-lapse geophysical investigations over a simulated urban clandestine grave. https://core.ac.uk/download/28874732.pdf (accessed on 12th July 2025).
8. Donoghue, H. D., Fratpietro, R., Gibson, S., et al. (2009). Molecular exploration of the first-century tomb of the shroud in Akeldama, Jerusalem. https://core.ac.uk/download/1687724.pdf (accessed on 12th July 2025).
9. Duffy, E., Duffy, E., Elliott, J., et al. (2023). Fragmented skeletonised remains: Paget's disease as a method of biological profiling using radiography. https://core.ac.uk/download/552803760.pdf (accessed on 12th July 2025).
10. Frelat, M., Halazonetis, D., Karell, M. A., et al. (2016). A novel method for pair-matching using three-dimensional digital models of bone: Mesh-to-mesh value comparison. https://core.ac.uk/download/305118311.pdf (accessed on 12th July 2025).
11. Ho, K. C., Jentzen, J., Johnson, L. T., Palermo, et al. (1994). Destructive hostility: The Jeffrey Dahmer case: A psychiatric and forensic study of a serial killer. https://core.ac.uk/download/213059368.pdf (accessed on 12th July 2025).
12. Klinkner, M. J. (2008). Forensic science for Cambodian justice. https://core.ac.uk/download/4897044.pdf (accessed on 12th July 2025).
13. Klinkner, M. J. (2008). Proving genocide? Forensic expertise and the ICTY. https://core.ac.uk/download/4897043.pdf (accessed on 12th July 2025).
14. Klinkner, M. J. (2009). Forensic science expertise for international criminal proceedings: An old problem, a new context and a pragmatic resolution. https://core.ac.uk/download/4897045.pdf (accessed on 12th July 2025).

15. Krey, I., Platzer, K., Esterhuizen, A., Berkovic, S. F., Helbig, I., Hildebrand, M. S., Lerche, H., et al. (2022). Current practice in diagnostic genetic testing of the epilepsies. *Epileptic Disorders, 24*, 765–786. https://doi.org/10.1684/epd.2022.1448 (accessed on 12th July 2025).
16. Lofthouse, A., & Wilkinson, C. (2025). The use of craniofacial superimposition for disaster victim identification. https://core.ac.uk/download/42477690.pdf (accessed on 12th July 2025).
17. Morgan, J. (2023). Wrongful convictions and claims of false or misleading forensic evidence. *Journal of Forensic Sciences, 68*, 908–961. https://doi.org/10.1111/1556-4029.15233 (accessed on 12th July 2025).
18. Opeskin, B., Weisbrot, D., & Breen, K. (2025). Essentially yours: The protection of human genetic information in Australia. https://core.ac.uk/download/pdf/30672952.pdf (accessed on 12th July 2025).
19. Perkins, H., Hughes, T., Forrest, A., & Higgins, D. (2024). 3D dental records in Australian dental–A hidden gold mine for forensic identification. *Australian Journal of Forensic Sciences, 57*, 322–339. https://www.semanticscholar.org/paper/c60473caa322729249ab7c6164fb326bbbe0aa80 (accessed on 12th July 2025).
20. Piraianu, A. I., Fulga, A., Mușat, C. L., Ciobotaru, O. R., Poalelungi, D. G., Stamate, E., Ciobotaru, O. C., et al. (2023). Enhancing the evidence with algorithms: How artificial intelligence is transforming forensic medicine. *Diagnostics, 13*, 2992–2992. https://doi.org/10.3390/diagnostics13182992 (accessed on 12th July 2025).
21. Ramey, S., & Savage, H. (2018). "Is this my great aunt?": An analysis of human skeletal remains to construct a biological profile. https://core.ac.uk/download/267588247.pdf (accessed on 12th July 2025).
22. Sansola, A. (2015). Postmortem iris recognition and its application in human identification. https://open.bu.edu/bitstream/2144/13975/8/Sansola_bu_0017N_11536_web.pdf (accessed on 12th July 2025).
23. Stein, D. J., Shoptaw, S., Vigo, D., Lund, C., Cuijpers, P., Bantjes, J., Sartorius, N., et al. (2022). Psychiatric diagnosis and treatment in the 21st century: Paradigm shifts versus incremental integration. *World Psychiatry, 21*, 393–414. https://doi.org/10.1002/wps.20998 (accessed on 12th July 2025).
24. Zahrani, A. A. (2024). Current trends in the methods of identification in forensic dentistry: A review of literature. *International Journal of Community Medicine and Public Health*. https://www.semanticscholar.org/paper/3c547bd38445fd67e0d984c7e926aba67b304070 (accessed on 12th July 2025).

FORENSIC ANTHROPOLOGY

14

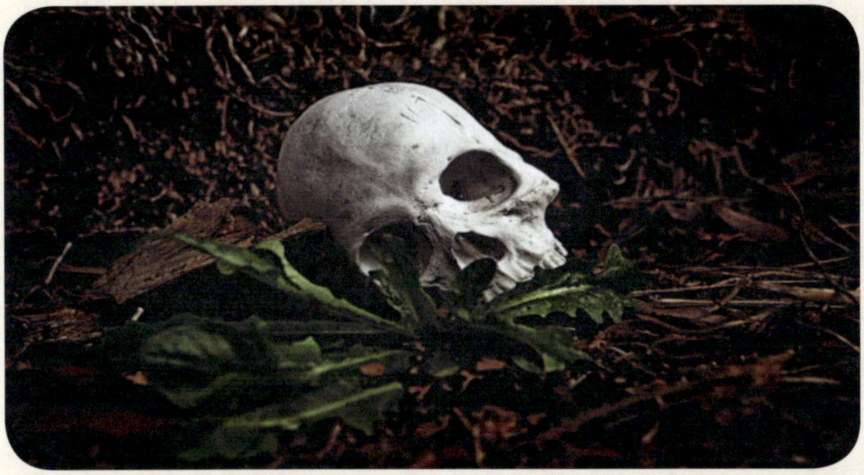

LEARNING OBJECTIVES

After studying this chapter, you will be able to:

1. Understand the role of forensic anthropologists;
2. Know the techniques and methods essential for the identification of human remains;
3. Describe the challenges of forensic anthropology;
4. Describe the future directions of forensic anthropology.

Introduction

Forensic anthropology is an essential field at the intersection of law and science that is asked to identify and examine human remains in legal cases. Forensic anthropologists use biological and anthropometric methods in an attempt to ascertain age, sex, ancestry, and height, as well as other characteristics relevant to the identification of remains. Forensic anthropology is especially important in mass disaster cases, murder, and historical investigation, where more typical means of identification, like fingerprints or DNA, are not applicable. This experience in forensic anthropology provides the foundation for what is required to understand the intricate techniques and methodologies employed to further solve complex cases of unidentified human remains, and it provides one with a vision for what moves the science of forensic anthropology along. Advances in isotopic analysis have changed the way forensic anthropologists can ascertain the geographic origins of unidentified remains, particularly when other forms of identification fail. Techniques such as stable oxygen and strontium isotope analysis enable scientists to make educated guesses about the geographic histories of people from chemical signatures that show up in their teeth. For instance, research identified significant differences in isotopic values between Colombian and New England populations, which indicate that isotopic techniques are capable of linking remains to a specific population. Such findings indicate the ability of forensic anthropology, as evidenced through the creation of isoscapes that have the potential to assist in long-term conflict and migration-related cases (Eck et al., 2017). This more subtle understanding of geographic origin is an important milestone in the identification process, further demonstrating the worth of forensic anthropology in yesterday's and today's worlds.

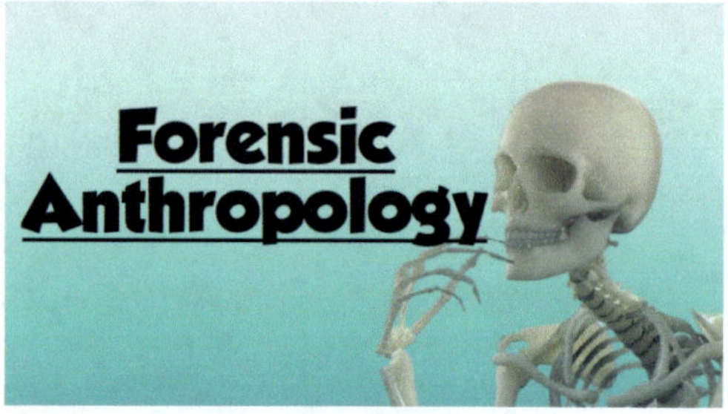

Figure 14.1. Forensic anthropology.

Source: https://blogger.googleusercontent.com/img/b/R29vZ2xl/AVvXsEjYiSeu2E1R6MZQARrYVLs88De-W-Q7Hk91fWLK-5P XxdlzlPim0OLwvJ_q0FCN9FVYj_gmEIF Qbu5R NyLEJRVq w1HzITEsUROBuMnUQE XkDSJSHkpo9lK_pK57sD3wTiJP DG73YEsItnJrR WZj8tLPn9pBhtx3DBEoU LOF CJ00q SC9nDRjyP-dguHlwkec/s1280/Photo_1618581045571.png.

Combined with isotopic analysis, the integration of advanced imaging technology into forensic anthropology increases the field's capability to analyze skeletal remains. Multi-modal imaging technologies, such as high-resolution X-ray computed tomography, allow scientists to see inside bones without causing them any harm and revealing critical information about the status and history of remains. Institutions such as the University of Texas High-Resolution X-ray CT Facility demonstrate how various scientific disciplines converge through interdisciplinarity, facilitating the development of forensic science (Ahmed et al., 2017). With these technologies, forensic anthropologists can extract information about trauma, pathologies, and taphonomy processes that can be utilized to guide investigations. All these advancements together illustrate the evolving dynamics of forensic anthropology, with it growing in sync with technological progress and making an invaluable contribution to the quest for justice (Figure 14.1).

Definition of Forensic Anthropology

Forensic anthropology is the intersection of forensic science and anthropology, focusing on the identification of human remains in the legal context. The field is about the application of skeletal analysis and anthropological data in the assistance of legal investigation, particularly in cases of suspected criminal acts or mass tragedies. Forensic anthropologists apply a number of techniques to make age, sex, ancestry, and stature estimations on unknown individuals, a valuable piece of information that can be used to narrow down identities in investigations. Given the sheer variety found in human skeletal variation, experts in this line of work must possess a solid understanding of how populations differ, thus their capacity to interpret data pertinent to remains found in forensic situations accurately. In addition to identification, forensic anthropology also has the task of providing evidence that assists in legal cases. The process involves thorough analysis of the skeletal information and comparison to biological as well as historical contexts for the creation of victim profiles. The challenge of forensic anthropology can be illustrated through some examples, such as war crimes or mass graves, in which skeletal remains are generally fragmented, and the conditions of analysis are subpar. Through the application of robust techniques using osteological analysis, forensic anthropologists can reconstruct events surrounding death and therefore contribute to what has been termed 'forensic truth' in forensic environments.

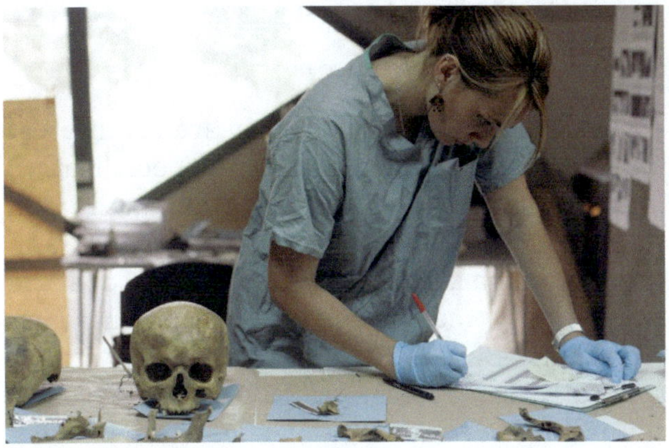

Figure 14.2. Understanding forensic anthropology.

Source: https://cdn.britannica.com/92/91892-050-43C2CBD8/Forensic-anthropologist-human-skull-grave-Bosnia-and-2005.jpg.

As much as the practice requires scientific discipline, it also requires enhanced ethical scrutiny due to the fact that forensic anthropologists work with sensitive social implications and the victims' families, maximizing the profession's sole function in contemporary forensic science (Klinkner et al., 2008). Apart from this, forensic anthropology also has a number of sub-disciplines that enhance its efficacy in answering forensic questions. For instance, age estimation remains a core topic, where techniques such as observing the closure of the Spheno-occipital synchondrosis are critical indicators of biological age in a specimen. Studies indicate that the closures can greatly differ with gender, thereby enhancing the efficacy of age estimation methods (Mangiulli et al., 2018). Such advancement within the discipline is needed, as it not only improves the accuracy of forensic analysis but also provides important information in reconstructing the life histories of unidentified dead individuals. Hence, by interdisciplinary collaboration and constant research, forensic anthropology is an active discipline that remains abreast of both scientific progress and the changing law (Figure 14.2).

Importance in the Criminal Justice System

Forensic anthropology's inclusion in the criminal justice system is crucial to enhance investigation effectiveness and accuracy. The discipline focuses on the application of anthropological methods to human remains, which plays a critical role in the majority of cases, such as homicide, mass disasters, and missing persons mysteries. Analysis of skeletal remains allows forensic anthropologists to convey significant information, including the age, gender, ancestry, and stature of the victim. Such biological profiles significantly increase the potential for a successful identification of victims, thus assisting law enforcers in their pursuit of justice.

Secondly, as forensic anthropology expands, there is a need to adopt new methods and technology, which are important in addressing contemporary challenges in the field and meeting the requirements of the justice system (Roux et al., 2021). In recent years, the integration of artificial intelligence (AI) techniques in forensic anthropology has added new channels for human identification and examination.

The computer-based methods have the capacity to support traditional methods with sophisticated instruments for biological profile approximation and comparative analysis through imaging techniques. Machine learning and computer vision AI techniques are offering assistance in revolutionary facial reconstruction, trauma analysis, and even pathology assessment (Mesejo et al., 2020). These advancements make it possible for forensic anthropologists to increase the precision and reliability of findings, making them a more vital part of the criminal justice system. This kind of contribution not only improves case-solving potential but also upholds public confidence in the integrity of forensic science.

Furthermore, forensic anthropology is more than identification: it has crime prevention and legal culpability implications. By systematically breaking down human remains and contributing to a holistic understanding of victimization patterns, forensic anthropologists can yield information that directs criminal investigations and prevention initiatives. This forward-thinking in criminal justice works to provide law enforcement with resources to identify and analyze patterns of violent crime.

In addition to this, collaboration between forensic anthropologists and law enforcement can also establish an educational and awareness culture regarding best practices so that investigation methods remain aligned with the latest scientific developments (Roux et al., 2021). Thus, the integration of forensic anthropology in the criminal justice system not only facilitates the solution of cases effectively but also promotes the values of justice and public security (Figure 14.3).

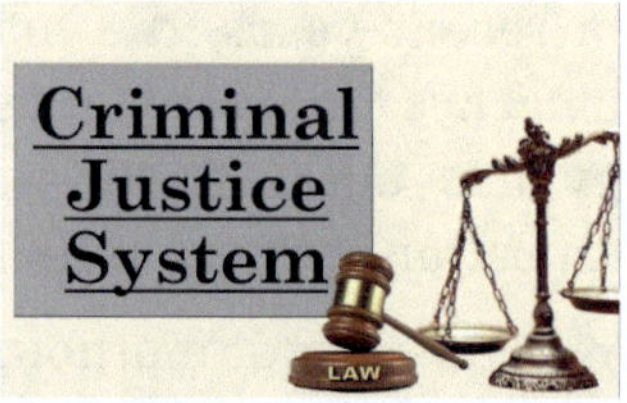

Figure 14.3. Criminal justice system.

Source: https://i.ytimg.com/vi/DxwQLrXhS0M/maxresdefault.jpg.

14.1. Role of Forensic Anthropologists

Learning Outcome

1. Identify human remains.
2. Understand the analysis of skeletal trauma.
3. Determine the age, sex, and ancestry in forensic anthropology.

Forensic anthropologists are an area of interest in the forensic science field, with specialization in the analysis and identification of human skeletons. Their services play a critical role in court cases, particularly where the cause of death is a mystery, mass tragedies, or human rights violations. Based on various methods, these specialists can determine age, sex, ancestry, and stature from skeletal remains, therefore offering crucial input for ongoing investigations. The work of the forensic anthropologist does not stop at identification; they also recover human remains at crime scenes and can be considered expert witnesses in the legal process. This range of activities is a testament to the significance of the role in bridging the gap between anthropology, biology, and the law to provide justice to the dead and their families. Apart from their contribution to analysis, forensic anthropologists also participate in broader scientific research projects and public awareness campaigns. Their findings and procedures are typically key elements for the creation of both forensic and archaeological sciences. Moreover, through workshops and lectures, the specialists educate law enforcement officials and medical examiners about the importance of proper recovery techniques and preservation of evidence. It is significant to interdisciplinary cooperation in this area because information from forensic anthropology can be applied to inform criminal justice practice and cadaver studies. By doing so, forensic anthropologists not only improve the validity of death investigations but also enhance the knowledge of human remains, leading to improved criminal investigations and methods. The role of forensic anthropologists is also highlighted when viewed from the perspective of their work for social justice. In most environments, especially for issues concerning marginalized communities or atrocities of the past, forensic anthropologists become voices for the dead, aiming to restore dignity for victims who are unidentified or forgotten. Their work enables mass grave exhumations, occasionally associated with human rights violations, as a critical move toward accountability and recovery for affected communities. By applying their anthropological knowledge to these sensitive matters, they provide valuable conclusions that can aid legal cases against perpetrators and further the historical record of abuses suffered by specific communities. This is where their work serves to underscore the broader social significance of forensic anthropology and broach its potential to guarantee reconciliation and sensitization of the people, thus elevating the discipline's relevance within contemporary legal and anthropological discourse (Figure 14.4).

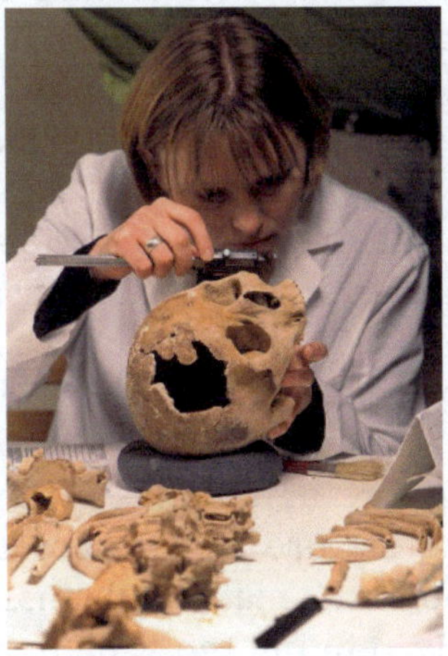

Figure 14.4. Role of forensic anthropologists.

Source: https://wp.stu.ca/forensicscience/wp-content/uploads/sites/22/2015/04/Forensic-Anthropology-forensic-anthropology-6380688-1200-1783-689x1024.jpg.

14.1.1. Identification of Human Remains

The determination of human remains is a critical aspect of forensic anthropology that is a synergy of scientific investigation and legal necessity. Several techniques, such as osteological analysis, enable forensic anthropologists to establish age, sex, ancestry, and stature from the bones, thus constructing a biological profile for identification purposes. As long as remains are available, this skeletal analysis may prove crucial, particularly when bodies are found in stages of advanced decomposition or destruction. Digital imaging technologies also enhance the ability to investigate skeletal features, which allows anthropologists to reconstruct trauma histories and differentiate human from non-human remains. The dynamic process of interaction between technological innovation and traditional approaches highlights the dynamic process of forensic anthropology in its quest to reconstruct the identities of the dead in challenging circumstances. In forensic anthropology, the use of dental analysis in human remains identification has emerged very prominently. Dental records are often able to provide crucial information, as teeth are some of the hardest tissues of the human body and tend to persevere under more trying conditions than other tissues. The unique characteristics of an individual's dental structure, including the patterns of wear and restorations, make possible positive identification, particularly when other means are met with failure. Use of technology, such as in dental radiography and advanced imaging techniques, also contributes to this identification process with the provision of realistic representations of dental features. From the efforts by Prokurat et al. (2024), the methods have been observed to reconstruct identities even in cases of mutilation or degradation. This multi-disciplinary intervention, which involves combining dental analysis and forensic anthropology, is a clear case of how various methodologies can collaborate in enhancing investigation findings. The methodological scope of forensic anthropology extends beyond bone and dental analysis to encompass cultural and archaeological inference, as emphasized by Valera (2024). Examination of burial ritual, grave goods, and contextual information surrounding the remains can inform the identity and cause of death. These cultural elements not only aid in the identification of individuals but also provide critical context for understanding the sociocultural dynamics of forensic cases. For instance, some burial practices are indicative of cultural identity or socioeconomic status, which can aid in the identification process. Furthermore, interdisciplinary studies, incorporating genetics and anthropology, enable better comprehension of biological and cultural elements involved in human identification processes. This collaborative structure emphasizes the utilitarian role of forensic anthropology in meeting complexities in human remains identification, particularly underlining its central role in modern investigative strategies (Figure 14.5).

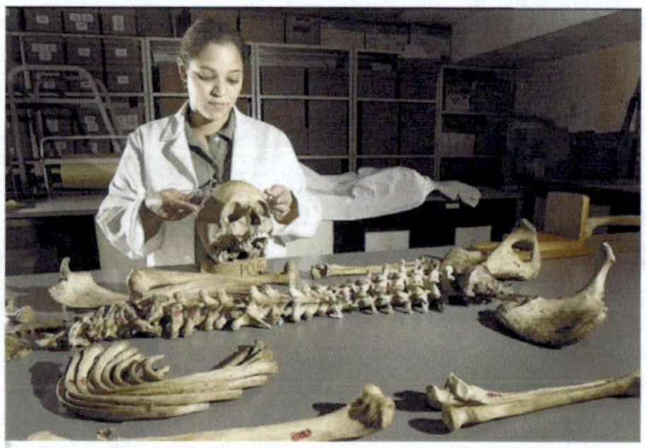

Figure 14.5. Identification of human remains.

Source: https://www.gainesville.com/gcdn/authoring/2003/10/24/NTGS/ghows-LK-f8e1d9a4-0159-4789-bbb3-9250c29a0228-361646e1.jpeg?width=660&height=446&fit=crop&format=pjpg&auto=webp.

14.1.2. Analysis of Skeletal Trauma

Skeletal trauma analysis is an important aspect of forensic anthropology, particularly in victim identification processes. The skeletal remains are thoroughly examined by forensic anthropologists to differentiate between pre-, peri-, and postmortem traumas. The discrimination between them not only assists in the construction of a timeline of events that contributed to the demise of an individual but also enhances the analysis in the context of the chronology of traumatic events. The information obtained through trauma analysis can shed light on patterns that are suggestive of violence, accidents, or chronic injuries associated with medical conditions. For example, knowing the category and severity of the trauma can give pertinent background when it comes to deciding if a death occurred due to foul play or other external causes. With advancing forensic technology, the use of trauma analysis goes further, more complex, but more dependable in reaching effective conclusions from skeletal remains, ultimately assisting victim identification procedures in complex investigations. In criminal or mass-disaster investigation circumstances, the contribution of trauma analysis is all the more significant. Forensic anthropologists collaborate with other forensic professionals and apply a range of methodologies to analyze skeletal remains. A full examination typically combines anthropological data with other forensic data, for example, DNA profiles and dental records. This multi-disciplinary practice not only enhances the overall effectiveness of victim identification but also promotes collaboration among various forensic disciplines. For example, the use of skeletal analysis techniques can determine important identifiers such as age, sex, ancestry, and stature of the deceased, further narrowing potential matches in missing persons databases. By refining these methods, forensic anthropologists will be better equipped to address the challenges of unidentified remains in mass casualty incidents, offering diverse insights to support investigative and legal situations. The usefulness of trauma analysis is also validated through application to case studies of rare antemortem injuries. A case, for instance, described how the combination of anthropological and imaging analysis buttressed an unusual pattern of skeletal trauma dating back to a person. The patient, believed to have been missing for years, had a past medical history of massive injuries to the right femur, including a high fall fracture and another gunshot injury. This is an elegant example of the manner in which comprehensive skeletal analysis can yield highly useful information in the history of a patient and assist positively in the process of identification. The ability to decipher the nature of such traumatic events through skeletal examination not only facilitates victim identification but also informs us more about the life histories of the person, thus pointing out the extensive contribution of forensic anthropology in breaking down complex human histories in trauma analysis (Garg, 2024; Petaros et al., 2024) (Figure 14.6).

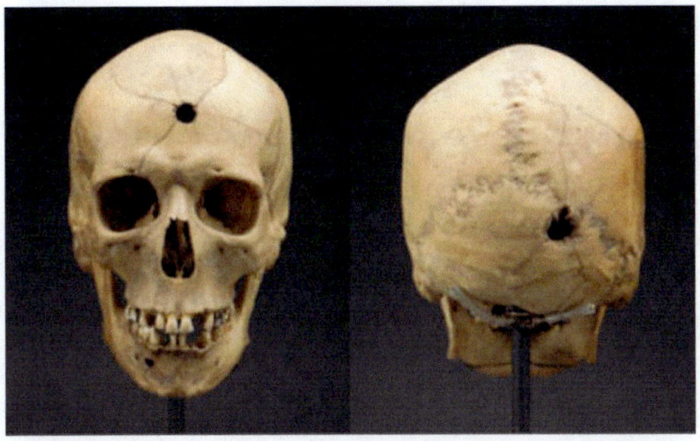

Figure 14.6. Analysis of skeletal trauma.

Source: https://pressbooks.ccconline.org/ppscant2315introtoforensicanthropology/wp-content/uploads/sites/131/2023/04/image3.png.

14.1.3. Determination of Age, Sex, and Ancestry

The determination of age, sex, and ancestry in forensic anthropology lays the groundwork for human identification, significantly enhancing the capacity to resolve criminal cases and shedding considerable light on past populations. Age at death can be determined nearly exclusively through the analysis of the skeleton, as bones go through certain morphological changes during an individual's lifetime. For example, the dental eruption sequence can provide age indicators in juveniles, while the condition of the pubic symphysis will give information regarding older age categories.

The above techniques are not without some restrictions, though; there is variability within and among persons, as well as environmental effects, which can jeopardize the accuracy of age estimations. Hence, forensic anthropologists must employ a combination of techniques and be aware of the context-dependent complexities that govern the skeletal aging processes. Sex determination is similarly crucial to the process of identification and involves assessing sexually dimorphic attributes in the skeleton. Pelvic structure and cranial variation allow forensic anthropologists to make educated conclusions about an individual's biological sex, yet these conclusions need to take into account population-specific sexual dimorphism as well. As stated, recent studies have pointed out the need for varying standards across populations, proving the importance of localized techniques for sex estimation.

More sophisticated techniques, such as the employment of medical imaging and advanced statistical techniques, have been found to be valuable assets. Not only do these techniques develop further the former paradigms for sex determination, but they also necessitate a critical debate concerning the moral implications of such assessments, particularly within the context of the interface between sex and gender in forensic anthropology (Curate, 2022). Ancestry identification, another significant function of forensic anthropology, is identifying genetic and phenotypic characteristics enabling the tracing of lineage and place of origin. Not only does this aid in suspect identification by law enforcement units, but it also improves the understanding of migration pathways and population diversity in past ages. Forensic anthropologists utilize cranial and postcranial measurements, along with modern genetic testing, to identify the probable ancestry of skeletal remains. The application of chemometric approaches is also promising in optimizing the interpretation of evidence and analytical techniques, further increasing the potential for ancestry determination in forensic practice (Sauzier et al., 2021). By the integration of classical morphological techniques with contemporary scientific advancements, forensic anthropology is constantly evolving, offering a more advanced and integrated approach to determination of age, sex, and ancestry (Figure 14.7).

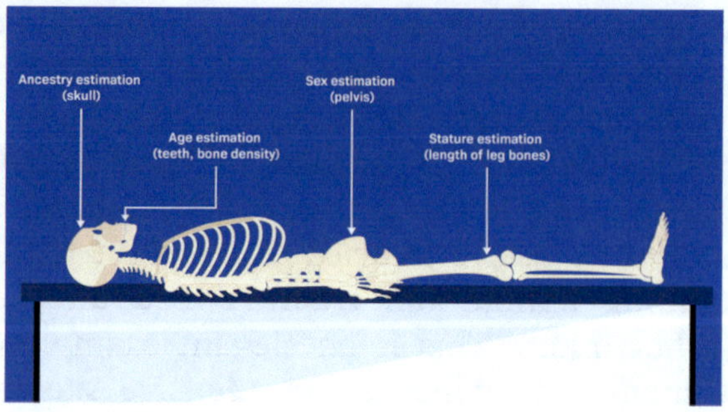

Figure 14.7. Forensic anthropologists analyze specific parts of a deceased person's skeleton to estimate ancestry, age, sex, and stature.

Source: https://api.www.labxchange.org/api/v1/xblocks/lb:LabXchange:18c58947:html:1/storage/v6_c1_p2_a8-_-text-image-_-case-study-the-complexities-of-ancestry-estimation-in-forensic-anthropology-_-rdeise-_graphic-updates_c1_p2_a8-021698756265658-4121b89dcb42bcc0ee202ad32ed5298a.png.

Test Your Knowledge

1. Which biological traits can forensic anthropologists determine using osteological analysis?
2. What is the primary goal of analyzing skeletal trauma in forensic anthropology?

14.2. Techniques and Methods

Learning Outcome

1. Understand the osteological analysis.
2. Integrate DNA analysis.
3. Describe the use of technology in forensic anthropology.

Forensic anthropology employs a variety of techniques and methods that are key to human identification in forensic cases. One of the most prominent methods is analysis of skeletal remains, which yields informative details about an individual's sex, age, ancestry, and height. The techniques have been enhanced in recent times, particularly in skull-derived sex estimation. A scoping review of the literature from 2020 to 2024 investigated this subject, finding relevant keywords to this topic and stressing the use of anatomical sites, modalities, and character types (Wang et al., 2024). Categorization of these studies provides a solid basis for future studies, extending knowledge of the intricate methods used in forensic anthropology. 3D medical imaging has revolutionized conventional methods of sex estimation from human skeletons. This new method enables forensic anthropologists to study the human skull with improved precision and reliability. Advanced computer vision methods have been integrated into the studies, leading to improvements in the efficiency and accuracy of sex estimation (Wang et al., 2024). The implications of these advances extend beyond mere identification; they permit a more nuanced understanding of human variation in forensic contexts. The process is centered on technology in forensic anthropology, an art-science field that guarantees adherence to appropriate ethical procedures while pursuing justice in the form of court cases. Furthermore, forensic anthropology is a multidisciplinary practice involving the use of physical anthropology, cultural anthropology, and archaeology, as highlighted in contemporary literature. This broad spectrum avails practitioners with diverse skills and methods in dealing with cases. For instance, when a corpse is excavated, forensic anthropologists typically employ taphonomic analyses to determine the conditions of decay and the environment in which the corpse was discovered. Such integrated approaches are essential for the determination of timelines and context in relation to death. By combining different disciplines, forensic anthropology not only facilitates the identification of remains but also strengthens the overall knowledge in the fields of human behavior and social contexts in relation to death, thus assisting the judicial process in a scientifically sound way.

14.2.1. Osteological Analysis

Osteological analysis forms the building block of the field of forensic anthropology, bridging biological and cultural data attained from bones to advance legal investigation and historical understanding. By meticulous observation of human bones, forensic anthropologists can infer valuable biological profiles such as age, sex, ancestry, and stature. The precision of age estimation, in particular, has undergone enhancement owing to traditional osteological methods that observe morphological changes in bones, such as the closure of cranial sutures and deterioration of the pubic symphysis. Additionally, the application of new technologies like CT and laser scanning enhances the analysis of skeletal elements to better comprehend bones that have not hitherto been factored in. Therefore, osteological analysis not only aids forensic practice but also aids archaeological comprehension, demonstrating its multi-faceted use in the understanding of human history and society (Acsádi et al., 2016). Further, osteological analysis is crucial in the diagnosis of pathological conditions diagnosed in skeletal remains to expose clues concerning the lifestyle and health of ancient human populations. By analyzing degenerated bones, forensic anthropologists are able to ascertain remnants of diseases, trauma, and nutrient deficiency that have plagued the individuals throughout their lifetime. For instance, analysis of bones at sites like the Tomb of the Shroud in Jerusalem demonstrates how genetic analysis on human bones, combined with osteological evaluations, allows researchers to establish kinship relationships and identify the presence of specific pathogens, such as *Mycobacterium tuberculosis* and *Mycobacterium leprae*. This cross-disciplinary research demonstrates the value of osteological methods in producing informative narratives about health issues and social impacts of historical eras, thus enriching human biology and historical migration dynamics (Donoghue et al., 2009). The scope of osteological analysis extends beyond identification; it is a dynamic process of reconstructing life activities and death practices surrounding burial. The meticulous analysis of skeletal assemblages allows researchers to make connections between past socio-political organizations and individual identities. Through the reconstruction of burial practices and the analysis of how the human remains were treated, forensic anthropologists are able to gather information regarding customs, social status, and even the socio-religious connotations surrounding death among ancient societies. The persistent growth of reference databases, particularly those derived from the most recent imaging techniques, continues to enhance the accuracy of these analyses, with the consequence that the interpretation of skeletal remains is informed by current scientific standards. As forensic anthropology evolves further, incorporation of osteological analysis remains paramount in piecing together the complex tapestry of human life, propelling thus scientific inquiry as well as heritage (Acsádi et al., 2016) (Figure 14.8).

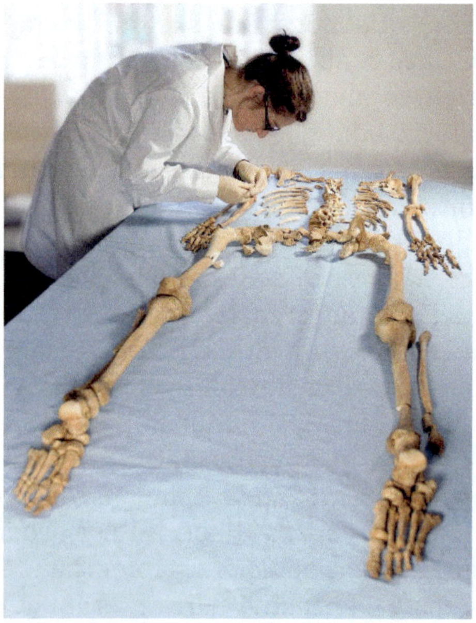

Figure 14.8. Osteological analysis.

Source: https://museumcrush.org/wp-content/uploads/2016/08/osteological-analysis2-1.jpg.

14.2.2. DNA Analysis and Its Integration

In forensic anthropology, DNA analysis is a significant breakthrough in the technologies used for identifying humans. Although skeletal analysis with conventional methods provides rudimentary information on age, sex, and ancestry, the specificity and accuracy of DNA profiling contribute immensely to such information. Since genetic technologies have improved, forensic scientists can now extract and analyze DNA even from highly degraded biological samples. This integration not only increases the accuracy of individual identification but also assists in confirming findings based on anthropological examination. Moreover, DNA analysis is an extremely powerful tool to connect individuals with crimes or incidents, as evidenced by its increasing application to cold cases, thus pushing the field of forensic anthropology to a new era of scientific rigor and validity. DNA analysis is most significant in cases where identification by conventional means is impossible, such as in mass death or trafficking of humans. Conventional methods are made useless in circumstances involving widespread decomposition or mutilation. Forensic anthropologists can utilize DNA recovery from bone or teeth to identify victims even in complex cases where victims have only provided partial remains. Besides, as indicated in an analysis of human trafficking, the integration of DNA analysis with emerging technologies, like artificial intelligence, enhances victim identification efficacy. The integration of these technologies not only broadens the boundaries of forensic investigation but also highlights the necessity of continuous innovation and collaboration among forensic fields (Aiswarya, 2025). Here, DNA analysis is not only an adjunct technique but also a foundation for carrying on the practice and use of forensic anthropology. Despite its revolutionary promise, using DNA analysis in forensic anthropology is not without problems. Contamination, compromised samples, and ethics of dealing with genetic data emphasize the requirement of strict standards and procedures. Accurate DNA profiling requires the collaboration of molecular biologists and forensic anthropologists with the aim of reinforcing methodologies that are robust and reproducible. Moreover, although DNA analysis raises personal identification, it can complicate investigations with its power to provide more questions than answers, particularly for the situation of mixed DNA profiles or population stratification. Consequently, although the forensic scenario is strengthened by DNA technology's accuracy, experts must be prudent about the implications of its use in the justice system. Subsequently, sustained training and education in both DNA and forensic anthropology are essential to make proper use of its full potential (Anwar ul Haq et al., 2025) (Figure 14.9).

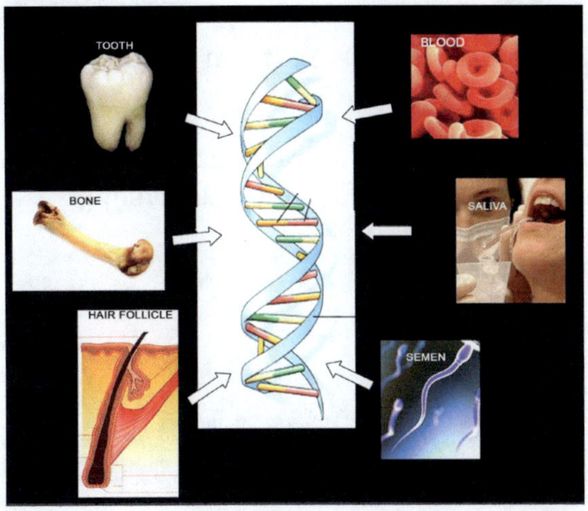

Figure 14.9. Sources of DNA for forensic analysis.

Source: https://www.researchgate.net/profile/Muruganandhan-Jayanandan/publication/51737474/figure/fig1/AS:203014913695748@1425413935690/Sources-of-DNA-for-forensic-analysis.png.

14.2.3. Use of Technology in Forensic Anthropology

The use of technology in forensic anthropology has transformed the approach used in skeletal recovery and analysis. The utilization of high-tech imaging techniques, including computed tomography (CT) and magnetic resonance imaging (MRI), enables anthropologists to view and assess the interior of bones without breaking them. The methods are utilized for analyzing skeletal remains without harming them, facilitating greater ease of thorough examination of skeletal pathology and trauma. Further, technology in 3D scanning and printing has revolutionized the way anthropologists record and reconstruct bone morphology. Not only is this more accurate and reliable, but it also allows for the creation of physical models that can be used for additional study and public education. With technology increasingly being adopted in forensic anthropology, the production of accurate, reproducible data sets will enable experts to collaborate, thus reducing the validity and reliability of forensic interpretation of human identity and trauma assessment. DNA analysis is extremely important in forensic anthropology, particularly where the skeletal remains are fragmented or have deteriorated. Techniques such as mitochondrial DNA sequencing, particularly effective in the retrieval of genetic information from poorly preserved remains, provide critical information on the identification of remains (Lacasella et al., 2025). Moreover, the application of autosomal DNA analysis has widened the scope of forensic identification to enable anthropologists to identify genetic relationships and confirm individual identities. New technological developments in forensic DNA, including the development of new methods of extraction and the ability to analyze infinitesimal quantities of biological samples, significantly enhance the accuracy of forensic analysis. This advance is essential in mass disaster scenarios as well as criminal cases in which conventional means of identification fail to identify the remains, further illustrating the synergistic harmony between molecular genetics and forensic anthropology. The convergence of these technologies underscores the necessity of continuous research in forensic methods to remain abreast of challenges. Outside of DNA analysis, dental forensics is an area of special significance where technology enhances the competence of forensic anthropology. Digital imaging technologies, including intraoral scanners and radiographic methods, have significantly enhanced the accuracy and efficiency of identifying human remains from dental records. Dental examinations are able to recognize one-of-a-kind identifier patterns, aiding in determining age and identity (Prokurat et al., 2024). Furthermore, forensic odontology's evolution continues to expand in tandem with anthropological techniques, employing computer-aided image analysis and biometric comparison to advance evidence. Integrating dental forensic analysis with other forensic sciences increases the integrity of the overall investigative process, enabling extensive examination of both skeletal and dental remains. As technology continues to evolve, forensic anthropology will increasingly rely on interdisciplinary techniques, utilizing emerging tools and techniques that further the field's ability and pursuit of human identification accuracy (Figure 14.10).

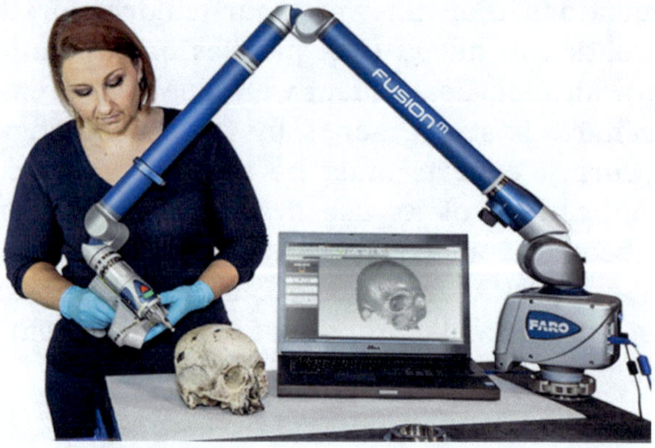

Figure 14.10. 3D Scan Arm for forensic anthropology.

Source: https://www.3printr.com/wp-content/uploads/2016/08/faro_3d_scanarm.jpg.

Test Your Knowledge

1. What is osteological analysis?
2. What is the use of technology in forensic anthropology?

14.3. Challenges in Forensic Anthropology

Learning Outcome

1. Understand the complex interplay between decomposition and environmental factors.
2. Describe the limitations of current techniques.
3. Describe the legal and ethical challenges in forensic anthropology.

Forensic anthropology, as expansive as its potential for clarifying human remains is, is confronted by a series of issues that make it more difficult to be effective in criminal proceedings. One of the greatest concerns is interpreting skeletal trauma and its impact on cause-of-death determination. The nuanced interaction between trauma—either via foul intent or environmental factors—adds depth of complication to a forensic anthropologist's examination. More complicating the issue further is skeletal preservation variability, which can mask significant markers. In various settings, like cold cases compared to newer cases, the level of decomposition and environmental factors can severely hamper the forensic anthropologist's ability to come to definitive conclusions. In general, these restraints make it imperative that there is a multidisciplinary approach, necessitating teamwork with forensic pathologists and law enforcement in order to improve interpretive precision around skeletal remains. Another serious concern arises from the accuracy of isotopic analysis employed to track unknown skeletal remains to their origin. Forensic anthropology employs multi-isotopic techniques in order to obtain information about geographic origin, and environmental factors may skew such analyses. Stable oxygen and strontium isotope ratios, for instance, yield results that vary depending on the geology and hydrology of the areas concerned. A geospatial comparison of human remains from New England and Colombia revealed strong geo-location differences through isotopic analysis, showing the potential of the method for forensic investigation (Eck et al., 2017). The underlying complexity of interpreting such ratios does mean that the need for contextualizing evidence in the broader socio-environmental landscape is emphasized. Therefore, forensic anthropologists must accurately keep track of these nuances so that there is no misinterpretation, which would nullify the strength of evidence presented in court proceedings. Finally, the application of an expert witness under forensic anthropology introduces new challenges, primarily to legal systems. The admissibility and credibility of forensic science evidence in the courtroom are disputable because the majority of judges and juries would not possess a comprehensive understanding of forensic science techniques. As is evident in international criminal trials, the intersection between science and law requires the presentation of forensic expertise, particularly on mass graves, explained and put forward during the trial. Problems tend to occur during cross-examinations, when the opposing attorney will attempt to undermine the validity of the forensic evidence (Klinkner et al., 2009). As such, it is necessary for forensic anthropologists to present their methodologies in an understandable manner and address counter-expertise tactfully. The complexity of this interaction not only influences specific cases but also shapes the continually shifting environment of forensic anthropology in the courtroom, thereby influencing public trust and perceived legitimacy of forensic evidence.

14.3.1. Decomposition and Environmental Factors

When dealing with forensic anthropology, understanding the complex interaction between the environment and decomposition is critical in order to determine the postmortem interval (PMI) with precision. Decomposition is a series of biological and chemical processes occurring after death, and it can be very diverse depending on the environment's influence. Microbial activity is influenced by temperature, humidity, and soil type, and this plays a critical part in breaking down human remains. Forensic anthropologists are also increasingly aware that these environmental conditions, aside from controlling the rate of decay, complicate standardization of PMI estimation methods. The need for an extremely subtle understanding of such interactions works to highlight the importance of intense scientific research within the field, as existing methodologies are primarily muddled by variation in environmental conditions, and, therefore, extensive data-gathering and analysis in forensic cases, as established in Weisensee et al. (2024). Existing advancements in microbial ecology provide significant perspectives on processes of decomposition and the impact of environmental conditions on them. Succession of microbial colonization, or sequential colonization of decomposers, is an up-and-coming area of development for PMI estimation methods. The initial occurrence and development changes of microbial communities are in relation to decomposition stages, which verifies that environmental conditions like soil pH and ambient temperature can significantly influence microbiological activity. In particular, studies that utilized machine learning models have sought to integrate microbial information with environmental conditions, which have shown the promise to enhance PMI estimates exponentially. However, such uses are riddled with complexities since they typically lack consistency with high rates of error due to varying sampling techniques and environmental changes, necessitating a more consistent mode of data gathering and analysis, highlighted by Allison et al. (2024). As forensic anthropology advances, incorporating environmental considerations into the studies of decomposition is becoming increasingly important in the quest to improve estimation processes.

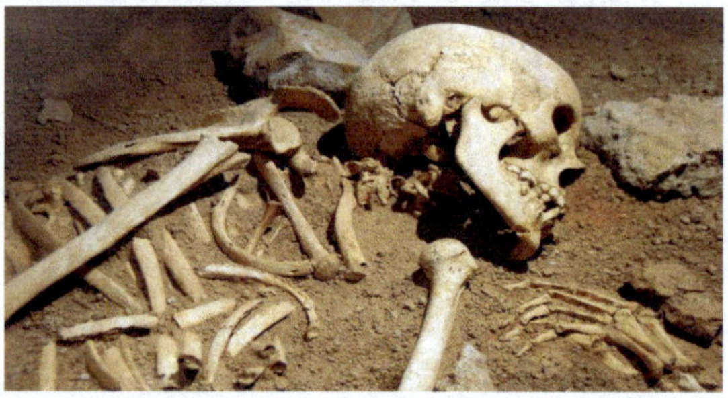

Figure 14.11. Human decomposition.

Source: https://images2.minutemediacdn.com/image/upload/c_fill,w_1440,ar_1440:810,f_auto,q_auto,g_auto/shape/cover/sport/544706-istock-91781076-b0d3246ec470628eb3312503cf90fee2.jpg.

The convergence of microbial analysis with environmental information can further our knowledge of decomposition processes and their application to forensic investigation. For example, research reveals that the incorporation of environmental variables can lower rates of prediction errors, especially when models compare particular microbial taxa. This would imply that the use of a broad range of variables could lead to more accurate and reliable PMI estimates. Indeed, applying a multi-disciplinary approach involving concepts from environmental biology, ecology, and data science can make forensic anthropology better. Lastly, by solving the limitations including current PMI estimation methods by emphasizing environmental aspects, the field can serve both justice and the sciences better, paving the way for novel forensic applications, which are critical as examined in (Weisensee et al., 2024) and (Allison et al., 2024) (Figure 14.11).

14.3.2. Limitations of Current Techniques

The discipline of forensic anthropology, as much as it is evolving with technology, remains severely hindered by the problems with current methods. Foremost among these is the utilization of several types of identification that default to general categories when individualization is not an option. As per a recent study, forensic methods such as fingerprinting and hair analysis can produce general categorizations like race or ethnicity rather than positive identification. This practice of collective identification, while pragmatically appearing, suppresses the line dividing scientific investigation from societal categorization.

Such limitations demand a more nuanced discrimination between individual and collective phenomena, posing ethical challenges in the application of forensic evidence within criminal justice proceedings, with the risk of reinforcing stereotypes or bias embedded within these broad categories (Cole et al., 2020). Besides, the accuracy of forensic techniques is also tainted by validity and reliability issues of the respective methodologies employed. The construction of forensic science is often met with reluctance in the form of obtaining worldwide acceptance from other disciplines. For instance, DNA was validated by both the scientific and legal worlds, but methods like bite mark analysis and microscopic hair comparison have been questioned because they are prone to human error and vary in their outcome. Such inconsistencies confirm that all forensic specialties remain under continuous review and evaluation for validity and reliability. The requirement of flawless forensic evidence, as noted by policy discussions regarding the use of the death penalty, underscores the core interests of flawed methodologies liable to lead to wrongful convictions and compromise justice delivery (Wheeler et al., 2016). The confines of current forensic practice become even more significant in light of their potential impact on vulnerable populations. The application of group categorization on the basis of race or ethnicity may continue to feed into the prejudices within the justice system. As forensic anthropology continues to evolve further, its methods must not only be questioned for their scientific validity but also for the implications of their application on society. Science and society are inextricably linked in forensic anthropology, and therefore, methods have to be transparent and equitable so that they do not perpetuate inequalities. Solving these ethical problems is crucial in developing a more equitable and credible forensic paradigm, enabling professionals to preserve the integrity of their information while promoting the ideals of a just justice system (Cole et al., 2020).

14.3.3. Legal and Ethical Issues

The union of legal systems and forensic anthropology introduces a treasure trove of legal and ethical issues that experts must contend with. Forensic anthropologists' work may be more than mere examination of the remains; they usually serve as expert witnesses in court cases whose conclusions can have significant impacts on the outcomes of trials. One of these essential aspects concerns the admissibility of forensic evidence, which has been tested at times under varied tests of law across varied jurisdictions. The expert opinion has its credibility based on the scientific methods applied as well as on legal tools governing their usage, as exemplified in international criminal proceedings concerning mass graves. It is by maintaining strict cross-examination and adherence to accepted standards of methodology that forensic anthropologists can maintain their evidence intact and valid within the legal system (Klinkner et al., 2009).In addition, ethical problems in forensic anthropology are compounded by the sensitivity of the delicate cases that these experts typically handle. When handling human remains, ethical obligations call for utmost respect towards the victims and their families.

This involves matters of consent, cultural sensitivity, and re-traumatization of violent crime-affected communities. Pursuit of truth and justice must be balanced against the ethical imperative to handle remains with respect and dignity. Advocating for their participation in conflict resolution and associated activities, anthropologists advance their inclusion, and ethical issues consequently take center stage. Researchers must navigate these complex dynamics while working toward gaining trust in the affected communities, a reflection of heightened interaction and sensitivity with forensic science (Dorshimer et al., 2019).

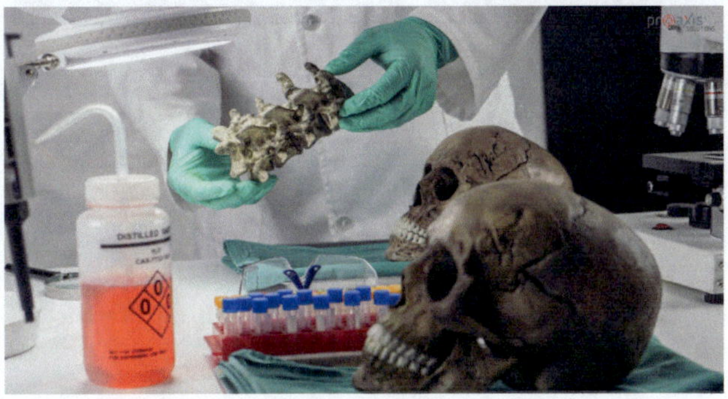

Figure 14.12. Legal systems and forensic anthropology.

Source: https://media.licdn.com/dms/image/v2/D4D12AQHXecsZNtT-ag/article-cover_image-shrink_720_1280/article-cover_image-shrink_720_1280/0/1721170888768?e=2147483647&v=beta&t=A6Fj4FpR4aGEktstV94OFqQynK2bT6FZEJjX-WQToaQ.

It also gets into legal and ethical dimensions in the combination of forensic anthropology with international law, especially in cases of human rights abuses. As forensic specialists provide evidence to international criminal courts, they must deal with challenges of responding to the implications of their findings in an international legal environment. The environment ordinarily poses a challenge in the form of sensitivity to the power dynamics involved in speaking for oppressed or victimized groups, and this makes forensic work difficult. Therefore, anthropologists must take seriously the extent to which their work will impact after the study is over, considering the possibility of influence on legal proceedings and humanitarian efforts. Responsibility to both the scientific community and the broader socio-political world is key to maintaining the integrity of forensic anthropology, thereby upholding the necessity for ethics and legality debates in the field (Klinkner et al., 2009; Dorshimer et al., 2019) (Figure 14.12).

Test Your Knowledge

1. Which environmental factors affect the rate of decomposition?
2. What role do forensic anthropologists often play in legal proceedings?

14.4. Future Directions

Learning Outcome

1. Discuss the technological and methodological advancements in forensic anthropology.
2. Describe the interdisciplinary collaboration of forensic anthropology.
3. Understand the potential for growth in forensic anthropology.

With the development of forensic anthropology, one of the most promising avenues for future study is the application of isotopic analysis in the identification of charred skeletal remains. Routine methods are unable to withstand the extremity of conditions involved in fire and arson cases, wherein identification becomes virtually impossible. The use of strontium, oxygen, and carbon isotope analysis has the ability to enhance the biological profile of human remains that are impacted by such conditions. Specifically, the analysis of oxygen isotopes could yield data regarding the temperature exposure to which remains were subjected, whereas strontium isotopes can track the geographical movement of a person. With the increasing significance of these techniques in forensic use, researchers still need to explore the impact of heat on isotopic composition, consequently advancing the understanding of where environmental conditions and skeletal biology meet (Coster et al., 2024). Another advanced field in forensic anthropology is applying human osteological documented collections (DCs) as fundamental instruments to further improve research techniques. These data sets are a core database for hypothesis-based age and sex estimation techniques, and human remains morphological variability. As testified by the considerable volume of publications regarding DCs in recent years, DCs are now more and more accepted as valuable resources to forensic science. Bibliometric analysis reveals a positive correlation between the evolution of such collections and the enhancement of biological profiling in forensic anthropology. Research-intensive institutions, such as those in the United States and Portugal, are likely to shape the future of this field, with opportunities for new types of research collaboration and increased understanding of human identification procedures (Alves-Cardoso et al., 2022). Finally, forensic anthropology's future may also be contingent upon the integration of interdisciplinary approaches that draw from new technologies, genetics, and data science.

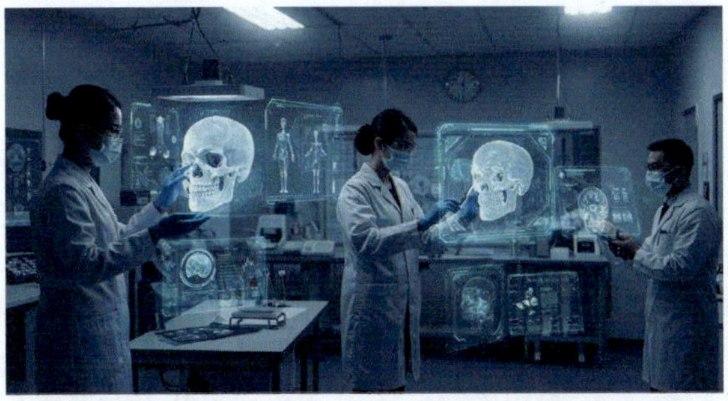

Figure 14.13. Future directions of forensic anthropology.

Source: http://www.forwardpathway.us/wp-content/uploads/2025/04/AI_Forensic_Anthropology_Lab.jpg.

Since the field aims to refine human identification techniques, these technological innovations have the potential to redefine forensic practice. Genetic analysis, for instance, would complement skeletal assessment through molecular data that provides a richer biological footprint. Furthermore, data analytics can enhance the capacity to detect patterns within large sets of data to provide more accurate identification. Through interdisciplinary collaboration, forensic anthropology can take advantage of these new technologies to resolve complex cases and further enhance the effectiveness of human remains identification in judicial and humanitarian cases. Adhering to these interdisciplinary methods is bound to open up new vistas in the quest for accuracy and reliability in forensic examination (Figure 14.13).

14.4.1. Advancements in Technology and Methodology

Technological innovation has significantly transformed the field of forensic anthropology, enhancing methodology and human identification performance. One improvement is the integration of artificial intelligence (AI) into forensic practice, which has enhanced data analysis and pattern recognition ability. Processes such as machine learning algorithms have enhanced the process of analyzing skeletal remains, making it possible to determine age, sex, and ancestry at a quicker and more accurate rate. Applications of convolutional neural networks in forensic anthropology, for instance, have increased precision in the identification of morphological traits, allowing forensic anthropologists to be in a position to provide more informed testimony in investigations. Further development in AI will further increase its ability to assist forensic experts in making predictions about skeletal remains, leading to improved outcomes in victim identification and understanding of elements that are central in criminal investigations (Agrawal et al., 2022). In addition to AI, advances in imaging technologies have also played a crucial role in the history of forensic anthropology. Techniques such as computed tomography (CT) and three-dimensional (3D) modeling now enable full scanning of skeletal systems, making comprehensive analyses possible without invasive testing. These developments not only allow for accurate reconstruction of the human remains but also allow forensic anthropologists to create virtual representations that are shareable with law enforcement and the legal sector. The enhanced visualization ability allows forensic specialists to gain greater insight into trauma and pathology since it permits them to look at skeletal remains in various positions. Besides, the use of such imaging techniques with AI provides enhanced detection of intricate details that might otherwise be overlooked, hence enhancing the robustness of forensic research (Marcello et al., 2021). Moreover, methodological advancements in forensic anthropology involve interdisciplinary assessment to include genetic analysis within the realm of usual skeletal analysis. Increasing reliance on nuclear and mitochondrial DNA analysis helps to confirm identity and establish biological connections of remains, making such methods highly useful for application in forensic analysis. Forensic anthropologists have been able to utilize even trace amounts of DNA from bone as genetic technology advances, further broadening the potential of human identification and person-of-interest identifications. The seamless merging of genetic data with anthropological data builds a denser, broader image of cases and allows for more robust inferences regarding the identity and past of human remains. The fusion underscores the transformative value of emerging technologies and techniques in forensic anthropology and leads to increased investigative effectiveness and accuracy in a field in continuous evolution to address new challenges and studies (Agrawal et al., 2022).

14.4.2. Interdisciplinary Work

Interdisciplinary collaboration is the lifeblood of forensic anthropology, introducing a rich intersection of various disciplines such as archaeology, biology, and law. Interdisciplinary collaboration enhances the effectiveness of investigations, especially in complex cases of human remains. Forensic anthropologists work collaboratively with law enforcement agencies, legal practitioners, and humanitarian organizations, marrying disparate skill sets to respond to challenging issues surrounding death and identity. By combining techniques from a range of disciplines, experts are better able to analyze skeletal remains, reconstruct biological profiles, and contribute to broader sociopolitical narratives, such as those related to historical injustices. Application of such an interdisciplinary method is well exemplified where archaeological methods are used in forensic settings to facilitate meticulous excavation and recovery of context, basic principles within legal settings. In addition, the application of exhumation in forensic anthropology demonstrates the need for multidisciplinary cooperation. Exhumation is the legally permitted recovery of remains, which sets it apart from other forms of excavation or disinterment. As part of their routine forensic casework, such units as CEMEL, the Medico-Legal Centre of the Ribeirão Preto Medical School-University of São Paulo, have collaborations ranging from local to regional to global levels. Alliances like these enhance the capacity to conduct scientific investigation and facilitate humanitarian research, particularly in contexts where fatalities are blended with political and historical evolution, that is, Brazil's civil-military regime of 1964–1985. Through interdisciplinary cooperation of this type, forensic anthropology not only becomes a tool for legal justice but also a means for social healing and the search for truth. The interdisciplinarity of forensic anthropology continues into areas of study that overlap with public health, ethics, and social justice. By engaging with experts in other fields, forensic anthropologists can address not only the physical dynamics of death, but also the ethical dimensions of how to treat human remains. This is critical in the context of humanitarian work where the objective is to maximize respect and dignity for the deceased while attempting to verify facts about a historic atrocity. The coordination resulting from organizations involved in exhumation activities allows for a complete understanding of the social dynamics of forensic cases. Consequently, these partnerships increase the strength of forensic anthropology in a way that it can serve as a general scientific and humanitarian tool in the judicial and social sphere, ultimately maximizing the impact of the field on society in general (Figure 14.14).

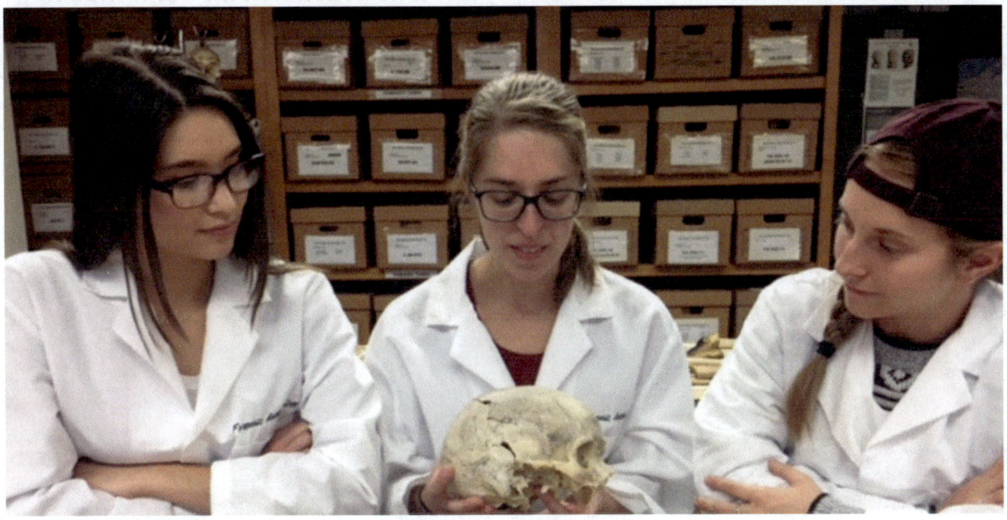

Figure 14.14. Interdisciplinary collaboration.

Source: https://i0.wp.com/anthropology.msu.edu/wp-content/uploads/2018/05/Mari-Elena-Alex-final-2.jpg?resize=640%2C329&ssl=1.

14.4.3. Potential for Growth in Forensic Anthropology

The field of forensic anthropology holds great potential for growth as it increasingly utilizes contemporary technologies and techniques. An especially fascinating direction of growth is the application of artificial intelligence (AI) to forensic analysis. AI techniques can enhance age estimation precision, identification techniques, and skeletal evidence interpretation by applying machine learning and neural network algorithms to analyze vast datasets of historical and contemporary cases. This forensic anthropology development mirrors changes in other fields where interdisciplinary work improves the findings of research. Advanced algorithms and computational models can be of help to forensic anthropologists in offering real-time analysis that is critical during investigation, and thus expanding their advisory role and potential contribution to trials. Ongoing research into AI's role in forensic applications is one instance of the general trend of interdisciplinary collaboration driving research and relevance to the legal system (Marcello et al., 2021). Further, the growth of increased understanding of biological markers and their forensic relevance foreshadows numerous avenues for development for age estimation methods as well as in evaluating human remains across contexts. Contemporary trends point towards significant advances in histological techniques, enabling more precise assessment of bone and dental age estimates with increased accuracy and demonstrating the potential for methodological improvement in forensic anthropology (Douglas et al., 2019). With literature growing to address concerns such as taphonomic influence and population variability, forensic anthropologists can increasingly engage confidently with the nuances of cases involving mixed demographics. The modification of procedures to include biochemical tests and high-tech techniques provides the potential for further refinement of existing practices. Through ongoing research and engagement with other scientific disciplines, forensic anthropology can adapt and modify, keeping its processes and analysis up-to-date with the latest forensic examinations. As forensic anthropology continues to develop, it is increasingly important that practitioners understand ethical concerns and the impact of their work on society. Greater emphasis on culturally sensitive practice and the terms of a diverse population for forensic investigation will enhance the discipline's utility as well as its ethical credibility. Building bridges between social science investigators and forensic anthropologists can make bridges of understanding between research and community views, as well as their expectations regarding forensic practice. This combined approach could further lead to more inclusive practices that are attuned to various cultural viewpoints and strengthen collaboration with law enforcement agencies and the judicial system. Ultimately, as forensic anthropology seizes these opportunities for expansion, its practitioners will likely be part of providing justice and illumination in the growing world of human remains cases (Marcello et al., 2021).

Test Your Knowledge

1. How has artificial intelligence (AI) contributed to forensic anthropology?
2. What types of DNA are commonly used in forensic anthropology?

SUMMARY

In the synthesis of forensic anthropology's functions in identification, it can be clearly seen that the field is essential to legal investigation and to humanitarian action. The synthesis of various forensic sciences, including anthropology, odontology, and molecular genetics, enhances the' credibility and dependability of identifications in complex cases, such as mass disasters or highly decomposed remains. Recent advancements in dental analysis techniques, as underscored by the increased emphasis on dental examinations, place significant emphasis on the unique identifiers obtainable from dental records and attributes. Forensic anthropology, as such, not only aids in resolving crimes but also facilitates the recovery of identities and maintains the dignity of victims under unfavorable circumstances, a goal of paramount consideration in milestone research (Prokurat et al., 2024). On top of that, the convergence of the different forensic specialists adds even more to the field, creating a multidisciplinary platform required for coping with human identification complexity. For instance, the convergence of anthropological knowledge with forensic odontology and radiological techniques allows complete investigations taking into account various contexts, from criminal to archaeological cases. This cohesive framework is critical in addressing the complex issues of forensic investigation, particularly those concerning cadavers through decomposition phases. The rigorous standards of methods established through the process provide forensic investigators with the tools that enable them to approach and understand every case effectively, showing the critical role of integrated experience in forensic anthropology (Gualtieri et al., 2024). Lastly, the practice and study of forensic anthropology are not only mentally stimulating but also ethically beneficial, as they support the broader aim of justice. The findings and procedures to be learned from this field transcend identification; they strive to recognize the social and legal consequences of the analysis of human remains in facilitating justice to victims and their loved ones. Continued research and development in forensic anthropology will be critical to remaining current with ongoing challenges as well as improving investigatory techniques. Pursuing an evolving role, the creation of forensic techniques will definitely improve practitioners' capabilities such that the valuable contributions of forensic anthropology continue to remain a core part of human rights and legal issue understanding and resolution in the years ahead (Prokurat et al., 2024).

Forensic anthropology constitutes a central interface between legal investigation and the biological sciences, as directed towards the requirement for accurate human identification. Salient points establish that conventional means of identification can prove ineffective where circumstances are complex, as in instances of mass disaster or highly burned or decomposed bodies. As evidenced in available studies, new methods such as the shadow positioning technique have significantly improved skeletal identity determination in the context of adversity in the environment. Such cases indicate the importance of medical image comparisons, with specific reference to the fact that successful forensic anthropology does not solely depend on traditional methods but also utilizes the integration of technology in order to enhance identification. Where decomposition complicates identification, it is then necessary to employ medical observations as primary identifiers rather than auxiliary ones, thus confirming the broadness of forensic anthropology in the human context (Lemos et al., 2024). At its core is an estimation of the postmortem interval (PMI), an element of paramount significance in the identification of remains, as well as providing a legal timeline. The research showing the integration of radiocarbon dating techniques has broadened the forensic arsenal, providing crucial information that assists in corroborating archaeological information as well as legal proceedings. Other case studies have illustrated how bomb-pulse dating can pinpoint ranges of years for death and birth, lending significant background to skeletal material otherwise anonymous. This double purpose, as both archaeologically relevant and medically significant, has the functional role of bridging the gap between historical analysis and the forensic demands of the present. The implications of such advancements are a reflection of the necessity for ongoing advancement in techniques employed by forensic anthropologists, hence increasing the overall efficiency of the field in human identification (Bertrand et al., 2024). Second, the engagement between traditional forensic procedures and emerging technologies operates to underscore the interdisciplinary emphasis of forensic anthropology. As the case studies show, advances in radiocarbon dating and imaging not only enhance identification techniques but also increase the knowledge of human remains from physical descriptions. The integration of DNA analysis and radiocarbon dating ensures a broader biological profile, capable of validating or negating initial hypotheses regarding identity and cause of death. This integrated process of human identification calls for cooperation between law enforcement, archaeologists, and forensic anthropologists, highlighting the variety of applications of forensic science in the criminal justice system. Finally, these points make it clear that both the disciplines of forensic anthropology and archaeology not only overlap with one another but are also crucial to developing humane justice through conscientious scientific research (Bertrand et al., 2024).

KEY TERMS FROM THIS CHAPTER

- Biology
- Forensic anthropology
- Human remains
- Legal system
- Mass graves
- Osteological analysis
- Social justice
- Criminal justice system
- Homicides
- Human rights violations
- Mass disasters
- Mystery deaths
- Skeletal trauma
- Spheno-occipital synchondrosis

CRITICAL THINKING QUESTIONS

1. **What is the primary focus of forensic anthropology?**
   a. Study of diseases in ancient populations
   b. Identification of unknown human skeletal remains
   c. Analysis of toxic substances in tissues
   d. Examination of dental records
2. **Which part of the skeleton is most reliable for determining sex?**
   a. Skull
   b. Humerus
   c. Tibia
   d. Pelvis
3. **The estimation of age in adult human remains is commonly done by analyzing:**
   a. Number of teeth
   b. Closure of cranial sutures
   c. Epiphyseal fusion
   d. Length of long bones
4. **Which bone is best suited for stature estimation in forensic anthropology?**
   a. Skull
   b. Femur
   c. Radius
   d. Clavicle
5. **Forensic anthropologists use the "ancestry estimation" technique primarily to determine:**
   a. Time since death
   b. Cause of death
   c. Biological origin based on skeletal traits
   d. Pathological conditions in bones

Short Answer Questions

1. What is forensic anthropology?
2. In what type of situation are forensic anthropologists particularly crucial?
3. What term is used to describe the reconstruction of events related to death through forensic anthropology?
4. Which traits can a forensic anthropologist typically estimate from skeletal remains?
5. In what types of cases are forensic anthropologists especially valuable?

Answer to Critical Thinking Questions

1. (b) 2. (d) 3. (b) 4. (b) 5. (c)

REFERENCES

1. Acsádi, G., Knüsel, C. J., Leth, P. M., Lynnerup, N., Lynnerup, N., Rühli, F. J., Ubelaker, D. H., et al. (2016). Evaluating osteological ageing from digital data. https://core.ac.uk/download/76945934.pdf (accessed on 12th July 2025).
2. Agrawal, P., & Nikhade, P. (2022). Artificial intelligence in dentistry: Past, present, and future. *Cureus*. https://doi.org/10.7759/cureus.27405 (accessed on 12th July 2025).
3. Ahmed, F., & Maisano, J. (2017). ToScA North America (6–8 June 2017, The University of Texas, Austin, TX) Program. https://core.ac.uk/download/211334283.pdf (accessed on 12th July 2025).
4. Aiswarya, G. R. (2025). Advancing forensic approaches to human trafficking: The role of dental identification. *Journal of Forensic Science and Research*. https://www.semanticscholar.org/paper/00cbc987fe5ecb74c64c27671a594767043d2cc4 (accessed on 12th July 2025).
5. Alves-Cardoso, F., & Campanacho, V. (2022). The scientific profiles of documented collections via publication data: Past, present, and future directions in forensic anthropology. *Forensic Sciences*. https://www.semanticscholar.org/paper/bfddbab24dab2c9451ea4605a23c17f99637da36 (accessed on 12th July 2025).
6. Arrabaça, F., Castro Pinheiro, M. E., da Silva, R., et al. (2017). Procedural and political aspects of forensic exhumation in Brazil. https://core.ac.uk/download/80693793.pdf (accessed on 12th July 2025).
7. Barrett, L. F., Adolphs, R., Marsella, S., Martínez, A. M., & Pollak, S. D. (2019). Emotional expressions reconsidered: Challenges to inferring emotion from human facial movements. *Psychological Science in the Public Interest, 20*, 1–68. https://doi.org/10.1177/1529100619832930 (accessed on 12th July 2025).
8. Bertrand, B., Clauzel, T., Richardin, P., Bécart, A., Morbidelli, P., Hédouin, V., & Marques, C. (2024). Application and implications of radiocarbon dating in forensic case work: When medico-legal significance meets archaeological relevance. *Forensic Sciences Research, 9*. https://www.semanticscholar.org/paper/f71993cf5ce191e912a2544c0785fd34c10cccce (accessed on 12th July 2025).
9. Cole, S. A. (2020). Individual and collective identification in contemporary forensics. https://core.ac.uk/download/323082704.pdf (accessed on 12th July 2025).
10. Curate, F. (2022). The estimation of sex of human skeletal remains in the Portuguese identified collections: History and prospects. *Forensic Sciences, 2*, 272–286. https://doi.org/10.3390/forensicsci2010021 (accessed on 12th July 2025).
11. da Silva, R., Evison, M., Francisco, R., et al. (2017). Forensic investigation, truth and trust in the context of transitional justice in Brazil. https://core.ac.uk/download/80693795.pdf (accessed on 12th July 2025).
12. De Coster, M., Ammer, S., Laning, T., & Kootker, L. (2024). The relevance of Sr–O–C isotope analysis on burnt human skeletal remains in archaeological and forensic contexts: A review and future directions. *WIREs Forensic Science*. https://www.semanticscholar.org/paper/b3687b6f45225d1872efc72e438e9a8c9b54ed18 (accessed on 12th July 2025).
13. Donoghue, H. D., Fratpietro, R., Gibson, S., et al. (2009). Molecular exploration of the first-century tomb of the shroud in Akeldama, Jerusalem. https://core.ac.uk/download/1687724.pdf (accessed on 12th July 2025).

14. Dörk, T., Hummel, S., Klintschar, M., et al. (2020). Genome-wide SNP typing of ancient DNA: Determination of hair and eye color of Bronze Age humans from their skeletal remains. https://core.ac.uk/download/288618847.pdf (accessed on 12th July 2025).

15. Dorshimer, E. G. (2019). What can anthropologists do? Applied anthropology in a conflict-ridden world. https://cupola.gettysburg.edu/cgi/viewcontent.cgi?article=1791&context=student_scholarship (accessed on 12th July 2025).

16. Eck, C. J. (2017). Using oxygen isotope analysis and a multi-isotopic approach in determining the region of origin of human remains. https://open.bu.edu/bitstream/2144/23783/5/Eck_bu_0017N_12708.pdf (accessed on 12th July 2025).

17. Garg, V. (2024). The role of forensic anthropology in mass disasters. *Open Access Journal of Criminology Investigation & Justice*. https://www.semanticscholar.org/paper/19a325e2ab197a68578250b12ae016c7cbef559c (accessed on 12th July 2025).

18. Gualtieri, S., Sacco, M. A., Galassi, F., Varotto, E., Tarallo, A. P., Verrina, M. C., Tarda, L., et al. (2024). The fascinating world of forensic sciences: Multidisciplinary approaches in human remains and the role of forensic pathology in Calabrian experience. *Cureus, 16*. https://www.semanticscholar.org/paper/ed33b8bb69c89efa9b8ffd3c31e718d1c3fd3b80 (accessed on 12th July 2025).

19. Haq, A. ul, & Siddiqui, N. (2025). Radiological assessment of sinus morphology for forensic identification. *Insights-Journal of Health and Rehabilitation*. https://www.semanticscholar.org/paper/fe09c5c78d7c6545c1764b3409ff5919935d554a (accessed on 12th July 2025).

20. Huang, J., Gates, A. J., Sinatra, R., & Barabási, A. L. (2020). Historical comparison of gender inequality in scientific careers across countries and disciplines. *Proceedings of the National Academy of Sciences, 117*, 4609–4616. https://doi.org/10.1073/pnas.1914221117 (accessed on 12th July 2025).

21. Kayser, M. (2017). Forensic use of Y-chromosome DNA: A general overview. *Human Genetics, 136*, 621–635. https://doi.org/10.1007/s00439-017-1776-9 (accessed on 12th July 2025).

22. Klinkner, M. J. (2008). Proving genocide? Forensic expertise and the ICTY. https://core.ac.uk/download/4897043.pdf (accessed on 12th July 2025).

23. Klinkner, M. J. (2009). Forensic science expertise for international criminal proceedings: An old problem, a new context and a pragmatic resolution. https://core.ac.uk/download/4897045.pdf (accessed on 12th July 2025).

24. Lacasella, G. V., Signorini, L., Ballini, A., Bizzoca, M. E., Musella, G., Lo Muzio, E., Cirulli, N., et al. (2025). Forensic odontology: A comprehensive review of advances and applications in dental forensic medicine. *Minerva Dental and Oral Science*. https://www.semanticscholar.org/paper/e9ede6ec39db3beac845df16b3a7bc91cf3af254 (accessed on 12th July 2025).

25. Lemos, Y. V., Furtado, A. N., Lima, A. Z., Dionísio, A. S., Araújo, R. M., & Cunha, E. (2024). Human identification by medical findings in a forensic anthropology context. *Forensic Sciences Research, 9*. https://www.semanticscholar.org/paper/eca79c431baaa4cab16f4b7b04a0c386271c89e6 (accessed on 12th July 2025).

26. Lynteris, C. (2019). Human extinction and the pandemic imaginary. https://doi.org/10.4324/9780429322051 (accessed on 12th July 2025).

27. Mangiulli, T., & Messineo, D. (2018). New method in the age estimation by the spheno-occipital suture. 3D cone-beam CT application. https://core.ac.uk/download/160051940.pdf (accessed on 12th July 2025).
28. Mariani, M. M., Perez-Vega, R., & Wirtz, J. (2021). AI in marketing, consumer research, and psychology: A systematic literature review and research agenda. *Psychology and Marketing, 39*, 755–776. https://doi.org/10.1002/mar.21619 (accessed on 12th July 2025).
29. Mason, A. R., McKee-Zech, H. S., Steadman, D., & DeBruyn, J. (2024). Environmental predictors impact microbial-based postmortem interval (PMI) estimation models within human decomposition soils. *PLOS ONE, 19*. https://www.semanticscholar.org/paper/623ed6fbe5e4e206db7602262b9fb537a7b42495 (accessed on 12th July 2025).
30. Mesejo, P., Martos, R., Ibáñez, Ó., Novo, J., & Ortega, M. (2020). A survey on artificial intelligence techniques for biomedical image analysis in skeleton-based forensic human identification. *Applied Sciences, 10*, 4703–4703. https://doi.org/10.3390/app10144703 (accessed on 12th July 2025).
31. Petaros, A., Lindblom, M., & Cunha, E. (2024). Combining anthropology and imaging to reconstruct antemortem trauma for identification purposes. *Forensic Sciences Research, 9*. https://www.semanticscholar.org/paper/49772c70a73a262ff5077d2aca79116ca933f28d (accessed on 12th July 2025).
32. Prokurat, M., Słomian, M., Grudnik, K., Grudnik, M., Jagielski, M., Budzik, M., Lau, K., et al. (2024). The role of dentistry in forensic medicine: The process of human remains identification. *Polski Merkuriusz Lekarski: Organ Polskiego Towarzystwa Lekarskiego, 52(4)*, 466–471. https://www.semanticscholar.org/paper/490b406d1965e7f513844e1be4a4333e1d66ef46 (accessed on 12th July 2025).
33. Rossi, P. J. (2010). Reading Kant from a Catholic horizon: Ethics and the anthropology of grace. https://core.ac.uk/download/213084152.pdf (accessed on 12th July 2025).
34. Roux, C., Willis, S., & Weyermann, C. (2021). Shifting forensic science focus from means to purpose: A path forward for the discipline? *Science & Justice, 61*, 678–686. https://doi.org/10.1016/j.scijus.2021.08.005 (accessed on 12th July 2025).
35. Sauzier, G., van Bronswijk, W., & Lewis, S. W. (2021). Chemometrics in forensic science: Approaches and applications. *The Analyst, 146*, 2415–2448. https://doi.org/10.1039/d1an00082a (accessed on 12th July 2025).
36. Ubelaker, D. H., & Khosrowshahi, H. (2019). Estimation of age in forensic anthropology: Historical perspective and recent methodological advances. *Forensic Sciences Research, 4*, 1–9. https://doi.org/10.1080/20961790.2018.1549711 (accessed on 12th July 2025).
37. Valera, E. E. (2024). Forensic anthropology: Challenges and scopes. *Forensic Research & Criminology International Journal*. https://www.semanticscholar.org/paper/405ec848ab4d9f49a52b9672367a64a902c16396 (accessed on 12th July 2025).
38. Wang, X., Liu, G., Wu, Q., Zheng, Y., Song, F., & Li, Y. (2024). Sex estimation techniques based on skulls in forensic anthropology: A scoping review. *PLOS ONE, 19*. https://www.semanticscholar.org/paper/589af52923518dc50a65f22ea3b9e64dcf836275 (accessed on 12th July 2025).

EMERGING TECHNOLOGIES IN FORENSIC PATHOLOGY

15

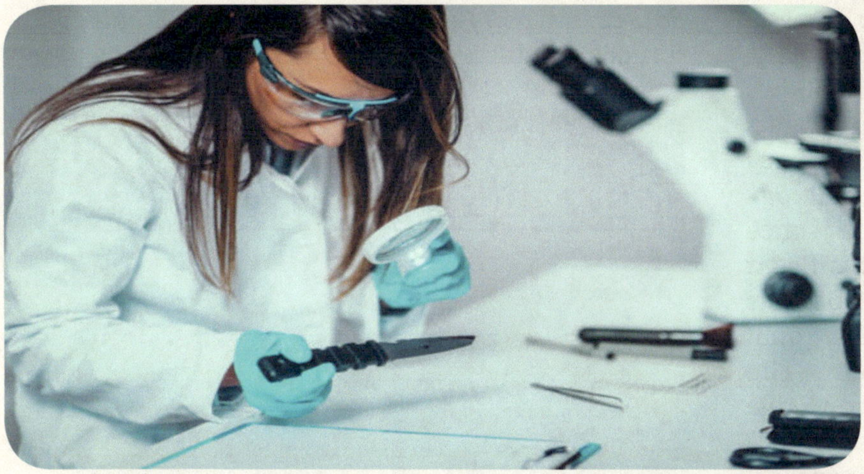

LEARNING OBJECTIVES

After studying this chapter, you will be able to:

1. Know the digital imaging techniques;
2. Describe the molecular biology advances;
3. Understand the artificial intelligence in forensics;
4. Describe the biometric technologies;
5. Understand the chemical analysis innovations.

Introduction

The field of forensic pathology has seen revolutionary improvements as new technologies revolutionize techniques and outcomes. Advances in fields such as digital autopsy equipment, more sophisticated imaging platforms, and genetic analysis technology are increasingly pivotal in the clinical and legal arenas. These technologies, beyond improving the speed and precision of postmortem examinations, also enable cause and manner of death to be better determined. When forensic pathologists examine these tools, they are confronted with ethical and practical concerns that need careful consideration, particularly in the area of the impact of new data and the preservation of historical methodologies. The overlap between technology and more traditional forensic methods highlights the need for ongoing training and flexibility within the field so that practitioners are equipped to apply these new technologies in the best possible way. The employment of technology by forensic pathology most often refers to significant ethical and legal questions worth investigating. As highlighted in the context of genetic data, the application of advanced genetics to forensic analysis must consider not only the scientific benefits but also potential ramifications for privacy, consent, and computer security. The (Opeskin et al., 2025) study indicates the widespread implications that result from the collection and interpretation of biological data, hence the adoption of strict ethical standards by forensic pathologists. The standards are crucial in guiding investigators and researchers in addressing the nuanced complexity that is associated with genetic testing in the field of forensic investigation. Also, establishing explicit ethical parameters allows for a justifiable process that reconciles the rights of the individual with optimizing the efficiency of forensic analyses to ensure that technology advancements serve the greater good in justice and public safety. Another extremely significant aspect of emerging technologies in forensic pathology is their potential for educational enhancement and public involvement. The need for openness and accessible knowledge then becomes critical, especially when the complexities of forensic science increase. Anatomical museums, as briefly touched on in a number of cases, are a good example of problems and challenges faced when trying to communicate progress in forensic science to diverse audiences. The results discussed by Ballestriero et al. (2019) regarding the historical evolution of medical science bring out the relevance of aesthetic and ethical considerations in these museums. As forensic pathology adopts increasingly modern technology, an increasing need exists to educate the public regarding the science behind such advances. Not only does it strip away the mystique surrounding forensic investigative procedures, but it also elicits a higher appreciation of the scientific methodology involved, leading to a more advanced society as a whole in forensic practices and their implications (Figure 15.1).

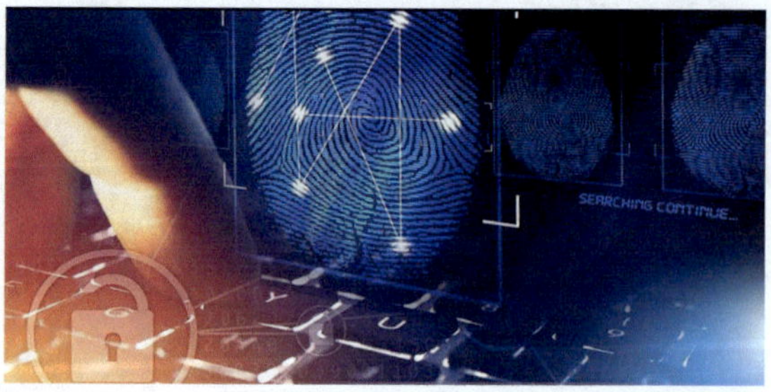

Figure 15.1. Technology trends shaping the future of the forensics industry.

Source: https://blog.bccresearch.com/hubfs/forensics-industry.webp.

15.1. Digital Imaging Techniques

Learning Outcome

1. Describe the high-resolution imaging.
2. Know the 3D imaging and reconstruction technologies in forensic pathology.
3. Describe the virtual autopsy applications.

In the last decade, digital imaging technologies have been at the forefront of forensic pathology. Perhaps the most important development is virtual autopsy or virtopsy, which employs high-throughput imaging technologies such as multi-slice computed tomography (MSCT) and magnetic resonance imaging (MRI). With such technologies, forensic pathologists are able to conduct non-invasive autopsies to determine cause and manner of death with extremely high levels of accuracy. Research has established that virtopsy is as good as the traditional autopsy methods, providing a compelling substitute that is responsive to cultural beliefs regarding post-mortem investigation. The application of three-dimensional body surface scanning adds further to the potential for inspecting and documenting autopsy lesions, thereby providing a comprehensive overview of the forensic investigation. With forensic sciences embracing these techniques, imaging integration should enhance the quality and velocity of autopsy practice. Moreover, digital imaging innovation is not specific to the human body but also has gained wider application in veterinary pathology. Since virtopsy techniques were established, there exists a prospect of applying these imaging modalities in animal necropsies, though a field that continues to be under-explored. The ability to see internal configurations without the necessity of invasion may ultimately feed into better diagnostic precision in veterinary medicine and further extend the benefits of digital imaging techniques. The flexibility and effectiveness of devices like MSCT and MRI in identifying fractures and soft tissue diseases suggest a promising future for the utilization of virtopsy techniques in veterinary clinics. As forensic pathology advances, ongoing development and application of these technologies could be a keystone to increasing diagnostic capability in human as well as animal investigations. While there is a rosy future for digital imaging techniques, their widespread adoption by the forensic pathology community is still daunting. One of the largest challenges is the training and qualification required by forensic pathologists to operate these advanced imaging technologies efficiently. Apart from that, utilization of these technologies requires a heavy resource outlay for equipment and infrastructure, which could present financial barriers, especially in low-resource settings. The evolving face of laboratory medicine predicts the growing significance of these imaging modalities, as evidenced through recent literature, by highlighting the economic factors and social developments guiding future applications (Fortina et al., 2015). Since the field addresses all these matters, ongoing education and research expenditure will be needed to maximize the potential of digital image technology in forensic investigation so that it complements and does not substitute traditional practice and offers end-to-end solutions for complex forensic challenges (Figure 15.2).

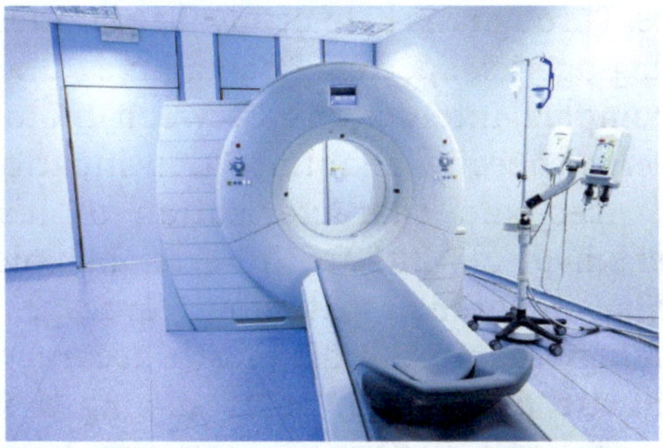

Figure 15.2. Digital forensic pathology.

Source: https://www.azolifesciences.com/images/Article_Images/ImageForArticle_1273_17080111203803016.jpg.

15.1.1. High-Resolution Imaging

High-resolution imaging is a new breakthrough in forensic pathology that allows for more detail and clarity than traditional methods often offer. Virtopsy is one such breakthrough that particularly stands out, employing newer imaging technologies such as multi-slice computed tomography (MSCT) and magnetic resonance imaging (MRI) to make a non-destructive examination of postmortem changes. The virtopsy technique makes it possible for forensic pathologists to visualize anatomical structures in three dimensions, which enables valuable information regarding cause and manner of death. Current studies have enhanced the effectiveness of virtopsy to be equivalent to conventional autopsy techniques in diagnosing autopsy lesions, which makes forensic conclusions more valid and minimizes ethical issues with invasive procedures (Bakar et al., 2012). In addition to virtopsy, spectral imaging has also fallen under the spotlight of forensic investigation, enhancing the capability for long-term pathological review. With its capacity to quantify greater than one parameter at a time on both a molecular and cellular basis, spectral imaging offers a rainbow of diagnostics unavailable through other imaging means. Through the help of advanced optics and labeling agents, spectral imaging may uncover the complex interactions between biological markers, thereby enabling identification of substances and characterization of lesions (Beechem et al., 2012). Hitherto unexploited potential in forensic pathology leverages this technology to improve diagnostic accuracy and prognostic capabilities, establishing a more comprehensive perspective on the cause of death.

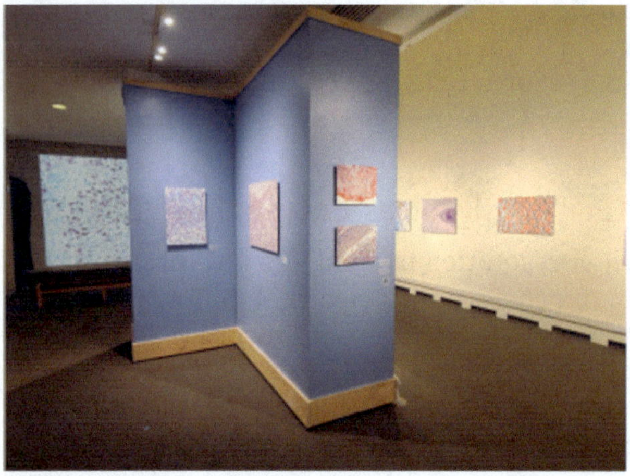

Figure 15.3. Histological images captured using high-resolution imaging were displayed as part of the death under glass exhibition at the Stedman gallery at Rutgers-Camden.

Source: https://cdn.sanity.io/images/f5b6mtfn/selectscience-prod/3570a85730fc8adc79c7b38a572a20347faa756e-350x262.png?w=828&q=75&fit=clip&auto=format.

The future of high-resolution imaging in forensic pathology is to keep expanding as the technologies evolve. The use of virtopsy and spectral imaging is poised to transform the field by way of an effective and ethical method of substituting traditional autopsy practice. As these techniques become increasingly sophisticated, forensic scientists may find that they not only offer increased diagnostic power but also improved training potential, allowing novice practitioners to learn from exquisitely detailed images of pathological conditions. The challenge now will be to bring these advanced techniques readily available and adequately integrated into routine forensic practice so that all specialists are able to use these new tools for better forensic outcomes (Bakar et al., 2012; Beechem et al., 2012) (Figure 15.3).

15.1.2. 3D Imaging and Reconstruction

Application of 3D imaging and reconstruction technology within forensic pathology represents a significant milestone in the functionality of crime scene analysis and documentation. Such technology permits users to create precise three-dimensional representations of physical environments and objects, and such representations assist forensic analysts in capturing precise details that would not be easily captured with standard two-dimensional methods. As elucidated, the advancement of forensic imaging technology has been complemented by enhanced data acquisition processes. 3D imaging allows for remote inspection through the application of extended reality technologies, which are particularly important for crime scene reconstruction and courtroom presentations. Furthermore, the increased portability of 3D scanning equipment makes forensic examiners capable of conducting on-site inspections quickly and safely, significantly improving their capacity for evidence collection and analysis while not contaminating the scene (Llerena et al., 2024). In recent years, several scanning technologies such as laser scanning and photogrammetry have emerged at the forefront of the growing field of non-contact forensic imaging. These technologies have developed to such an extent that experts can acquire precise spatial data without physically contacting the crime scene. Utilization of these methods in forensic investigation not only enhances the accuracy of data collection but also allows for the reconstruction of scenes difficult to envision otherwise. As pointed out, such methods have been priceless in preserving the context of a crime scene, which is extremely crucial in legal proceedings.

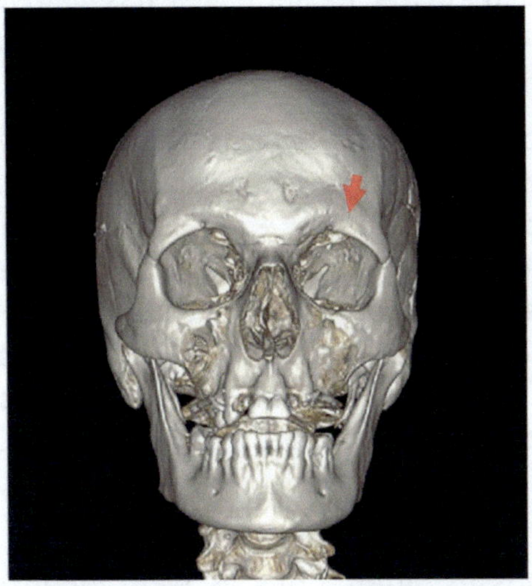

Figure 15.4. 3D Reconstruction of the skull (multidetector computed tomography scan before autopsy), showing the front side of the skull before autopsy. No fracture is visible on the left frontal bone, above the left orbit (red arrow).

Source: https://www.researchgate.net/publication/373073742/figure/fig5/AS:11431281183553328@1692925649284/D-Reconstruction-of-the-skull-multidetector-computed-tomography-scan-before-autopsy.png.

The application of digital, three-dimensional models of crime scenes also enables more effective collaboration and communication among law enforcement, counsel, and juries, which translates into more knowledge-driven decision-making during the course of investigations and trials (Carew et al., 2019). Additionally, the use of 3D imaging in forensic pathology has some hurdles to overcome in order to achieve its full potential. While the technology has greatly improved documentation and analysis of crime scenes, overdependence on advanced imaging equipment and computer software can serve as a deterrent to some forensic practitioners. Training and mastery of such technologies are necessary to interpret and analyze data appropriately, thereby making ongoing education in forensic sciences necessary. With the constant development of the field, it is necessary to address these challenges in an effort to optimize the effectiveness of 3D imaging techniques. Overall, the combination of these technologies holds the key to a deeper understanding of forensic evidence to a large degree, adding an essential contribution to criminal investigation reliability and accuracy (Llerena et al., 2024) (Figure 15.4).

15.1.3. Virtual Autopsy Applications

Virtual autopsy software convergence represents a paradigm shift in forensic pathology from the traditional invasive autopsy to advanced imaging technologies. Labeled virtopsy, this new method employs multi-slice computed tomography (MSCT) and magnetic resonance imaging (MRI) to create high-resolution three-dimensional anatomy models of the human body. These models allow forensic pathologists to examine autopsy lesions without being invasive, preserving body integrity, but still effectively determining cause and manner of death. Studies find that virtopsy is just as effective as traditional methods, possibly making it an appealing adjunct or even eventual replacement for autopsy. Application of these high-throughput imaging techniques not only enhances the credibility of forensic analysis but also enables enhanced documentation of findings, which is crucial to court trials and to victimized kin (Bakar et al., 2012). Beyond use in human autopsies, the principle of virtopsy can be applied in veterinary medicine too, opening new avenues for research as well as clinical practice in the field. Given the absence of invasive procedures, virtual autopsy would be in a position to resolve animal welfare-related ethical issues and provide veterinarians with the latest diagnostic technology. As studies strive to address the potential of virtopsy in veterinary necropsy, its application would lead to increased knowledge of disease and public health interventions for zoonotic disease. With the improvement of technology, its limitations and challenges, such as the extravagant cost of acquiring advanced imaging equipment and the requirement of a specific training program, need to be assessed. Continuous research will strive to make virtopsy an essential component of human and animal forensic analysis (Bakar et al., 2012).

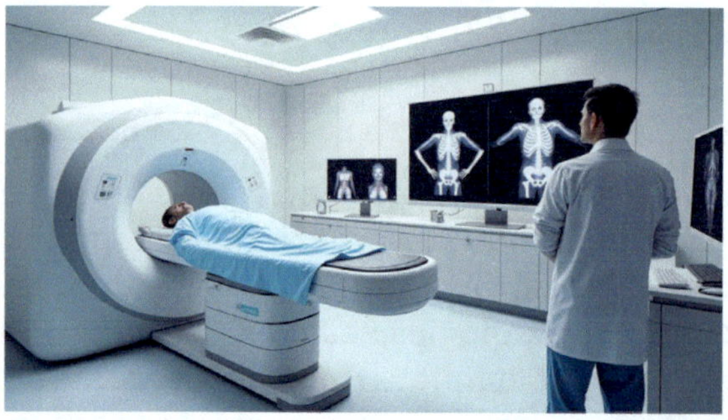

Figure 15.5. Virtual autopsy: Science behind digital post-mortem analysis.

Source: https://simplyforensic.com/wp-content/uploads/2025/04/Virtual_Autopsy.webp.

Further, emerging technologies applied in forensic pathology, including virtual autopsy software, have typically enhanced the pace and efficiency of crime scene investigation. Integration with advanced data analytics and extended reality technologies has allowed for faster and more accurate interpretation of evidence.

Forensic professionals increasingly leverage the digitalization of crime scenes to facilitate remote examination and cross-disciplinary collaboration. This shift not only accelerates investigative procedures but also offers more precise outputs, since electronic systems are capable of combining humongous data processed via artificial intelligence and machine learning techniques.

While huge potential lies in these tools, they possess limitations as well, for instance, the need for forensic specialists to catch up with fast-changing technology and to make sure that such advances assist rather than supplant human expertise in investigations (Figure 15.5).

Test Your Knowledge

1. What is high-resolution imaging?
2. What is the term used to describe a virtual autopsy in forensic pathology?

15.2. Molecular Biology Advances

Learning Outcome

1. Understand the DNA analysis in forensic pathology.
2. Describe the application of RNA sequencing in post-mortem studies.
3. Know the proteomics and its implications.

With the evolving world of forensic pathology, molecular biology has been able to revolutionize the analysis of biological evidence. With the integration of molecular tools such as polymerase chain reaction (PCR) and DNA sequencing, the identification of genetic traces from crime scenes has become simpler. The tools allow forensic scientists to analyze and isolate tiny DNA particles, leading to more precise and unique identification of perpetrators and victims. With the developing technology, the opportunity to use next-generation sequencing is an opportunity to detect not just single genetic markers but also to sequence entire genomes at speed. This new capacity generates the imperative for ongoing discussion of the ethical implications and validity of interpretation of data in forensic contexts, which emphasizes the imperative for ongoing research and innovation in molecular technologies for forensic examination of crime scenes (Fortina et al., 2015). In addition to facilitating processes of identification, molecular biology technologies have opened up new avenues for understanding the context and chronology of events in forensic analysis. Techniques such as RNA sequencing can provide insights into gene expression profiles, which can be used by forensic pathologists to determine the time of death or assess the condition around the body prior to death. Further, these molecular techniques can help differentiate between ante-mortem and post-mortem changes, a task that is highly critical for accurate forensic assessments. The highly dynamic, evolving nature of such techniques mirrors an overall trend toward integrating progressively sophisticated biological data into forensic science. The continuous evolution between forensic needs and technological advancements highlights the importance of integrated training and inter-professional environments for forensic professionals, molecular biologists, and legal frameworks (Seaman et al., 2001). Although molecular biology's potential benefits in forensic pathology cannot be overstated, there exist challenges to their implementation. Contamination of samples, genetic privacy concerns, and the legitimacy of analytical procedures are some of the concerns that must be answered to uphold the integrity of forensic evidence.

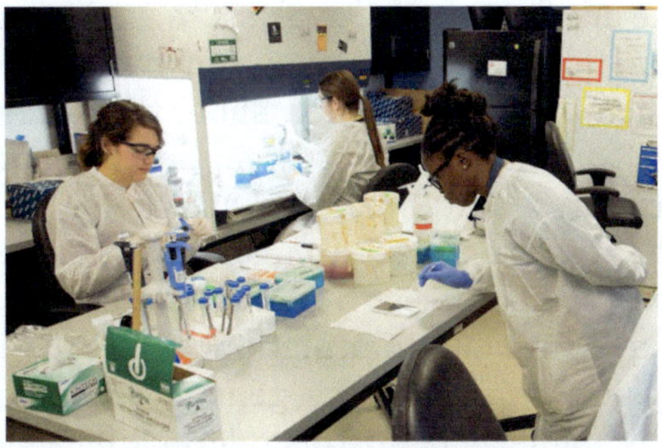

Figure 15.6. Molecular biology.

Source: https://forensicsciences.columbian.gwu.edu/sites/g/files/zaxdzs4771/files/image/3-MFSChemistry.jpg.

Molecular techniques have high demands for precision, since faulty interpretation will lead to wrongful convictions or failure to detect criminals. Forensic experts are also tasked with keeping up with fast-developing molecular technologies using plenty of resources and training. With advancing science, it will be imperative that the forensic scientists interface in an interdisciplinary manner, tapping into the skills of molecular biologists to enhance best practices and the application of these advances in legal contexts. Taking an integrated approach that includes the consideration of ethics will be essential to unlocking the full potential of molecular biology in forensic pathology (Fortina et al., 2015) (Figure 15.6).

15.2.1. DNA Analysis Improvements

The evolution of DNA analysis in forensic pathology is a seminal advancement in the accuracy and reliability of criminal investigations. The application of genetic polymorphism, for example, blood group antigens, has previously been utilized to signify the start of forensic genetics. Recent advances in molecular biology have revolutionized this field through the exploitation of new techniques that optimize the recovery and examination of DNA from various biological samples. These advances have opened up the area of forensic analysis to explore more in genetic information that can be utilized in enhancing the information about the deceased, as well as the cause of their death. As seen, the rapid evolution of forensic genetics has turned it into a cornerstone of modern forensic science, which not only solves crimes but also provides valuable information in medico-legal autopsies, improving the general efficiency of this discipline in identifying relevant information linked with the cause of death (Kozma et al., 2018). Also, the use of cutting-edge DNA profiling techniques has significantly improved post-mortem interval estimation in forensic science. Traditional PMI estimation has, in the past, been limited by environmental conditions at the time of recovery and the decomposition process. Advanced technologies, however, employ DNA analysis alongside other forensic processes, such as entomological analysis, to estimate a broader inference of the time of death. Current research aims at targeting the molecular process of decomposition and the ways genomic data can be exploited to give better estimates of post-mortem interval. By exploring how environmental conditions correlate with the degradation of biological tissues at a molecular level, forensic scientists are revolutionizing the methods to establish PMI, ultimately resulting in an informed reaction to unnatural fatalities (Jawad et al., 2019). Apart from streamlining PMI appraisal, developments in DNA analysis have also led to exploring non-human origins of biological matter for forensic research. A study of animal DNA, which has previously been given minimal attention, can be beneficial to incorporate useful evidence in complex crime scenes. As forensic genetics extends itself to the analysis of animal DNA, it opens up new paradigms of linking suspects to crime scenes through genetic trails left by animals. This multi-disciplinary strategy not only enhances the accuracy of forensic examinations but also promotes interdisciplinary cooperation among forensic entomologists, geneticists, and pathologists. With progress and evolution in this regard, the applications of non-human DNA analysis are increasingly recognized, providing innovative solutions in forensic pathology that can potentially improve the outcomes of criminal investigations and autopsy reports in the long run (Kozma et al., 2018) (Figure 15.7).

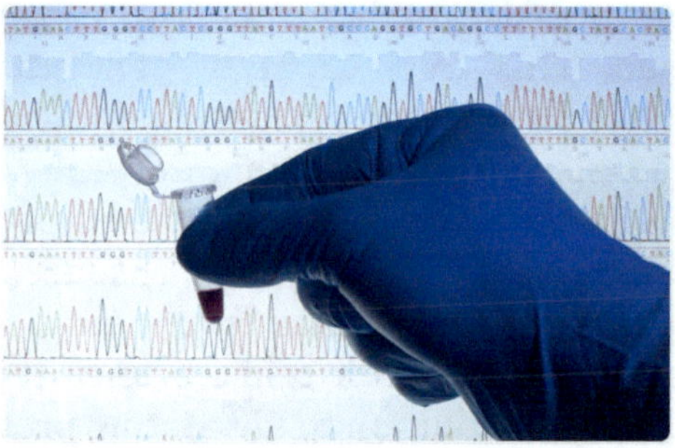

Figure 15.7. The future of forensic DNA analysis.

Source: https://www.azolifesciences.com/image-handler/picture/2021/4/shutterstock_129794300.jpg.

15.2.2. RNA Sequencing in Post-Mortem Studies

Utilization of RNA sequencing in post-mortem analysis represents a significant shift in the protocols followed under forensic pathology.

Historically, biological samples tested after death have relied mainly on protein and DNA analysis. However, the degradation of RNA following death offers a new opportunity to approximate the Post Mortem Interval (PMI) with increased accuracy. While DNA is quite stable over a period of time, RNA degrades quickly once the person has died, giving a shorter marker for the time since biological activity ceased. This rapid degradation can offer insight into the cellular and molecular changes occurring, allowing forensic experts to establish a timeline of events culminating in death and hence add to an understanding of the circumstances of the death, as recorded in the developing forensic practice (Kozma et al., 2018). In addition, with RNA sequencing, researchers can now investigate patterns of gene expression that may potentially reflect the physiological state of the individual at the moment of death. These patterns may be reflective of many possible factors, such as disease, trauma, or even temporary reactions to environmental changes. The analysis of specific forms of RNA, microRNAs and circRNAs, can provide crucial biomarkers that determine the biological processes that are taking place during the period leading to death. Current research has proved that such biomarkers can serve as sensitive markers for determining the cause and manner of death, bridging a knowledge gap between post-mortem changes as perceived today (Solanki et al., 2019). Also, the integration of RNA sequencing in forensic inquiry not only enhances the specificity of investigation but also promotes interdisciplinary research, bringing molecular biology into forensic science. The potential of using RNA sequencing is wide-ranging, particularly where it comes to the analysis of complex cases where other approaches may fall short. As sequencing technologies advance and develop, opportunities for high-throughput analysis become increasingly promising. It is possible for a complete picture of the biological landscape at the moment of death to be achieved so that forensic pathologists are better able to reconstruct events prior to death. This new technique can begin the detection of RNA from non-human sources, thus expanding forensic searches beyond human remains themselves, as intimated by recent research into environmental and microbial influences in decompositions (Kozma et al., 2018). Taking on these fresh advances in RNA technology, forensic pathology is about to guide a revolutionary era, creating new avenues for inquiry and eventually increasing justice in the legal framework (Figure 15.8).

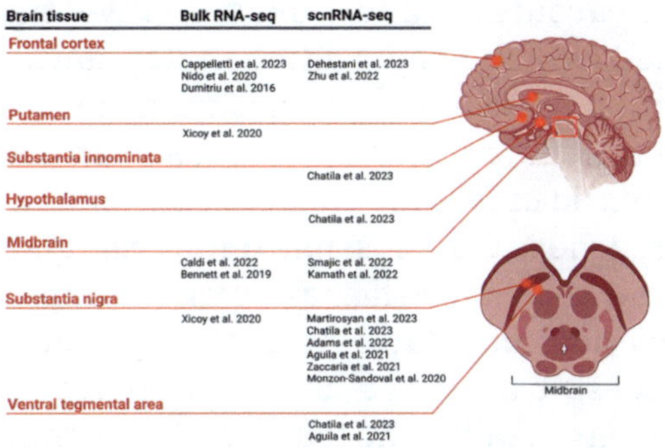

Figure 15.8. RNA sequencing (RNA-seq) studies on Parkinson's disease (PD). RNA-seq studies performed on human post-mortem brain tissue to study PD, which were reviewed herein. Studies are categorized by RNA-seq technology and brain tissue.

Source: https://www.researchgate.net/publication/379600007/figure/fig2/AS:11431281285238123@1729649141337/RNA-sequencing-RNA-seq-studies-on-Parkinsons-disease-PD-RNA-seq-studies-performed.png.

15.2.3. Proteomics and Its Implications

Proteomics, high-throughput protein and function analysis, is a significant technological advance for forensic pathology. Through the elucidation of protein expressions and interactions, proteomics offers unprecedented understanding of the molecular pathogenesis of disease and multiple mechanisms of body response. Forensic scientists can apply this technique to identify biomarkers that can indicate specific conditions or responses to traumatic insult and aid in the determination of cause and manner of death. Such specific molecular information will further enhance the validity of forensic testing by enabling discrimination between natural versus synthetic origins, thereby supporting legal and clinical conclusions based on scientific findings. The integration of proteomic data into forensic testing represents an advancement toward more accurate and focused investigative procedures and is yet another step toward the overall objectives of personalized medicine. One extremely interesting application of proteomics to forensic uses is the application to noninvasive approaches. One possible opportunity is the utilization of human hair as a carrier sample. Hair, which accommodates prolonged physiological changes, can serve as a biological clock reflecting health and pathological conditions over a long period. This non-invasive hair matrix allows forensic pathologists to monitor drug compliance, detect abuse of substances, and even identify diagnostic biomarkers, building a multidimensional report of the deceased. Because hair is primarily composed of keratin and associated proteins, identifying the proteomic signature in hair potentially opens up the possibility to reveal significant information often overlooked with other post-mortem methods. With the application of advanced high-throughput omics technology, the forensic community is able to significantly boost the diagnostic power of the field, revolutionizing traditional modes of pathology and legal inquiry (Adeola et al., 2018). Implications for the use of proteomics in forensic pathology are not just in the identification and characterization of substances but also extend to the broader context of precision medicine. By integrating proteomic data and artificial intelligence, forensic investigation can be rendered more accurate in terms of outcome prediction as well as the customization of strategies to a particular case. For instance, predictive modeling from protein expression profiles can be used to predict disease progression or recurrence in cases of death related to violent causes of chronic diseases. With the development of forensic science, proteomics and AI-based methods will be synergized, ushering in a new era of individualized case management wherein each investigation is augmented by the most relevant bio-molecular data available. Continuing research and collaboration among multidisciplinary experts will be key to overcoming the present challenges of privacy and moral standards, ultimately making the incorporation of these innovations into forensic work a reality (Allami et al., 2023) (Figure 15.9).

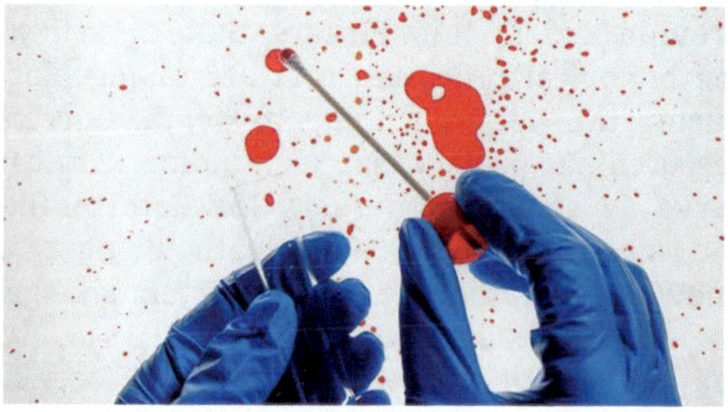

Figure 15.9. Forensic proteomics.

Source: https://cdn.labmanager.com/assets/articleNo/2680/aImg/40173/forensic-proteomics-a-ground-floor-opportunity-m.jpg.

Test Your Knowledge

1. What is DNA analysis in forensic pathology?
2. What is proteomics and its implications?

15.3. Artificial Intelligence in Forensics

Learning Outcome

1. Describe the AI algorithms for pattern recognition in forensic pathology.
2. Understand the predictive analytics in forensic investigations.
3. Learn about machine learning applications in case analysis.

The integration of artificial intelligence (AI) into forensic pathology is a milestone in the accuracy and efficiency of criminal investigations. With the enhancement of traditional forensic methods, AI systems can analyze enormous amounts of information—for example, crime scene images, fingerprints, and DNA profiles—faster than their human equivalents. This capability not only makes the analytical process easier but also minimizes human error, which is particularly significant in the high-stakes game of criminal justice. The predictive capability of AI can be used to identify possible suspects or link crimes that would otherwise remain unlinked. As AI advances, its uses in forensic pathology will also expand, offering valuable support in laboratory and court settings, thereby changing the face of forensic science. Moreover, the use of AI technologies puts forensic pathologists at the forefront of cutting-edge tools that are at the confluence of machine learning and actual application. For instance, image recognition tools can analyze pathology specimen patterns for irregularities that may even elude trained observers. Further, AI platforms, deployed through practices such as deep learning, can enhance the efficiency of facial recognition and biometric data processing. This not only helps in evidence gathering on stronger foundations but also facilitates a faster turnaround in investigations to deliver timely justice to victims. With these technologies becoming increasingly widespread in usage, only more will they further drive the effectiveness of forensic examinations and complement legal processes within an era dominated by rapid technological development (Llerena et al., 2024). While the advantages brought about by AI within forensics are many, impediments still abound that deserve strict analysis. Privacy concerns related to data collection and the ethical dilemmas of AI decision-making are foremost debated in legal and scientific communities. Moreover, the validity of inferences drawn by AI can be compromised when prejudiced datasets provide input to the algorithms. As forensic pathology increasingly employs these emerging technologies, it is important to formulate robust guidelines and standards for their use. As indicated by the past trends in laboratory medicine from more than a century of reviews, the journey to the integration of new technology must be navigated carefully so that the innovation is serving beneficial purposes in forensic inquiries without violating civil liberties (Fortina et al., 2015) (Figure 15.10).

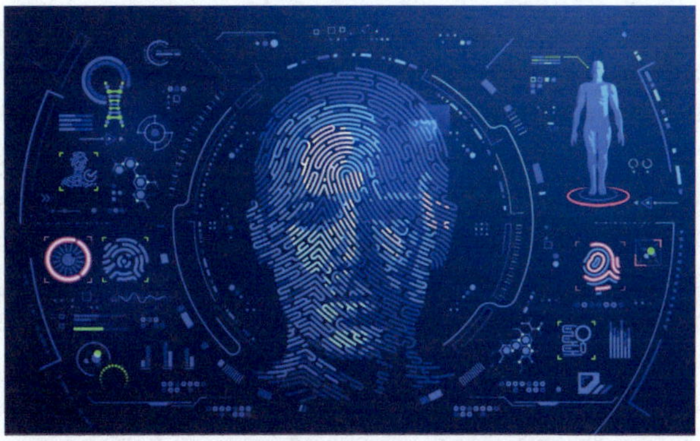

Figure 15.10. Artificial intelligence in forensics.

Source: https://www.azorobotics.com/images/Article_Images/ImageForArticle_744_17417757964241781.jpg.

15.3.1. AI algorithms for Pattern Recognition

The application of AI pattern recognition software in forensic pathology is a significant breakthrough in investigative work. The software is designed to sort through millions of data points to locate anomalies, patterns, and correlations that may not otherwise be apparent. With the aid of machine learning techniques, forensic scientists can enhance their analysis techniques and make more precise crime scene recreations and suspect identifications. As highlighted in recent literature, technology advancements provide forensic experts with improved apparatus that can digitize crime scenes and facilitate distant analysis, thereby comprehensively grasping intricate cases. Not only does this revolution enhance the efficiency of investigations, but it also guarantees the enforcer function of forensic experts, which allows them to focus on primary decision-making and strategic analysis rather than iterative data processing (Llerena et al., 2024). Further, AI's capacity to perform predictive analytics once again innovates forensic pathology. Algorithms can analyze historical crime data to forecast pending criminal activity and identify patterns that guide law enforcement policy. One recent study concluded that the use of AI-powered data processing dramatically enhances the accuracy and efficiency of investigative processes by revealing unseen correlations in enormous databases. This capability enables forensic pathologists to intervene proactively on the probable trends of criminal activity, facilitating preventive interventions. The transition towards AI-driven analytics is a paradigm shift in forensic evidence interpretation and utilization, stressing the need to adapt to new technology to achieve improved criminal investigative results (Alagarsundaram et al., 2023). Even with all the advantages of AI algorithms in spotting patterns, ethical concerns remain paramount to their application. Issues such as data privacy and algorithmic bias need close examination to ensure sufficient utilization of the technology and fair utilization. While AI can enhance investigative processes with efficiency and precision, it is important for there to be forensic experts keeping a close eye on ethical standards and the AI-driven decision-making process. Overcoming these issues will demand a collective effort to develop open algorithms and strong oversight systems. In the end, the harmony between technological innovation and ethical responsibility will determine the effective application of AI in forensic pathology in enhancing its credibility without compromising investigative integrity (Alagarsundaram et al., 2023) (Figure 15.11).

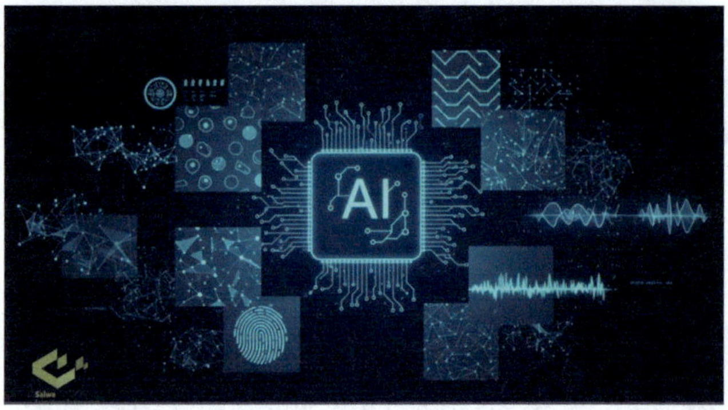

Figure 15.11. AI for pattern recognition.

Source: https://cdn3.saiwa.ai/Goals_of_Pattern_Recognition_06d047286d.webp.

15.3.2. Predictive Analytics in Forensic Investigations

Combining predictive analytics and forensic investigation is a groundbreaking step in the field of forensic pathology. Using machine learning and artificial intelligence, predictive analytics allows investigators to process enormous amounts of data very rapidly. This capacity revolutionizes the way cases are managed by law enforcement agencies, as it allows them to identify connections and patterns that may otherwise go unnoticed. As has been brought out in recent research, AI-powered analysis can potentially improve accuracy and efficiency in investigation procedures by allowing professionals to focus on higher-level and strategic decision-making tasks. With the possibility of accelerated data processing and evaluation, predictive analytics becomes a necessity for the determination of criminal behavior and dealing with the complexity involved in forensic investigations (Alagarsundaram et al., 2023). Besides, predictive analytics can also be used to support resource deployment in forensic groups to guarantee the optimal distribution of people and technology to focus on high-risk areas. Using machine learning models such as Gaussian Naive Bayes, Decision Tree Classifier, and Random Forest Classifier, forensic investigators can easily predict crime patterns with extremely high accuracy. Not only do such models allow for the identification of potential criminal activities, but they also enhance overall forensic investigation operation effectiveness. With data privacy and ethics remaining a top concern, it is necessary to ensure that such predictive models reduce bias and adhere to ethical practices. Careful calibration and validation of such models also contribute to a shifting paradigm in which technology enhances investigative outcomes (Alagarsundaram et al., 2023). The potential of predictive analytics to transform forensic investigations is most realized in its ability to address high-faceted, complex cases. Through the application of sophisticated analytical tools, forensic pathology can overcome the conventional methods by relying on data-driven intelligence to guide its investigative strategy. The research being conducted currently in the field, as highlighted in platforms like the SDSU Data Science Symposium, is to unveil the potential of the technologies to address criminal phenomena. This advancement marks a paradigm shift in forensic practice, enabling law enforcement agencies to effectively address complicated cases. Eventually, the integration of newer technologies like predictive analytics will revolutionize the scope of forensic investigations, ushering in a new era of justice.

15.3.3. Machine Learning Applications for Case Analysis

The application of machine learning tools in the analysis of cases is revolutionizing the field of forensic pathology, as it offers enhanced analytical capability that traditional methods cannot. Machine learning algorithms take massive amounts of data and evaluate patterns and variations that could be missed by human investigators. These computational abilities allow forensic pathologists to effectively analyze complex cases, which ultimately leads to timely and accurate results. For example, predictive model techniques can test case data from previous experience so that specialists can predict probable findings from past experiences. Thus, not only does diagnostic power increase with machine learning, but it also facilitates the unveiling of strong evidence that might have resulted in radical changes in court cases. Moreover, machine learning algorithms are most capable of processing various types of data, such as imaging and genetic data, that are increasingly frequent in forensic examination. Advanced image recognition software, part of machine learning, is utilized to analyze forensic images to facilitate the detection of subtle details in photographs or scans, which may be proof of murder.

With the help of these technologies, forensic pathologists are able to enhance visual inspection so that there can be a clearer interpretation of evidence. In addition, with the deluge of genomic data in forensic environments, machine learning can assist in breaking down complex genetic data to connect suspects and crime scenes, which is a classic example of its breadth of application in case analysis. This ability to integrate different forms of data echoes the transformative power of machine learning for forensic pathology.

Regarding the broader impact of such innovation, both the ethical and pragmatic implications of using machine learning technology in the analysis of forensic cases need to be addressed. As the technologies become more integral to the investigative process, concerns with data privacy and algorithmic transparency emerge. Machine learning tools bring an awareness of the limitations and biases in data-driven decision-making that need to be understood. Forecasts and interpretations made by such systems must be critically evaluated in order to avoid misinterpretations that could jeopardize justice. The continuous evolution of forensic practice through machine learning thus requires a balanced approach in such a manner that while the benefits are maximized, the ethical aspects are firmly tackled, finally achieving a responsible incorporation of such new technologies in forensic pathology (Figure 15.12).

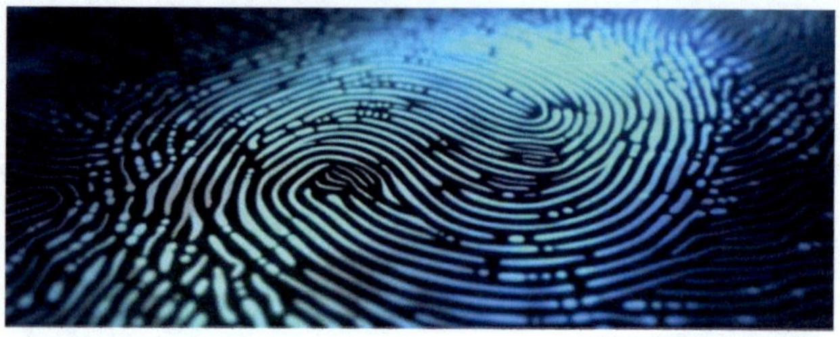

Figure 15.12. Machine learning helps fingerprint PFAS to build effective remediation plans.

Source: https://www.wsp.com//-/media/insights/global/image/2024/machine-learning-helps-fingerprint-pfas/machine-learning-for-pfas-fingerprinting-thumbnail.jpg?h=221&w=564&hash=A4B17E988C04552F37CFC2A4F3B91AF5.

Test Your Knowledge

1. Which technologies power predictive analytics in forensic investigations?
2. Which machine learning models are mentioned as useful in predicting crime patterns?

15.4. Biometric Technologies

Learning Outcome

1. Understand the advancements in fingerprint analysis.
2. Integrate the facial recognition software within forensic pathology.
3. Describe the iris and retinal scanning techniques.

As the environment of forensic pathology evolves, biometric technologies are becoming more crucial as they possess the ability to enhance investigative efficacy and precision. Biometric methods like fingerprinting, facial recognition, and iris scans provide crime and enforcement agencies and forensic examiners with new means of rapidly and accurately verifying identity. These technologies allow for systematic gathering and analysis of biometric information to facilitate robust connections between suspects and crime scenes. Moreover, advancements in machine learning approaches and artificial intelligence (AI) have significantly increased the accuracy of biometric systems, which helps to decrease errors by humans and ensure that results from investigations are not only credible but also admissible in court. This technology development is evidence of a paradigm shift in forensic investigation, which suggests that the application of biometric technologies has the potential to facilitate a scientific procedure within criminal justice, and is a reflection of how technological development continues to shape forensic procedures (Llerena et al., 2024). The application of biometric technologies in forensic pathology also comes with some challenges that need to be addressed for effective implementation. To start with, there are privacy concerns surrounding the gathering and storing of biometric data, with citizens increasingly sensitive to monitoring and concerns over data protection. Secondly, biometric systems can be prone to errors based on external factors or changes in individuals' biology, leading to potential identification errors. Adequate training and protocols should prevent such risks and create best practices within forensic units. As emphasized by existing research, large-scale use of biometric technologies involves surmounting such challenges to utilize their application in forensic examination effectively. This concomitant focus on innovation and caution reflects the appeal for ethical utilization of emerging technologies so that progress is channeled toward justice without encroaching on the rights of citizens (Martínez Hinarejos et al., 2011). Apart from solving problems, the future of forensic pathology biometric technologies holds high promise for future innovations through collaborative research. The establishment of networks in speech and audio processing, as in the case of Spain, is a fine example of how multidisciplinary approaches can fuel innovation in biometric methods (Martínez Hinarejos et al., 2011). Interoperability through the collaboration of technical experts, law enforcement officers, and universities can stimulate developments in biometric algorithms and capabilities for real-time analysis. In addition, with the development of the Internet of Things (IoT) day by day, the possibility of remote analysis and real-time data collection becomes a big plus for forensic investigations. A focus on collaboration and the exchange of knowledge among various stakeholders can promote the development of more sophisticated biometric technologies, in response to growing demands for accuracy and effectiveness in forensic pathology, eventually redefining the context for criminal investigation (Llerena et al., 2024) (Figure 15.13).

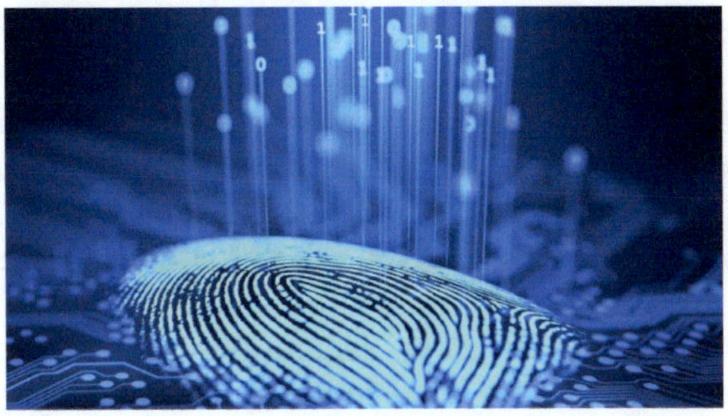

Figure 15.13. Biometric technology.

Source: https://www.manufacturingtodayindia.com/cloud/2024/04/16/Biometric-Technology-1.jpg.

15.4.1. Fingerprint Analysis Advancements

The last few years have seen advancements in the analysis of fingerprints significantly contribute to the strength of forensic science, enabling more precise and reliable criminal suspect identification. Traditional fingerprint analysis, while beneficial, was limited by the precision and quality of impressions taken at crime scenes. Technologies such as automated fingerprint identification systems (AFIS) improved the process by allowing police forces to rapidly compare fingerprints against vast databases to increase the chances that suspects are identified promptly. Additionally, the use of artificial intelligence in the systems has improved the ability to differentiate patterns and minutiae in fingerprint records, which is important to authenticate identities in complex cases. Such technological innovation not only increases the validity of investigations but also encourages greater confidence in the forensic process as a whole, showing the evolution of fingerprint analysis in current forensic pathology. Further innovations in fingerprint analysis have been made at the interface of biochemistry and technology, that is, with chemical detection methods. Techniques such as cyanoacrylate fuming and the use of advanced luminescent dyes allow latent fingerprints to be visualized more effectively by forensic experts. It has been found that these procedures prove helpful, especially where prints are recovered from challenging surfaces or regular methods fail. The application of the new methods is consistent with the trend for greater use of an interdisciplinary model for forensic analysis, as outlined in more recent literature. With the combination of technology and enhanced chemical methods, forensic investigators can yield superior and more identifiable prints, thus leaving valuable evidence in criminal matters.

The success of such innovations informs us of the necessity of ongoing research and development in forensic fingerprint analysis and its invaluable role in the solving of criminal cases, as discussed in Llerena et al. (2024). Further, fingerprint analysis is more than merely identification; there is a need to understand the broader crime trend landscape and criminality. Emerging technologies that use data analytics provide crime trend data from fingerprints. Forensic experts are able to correlate crimes with potential suspects by reviewing large quantities of fingerprint data, thereby facilitating proactive prevention of crime. Further, the study of fingerprint characteristics as precursors to certain behavior or classifications is a field to be explored further. This inter/multidisciplinary approach to fingerprint analysis not only provides additional thrust to its use in criminal justice but also supports overall forensic investigations. As outlined in recent literature, the evolution of fingerprint analysis indicates the gradual addition of the latest technologies to forensic pathology, demonstrating the way that improvements in science will continue to transform centuries-long practices and procedures (Kozma et al., 2018) (Figure 15.14).

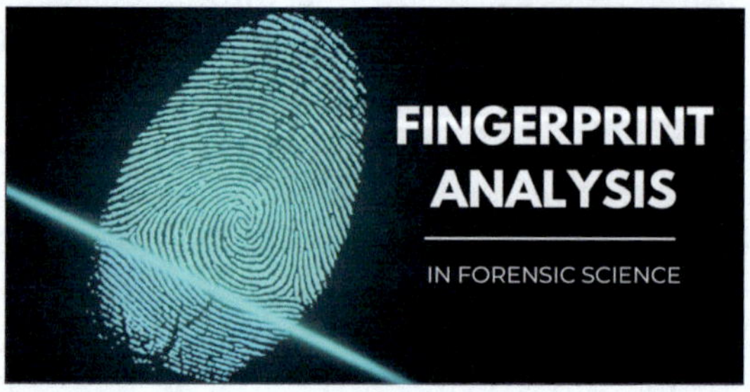

Figure 15.14. Fingerprint analysis in forensic science.

Source: https://lifs.co.in/images/LBS/lifs/blog/fingerprints-analysis-in-forensic-science.webp.

15.4.2. Facial Recognition Software

The use of facial recognition software in forensic pathology has been a great leap forward in identification, where criminal investigations are underway. The technology allows for speedy examination of the biometric features, thereby enabling forensic specialists to match suspects with images from surveillance or video recordings with ease. As revealed from numerous studies, the portability of facial recognition systems allows for on-site analysis, thereby enhancing the speed and accuracy of the investigation. The virtualization of crime scenes also exacerbates the efficient use of this technology by creating access and analysis through remote locations with the help of extended reality technologies, which have been shown to present accurate conclusions about the state of a crime (Llerena et al., 2024). Therefore, the increasingly widespread application of facial recognition software represents a paradigm shift in forensic pathology that provides investigators with a valuable tool to assist their analyses without impairing their critical role in solving cases. However, while being full of promise, facial recognition software also presents limitations, most notably its ethical pitfalls and risks associated with misidentification. Application of such technology raises doubt about the validity of expert identification evidence, particularly in the presence of rigorous legal testing. Empirical research has called attention to the inadequacy of existing protections under the adversarial model of trial, with the suggestion that traditional admissibility jurisprudence was unable to provide accused individuals with a sufficient level of protection against wrongful conviction on grounds of facial mapping evidence (Biber et al., 2009). Thus, the issues demand a strict examination of the techniques and technical specifications used in facial recognition software. It is crucial that such systems be used judiciously and transparently so that their integrity within the justice system is maintained and ultimately public trust in forensic practices is achieved.

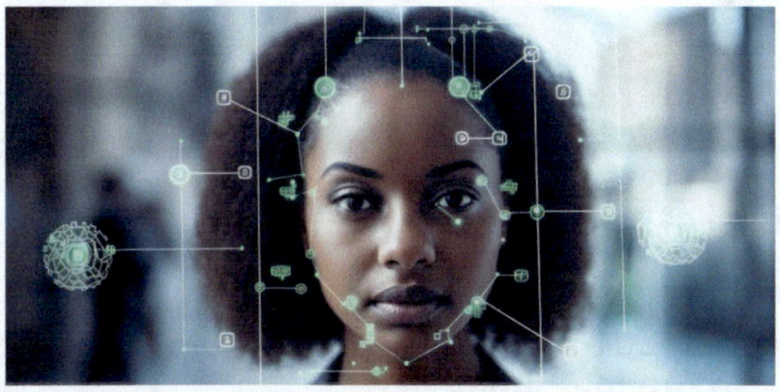

Figure 15.15. Facial recognition technology.

Source: https://www.envistaforensics.com/media/f4tiacr3/adobestock_628144110.jpeg?anchor=center&mode=crop&width=900&height=447&rnd=133456721744330000&format=webp&quality=80.

Also, the changing nature of facial recognition software means that law enforcement and forensic scientists must continually revise and update themselves. As technology improves, the need to ensure that practitioners understand the nuances of such tools and the ethical implications of their use becomes more pressing. Ongoing education can help counter the risks of misuse and misinterpretation of data gathered by facial recognition tools, protecting the importance of rigorous standards and best practices in forensic pathology. In addition, research and development in this area should target making facial recognition technology more precise and reliable. By harmonizing technological advancement with ethical backing and legal protection, the forensic pathology community can harness the power of facial recognition software while preventing encroachment on the rights of individuals who appear in criminal cases (Llerena et al., 2024) (Figure 15.15).

15.4.3. Iris and Retinal Scanning Techniques

Iris and retinal scanning technologies are a significant advancement in biometric identification, particularly relevant to emerging technologies in forensic pathology. These technologies use the very unique patterns in the iris and retina of an individual's eye, developed early in life and not thereafter altered. Iris scanning captures a precise pattern of the iris, such as color transition and identifying rings, and retinal scanning scans the pattern of blood vessels within the retina. Both are of high accuracy, typically more than that obtained by traditional fingerprinting and face recognition technology. Their application in forensic uses has the potential to accelerate suspect identification for criminal cases, enhancing police and judicial efficiency. By incorporating iris and retinal scanning technology into forensic processes, agents can have a more secure and reliable identification process that minimizes the possibility of human error or identity misrepresentation. Furthermore, the inclusion of iris and retinal scanning in forensic practice also raises some ethical and privacy concerns that need to be addressed. As biometric data gathering is becoming increasingly popular, issues of consent, data storage, and abuse are being raised. Investigative applications necessitate rigid rules and regulations to ensure that biometric information is not used other than authorized, which can infringe upon the rights of individuals. Secondly, the reliability of such methods under various conditions, such as dim illumination or obstructed observation, also demands further research and testing to ensure that they are fail-safe. Ongoing debate under the ethical and legal standards of forensic science is required to develop procedures that protect individuals but allow law enforcement officers to utilize modern technology. Sustained balancing of the development of technology and privacy rights of the individual remains a constant challenge as these techniques advance in application. Development and use of iris and retinal scanners also reflect the growing importance of interdisciplinarity in forensic science. Infrastructure such as the Boston University Photonics Center has played a significant role in advancing optical technology, which enhances the efficacy of biometric systems (Center TBUP, 2015). Research initiatives focused on enhancing image capture and processing techniques can further improve the accuracy of iris and retinal scans. Moreover, collaborative efforts among scientists, legal experts, and law enforcement professionals will ensure that new technologies not only fulfill technological needs but also social implications. By adopting an integrated approach towards technology development in forensic pathology, stakeholders can establish a framework that facilitates innovation while ensuring ethical practices and public confidence. Continued investment in research and inter-disciplinary collaboration will in the end be essential as iris and retinal scanning technologies prove to be valuable assets in the pursuit of justice and accountability (Center TBUP, 2015) (Figure 15.16).

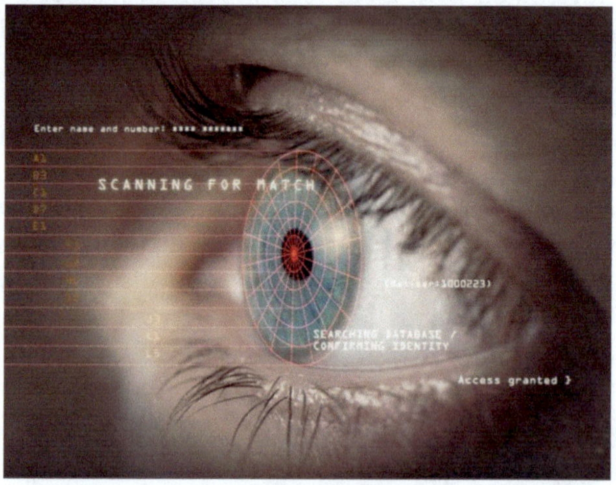

Figure 15.16. Iris and retina scanning.

Source: https://cdn.wccftech.com/wp-content/uploads/2014/07/6a0120a5580826970c019b001ea028970c-800wi.jpg.

Test Your Knowledge

1. What major innovation has improved the speed and accuracy of fingerprint matching?
2. What chemical technique helps reveal latent fingerprints?

15.5. Chemical Analysis Innovations

Learning Outcome

1. Describe the mass spectrometry in toxicology.
2. Know the applications of gas chromatography.
3. Describe the novel methods for drug detection.

The practice of chemical analysis research has become increasingly important in the world of forensic pathology, offering technologies that heighten the accuracy and effectiveness of investigations. Modern techniques of chemical analysis, such as mass spectrometry and gas chromatography, have revolutionized the detection of substances at trace levels. These advances enable the identification of toxic chemicals, drugs, and other substances of relevance to crime scenes. Considering the intricacy of samples, the accuracy of these techniques guarantees that forensic experts are capable of offering consistent evidence that is critical in legal proceedings. Analyzing the path of laboratory medicine, it is evident that past assumptions have underestimated the capacity for such innovation to revolutionize forensic analysis considerably (Fortina et al., 2015). The current tide of technological development emphasizes a shift to more complex, sophisticated techniques in laboratory settings. In the new field of forensic pathology, advancements in chemical analysis are founded on integrating cross-cutting technologies that enhance the investigative process. For instance, advances in portable analytical equipment now facilitate forensic examiners to examine evidence in real-time on-site, which significantly accelerates the process of gathering evidence. These technologies not only save time but also improve overall findings reliability by reducing the risk of contamination. Furthermore, the new use of machine learning and artificial intelligence in these chemical examinations enables easier interpretation of the data, allowing for a better understanding of complex cases (Llerena et al., 2024). By facilitating quicker decisions, such technologies allow forensic pathologists to make more precise conclusions, and thus they are a major force behind modern justice systems. Forensic pathology's future will likely see still more integration of innovations in chemical analysis as technology continues to progress. Digital twin technology and enhanced spectral imaging are expected to introduce increased insight into forensic evidence. These technologies provide forensic scientists with never-before-seen abilities to visualize crime scenes and chemical structures in three dimensions, resulting in enhanced situational awareness. Second, the ability to create digital replicas of evidence enables forensic practitioners to perform more rigorous analyses without actually touching fragile materials. As forensic pathology takes on these innovations, science and law alike will have to adapt so that ethical standards and accuracy are maintained at all times. In the end, the relentless pursuit of innovation in chemical analysis will continue to aid the efficacy of forensic investigation, setting ever-higher standards in the field (Fortina et al., 2015; Llerena et al., 2024).

15.5.1. Toxicology Using Mass Spectrometry

Mass spectrometry has been a useful analytical tool in the field of toxicology, particularly in forensic pathology. The analytical technique is very sensitive and specific and can be employed to detect and quantify a large number of substances, including drugs and poisons, in body fluids. With increasingly complicated forensic cases, the need for precise analytical techniques has accelerated the application of mass spectrometry in routine toxicological analysis. Its trace-level sensitivity allows forensic scientists to recover critical evidence that can have a profound impact on legal conclusions. Moreover, advances in mass spectrometry technology, for example, high-resolution mass spectrometers, have extended the limits for the identification of new psychoactive substances and novel poisons that more traditional methods can miss. As a result, mass spectrometry not only enhances toxicological screening precision but also delivers an enhanced chemical exposure profile in forensic samples. The versatility of mass spectrometry extends beyond identification; it is also essential for identifying complex mixtures and metabolites. In toxicology analysis, drug metabolism research can provide information about a victim's or a suspect's history of drug abuse. Through the use of techniques such as liquid chromatography-tandem mass spectrometry (LC-MS/MS), forensic toxicologists can delineate metabolic pathways by identification of parent compounds and their metabolites in body fluids like blood and urine. This is highly important in cases of drug abuse and can have a bearing on treatment in medicine. In addition, the ability to conduct pharmacokinetic studies with the assistance of mass spectrometry allows forensic scientists to further assess the time course of drug action and its relevance to particular cases. Such information encourages a better appreciation of toxicity and its effects on public health and the criminal justice system. Last but not least, the advances in mass spectrometry techniques, for example, the ability to use non-invasive sampling, have significantly changed toxicological assessments. The availability of using human hair analysis, say, is reflective of this trend towards less invasive techniques. Hair samples can be employed to generate a substance exposure history over a long time, offering an added benefit over the typical biological matrices. Forensic toxicologists are able to build a substance use chronology with this process, while being less invasive than blood or urine screening. New research is increasingly centered around using hair-based omics technologies, as discussed in a number of studies highlighting their potential in disease diagnosis and precision medicine. Integration of these newly arising mass spectrometry instruments in forensic toxicology will intensify the level of investigation as well as enhance the precision of findings in forensic investigations, which ultimately will translate into more informed and fair decisions within the judicial process (Capiau et al., 2016; Adeola et al., 2018) (Figure 15.17).

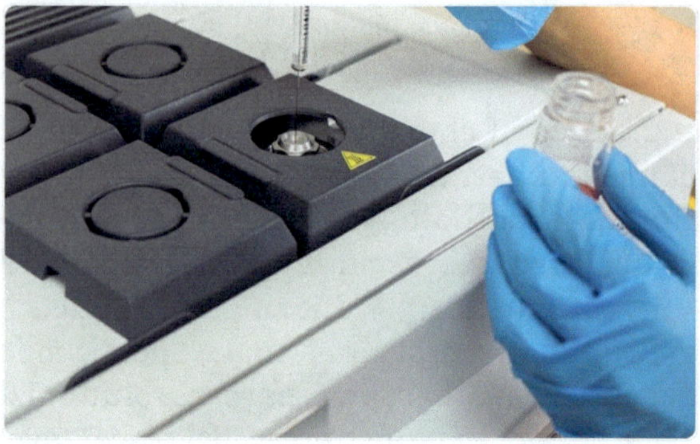

Figure 15.17. Mass spectrometry as a tool in forensic science.

Source: https://www.news-medical.net/image-handler/ts/20190524055716/ri/673/picture/2019/5/By_Lerner_Vadim-1.jpg.

15.5.2. Gas Chromatography Applications

Gas chromatography (GC) is one of the cornerstones of forensic pathology, more so in the analysis of volatile and semi-volatile compounds. Since GC is capable of sorting out complex mixtures at high resolution, trace material may be identified by forensic examiners in such samples as biological fluids and tissues. This specificity can be a godsend in solving crimes, wherein traces of drugs or poison are more than sufficient to yield much information in a case. Furthermore, the combination of mass spectrometry (MS) with gas chromatography (GC-MS) improves sensitivity and specificity of analysis in a bid to identify low-concentration analytes. With forensic applications expanding and evolving further, the use of GC-MS is gaining prominence in the discipline due to the fact that it has been established to provide qualitative and quantitative data required for legal judgments, cementing its pivotal role in contemporary forensic science. In the past few years, new psychoactive substances (NPS) have been a major challenge for forensic pathology. The obstacle has been overcome using gas chromatography after modifying it with the aid of newer methodologies that allow for the identification of the substances in biological matrices. For instance, GC coupled with high-resolution mass spectrometry can effectively identify urine or serum samples for the detection of NPS and their metabolites. In this, the application of systematic screening workflows is invaluable, as it eases the work of detecting such unstable compounds. These advances in GC methods have ensured that forensic laboratories remain at the forefront in drug analysis, providing invaluable information to assist in explaining trends in consumption and potential toxicological effects as a result of exposure to NPS, thereby enhancing public safety and health. Also important is the ability to analyze challenging environmental samples using gas chromatography in forensic science related to chemical exposure or contamination accidents. For the detection of arson or toxic chemical leakage, GC can trace out the presence of accelerants or toxic pollutants that may be present in soil or air samples. The enhanced sensitivity of modern gas chromatography devices allows forensic scientists to trace even the most elusive drugs that may be instrumental in verifying timelines or origins of contamination. With forensic pathologists integrating gas chromatography with other advanced techniques such as high-precision mass spectrometry (precise-mass mass spectrometry) (Capiau et al., 2016) and the qualitative screening protocols for NPS (Bijlsma et al., 2015), the horizon of forensic investigations unfolds, an era in which advanced analytical equipment enhances the efficacy of criminal justice and public safety activities (Figure 15.18).

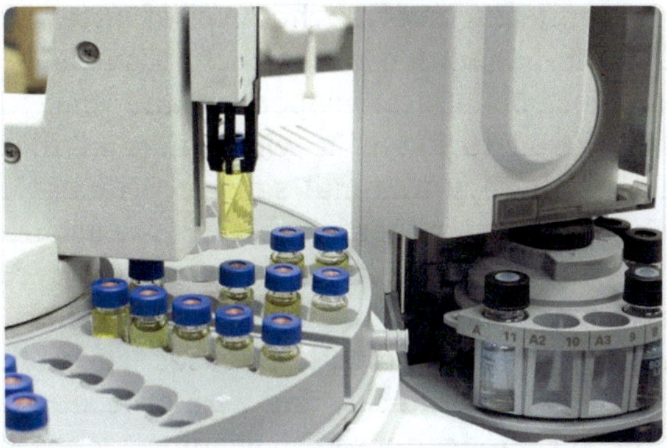

Figure 15.18. Applications of gas chromatography.

Source: https://www.news-medical.net/image-handler/ts/20201022050928/ri/673/picture/2020/10/shutterstock_51050179.jpg.

15.5.3. Novel Methods for Drug Detection

Forensic pathology has been greatly boosted by new drug detection technologies, particularly the inclusion of biomarker analysis. Traditional drug testing technologies rely on samples from blood or urine, which may not give the whole picture of the individual's drug consumption or the timing of consumption. New technologies that are intended to examine microRNAs and other biomarkers in body fluids have a number of benefits. For example, some microRNAs have been identified as potential non-invasive biomarkers of renal cell carcinoma whose levels have been found to vary in the urine of patients with respect to healthy subjects. This not only aids diagnosis, but can also be utilized in the forensic analysis of drug use to demonstrate how a specific biomarker will signal exposure and how drugs affect the organism (Carbone et al., 2017). Another very promising approach is the utilization of novel biosensors that utilize nanotechnology to achieve more sensitive drug detection. These biosensors have high sensitivity as well as specificity and hence are able to detect drugs at much lower concentrations compared to traditional methods. Recent developments involve the use of inter alia graphene-based sensors, which possess very good electrochemical properties, and therefore can be used to detect a wide range of illegal drugs with very minimal sample preparation. Such technology not only enhances the accuracy of drug testing in forensic use but also cuts down the timeframe for getting results, thereby simplifying drug-related legal cases. The ability to identify drugs quickly and with precision has significant implications for law enforcement and drug-related public health activities, creating the prospect of more effective interventions in drug crime (Fortina et al., 2015). Furthermore, the advent of liquid chromatography-mass spectrometry has profoundly impacted the practice of drug detection in forensic pathology. The method can detect various drugs and their metabolites in intricate biological matrices in one go. The advancement of these analysis methods allows forensic scientists to obtain detailed drug profiles, which can be a critical factor in establishing drug use timelines or in exploring contexts of poly-drug use. In addition, the constant advancement in sample preparation techniques, such as solid-phase microextraction, also boosts the efficiency and precision of drug detection. As forensic pathology continues to evolve, the integration of these emerging methods is bound to enrich our information on drug cases as well as improve the general efficacy of forensic examination (Carbone et al., 2017).

Test Your Knowledge

1. What is mass spectrometry?
2. What are the applications of gas chromatography?

SUMMARY

In summarizing the quest for next-generation technology in forensic pathology, it is evident that advances have revolutionized the field in a spectacular manner. Techniques such as virtual autopsies, or virtopsy, are indicative of a new paradigm that moves towards non-invasive technologies to enhance the precision and effectiveness of autopsy procedures. With the application of three-dimensional body surface scanning, multi-slice computed tomography, and magnetic resonance imaging, it is now possible for forensic scientists to identify causes of death with increased accuracy without employing traditional invasive methods. Aside from this new methodology paying respects to family wishes regarding the handling of the dead, it also provides us with an understanding of forensic inquiry, pinpointing the ethical issues relating to modern pathology practices (Bakar et al., 2012). Second, the development of non-invasive biomarkers, and indeed in cancer diagnosis, provides an illustration of how technology can revolutionize patient management in forensic pathology. For instance, deregulation of some miRNAs in renal cell carcinoma holds promise for novel diagnostic technologies beyond standard tissue biopsies. Studies indicating that miR-210-3p is strongly upregulated in urine from patients point to a key advance towards less invasive, if extremely sensitive, approaches to disease monitoring and measurement of treatment response. The use of such biomarkers not only makes diagnosis processes easier but also comes within enhanced practice concerning patients' comfort and quality of care, which touches on the central synergy between technology and humane practice in forensic pathology (Carbone et al., 2017). In the end, the future of forensic pathology is marked by tremendous advancement thanks to technology, which enhances diagnostic abilities while maintaining ethical practices. Although virtopsy provides an enhanced, more dignified way of conducting post-mortem examination, the promise of non-invasive biomarkers is the key to real advances in the control and research of disease. These new technologies are instruments, yet represent a paradigm shift in how forensic pathology intersects with legal and medical processes. In the future, continued investment in research and development will be necessary to ensure the adoption of these technologies. This will guarantee that forensic pathology keeps developing responsibly, ultimately contributing to judicial proceedings and public health in the face of the increasingly complex environment of contemporary medicine.

The use of advanced technology in forensic pathology is transforming traditional techniques, creating a revolutionary movement towards more efficient and accurate investigative procedures. One of the best examples can be seen in the discipline of next-generation sequencing (NGS), and more directly, clinical metagenomic next-generation sequencing (mNGS). The new process allows forensic pathologists to conduct extensive analysis of microbial and host genomic material. By the facilitation of rapid identification of pathogens in forensic samples, mNGS streamlines identification processes and potentially reveals hidden connections between human health and microbial communities. By closing the gap between research use and clinical application, the use of this technology in forensic pathology can potentially offer greater diagnostic accuracy and the ability to solve complex infectious disease cases, emphasizing the necessity to investigate this subject further (Chiu et al., 2019). Furthermore, imaging technology has revolutionized the documentation and analysis of forensic evidence. High-resolution 3D imaging, for instance, allows forensic analysts to perform intricate crime scene reconstructions that can be analyzed in different dimensions. This capability not only aids in the documentation of evidence in the courtroom but also strengthens the investigation process through improved visualization of the spatial relationship between various components in the scene. Furthermore, the use of remote sensing technologies enables forensic teams to examine crime scenes without bodily contortion. Advances in technology, such as extended reality (XR) applications, enable immersive environments where experts can perform data analysis remotely, thereby showcasing the potential of technology in promoting teamwork and enhancing situational awareness in investigations (Llerena et al., 2024). Moreover, the application of artificial intelligence (AI) and machine learning (ML) technologies in forensic pathology offers great improvements in analyzing data and recognizing patterns that may not be immediately apparent to human examiners. These technologies can process massive amounts of data from biometric databases and forensic data at high speed and deliver improved accuracy in suspect or victim identification. Artificial intelligence-based algorithms assist in automating routine tasks, thereby enabling forensic technicians to spend more time on advanced analyses that require human intervention. With such technologies on the rise, forensic specialists will most probably encounter new challenges, such as the challenge of ethical reasoning and the demand for strict validation processes. Still, the possibility of adopting AI and ML in forensic pathology indicates the necessity of a strategic approach towards integrating these technologies into existing systems (Llerena et al., 2024).

KEY TERMS FROM THIS CHAPTER

- Artificial intelligence
- Deep learning
- DNA sequencing
- High-resolution imaging
- Magnetic resonance imaging
- Multi-slice computed tomography
- Proteomics
- Criminal justice
- Digital autopsy
- Genetic material
- Machine learning
- Molecular biology
- Predictive analytics
- RNA sequencing

CRITICAL THINKING QUESTIONS

1. **What is a "virtopsy"?**
   a. A simulated murder investigation
   b. A virtual reconstruction of the crime scene
   c. A non-invasive autopsy using imaging techniques
   d. An online database of forensic case reports
2. **Which imaging modality is most commonly used in virtual autopsies to detect skeletal injuries?**
   a. MRI
   b. PET scan
   c. CT scan
   d. Ultrasound
3. **One of the main advantages of using MRI in forensic pathology is:**
   a. Bone density evaluation
   b. Detailed visualization of soft tissue structures
   c. Detection of metal fragments
   d. Assessing blood alcohol levels
4. **Artificial intelligence (AI) is increasingly used in forensic pathology for:**
   a. Replacing autopsy personnel
   b. Automating toxicology tests
   c. Image analysis and pattern recognition in autopsy imaging
   d. Determining time of death using astrology
5. **Which molecular technique helps in estimating the postmortem interval (PMI)?**
   a. Western blotting
   b. Microbiome analysis
   c. X-ray diffraction
   d. Hemagglutination test

Short Answer Questions

1. What is one major advantage of emerging technologies in forensic pathology?
2. What type of technologies are transforming traditional forensic pathology practices?
3. Which imaging modalities are commonly used in virtopsy?
4. Which molecular technique has significantly improved the ability to analyze small quantities of DNA in forensic investigations?
5. What AI technique is particularly effective in improving facial recognition and biometric analysis?

Answer to Critical Thinking Questions

1. (c) 2. (c) 3. (b) 4. (c) 5. (b)

REFERENCES

1. Adeola, H. A., Arowolo, A. T., Khumalo, N. P., et al. (2018). Human hair as a testing substrate in the era of precision medicine: Potential role of 'omics-based approaches. https://core.ac.uk/download/322437132.pdf (accessed on 12th July 2025).
2. Alagarsundaram, P. (2023). AI-powered data processing for advanced case investigation technology. https://core.ac.uk/download/622609901.pdf (accessed on 12th July 2025).
3. Allami, R. H., Fatima, G., & Yousif, M. G. (2023). Integrative AI-driven strategies for advancing precision medicine in infectious diseases and beyond: A novel multidisciplinary approach. http://arxiv.org/abs/2307.15228 (accessed on 12th July 2025).
4. Ballestriero, R., Cusella, G., Monza, F., et al. (2019). New life to Italian university anatomical collections: Desire to give value and open museological issues. Cases compared. https://core.ac.uk/download/201724876.pdf (accessed on 12th July 2025).
5. Beechem, J., Levenson, R., & McNamara, G. (2012). Spectral imaging in preclinical research and clinical pathology. https://core.ac.uk/download/323068082.pdf (accessed on 12th July 2025).
6. Biber, K., Edmond, G., Kemp, R. I., et al. (2009). Law's looking glass: Expert identification evidence derived from photographic and video images. https://opus.lib.uts.edu.au/bitstream/10453/10446/1/2008003470OK.pdf (accessed on 12th July 2025).
7. Bijlsma, L., Covaci, A., Hernandez, F., et al. (2015). A data-independent acquisition workflow for qualitative screening of new psychoactive substances in biological samples. https://core.ac.uk/download/61463348.pdf (accessed on 12th July 2025).
8. Capiau, S., Stove, C., & Velghe, S. (2016). Opening the toolbox of alternative sampling strategies in clinical routine: A key role for (LC-)MS/MS. https://core.ac.uk/download/84043363.pdf (accessed on 12th July 2025).
9. Carbone, A., Costantini, M., Di Carlo, A., et al. (2017). Secreted miR-210-3p as non-invasive biomarker in clear cell renal cell carcinoma. https://core.ac.uk/download/98350355.pdf (accessed on 12th July 2025).
10. Carew, R. M., & Errickson, D. (2019). Imaging in forensic science: Five years on. https://core.ac.uk/download/188365686.pdf (accessed on 12th July 2025).
11. Chiu, C. Y., & Miller, S. A. (2019). Clinical metagenomics. https://core.ac.uk/download/323062552.pdf (accessed on 12th July 2025).
12. Fortina, P., Kricka, L. J., Park, J. Y., & Polsky, T. G. (2015). The future of laboratory medicine – A 2014 perspective. https://core.ac.uk/download/54509579.pdf (accessed on 12th July 2025).
13. Gheorghe, A., Badiu, D. C., Dumitru, A., et al. (2019). Ethical aspects in managing patients diagnosed with digestive cancers: A review of literature. https://core.ac.uk/download/216811031.pdf (accessed on 12th July 2025).
14. Hübner, D., & White, L. (2016). Neurosurgery for psychopaths? An ethical analysis. https://core.ac.uk/download/131208688.pdf (accessed on 12th July 2025).
15. Jawad, M., Khalid, M., Mona, S., et al. (2019). Forensic entomology: A comprehensive review. https://core.ac.uk/download/268082179.pdf (accessed on 12th July 2025).

16. Kozma, Z., Pádár, Z., & Zenke, P. (2018). Forensic DNA technological advancements as an emerging perspective on medico-legal autopsy: A mini review. https://core.ac.uk/download/322434894.pdf (accessed on 12th July 2025).

17. Llerena, C., Unda, F., Jiménez, G., Gómez Moreno, et al. (2024). Technology in forensic sciences: Innovation and precision. https://core.ac.uk/download/622341556.pdf (accessed on 12th July 2025).

18. Martínez Hinarejos, C. D., Ortega, A., & San Segundo Hernández, R. (2011). Review of research on speech technology: Main contributions from Spanish research groups. https://core.ac.uk/download/148660995.pdf (accessed on 12th July 2025).

19. Mathematics & Statistics, Department of. (2022). 2022 SDSU Data Science Symposium presentation abstracts. https://core.ac.uk/download/519731171.pdf (accessed on 12th July 2025).

20. Office of Continuing Legal Education at the University of Kentucky College of Law. (2002). Scientific, technical, and forensic evidence. https://core.ac.uk/download/232583377.pdf (accessed on 12th July 2025).

21. Opeskin, B., Weisbrot, D., & Breen, K. (2025). Essentially yours: The protection of human genetic information in Australia. https://core.ac.uk/download/pdf/30672952.pdf (accessed on 12th July 2025).

22. Seaman, W., & Whitehouse, J. H. (2001). Florida marine biotechnology: Research, development, and training capabilities to advance science and commerce. https://core.ac.uk/download/11016354.pdf (accessed on 12th July 2025).

23. Solanki, M. (2019). Microbiome biomarkers – Postmortem interval. https://core.ac.uk/download/222929135.pdf (accessed on 12th July 2025).

24. The Boston University Photonics Center. (2015). The Boston University Photonics Center annual report 2014–2015. https://open.bu.edu/bitstream/2144/29753/1/Photonics-Center-Annual-Report-2015-final.pdf (accessed on 12th July 2025).

25. Zakaria, A. B., Zuki, Md, Ibrahim, M., Okene, A., Mustapha, M., & Noordin, M. (2012). Applicability of virtopsy in veterinary practice: A short review. https://core.ac.uk/download/42992189.pdf (accessed on 12th July 2025).

INDEX

N

O

P